Dyslexia: Diagnosis and Treatment

Dyslexia: Diagnosis and Treatment

Edited by Andy Parker

hayle
medical
New York

Hayle Medical,
750 Third Avenue, 9th Floor,
New York, NY 10017, USA

Visit us on the World Wide Web at:
www.haylemedical.com

ISBN: 978-1-63241-492-2

The publisher's policy is to use permanent paper from mills that operate a sustainable forestry policy. Furthermore, the publisher ensures that the text paper and cover boards used have met acceptable environmental accreditation standards.

Printed in China.

Cataloging-in-Publication Data

Dyslexia : diagnosis and treatment / edited by Andy Parker.
p. cm.
Includes bibliographical references and index.
ISBN 978-1-63241-492-2
1. Dyslexia. 2. Dyslexia--Diagnosis. 3. Dyslexia--Treatment.
I. Parker, Andy.
RC394.W6 D97 2018
616.855 3--dc23

Table of Contents

Preface VII

Chapter 1 **Postural Control is not Systematically Related to Reading Skills: Implications for the Assessment of Balance as a Risk Factor for Developmental Dyslexia** 1
Håvard Loras, Hermundur Sigmundsson, Ann-Katrin Stensdotter, Joel B. Talcott

Chapter 2 **Prevalence and Associated Risk Factors of Dyslexic Children in a Middle-Sized City of China** 9
Zhao Sun, Li Zou, Jiajia Zhang, Shengnan Mo, Shanshan Shao, Rong Zhong, Juntao Ke, Xuzai Lu, Xiaoping Miao, Ranran Song

Chapter 3 **Cognitive Profile of Students who Enter Higher Education with an Indication of Dyslexia** 19
Maaike Callens, Wim Tops, Marc Brysbaert

Chapter 4 **Grey Matter Alterations Co-Localize with Functional Abnormalities in Developmental Dyslexia** 33
Janosch Linkersdörfer, Jan Lonnemann, Sven Lindberg, Marcus Hasselhorn, Christian J. Fiebach

Chapter 5 **Subtle Increases in Interletter Spacing Facilitate the Encoding of Words during Normal Reading** 43
Manuel Perea, Pablo Gomez

Chapter 6 **New Insights on Developmental Dyslexia Subtypes: Heterogeneity of Mixed Reading Profiles** 50
Rachel Zoubrinetzky, Frédérique Bielle, Sylviane Valdois

Chapter 7 **The Zebrafish Orthologue of the Dyslexia Candidate Gene *DYX1C1* is Essential for Cilia Growth and Function** 65
Gayathri Chandrasekar, Liselotte Vesterlund, Kjell Hultenby, Isabel Tapia-Páez, Juha Kere

Chapter 8 **Dyslexia Impairs Speech Recognition but can Spare Phonological Competence** 76
Iris Berent, Vered Vaknin-Nusbaum, Evan Balaban, Albert M. Galaburda

Chapter 9 **Position of Neocortical Neurons Transfected at Different Gestational Ages with shRNA Targeted against Candidate Dyslexia Susceptibility Genes** 91
William T. Adler, Maryann P. Platt, Alison J. Mehlhorn, Joshua L. Haight, Timothy A. Currier, Mikel A. Etchegaray, Albert M. Galaburda, Glenn D. Rosen

Chapter 10 **Differences in Brain Function and Changes with Intervention in Children with Poor Spelling and Reading Abilities** 100
Daniela Gebauer, Andreas Fink, Reinhard Kargl, Gernot Reishofer Karl Koschutnig, Christian Purgstaller, Franz Fazekas, Christian Enzinger

Chapter 11 **Speech Sound Processing Deficits and Training-Induced Neural Plasticity in Rats with Dyslexia Gene Knockdown** 109
Tracy M. Centanni, Fuyi Chen, Anne M. Booker, Crystal T. Engineer, Andrew M. Sloan, Robert L. Rennaker, Joseph J. LoTurco, Michael P. Kilgard

Chapter 12 **Evidence for Deficits in the Temporal Attention Span of Poor Readers** 123
Troy A. W. Visser

Chapter 13 **Association of the *DYX1C1* Dyslexia Susceptibility Gene with Orthography in the Chinese Population** 130
Yuping Zhang, Jun Li, Twila Tardif, Margit Burmeister, Sandra M. Villafuerte, Catherine McBride-Chang, Hong Li, Bingjie Shi, Weilan Liang, Zhixiang Zhang, Hua Shu

Chapter 14 **The Effect of Learning on Feedback-Related Potentials in Adolescents with Dyslexia: An EEG-ERP Study** 137
Dror Kraus, Tzipi Horowitz-Kraus

Chapter 15 **Segregation of Lexical and Sub-Lexical Reading Processes in the Left Perisylvian Cortex** 147
Franck-Emmanuel Roux, Jean-Baptiste Durand, Mélanie Jucla, Emilie Réhault, Marion Reddy, Jean-François Démonet

Chapter 16 **Immaturity of the Oculomotor Saccade and Vergence Interaction in Dyslexic Children: Evidence from a Reading and Visual Search Study** 157
Maria Pia Bucci, Naziha Nassibi, Christophe-Loic Gerard, Emmanuel Bui-Quoc, Magali Seassau

Chapter 17 **Strategy Choice Mediates the Link between Auditory Processing and Spelling** 165
Tru E. Kwong, Kyle J. Brachman

Chapter 18 **Episodic Future Thinking in Semantic Dementia: A Cognitive and fMRI Study** 176
Armelle Viard, Pascale Piolino, Serge Belliard, Vincent de La Sayette, Béatrice Desgranges, Francis Eustache

Chapter 19 **The Effect and Mechanism of Growth Hormone Replacement on Cognitive Function in Rats with Traumatic Brain Injury** 198
Hao Zhang, Mengqi Han, Xiaonian Zhang, Xinting Sun, Feng Ling

Permissions

List of Contributors

Index

Preface

The purpose of the book is to provide a glimpse into the dynamics and to present opinions and studies of some of the scientists engaged in the development of new ideas in the field from very different standpoints. This book will prove useful to students and researchers owing to its high content quality.

Dyslexia is a learning disability which mainly occurs in children. It can also occur in adults because of an injury or an illness like dementia. Difficulty in reading quickly, pronouncing words aloud, spelling words and comprehending them are all conditions associated with dyslexia. This book presents researches and studies performed by experts across the globe related to the diagnosis and treatment of dyslexia. For all readers who are interested in the subject of dyslexia, the case studies included in this book will serve as an excellent guide to develop a comprehensive understanding.

At the end, I would like to appreciate all the efforts made by the authors in completing their chapters professionally. I express my deepest gratitude to all of them for contributing to this book by sharing their valuable works. A special thanks to my family and friends for their constant support in this journey.

Editor

Postural Control Is Not Systematically Related to Reading Skills: Implications for the Assessment of Balance as a Risk Factor for Developmental Dyslexia

Håvard Loras[1], Hermundur Sigmundsson[1,2], Ann-Katrin Stensdotter[2], Joel B. Talcott[3]*

1 Sør-Trøndelag University College, Trondheim, Norway, **2** Norwegian University of Science and Technology, Trondheim, Norway, **3** Aston Brain Centre, School of Life and Health Sciences, Aston University, Birmingham, United Kingdom

Abstract

Impaired postural control has been associated with poor reading skills, as well as with lower performance on measures of attention and motor control variables that frequently co-occur with reading difficulties. Measures of balance and motor control have been incorporated into several screening batteries for developmental dyslexia, but it is unclear whether the relationship between such skills and reading manifests as a behavioural continuum across the range of abilities or is restricted to groups of individuals with specific disorder phenotypes. Here were obtained measures of postural control alongside measures of reading, attention and general cognitive skills in a large sample of young adults ($n = 100$). Postural control was assessed using centre of pressure (CoP) measurements, obtained over 5 different task conditions. Our results indicate an absence of strong statistical relationships between balance measures with either reading, cognitive or attention measures across the sample as a whole.

Editor: Frederic Dick, Birkbeck College, United Kingdom

Funding: Ths study was supported by a studentship grant from the Faculty of Health Education and Social Work at Sør-Trøndelag University College. The funders had no role in study design, data collection and analysis, decision to publish, or preparation of the manuscript.

Competing Interests: The authors have declared that no competing interests exist.

* E-mail: j.b.talcott@aston.ac.uk

Introduction

Developmental disorders are typically defined when a child experiences failure in attaining age-appropriate levels of achievement in one or more specific cognitive or behavioural domains. These deficits in achievement occur in the absence of other obvious endogenous or exogenous causes, which results in diagnoses weighted heavily by exclusionary compared to inclusionary criteria.

Reading disorder, or developmental dyslexia, is defined by achievement of reading skills that are considerably lower than would be expected from the profile of measured abilities in other cognitive domains, when neurological and sensory function is normal, and other socio-cultural factors, including access to education, are at least adequate [1]. Dyslexia is highly heritable; approximately half of the population variance in reading skills and deficits thereof can be attributed to genetic factors [2–4]. These risks explain a similar proportion of phenotypic variance, irrespective of whether reading is assessed with a continuous measure or as a categorical phenotype, suggesting that the same genes impact upon common cognitive skills that constrain reading achievement in both normal and atypical development [4,5].

Deficits in the representation and cognitive processing of phonological information are recognized as core risk factors for the genesis of poor reading ability across the lifespan [6,7]. In preliterate children, phonological awareness skills strongly predict future reading skill across a broad age and ability range [8]. Despite the prominence of phonological deficits as a potent risk factor [6–9], the phenotype of dyslexia often encompasses a broad constellation of information processing deficits that extend well-beyond the phonological domain [10–12]. One of these areas is in motor control, where previous studies have reported difficulties in measures of balance and posture that are associated both with dyslexia [13–18] and with reading skills across the range of abilities in the general population [19]. Nicolson, Fawcett & Dean [20] proposed that the apparent link between balance and reading in dyslexia may result from mild impairment of the development and functioning of the cerebellum. This hypothesis suggests that cerebellar dysfunction in dyslexia impairs not only motor control and coordination, but also limits the extent to which cognitive skills such as reading can be learned and automated. Several empirical studies of dyslexia have reported differences in cerebellar morphology [21] and neurochemistry [22] consistent with this hypothesis. Some current neuropsychological screenings for dyslexia risk incorporate measures of balance or of other motor skills as subscales for the prospective assessment of disability risk [23,24].

An important consideration in the evaluation of measures of posture and balance for the assessment of *specific* risk for dyslexia, however, centres on the ability of such assessments to discriminate between individuals at risk for reading difficulties from those without impairments and those with other developmental disorders. Deficits in motor control may also be associated with other disorder phenotypes, such as ADHD [25] and developmental coordination disorder (DCD) [26], both of which have particularly high diagnostic co-morbidity with dyslexia. The overlap between these disorders is high enough to suggest that they share underlying risk factors, yet a demonstration of the positive predictive value of deficits in posture and balance for ascribing specific risk for dyslexia relies on the demonstration of co-variance between motor function and the core symptom of dyslexia, namely poor reading skill. The research in this area is equivocal; few studies have sufficiently examined these relationships with continuous variables of reading and posture in typically developing readers, particularly with measures that are both objective and sufficiently sensitive (cf., [16,18,27–29]).

In a series of case-control studies, Fawcett, Nicolson and colleagues [30,31] reported that difficulties in motor skills, and particularly measures of balance, provided high diagnostic sensitivity for dyslexia. They demonstrated that the majority of adults with dyslexia but only a small proportion of the control group showed at risk performance on a balance measure [30]. In children, similar discriminative validity was reported [31]. Several other studies have reported contrasting findings, however. Ramus et al. [27] reported that only about a quarter of adults with dyslexia could be described as having abnormal balance performance. Wimmer, Mayringer and Rayberger [32] also presented negative evidence and suggested that the presence of balance deficits in dyslexia may be better explained by the effects of an often unmeasured third variable, namely the presence of co-morbid developmental disorders, and specifically ADHD.

In an attempt to reconcile this apparently conflicting literature, Rochelle and Talcott [33] conducted a meta-analysis to quantitatively assess the evidence for a balance deficit in dyslexia. Effect-size estimates for balance measures, obtained from 15 case-control studies, revealed overall strong effects between groups ($d = .64$) but with highly inhomogeneous effect-sizes across studies. Moderator variable analyses suggested that the variability in effect-sizes in the population of studies was strongly modulated ($r = \sim 0.8$) by the probable presence of co-morbid but often unmeasured ADHD symptoms in the samples, but much less so with variability in measures of reading and component skills. In a follow-up study Rochelle, Witton & Talcott [29] experimentally replicated this effect, showing that balance measures co-varied substantially with ADHD symptoms, but not with measures of reading skill, in a between-group comparison of good and poor adult readers.

In this study, we investigated the association between measures of postural control, reading, attention, and cognitive ability in a large opportunity sample of young adults. We obtained measurements of centre of pressure (CoP) for 5 different standing balance conditions, using a force plate to acquire postural displacements in real time. CoP measures of postural sway provide sensitive and objective assessment of balance and were used as predictors of the reading and cognitive constructs that comprise the core symptom dimensions in dyslexia.

Materials and Methods

Participants

The experimental procedures were initiated following approval of the protocol by the central regional ethics committee for medical research (REC Central). All subjects provided written consent prior to participating in the study and all procedures were carried out in accordance with the code of Ethics of the World Medical Association (Declaration of Helsinki).

The participants ($n = 100$), including 37 men and 63 women, were recruited from a college community in Norway. All were neurologically healthy adults, with a mean age of 22.6 years (SD 2.6) across the entire sample.

Table 1. Descriptive statistics for the participant sample ($n = 100$) on the study measures.

Variable (unit)	Mean (SD)	Min-Max
Age (years)	22.6 (2.6)	19–33
Ravens Matrices (raw score)	52.4 (4.5)	38–60
Symbol Search (raw score)	39.1 (6.3)	27–57
Digit Symbol (raw score)	88.2 (13.6)	52–126
Rapid Naming (s)	26.0 (4.7)	18.7–43.6
WordChains (raw score)	59.1 (11.0)	34–90
ASRS (score)	28.6 (6.9)	16–60
Normal Standing ML	1.46 (.66)	.52–3.99
AP	4.36 (1.65)	1.89–10.68
Feet Together ML	5.09 (1.26)	2.85–9.64
AP	5.62 (2.09)	2.44–12.82
Semi-tandem ML	6.15 (1.23)	3.18–10.22
AP	5.04 (1.64)	2.45–10.47
Tandem ML	6.90 (1.35)	4.10–13.04
AP	7.25 (3.97)	2.55–23.11
Right ML	7.91 (3.54)	4.73–26.85
AP	9.13 (3.97)	4.82–29.87
Left ML	7.50 (3.07)	4.05–23.92
AP	8.84 (2.77)	3.61–21.18

Postural displacements during the recording epochs are expressed in standard deviation units of displacement in millimetres for the centre of pressure in the medio-lateral (ML) and anterior-posterior (AP) axes. s: seconds.

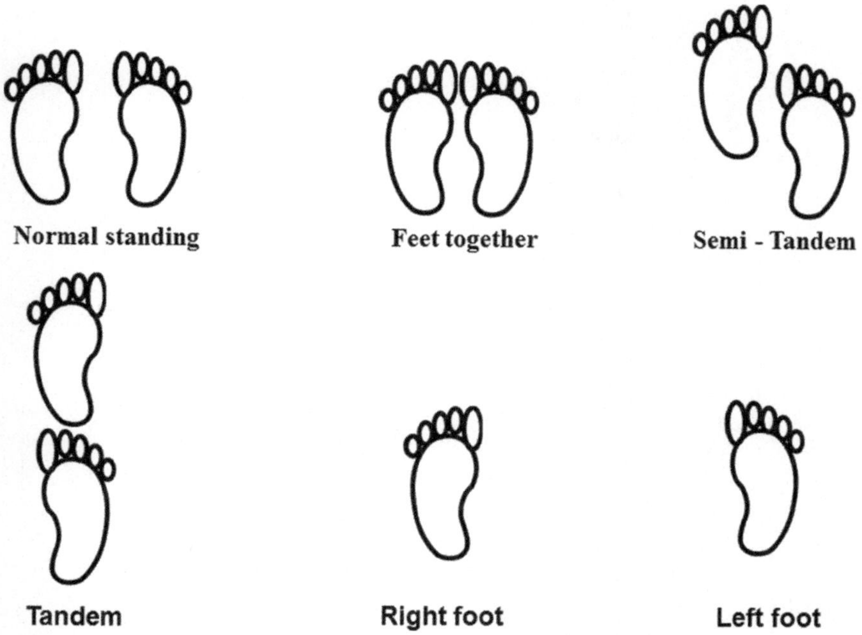

Figure 1. Schematic diagram of the postural control conditions employed in this study.

In their meta-analysis, Rochelle and Talcott [33] reported average correlations between balance and reading skill of .31 and a mean *d* effect size of .64 (*r* effect-size equivalent of .41) for between-group comparisons of groups with and without dyslexia. Using these effect-size estimates, the statistical power of this study ($n = 100$) is in excess of 80% for detection of correlations at .3 and above and in excess of 90% for correlations .4 and higher.

Stimuli

Cognitive measures. Participants were assessed on a battery of psychometric constructs, including the Digit Symbol-Coding and Symbol Search subtests of the Wechsler Adult Intelligence scales [34], and non-verbal reasoning using the Raven's progressive matrices [35]. We also administered the Rapid Naming measure from the Dyslexia Adult Screening Test (DAST) [24]. Raw scores on all the cognitive measures were obtained as measures of individual performance for use in subsequent statistical analyses.

Participants also completed a self-report measure of ADHD-symptoms: the World Health Organization adult self-report scale (ASRS 1.1) [36]. The ASRS includes 18 questions about the frequency of DSM-IV symptoms of adult ADHD over the past 6 months, using a 5-point Likert scale. The individual total score obtained across all 18 questions was used for further analysis.

Reading skill. Reading achievement was measured using *Wordchains* [37,38], a measure of fluency of word recognition. Wordchains provides a reliable and valid test of the speed and accuracy of word recognition skills across a large age range [37–39]. It avoids ceiling effects associated with measures based on accuracy only, which makes it particularly well-suited for the assessment of reading achievement in languages with more transparent orthographies such as Norwegian. This task has been validated against reading outcomes in both English and Scandinavian languages [39], with scores correlating highly with concurrent measures of reading skill [37,38] across a broad age and ability range.

Participants were given a booklet containing rows of Norwegian words presented in the form of 90 'chains' (for e.g., presentedformchains) and were given 4 minutes to divide as many chains as possible into their component words by drawing a line to designate the appropriate word boundaries (i.e., presented/form/chains). The number of correctly segmented words in the time allowed is adopted as the operational definition of performance. For the age of the adult participants in our sample, a raw score of 34 or lower corresponds to a standard score 1sd below the standardized population mean. Descriptive statistics for the participant samples on the test battery are shown in Table 1.

Postural stability. CoP across the anterior-posterior (AP) and medio-lateral (ML) planes was collected with a portable force platform (Good Balance, Metitur Ltd., Finland), equipped with a strain-gauge force-transducer in each corner. The platform was connected to a three-channel, direct-current amplifier and a 12 byte AD converter, linked via a Blue-tooth connection to a stationary computer where data were collected at a sampling rate of 200 Hz and stored with proprietary software. The platform was calibrated prior to each test session, including level positioning of the unit on the floor.

Static postural stability in 5 different quiet standing conditions was collected during separate one minute recording epochs [40,41]. Figure 1 provides a visual schematic of the balance conditions completed by participants. These included: (1) *Normal standing-* the participant's normal stance, including self-chosen angle of foot position and distance between the feet; (2) *Feet together-* the participant was instructed to place their feet closely together toe-to-toe; (3) *Semi-tandem-* the subject was instructed to place the heel of one foot alongside the big toe of the opposite foot; (4) *Tandem-* the heel of one foot was placed directly in front of the other with the big toe touching the heel of the forward foot; (5) *Stork stand-* the participants stood on either the right or left foot with the sole of the other foot against the side of the supporting knee. All standing conditions were performed without shoes, with arms folded across the chest and with eyes open. Participants were instructed to step onto the force platform and to remain still and

Table 2. Zero-order Pearson product-moment correlation coefficients between cognitive and postural sway measures.

	1 2	3	4	5	6	7	8	9	10	11	12	13	14	15	16	17	18
1. Ravens	**.20**	**.20**	.02	.09	.07	.05	.13	.05	.05	.14	.01	.02	**−.23**	.09	.10	.08	.01
2. SS		**.51**	**−.28**	**.50**	.05	.04	.04	.09	.08	.01	.03	.05	.03	.01	.06	**−.22**	.09
3. DSC			**−.41**	**.55**	.08	.05	.13	.05	.03	**−.23**	.01	.15	.02	.15	.09	.09	.04
4. RSN				**−.31**	.06	.16	.05	.10	.03	.04	.03	.11	.01	.02	.10	.12	.01
5. WC					.01	.06	.06	.02	.04	.04	.03	.05	.11	.04	.01	.07	.01
6. ASRS						**.21**	.08	.07	.12	**.24**	.13	−.07	**−.20**	−.12	**−.21**	.12	.06
7. Normal Standing ML							**.60**	**.39**	**.29**	.16	**.27**	.18	.07	.02	.02	**.20**	.18
8. AP								**.26**	**.41**	.19	**.36**	.12	**.24**	**.07**	.08	.05	.15
9. Feet Together ML									**.54**	**.39**	**.34**	**.27**	**.29**	.19	.13	**.38**	**.35**
10. AP										**.33**	**.48**	**.24**	**.42**	**.15**	.13	**.32**	**.46**
11. Semi-tandem ML											**.28**	**.44**	**.23**	.21	**.28**	**.33**	**.28**
12. AP												**.28**	**.28**	.16	.15	**.24**	**.33**
13. Tandem ML													**.48**	**.35**	**.43**	**.45**	**.43**
14. AP														.15	**.25**	**.32**	**.26**
15. Right ML															**.85**	**.27**	.17
16. AP																.19	.19
17. Left ML																	**.69**
18. AP																	

Significant correlations in bold ($p<.05$, not corrected). SS: Symbol search; DSC: Digit symbol coding; RSN: Rapid serial naming; WC: Word chains; ASRS: Adult ADHD Self Report Scale; ML: Medio-lateral; AP: Anterior-posterior.

Table 3. Results of the principal-component analysis of postural sway measures.

	Medio-lateral	Anterior-posterior
Normal Standing	.45	.59
Feet together	.70	.81
Semi-tandem	.69	.71
Tandem	.73	.64
Right	.50	.37
Left	.72	.64
Eigenvalue	2.46	2.47
Explained variance (%)	41.1	41.1

Factor loadings for each postural sway variable, including eigenvalues, and variance explained for the one-factor principal component solutions across each measurement plane.

relaxed in the given stance. After finding a comfortable position, the participant was asked to fix their gaze on a point placed on a wall 4m in front of them throughout the duration of each recording epoch.

Data analysis

Analyses of postural stability data were conducted in Matlab 7.12 (Mathworks, USA) with scripts provided by Duarte & Freitas [42]. Raw signals containing CoP displacements were filtered with a low pass, 10 Hz, second order, zero-phase Butterworth filter and detrended. Consistent with previous research (for e.g., [29]), we calculated the standard deviation of the ML and AP CoP displacements as dependent measures of postural sway.

Results

As shown in Table 2, zero-order, parametric correlations between postural sway and cognitive variables did not exceed $r = .23$ ($p = .024$; Ravens and AP sway in the Tandem condition), and there were no significant relationships (maximum $r = .16$, $p > .05$) between postural sway and the WordChains or RAN measures. These data provide no evidence of any consistent pattern of association between reading and postural control variables.

The significant correlations observed between postural sway variables (see Table 2), coupled with inspection of anti-image matrices, Kaiser-Meyer-Olkin measures of sampling adequacy exceeding .6 and a significant Bartlett's test of sphericity ($p < 0.001$), indicated that the covariance within ML or AP sway measures were factorable. Principal components analyses for the sway measures in each plane resulted in similar one-factor solutions, supported by inspection of scree plots and the presence of a single eigenvalues exceeding 1. Monte Carlo simulation (6 variables, 100 subjects, 1000 replications) confirmed that only these single factors in each solution had eigenvalues larger than would be expected for randomly generated data. The factor loadings of all the tasks, eigenvalues and total explained variances for the one-factor PCAs of postural sway measures are presented in Table 3. The one-factor solutions for each movement plane had moderate to relatively high loadings from all posture tasks (range .37–.81), which accounted for 41% of the total explained variance in each model.

Table 4 shows the correlations between the cognitive variables and the principal component of postural sway for each measurement plane. Consistent with the pattern of zero-order correlations presented in Table 2, there were neither significant nor strong statistical relationships between postural sway on the ML or AP axes and any of the cognitive or reading measures.

A plausible alternative explanation for the lack of statistical relationship between postural stability variables and cognitive or reading skills across the range of participant abilities is that deficits in posture are restricted to persons at the lower end of the performance continua on these measures. As a test of this hypothesis, we selected the individuals in the sample who scored at or below the 10th percentile on the WordChains ($n = 10$), ASRS ($n = 10$) or Raven's matrices ($n = 14$) and compared them to the remainder of the sample on the postural stability measures using non-parametric Mann-Whitney tests. There were no significant between-group differences on any postural control variable for the reading (WordChains, minimum $p = .063$) or non-verbal reasoning groups (Raven's, minimum $p = .060$). For the attention (ASRS) group, one significant between group effect was found for the semi-tandem task in the ML plane [$p = .022$]. The lack of consistent significant relationships between controls and extreme groups derived from the cognitive and reading measures was upheld when the same analyses were run for the principal components of postural sway across the two movement planes (minimum $p = .290$ for comparison of the attention groups on ML sway).

As a final test, we assessed whether a group with multiple instances of low scores on the reading, attention and non-verbal reasoning variables experienced postural control differences compared to controls. We identified individuals in the sample who had performance on more than one of the measures that fell below the 10th percentile. Non-parametric comparisons between groups with either multiple instances of low scores, one low score, or no such scores, were not significant across the different postural control conditions for either of the two planes of displacement. This lack of statistically significant relationship was repeated when the reduced principal component measures were used as the dependent measures.

Discussion

Postural control variables have been employed in test batteries for the assessment of specific risk of dyslexia. However, it remains unclear to what extent inter-subject variability on such measures captures individual differences in reading achievement, the primary diagnostic symptom of developmental dyslexia. Here we obtained measures of postural stability in 5 different experimental conditions, in parallel with psychometric measures of reading skill and other cognitive dimensions (e.g., ADHD symptoms) that may

Table 4. Pearson product-moment correlation coefficients between cognitive measures and principal components of postural sway measures.

	1	2	3	4	5	6	7	8
1. Ravens		**.20**	**.20**	.02	.09	.07	−.09	−.12
2. SS			**.51**	**−.28**	**.50**	.05	−.07	−.05
3. DSC				**−.41**	**.55**	.08	−.17	.03
4. RSN					**−.31**	.06	.14	−.02
5. WC						.01	−.03	−.03
6. ASRS							.18	.03
7. ML PC								**.68**
8. AP PC								

Significant correlations in bold ($p<.05$, not corrected). Abbreviations as for Table 2, except PC (principal component).

also statistically co-vary with motor control variables. Our data do not support the contention that measures of balance and reading skill are tightly correlated, at least in this non-clinical sample of young adults. Therefore, if reading impairment is the primary symptom upon which differential diagnosis of developmental dyslexia is to be made, then our results suggest that balance measures do not alone provide sensitivity sufficient for the assessment of specific dyslexia risk. Although our data do not support the existence of a substantial covarying relationship between reading and postural control variables, there are at least four alternative hypotheses that might explain both our pattern of results and the variability in the findings reported across previous studies in this area.

First, variability in posture and balance may only predict reading skills in children where performance in these domains has not yet reached asymptote via maturation or other developmental influences. Although our data do not address this alternative hypothesis directly, this explanation is in our view the least likely to adequately explain the inconsistency of findings for measures of balance and posture in dyslexia. Although, there are comparatively fewer studies of adults in the literature, the magnitude of between-group effect sizes for these studies are of similar magnitude to those found in studies of children [33]. Variability in the age of both the clinical and control participants was investigated as a moderating variable in the meta-analysis of Rochelle & Talcott [33], which showed that the age of participants was not a strong predictor of between-group effect sizes on balance measures.

Second, several studies have suggested that the presence of a balance deficit depends upon the paradigm used for its assessment, with difficult and dual-task paradigms more likely to yield significant group effects [43–45]. Larger between-group differences may result from the application of more difficult and complex paradigms, for example those involving sensory modulation [13], perturbation of the consistency of the standing surface [16], or the presence of a secondary, distractor task [44]. Dual task environments in particular have been argued to provide superior paradigms for measuring the ability to automate motor tasks, because the presence of the secondary task requires reallocation of attention resources away from the primary task (for e.g., postural control), resulting in performance decrements and thereby mitigating against ceiling performance. The effectiveness of dual tasks in this context has been interpreted by Nicolson and Fawcett [20] as evidence for impaired 'automaticity' of motor control in dyslexia. However, as Wimmer, Mayringer & Rayberger [32] argued, the impairment of performance in dual task conditions by participants with dyslexia may also result from the presence of ADHD symptoms such as inattention, given the additional load on attentional modulation in multiple task paradigms. We did not identify robust correlations between a self-report measure of ADHD symptoms and postural stability obtained for simple (i.e., not dual task) balance tasks in our non-clinical sample of adults. Nevertheless, previous studies have shown that the effects of task difficulty may interact with other participant attributes other than reading skill to impact upon the dependent measures of balance, for example if participants are selected for differences in attentional control variables [46], or where there are asymmetries of variability in attention skills within and/or between groups [15,47]. The assessment of co-occurring symptoms associated with other developmental disorders may be particularly important in clinical samples where the incidence of disorder comorbidity would be predicted to be much higher than in the general population.

Rochelle and Talcott [33] identified that systematic differences in task parameters did not account for significant variance in the magnitude of between-group effects for balance. Although the presence or absence of a dual task does not, therefore, appear to be a strong predictor of effect size in studies of dyslexia, one potential contributing factor to inter-study variability could be the sensitivity of the paradigm for measuring balance and particularly the extent to which the data are obtained through purely objective empirical measures. Measurements of fine grained and often subtle individual differences in adjustments of posture are afforded by technological developments in real-time motion detection. Yet, for pragmatic reasons, the measures of balance developed for use in clinical contexts, such as those embedded in current dyslexia screening batteries [23,24] are limited in their ability to provide precise and objective assessment of balance function. While more subjective measures of balance assessment may yield particularly large effect sizes (see for e.g., [30,31]) several previous studies have examined balance in dyslexia using objective, experimental paradigms with fine-grained sensitivity to detect subtle differences in postural control, with some reporting moderate positive effects [16,18,28], and others demonstrating an absence of significant differences between groups [27].

Third, it might be argued that balance and reading skills do not correlate in the population overall, but have a relationship that occurs only in individuals with the most severely impaired reading skills. Although it should be noted that none of our sample of young adults achieved a score greater than one standard deviation below the population norm on the reading measure, when our sample was stratified to investigate the hypothesis that balance deficits are only identified in individuals in the comparative tails of the sampling distributions, we found no significant between-group effects. Recent analyses, both of the behavioural phenotype of dyslexia and of reading disability genetics [48], support the hypothesis that dyslexia is best represented by the lower tail of the normal distribution of reading skills, rather than a discontinuity or qualitatively different syndrome. Although we did not obtain a clinical sample of individuals with dyslexia, the variability on the WordChains measure (see Table 1) suggests a wide-range of abilities that would be sensitive enough to reveal correlations between reading and postural control variables if they existed in the population.

Finally, balance may not be a specific risk factor for developmental reading disability but instead comprises a more general risk factor for delayed or atypical development in domains independent from reading [28,29,49]. Consistent with this hypothesis, Viholainen et al [28] showed that balance was poorly correlated with reading outcomes in a large sample of children with and without family risk for dyslexia. However, they also demonstrated differences in postural control variables between the at-risk and non-risk groups, suggesting that balance was related to dyslexia, but through third variables other than reading skill. Models of disorder co-morbidity increasingly point to the idea that developmental disorders are best represented by variability across multiple performance continua rather than manifesting as discrete, categorical phenotypes. Plomin & Kovacs [50] as well as other authors (for e.g., [48,49]) have suggested that the genetic risk factors for putatively different behavioural phenotypes are highly overlapping, and that the candidate genes are the same as those that mediate population variability on the same cognitive and behavioural skills. Diagnoses of the most common developmental disorders overlap at such a high rate that they almost certainly share underlying risk factors. Aside from dyslexia, balance deficits have been shown to occur in mathematics disorder [51], ADHD [25] and developmental coordination disorder (DCD) [52], (cf. [53]). All of these disorders diagnostically overlap with dyslexia by up to 50%, which is much higher than would be expected by the random co-occurrence of independent diagnostic entities with moderate prevalence rates (~5%) in the population.

Our results suggest that balance difficulties are not correlated directly with the primary symptom of dyslexia, namely reading skill. The absence of significant covariance with reading skill, but in the presence of the apparently higher incidence of deficits of postural control in dyslexia [33], is consistent with the alternative hypothesis that such symptoms may comprise part of a broader set of non-specific risk factors. Such non-specific deficits might be considered overlapping, bridge symptoms (for e.g., see 54) that provide links to identify co-morbid aspects of developmental disorders rather than to specific symptom features of any one diagnostic category. Alternatively, the link between dyslexia and deficits in postural control in some individuals may be explained by the presence of disorder comorbidity [32,33,51,52], with balance deficits more tightly associated with the co-occurring condition than with dyslexia.

Conclusions

Developmental dyslexia has been previously associated with deficits in balance and postural stability, but this relationship does not hold in a putatively normal population for the prediction of reading skills. The link between motor control and reading disability is therefore almost certainly accounted for by associations with processing domains other than reading, including those in which deficits are considered symptoms of other developmental disorders. Given the high diagnostic overlap between developmental disorders, symptoms of impairment in motor control may be better accounted for as non-specific symptoms that represent the overlapping dimensions of disability risk. Instead of using motor difficulties to promote diagnosis of dyslexia specifically, the appearance of such symptoms may provide indicators that additional assessment is needed in other cognitive and physiological domains.

Author Contributions

Conceived and designed the experiments: HL JT AS HS. Performed the experiments: HL. Analyzed the data: HL JT. Contributed reagents/materials/analysis tools: AS HS. Wrote the paper: HS JT.

References

1. American Psychiatric Association (2000) *Diagnostic and statistical manual of mental disorders (DSM IV-TR)*. Author, Washington, DC.
2. Olson RK (2002) Dyslexia: nature and nurture. Dyslexia 8: 143–159.
3. Paracchini S, Scerri T, Monaco A (2007) The genetic lexicon of dyslexia. Ann Rev Genomic Hum Genet 8: 57–79.
4. Williams J, O'Donovan MC (2006) The genetics of developmental dyslexia. Eur J Hum Genet 14: 681–689.
5. Paracchini S, Steer CD, Buckingham L, Morris AP, Ring S, et al. (2008) Association of the KIAA0319 dyslexia susceptibility gene with reading skills in the general population. Am J Psychiatry 165: 1576–1584.
6. van Ijzendoorn MH, Bus AG (1994) Meta-analytic confirmation of the nonword reading deficit in developmental dyslexia. Read Res Q 29: 267–275.
7. Rack JP, Snowling MJ, Olson RK (1992) The nonword reading deficit in developmental dyslexia: A review. Read Res Q 27: 28–53.
8. Bradley L, Bryant PE (1978) Deficits in auditory organisation as a possible cause of reading backwardness. Nature 271: 746–747.
9. Pennington BF, Van Orden GC, Smith SD, Green PA, Haith MM (1990) Phonological processing skills and deficits in adult dyslexics. Child Dev 61: 1753–1778.

10. Menghini D, Finzi A, Benassi M, Bolzani R, Facoetti A, et al. (2010) Different underlying neurocognitive deficits in developmental dyslexia: a comparative study. Neuropsychologia 48: 863–872.
11. Snowling M (2008) Specific disorders and broader phenotypes: The case of dyslexia. Q J Exp Psychol 61: 142–156.
12. Talcott JB, Witton C, Stein JF (2013) Probing the neurocognitive trajectories of children's reading skills. Neuropsychologia 51: 472–481.
13. Barela JA, Dias JL, Godoi D, Viana AR, de Freitas PB (2011) Postural control and automaticity in dyslexic children: The relationship between visual information and body sway. Res Dev Disabil 32: 1814–1821.
14. Brookes RL, Tinkler S, Nicolson RI, Fawcett AJ (2010) Striking the right balance: motor difficulties in children and adults with dyslexia. Dyslexia 16: 358–373.
15. Iversen S, Berg K, Ellertsen B, Tonnessen F (2005) Motor coordination difficulties in a municipality group and in a clinical sample of poor readers. Dyslexia 11: 217–231.
16. Moe-Nilssen R, Helbostad J L, Talcott JB, Toennessen FE (2003) Balance and gait in dyslexic children. Exp Brain Res 150: 237–244.
17. Patel M, Magnusson M, Lush D, Gomez S, Fransson P (2010) Effects of dyslexia on postural control in adults. Dyslexia 16: 162–174.
18. Stoodley CJ, Fawcett AJ, Nicolson RI, Stein JF (2005) Impaired balancing ability in dyslexic children. Exp Brain Res 167: 370–380.
19. Brookes R, Stirling J (2005). The cerebellar deficit hypothesis and dyslexic tendencies in a non-clinical sample. Dyslexia 11: 174–185.
20. Nicolson R, Fawcett A, Dean P (2001). Developmental dyslexia: the cerebellar deficit hypothesis. Trends Neurosci 24: 508–511.
21. Rae C, Harasty J, Dzendrowskyj T, Talcott J, Simpson J, et al. (2002) Cerebellar morphology in developmental dyslexia. Neuropsychologia 40: 1285–1292.
22. Rae C, Lee MA, Dixon RM, Blamire AM, Thompson CH, et al. (1998). Metabolic abnormalities in developmental dyslexia detected by ^{1}H magnetic resonance spectroscopy. Lancet 351: 1849–1852.
23. Fawcett AJ, Nicolson RI (2004) *The Dyslexia Screening Test-Junior (DST-J)*. London: Harcourt Assessment.
24. Fawcett AJ, Nicolson RI (1998) *The Dyslexia Adult Screening Test (DAST)*. London: Psychological Corporation.
25. Piek JP, Pitcher TM, Hay DA (1999) Motor coordination and kinaesthesis in boys with attention deficit-hyperactivity disorder. Dev Med Child Neurol 41: 159–165.
26. Sugden D, Kirby A, Dunford C (2008) Movement difficulties in children: developmental coordination disorder. International Journal of Disability, Development and Education 55: 93–96.
27. Ramus F, Rosen S, Dakin SC, Day BL, Castellote JM, et al. (2003). Theories of developmental dyslexia: Insights from a multiple case study of dyslexic adults. Brain, 126, 841–865.
28. Viholainen H, Aro M, Ahonen T, Crawford S, Cantell M, et al. (2011). Are balance problems connected to reading speed or the familial risk for dyslexia? Dev Med Child Neurol 53: 350–353.
29. Rochelle KSH, Witton C, Talcott JB (2009) Symptoms of hyperactivity and inattention can mediate deficits of postural stability in developmental dyslexia. Exp Brain Res 192: 627–633.
30. Nicolson RI, Fawcett AJ (1997) Development of objective procedures for screening and assessment of dyslexic students in higher education. Journal of Research in Reading 20: 77–83.
31. Nicolson RI, Fawcett A J (1995) Dyslexia is more than a phonological disability. Dyslexia 1: 37–45.
32. Wimmer H, Mayringer H, Rayberger T (1999) Evidence against the automatization deficit explanation of developmental dyslexia. J Learn Disabi, 32: 473–478.
33. Rochelle KS, Talcott JB (2006) Impaired balance in developmental dyslexia? A meta-analysis of the contending evidence, J Child Psychol Psychiatry 47: 1159–66.
34. Wechsler D (1999) *Manual for the Wechsler Adult Intelligence Scale-III*. New York: Psychological Corporation.
35. Raven J, Raven JC, Court JH (2000) *Manual for Raven's Standard Progressive Matrices*. San Antonio, TX: Harcourt Assessment.
36. Kessler RC, Adler L, Ames M, Demler O, Faraone S (2005) The World Health Organization adult ADHD self-report scale (ASRS): a short screening scale for use in the general population. Psychol Med 35: 245–256.
37. Høien T, Tonnessen G. (1997) Ordkjedetesten [Wordchains Test]. Stavanger, Norway: Lesesenteret.
38. Miller-Guron L (1999) *Wordchains: Word reading test*. Teachers guide. Windsor, UK: NFER-Nelson.
39. Miller-Guron LM, Lundberg I (2004) Error patterns in word reading among primary school children: a cross-orthographic study, Dyslexia, 10, 1, 44–60.
40. Era P, Sainio P, Koskinen S, Haavisto P, Vaara M, et al. (2006) Postural balance in a random sample of 7,979 subjects aged 30 years and over. Gerontology 52: 204–13.
41. Forseth AK, Sigmundsson H. (2003) Static balance in children with hand-eye co-ordination problems, Child Care Health Dev 29: 569–79.
42. Duarte M, Freitas S (2010) Revision of posturography based on force plate for balance evaluation, Braz J Phys Ther 14: 183–92.
43. Maki BE, McIlroy WE (1996) Influence of arousal and attention on the control of postural sway. J Vestib Res 6: 53–59.
44. Viera S, Quercia O, Michel C, Pozzo T, Bonnetblan F (2009) Cognitive demands impair postural control in developmental dyslexia: A negative effect that can be compensated. Neurosci Lett 462: 125–129.
45. Yap RL, van der Leij A. (1994) Testing the automatization deficit hypothesis of dyslexia via a dual-task paradigm. J Learn Disabil 27: 660–665.
46. Raberger T, Wimmer H. (2003) On the automaticity/cerebellar deficit hypothesis of dyslexia: balancing and continuous rapid naming in dyslexic and ADHD children. Neuropsychologia 41: 1493–1497.
47. Haslum M, Miles T. (2007). Motor performance and dyslexia in a national cohort of 10-year-old children. Dyslexia 13: 257–275.
48. Pennington BF (2006) From single to multiple deficit models of developmental disorders. Cognition 101: 385–413.
49. Bishop DVM (2002). Cerebellar abnormalities in developmental dyslexia: Cause, correlate or consequence? Cortex 38: 491–498.
50. Plomin R, Kovas Y. (2005) Generalist genes and learning disabilities. Psychol Bull 131: 592–617.
51. Lonnemann J, Linkersdoerfer J, Heselhaus V, Hasselhorn M, Lindberg S. (2011) Relations between balancing and arithmetic skill in children- Evidence of cerebellar involvement? J Neurolinguistics 24: 592–601.
52. Tsai CL, Wu SK, Huang CH (2008) Static balance in children with developmental coordination disorder. Hum Movement Sci 27: 142–53.
53. Geuze RH (2003) Static balance and developmental coordination disorder. Hum Movement Sci 22: 527–48.
54. Cramer AOJ, Waldorp LJ, van der Maas HLJ, Borsboom D (2010) Comorbidity: A network perspective. Behav Brain Sci 33: 137–150.

Prevalence and Associated Risk Factors of Dyslexic Children in a Middle-Sized City of China

Zhao Sun[1]☯, Li Zou[1,2]☯, Jiajia Zhang[3], Shengnan Mo[4], Shanshan Shao[1], Rong Zhong[2], Juntao Ke[2], Xuzai Lu[2], Xiaoping Miao[2], Ranran Song[1]*

1 Department of Maternal and Child Health, School of Public Health, Tongji Medical College, Huazhong University of Science and Technology, Wuhan, China, **2** Department of Epidemiology and Biostatistics and MOE Key Lab of Environment and Health, School of Public Health, Tongji Medical College, Huazhong University of Science and Technology, Wuhan, China, **3** Department of Epidemiology and Biostatistics, Arnold School of Public Health, University of South Carolina, Columbia, South Carolina, United States of America, **4** Office of Administration, Renmin Hospital of Wuhan University, Wuhan, China

Abstract

Background: There are many discussions about dyslexia based on studies conducted in western countries, and some risk factors to dyslexia, such as gender and home literacy environment, have been widely accepted based on these studies. However, to our knowledge, there are few studies focusing on the risk factors of dyslexia in China. Therefore, the aim of our study was to investigate the prevalence of dyslexia and its potential risk factors.

Methods: A cross-sectional study was conducted in Qianjiang, a city in Hubei province, China. Two stages sampling strategy was applied to randomly selected 5 districts and 9 primary schools in Qianjiang. In total, 6,350 students participated in this study and there were 5,063 valid student questionnaires obtained for the final analyses. Additional questionnaires (such as Dyslexia Checklist for Chinese Children and Pupil Rating Scale) were used to identify dyslexic children. The chi-square test and multivariate logistic regression were employed to reveal the potential risk factors to dyslexia.

Results: Our study revealed that the prevalence of dyslexia was 3.9% in Qianjiang city, which is a middle-sized city in China. Among dyslexic children, the gender ratio (boys to girls) was nearly 3:1. According to the *P*-value in the multivariate logistic regression, the gender ($P<0.01$), mother's education level ($P<0.01$), and learning habits ($P<0.01$) (active learning, scheduled reading time) were associated with dyslexia.

Conclusion: The prevalence rate of dyslexic children in middle-sized cities is 3.9%. The potential risk factors of dyslexic children revealed in this study will have a great impact on detecting and treating dyslexic children in China as early as possible, although more studies are still needed to further investigate the risk factors of dyslexic children in China.

Editor: Li-Min Huang, National Taiwan University Hospital, Taiwan

Funding: This research was supported by the National Natural Science Foundation of China, Project No. 81273092. The funders had no role in study design, data collection and analysis, decision to publish, or preparation of the manuscript.

Competing Interests: The authors have declared that no competing interests exist.

* E-mail: ranransong@gmail.com

☯ These authors contributed equally to this work.

Introduction

Reading is one of the most important approaches to acquire information in modern society. Developmental dyslexia is defined as a specific and significant impairment in reading ability that cannot be explained by deficits in intelligence, learning opportunity, motivation or sensory acuity [1] and it can occur in areas of basic reading skills, written expression, listening and speaking. It has great wide effect on children involving aspects such as education, career, communication and even health. Some studies demonstrated that the children or adolescents with reading disabilities reported more depress mood, scored higher on the measures of anxiety symptoms and more somatic complaints than youth without reading problems [2,3,4]. Other studies showed that the adolescents with dyslexia had higher rates of externalizing behavior problem, aggressive and delinquent behaviors compared with their peers who were normal readers [3,5,6]. The importance of research in dyslexia has been well known by educational, medical and social researchers.

Dyslexia is a vital and controversial issue around the world. In western countries, dyslexia has been studied widely during the last several decades. It is agreed that dyslexia is estimated to have a prevalence of 5% to 17% among school-age children [7]. Recently, one population-based birth cohort showed cumulative incidence rates of dyslexia varied from 5.3% to 11.8% depending on the formula used [8]. Whether the boys are more likely to be affected than girls is still in debate [8,9,10]. A longitudinal study found no significant difference in the prevalence of dyslexia in research-identified boys compared with research-identified girls. In contrast, they found more dyslexic boys among school-based samples [11]. Besides gender, other risk factors, such as parental education, home literacy, family history, have been investigated. Anne's study showed important differences between adolescents with and without dyslexia relating to psychosocial variables [12]. Moreover, Reanto's study demonstrated associations between dyslexia and gender, season of birth, and age at school entry in a large clinical sample of Italian children [13]. Research on dyslexia developed early and comprehensively in western countries.

However, the knowledge of Chinese dyslexia is limited compared with that in alphabetic language. It is worth pointing out that the results of dyslexia with alphabetic language cannot be generalized to the Chinese dyslexia, because the risk factors associated to dyslexia may differ across cultures and languages. Stevenson et al. found that dyslexia existed among Chinese, Japanese as well as American children [14]. It had been the time that people came to realize the issue existing in Chinese. There are some researches which focused on the cognitive profiles of Chinese dyslexic children in Hong Kong [15,16,17,18,19], and the similar work has been done in mainland China [20,21]. Researchers highlighted the importance of morphological awareness for learning to read Chinese and revealed that it might be a core theoretical construct. Although Chinese dyslexia have received more attentions than before, particularly in the brain function using brain imaging techniques [22,23,24] which advance in neurology, genetics and psychology, there are still gaps in epidemiological studies in China. Compared with the abundant studies on potential environmental factors of dyslexia and epidemiological survey in alphabetic language countries, research like present study in China is rare. To address the gap, we explored the prevalence rate of dyslexia and possible risk factors, including those related to school and family environment. The Dyslexia Checklist for Chinese Children (DCCC) based on the definition and diagnostic criteria of dyslexia in the Diagnostic and Statistical Manual of Mental Disorders fourth Edition (DSM-IV) was used to diagnose Chinese dyslexic children. This study aims to investigate the prevalence rate of dyslexic children in a middle-sized city and further our understanding of dyslexia which may be influenced by gender, nurture-ways from parents and home literacy environment.

Methods

Ethics statement

Written informed consents were obtained from all participants and the next of kin, caretakers, or guardians on the behalf of the participants involved in the study. Besides, the study was approved by the Ethical Committee of Medical Association of Tongji Medical College, Huazhong University of Science and Technology.

Study design and participants

This study was conducted in Qianjiang, a city located in the southeast of Hubei province, China, which has a population of 1,030,000 with the 2,004 square kilometers [25]. In 2011, there are about 37,927 students in the primary schools. From China census data (2011) [26], there are 657 cities in total China, and among them there are 370 (56.32%) cities defined as the middle-sized (country-level) cities based on the populations and economic status. Qianjiang is one of the 370 middle-sized cities in China, and therefore, results of current study can be generalized to other middle-sized cities. Since there are 22 districts in Qianjiang city and many primary schools in each district, we applied the two-stage sampling to randomly select 5 districts from 22 districts and 9 primary schools from these 5 districts.

All students of third- to sixth-grade in the selected schools were included. The child with dyslexia was recognized based on the following criteria: (a) The score of Dyslexia Checklist for Chinese Children (DCCC) was 2 standard deviations higher than the mean score. The DCCC is an ideal rating scale for Chinese dyslexia with well-established reliability and validity. It consists of 58 items which applied five degrees ranging in scale from 1 to 5 and requires parents to fill out each item according to his/her child's daily behavior. The higher score of DCCC corresponds to the worse reading ability. Referring to our norm of DCCC, the mean score and standard deviation were 105.7 and 33.0 respectively. (b) The score of Pupil Rating Scale Revised Screening for Learning Disabilities (PRS) was lower than 65 points. The PRS is a convenient tool widely used to undertake a diagnose of learning disability in China, containing a total of 24 items divided into five scopes such as listening comprehension, time and spatial judgments, social behavior, motion ability, memory and language ability. The head teacher was demanded to complete the scale depending on the students' performance at school. (c) Chinese language test was below the tenth percentile among all children in the same grade. (d) The intelligence quotient was above 80 assessed by Combined Raven's Test. (e) The child was not suffered from visual and auditory disorders or psychiatric diseases.

Data collection

Before data collection, we got the permission from all selected schools and informed consents from students and their parents or the next of kin, caretakers, or guardians on the behalf of participants who were invited to participant in the study.

The study was conducted between October 1 and October 31, 2011 by 2 researchers and 5 students with master's degree who are acquaint with the manual of each scale and experienced in epidemical survey. After explanation of our study aims by investigators, the PRS and DCCC scales were respectively completed by the head teachers and guardians depending on the written instruction of the scales. According to the criteria in our study, IQ≥80 was used as an exclusion rule for the subjects, which could be obtained from their medical history in schools. That is, all the subjects enrolled in this study had normal IQ (≥80) by Raven's test. The average score of two unified exams was applied to assess the Chinese language capacity of each student. Besides the scales, we required parents to complete a questionnaire containing three aspects: general information, children's reading habits and home literacy environment. Briefly, general information was collected including children's age, gender, height and weight, medical history, parental education, occupation and family economic status. With regard to children's reading habits, the items about scheduled time on watching TV and surfing internet, whether the children conducting activity reading, whether the children having scheduled reading time were established. Home reading environment was reflected by many items, such as the parents' attitude toward extracurricular reading, how much money spent on the extracurricular books, the frequency of buying books for children, whether the parents telling stories to their children from early childhood, whether the parents having a reading routine, whether the parents buying the books which their children favor.

Statistical analysis

A descriptive analysis was conducted using mean ± standard deviation (SD) for quantitative variables and frequencies for qualitative variables, respectively. Differences of quantitative or qualitative variables between dyslexic and non-dyslexic children were examined by t test or χ^2 test. The variables which were statistical significance in t test or χ^2 test were included in a multivariate logistic regression model. All P values were two-tailed with a significant level at 0.05 and all statistical analyses were carried out in SPSS 12.0.

Results

Participant characteristics

Totally, there are 6350 students from grade 3 to grade 6 in the selected schools, of which 5536 students returned their questionnaires. However, only 5063 questionnaires were completed, with a response rate of 91.5%. The descriptive statistics of the participants in our study were shown in Table 1. Of the 5063 participants, 2581 (51%) were boys and 2482 (49%) were girls. Their age ranged from 7 to 13 years, with a mean age of 9.4 years (SD = 1.2). With respect to the economic status, 946 (18.7%), 1638 (32.4%), 1909 (37.7%) and 570 (11.3%) families had income of >3000 RMB, 2000–3000 RMB, 1000–2000 RMB, <1000 RMB per month, respectively. Regarding parents' occupation, 25% fathers were professional technical staff and 26.9% mothers were classified as inconvenience, which meant that they had no jobs. According to fathers' education level, 10.1% of fathers had college diploma or above, 18.3% were junior college, 39.8% only completed senior high school or equal, and 31.9% finished junior high school or below. There were 41.1% of mothers with education of junior high school or below, which was the largest proportion among four levels. Mother with college diploma or above and junior college were 6.6% and 14.7% respectively (Table 1).

The prevalence rate of Chinese dyslexia in Qianjiang city

Among total 5063 participants, there were 195 individuals who suffered from dyslexia. The prevalence rate of dyslexia was 3.9% in primary schools in Qianjiang city. Of the 195 children with dyslexia, 146 (74.9%) were boys and 49 (25.1%) were girls, which suggested that the gender ratio of dyslexia was about 3:1 (boy:girl). The percentage of dyslexia in each grade was drawn in Figure 1. In 3rd grade, the percentages of boys and girls were 71.4% and 28.6%. Similarly, the percentages were 80.4% and 19.6%, 71.9% and 28.1%, 75% and 25% in 4th, 5th and 6th grades respectively.

The prevalence rate of dyslexia in different grades

As shown in Table 2, the prevalence rates of dyslexia from 3rd to 6th grades were 4.1%, 4.6%, 4.2% and 2.7% separately. There were significant differences on prevalence rates across four grades ($P<0.05$). According to the pair-wise comparisons, significant differences of prevalence rates only existed between 3rd and 6th, 4th and 6th, 5th and 6th grades ($P<0.05$).

Factors associated with Chinese dyslexia

Table 3 shows the potential risk factors of dyslexia based on the chi-square test. There was significant difference in gender between two groups ($P<0.05$). In dyslexic group, more boys (146, 74.9%) suffered from dyslexia than girls (49, 25.1%), while the number of boys and girls were similar in non-dyslexic group. The average age was 9.35 years for the dyslexia, and 9.39 years for non-dyslexia. The percentages of different economic levels in dyslexia group from high to low levels were 14.9%, 29.2%, 43.1%, 12.8% separately, which were similar to the percentages of non-dyslexia (18.8%, 32.5%, 37.5%, and 11.2%). There was no statistical significance in age and income of family between the two groups ($P>0.05$). Parents' educational level was significantly lower among the dyslexic children than that in non-dyslexia group ($P<0.05$). In

Table 1. Descriptive statistics of the participants (N = 5063).

Variables	N	%
Dependent variable: dyslexia		
Non-dyslexia	4868	96.1
Dyslexia	195	3.9
Gender		
Boy	2581	51.0
Girl	2482	49.0
Age(years), Mean ± SD	9.4±1.2	
Grade		
Grade three	1020	20.1
Grade four	1205	23.8
Grade five	1355	26.8
Grade six	1483	29.3
Variables of socioeconomic status, SES		
Income of family per month (RMB)		
①More than 3000 Yuan	946	18.7
②Between 2000 and 3000 Yuan	1638	32.4
③Between 1000 and 2000 Yuan	1909	37.7
④Less than 1000 Yuan	570	11.3
Occupation of father		
①Professional technical staff	1268	25.0
②Principal of institution and government	384	7.6
③The office staff	360	7.1
④Business staff	649	12.8
⑤Service staff	360	7.1
⑥Farming, forestry, fishery worker	407	8.0
⑦Production worker, transport worker and other related occupations	752	14.9
⑧Classification of inconvenience	883	17.4
Occupation of mother		
①Professional technical staff	611	12.1
②Principal of institution and government	153	3.0
③The office staff	350	6.9
④Business staff	767	15.1
⑤Service staff	873	17.2
⑥Farming, forestry, fishery worker	404	8.0
⑦Production worker, transport worker and other related occupations	543	10.7
⑧Classification of inconvenience	1362	26.9
Father's education level		
①Junior high school or below	1615	31.9
②Senior high school or equivalency	2014	39.8
③Junior college	925	18.3
④College diploma or above	509	10.1
Mother's education level		
①Junior high school or below	2079	41.1
②Senior high school or equivalency	1906	37.6
③Junior college	743	14.7
④College diploma or above	335	6.6

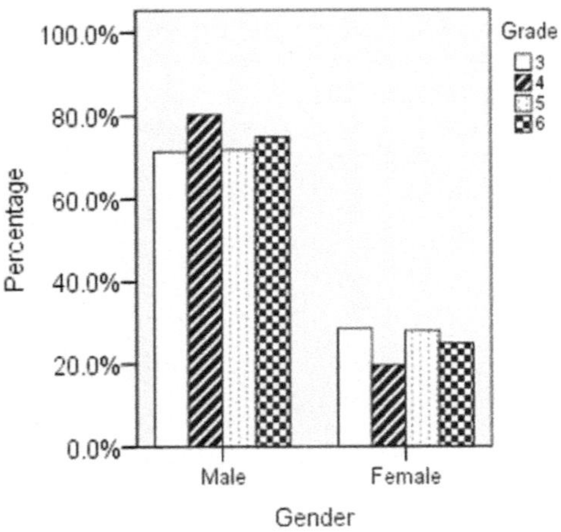

Figure 1. The distribution of dyslexia in grade and gender.

dyslexic group, fewer father received education of junior college (25, 12.8%) or above college (3, 1.5%), and fewer mother had attended the junior college (14, 7.2%) or above college (1, 0.5%) when compared with non-dyslexia group.

There was significant difference in parents' attitude regarding to surfing internet between two groups ($P<0.05$). More parents (54, 27.7%) chose to prohibit their children using internet in dyslexia group than those (862, 17.7%) in non-dyslexia group. Hours on watching TV were longer among the dyslexic children than among the non-dyslexia children ($P<0.05$). Among the dyslexic children, 15.4% of children watched TV 2–3 hours every day and 8.7% watched TV more than 3 hours, while they were 8.1% and 4.1% for the non-dyslexia, respectively. The dyslexic children were lack of active learning habit ($P<0.05$). In dyslexia group, fewer children had habit of active learning (18, 9.2%) and more children never learn actively (77, 39.5%) than those in non-dyslexic group.

Home literacy environment

There was significant association between dyslexia and home literacy environment ($P<0.05$). There were lower frequencies in parents' telling stories (5, 2.6%), encouraging the child to read extra-curricular books (108, 55.4%), buying the books which child was interested in in dyslexia group (51, 26.2%) compared with the non-dyslexia group. There were only 18.5% parents reading every day, which was lower than that in non-dyslexia group (1285, 26.4%). With regard to the children' scheduled reading time, there was a large percentage of children without fixed reading time in dyslexia group (156, 80%), whereas only 6.8% (2767) children had not fixed reading time in non-dyslexia group. Furthermore, the expenses of books varied. There were more parents spending money less than150 RMB on books every year for the dyslexic children (114, 58.5%) than those in non-dyslexia group (2196, 45.1%), and fewer parents (2, 1%) paid more than 500 RMB for books per year in dyslexia group than those in non-dyslexia group (190, 3.9%).

Multivariate logistic regression

There were significant associations between dyslexia and gender, parental education level, attitude to using internet, scheduled time on TV and internet, active learning and home literacy environment (Table 3). To estimate the effect sizes of these possible risk factors, we conducted a multivariate logistic regression analysis. Table 4 shows ORs and 95% CIs for the potential risk factors. From table 4, we could see that there was a significant difference in gender between two groups and the OR in boys who suffered from dyslexia was 2.3 times as high as that in girls. Low educational level of mothers was a risk factor for dyslexia (junior high school or below: OR = 12.1, 95% CI: 1.7–87.3; senior high school or equivalency: OR = 9.3, 95% CI: 1.3–67.4) compared with mothers with higher education level. Active learning had positive effect on dyslexia with OR being 0.1 and 0.3 among children who always or sometimes had active learning habit. For children with scheduled reading time, the OR to be dyslexic was 0.5 times as high as those children without scheduled reading time. Therefore, we concluded that dyslexia was significantly associated with child's gender, mother's education level, active learning, and scheduled reading time.

Risk factors associated with dyslexia for low and high grades students

We divided the subjects into low (3–4 grades) and high grades (5–6 grades). Based on Table 3, common risk factors for both grades include gender, parents' education level, scheduled time on watching TV and surfing internet, whether the children conducting active learning, whether the children having scheduled reading time, and expenses of buying books for children. There were several risk factors specific to low and high grades. For example, the factors including the frequency of parents telling stories to their children, parents buying extracurricular books for their children and parents buying new books, the parents' attitude toward extracurricular reading were significant associated with dyslexia in low grades. While parents' attitude toward surfing internet, and whether parents having a reading routine were found to be risk factors for high grades. We also conducted the multivariate logistic regression, and found that gender and whether the children conducting activity reading were related to dyslexia risk for both grades (Table 4).

Table 2. The prevalence rate of dyslexia in different grades[a].

Subjects	Grade	Dyslexia (n)	Non-dyslexia (n)	Prevalence rate (%)	x^2	P
All grades					8.053	0.045
	3	42	978	4.1		
	4	56	1149	4.6		
	5	57	1298	4.2		
	6	40	1443	2.7		

[a]There was significant differences between 3rd and 6th grades ($P=0.049$), 4th and 6th grades ($P=0.007$), 5th and 6th grades ($P=0.027$) in prevalence rates separately and no significant differences between 3rd and 4th grades ($P=0.544$), 3rd and 5th grades ($P=0.914$), 4th and 5th grades ($P=0.588$).

Table 3. Analytical statistics for the dyslexia and non-dyslexia groups.

Variables	Low grade				High grade				All subjects			
	Dyslexia (n = 98)	Non-dyslexia (n = 2127)	x^2	P	Dyslexia (n = 97)	Non-dyslexia (n = 2741)	x^2	P	Dyslexia (n = 195)	Non-dyslexia (n = 4868)	x^2	P
	n(%)	n(%)			n(%)	n(%)			n(%)	n(%)		
General information												
Gender			28.7	<0.05			18.6	<0.05			46.3	<0.05
Male	75 (77.0)	1039 (49.0)			71 (73.2)	1396 (50.9)			146 (74.9)	2435 (50.0)		
Female	23 (23.0)	1088 (51.0)			26 (26.8)	1345 (49.1)			49 (25.1)	2433 (50.0)		
Age[a]	8.4±0.7	8.3±0.7	−1.8	>0.05	10.2±0.8	10.2±0.7	−0.4	>0.05	9.35±1.2	9.39±1.2	0.5	>0.05
BMI[b]	16.8±2.8	16.8±4.2	−0.1	>0.05	17.1±3.5	17.7±3.0	−1.8	>0.05	17.25±2.9	16.94±3.8	−1.1	>0.05
Income of family per month			1.0	>0.05			4.3	>0.05			4.2	>0.05
①More than 3000 Yuan	15 (15.3)	387 (18.2)			14 (14.4)	530 (19.3)			29 (14.9)	917 (18.8)		
②Between 2000 and 3000 Yuan	31 (31.6)	696 (32.7)			26 (26.8)	885 (32.3)			57 (29.2)	1581 (32.5)		
③Between 1000 and 2000 Yuan	40 (40.8)	832 (39.1)			44 (45.4)	993 (36.2)			84 (43.1)	1825 (37.5)		
④Less than 1000 Yuan	12 (12.2)	212 (10.0)			13 (13.4)	333 (12.1)			25 (12.8)	545 (11.2)		
Father's education level			9.6	<0.05			16.5	<0.05			25.2	<0.05
①Junior high school or below	39 (39.8)	634 (29.8)			43 (44.3)	899 (32.8)			82 (42.1)	1533 (31.5)		
②Senior high school or equal	43 (43.9)	883 (41.5)			42 (43.3)	1046 (38.2)			85 (43.6)	1929 (39.6)		
③Junior college	13 (13.3)	387 (18.2)			12 (12.4)	513 (18.7)			25 (12.8)	900 (18.5)		
④College diploma or above	3 (3.1)	223 (10.5)			0(0)	283 (10.3)			3 (1.5)	506 (10.4)		
Mother's education level			17.2	<0.05			13.3	<0.05			29.3	<0.05
①Junior high school or below	52 (53.1)	823 (38.7)			56 (57.7)	1148 (41.9)			108 (55.4)	1971 (40.5)		
②Senior high school or equal	39 (39.8)	802 (37.7)			33 (34.0)	1032 (37.7)			72 (36.9)	1834 (37.7)		
③Junior college	7 (7.1)	334 (15.7)			7 (7.2)	395 (14.4)			14 (7.2)	729 (15.0)		
④College diploma or above	0 (0)	168 (7.9)			1 (1.0)	166 (6.1)			1 (0.5)	334 (6.9)		
Learning habits												
Times of surfing internet per week			4.6	>0.05			0.5	>0.05			3.2	>0.05
1 time or less	82 (83.7)	1608 (75.6)			68 (70.1)	1871 (68.3)			150 (76.9)	3479 (71.5)		
2–4 times	14 (14.3)	413 (19.4)			24 (24.7)	700 (25.5)			38 (19.5)	1113 (22.9)		
5–6 times	2 (2)	54 (2.5)			2 (2.1)	90 (3.3)			4 (2.1)	144 (3)		
7 times or more	2 (2)	52 (2.4)			3 (3.1)	80 (2.9)			3 (1.5)	132 (2.7)		
Hours of surfing per time			1.4	>0.05			0.9	>0.05			1.4	>0.05
Less than an hour	79 (80.6)	1614 (75.9)			60 (61.9)	1722 (62.8)			139 (71.3)	3336 (68.5)		
1–2 hours	16 (16.3)	439 (20.6)			28 (28.9)	829 (30.2)			44 (22.6)	1268 (26.0)		
2–4 hours	3 (3.1)	6 8(3.2)			8 (8.2)	165 (6.0)			11 (5.6)	233 (4.8)		
More than 4 hours	0 (0.0)	6 (0.3)			1 (1.0)	2 5(0.9)			1 (0.5)	31 (0.6)		

Table 3. Cont.

Variables	Low grade				High grade				All subjects			
	Dyslexia (n=98)	Non-dyslexia (n=2127)	x^2	*P*	Dyslexia (n=97)	Non-dyslexia (n=2741)	x^2	*P*	Dyslexia (n=195)	Non-dyslexia (n=4868)	x^2	*P*
	n(%)	n(%)			n(%)	n(%)			n(%)	n(%)		
Parents' attitude to surfing internet			1.5	>0.05			16.7	<0.05			13.9	<0.05
Ban internet access	23 (23.5)	403 (18.9)			31 (32.0)	459 (16.7)			54 (27.7)	862 (17.7)		
Surf internet only during vacation	28 (28.6)	597 (28.1)			30 (30.9)	861 (31.4)			58 (29.7)	1458 (30.0)		
Surf internet after school	45 (45.9)	1083 (50.9)			34 (35.1)	1362 (49.7)			79 (40.5)	2445 (50.2)		
Up to the child	2 (2.0)	44 (2.1)			2 (2.1)	59 (2.2)			4 (2.1)	103 (2.1)		
Scheduled time on watching TV and surfing internet			7.7	<0.05			16.3	<0.05			20.6	<0.05
Yes, the child can execute	57 (58.2)	1403 (66.0)			41 (42.3)	1677 (61.2)			98 (50.3)	3080 (63.3)		
No	15 (15.3)	385 (18.1)			27 (27.8)	603 (22.0)			42 (21.5)	988 (20.3)		
Yes, the child can't execute	26 (26.5)	339 (15.9)			29 (29.9)	461 (16.8)			55 (28.2)	800 (16.4)		
Hours on watching TV			13.5	<0.05			11.6	<0.05			24.1	<0.05
Less than an hour	41 (41.8)	1044 (49.1)			39 (40.2)	1285 (46.9)			80 (41.0)	2329 (47.8)		
1–2 hours	34 (34.7)	840 (39.5)			34 (35.1)	1104 (40.3)			68 (34.9)	1944 (39.9)		
2–3 hours	14 (14.3)	162 (7.6)			16 (16.5)	233 (8.5)			30 (15.4)	39 (8.1)		
More than 3 hours	9 (9.2)	81 (3.8)			8 (8.2)	119 (4.3)			17 (8.7)	200 (4.1)		
Frequency of parents watching TV with child			4.9	>0.05			1.0	>0.05			4.1	>0.05
Rarely	18 (18.4)	406 (19.1)			22 (22.7)	528 (19.3)			40 (20.5)	934 (19.2)		
Sometimes	68 (69.4)	1274 (59.9)			57 (58.8)	1617 (59.0)			125 (64.1)	2891 (59.4)		
Often	12 (12.2)	447 (21.0)			18 (18.6)	596 (21.7)			30 (15.4)	1043 (21.4)		
Active learning			90.3	<0.05			101.4	<0.05			194.2	<0.05
Yes	8 (8.2)	737 (34.6)			10 (10.3)	1104 (40.3)			18 (9.2)	1841 (37.8)		
Sometimes	50 (51.0)	1162 (54.6)			50 (51.5)	1391 (50.7)			100 (51.3)	2553 (52.4)		
Never	40 (40.8)	228 (10.7)			37 (38.1)	246 (9.0)			77 (39.5)	474 (9.7)		
Home literacy environment												
Frequency of parents telling stories			9.1	<0.05			3.2	>0.05			10.1	<0.05
Occasionally	56 (57.1)	999 (47.0)			53 (54.6)	1494 (54.5)			109 (55.9)	2493 (51.2)		
Sometimes	40 (40.8)	896 (42.1)			41 (42.3)	1035 (37.8)			81 (41.5)	1931 (39.7)		
Often	2 (2.0)	232 (10.9)			3 (3.1)	212 (7.7)			5 (2.6)	444 (9.1)		
How about parents encourage the child to read book extra-curricular			8.5	<0.05			4.2	>0.05			12.6	<0.05
Occasionally	16 (16.3)	192 (9.0)			13 (13.4)	246 (9.0)			29 (14.9)	438 (9.0)		
Sometimes	31 (31.6)	564 (26.5)			27 (27.8)	630 (23.0)			58 (29.7)	1194 (24.5)		

Table 3. Cont.

Variables	Low grade				High grade				All subjects			
	Dyslexia (n = 98)	Non-dyslexia (n = 2127)	x^2	*P*	Dyslexia (n = 97)	Non-dyslexia (n = 2741)	x^2	*P*	Dyslexia (n = 195)	Non-dyslexia (n = 4868)	x^2	*P*
	n(%)	n(%)			n(%)	n(%)			n(%)	n(%)		
Often	51 (52.0)	1371 (64.5)			57 (58.8)	1865 (68.0)			108 (55.4)	3236 (66.5)		
Frequency of parents buying the books child was interested in			11.7	<0.05			7.8	>0.05			18.6	<0.05
Occasionally	26 (26.5)	337 (15.8)			25 (25.8)	489 (17.8)			51 (26.2)	826 (17.0)		
Sometimes	46 (46.9)	920 (43.3)			47 (48.5)	1194 (43.6)			93 (47.7)	2114 (43.4)		
Often	26 (26.5)	870 (40.9)			25 (25.8)	1058 (38.6)			51 (26.2)	1928 (39.6)		
Frequency of parents buying new books			9.5	<0.05			7.2	>0.05			12.8	<0.05
Per week	0 (0.0)	48 (2.3)			2 (2.1)	92 (3.4)			2 (1.0)	140 (2.9)		
Per month	4 (4.1)	258 (12.1)			7 (7.2)	339 (12.4)			11 (5.6)	597 (12.3)		
Per term	13 (13.3)	320 (15.0)			19 (19.6)	414 (15.1)			32 (16.4)	734 (15.1)		
Every year	1 (1.0)	16 (0.8)			3 (3.1)	29 (1.1)			4 (2.1)	45 (0.9)		
Irregularly scheduled, buy when needed	80 (81.6)	1485 (69.8)			66 (68.0)	1867 (68.1)			146 (74.9)	3352 (68.9)		
Frequency of parents' reading			2.9	>0.05			10.9	<0.05			12	<0.05
Every day	18 (18.4)	534 (25.1)			18 (18.6)	751 (27.4)			36 (18.5)	1285 (26.4)		
Every week	50 (51.0)	1059 (49.8)			41 (42.3)	1310 (47.8)			91 (46.7)	2369 (48.7)		
Every month	30 (30.6)	534 (25.1)			38 (39.2)	680 (24.8)			68 (34.9)	1214 (24.9)		
Scheduled reading time			21.6	<0.05			17.8	<0.05			41.2	<0.05
Yes	13 (13.3)	770 (36.2)			26 (26.8)	1331 (48.6)			39 (20.0)	2101 (43.2)		
No	85 (86.7)	1357 (63.8)			71 (73.2)	1410 (51.4)			156 (80.0)	2767 (56.8)		
Expenses of buying books for child every year			8.7	<0.05			10.5	<0.05			16.6	<0.05
Less than 150 Yuan	55 (56.1)	962 (45.2)			59 (60.8)	1234 (45.0)			114 (58.5)	2196 (45.1)		
150–300 Yuan	28 (28.6)	871 (40.9)			28 (28.9)	1032 (37.7)			56 (28.7)	1903 (39.1)		
300–500 Yuan	14(14.3)	225 (10.6)			9 (9.3)	354 (12.9)			23 (11.8)	579 (11.9)		
More than 500 Yuan	1 (1.0)	69 (3.2)			1 (1.0)	121 (4.4)			2 (1.0)	190 (3.9)		

[a]Age was represented as mean ± standard deviation, *P* value was calculated by the *t* test.
[b]BMI was represented as mean ± standard deviation, *P* value was calculated by the *t* test.

Table 4. Multivariate logistic regression analysis of associated factors for dyslexia.

Subjects	Variables	OR (95%CI)	*P*
Low-grade			
	Gender		
	Female	1	
	Male	2.7 (1.7–4.4)	<0.001
	Active learning		
	Never	1	
	Yes	0.1 (0.0–0.2)	<0.001
	Sometimes	0.3 (0.2–0.5)	<0.001
High-grade			
	Gender		
	Female	1	
	Male	2.0 (1.2–3.1)	0.004
	Active learning		
	Never	1	
	Yes	0.1 (0.0–0.1)	<0.001
	Sometimes	0.3 (0.2–0.4)	<0.001
All subjects			
	Gender		
	Female	1	
	Male	2.3 (1.6–3.2)	<0.001
	Mother's education level		
	College diploma or above	1	
	Junior college	5.0 (0.7–38.5)	0.122
	Senior high school or equivalency	9.3 (1.3–67.4)	0.028
	Junior high school or below	12.1 (1.6–87.3)	0.014
	Active learning		
	Never	1	
	Yes	0.1 (0.1–0.2)	<0.001
	Sometimes	0.3 (0.2–0.4)	<0.001
	Schedule reading time		
	No	1	
	Yes	0.5 (0.4–0.8)	0.002

OR: odds ratio, CI: confidence interval.

Discussion

To our knowledge, the current study is one of the first studies focusing on the prevalence and risk factors for Chinese dyslexic children. Not only did we use the DCCC scale to evaluate the dyslexia among children, but also we considered their school and family environment. The main findings from this study were (1) The prevalence of dyslexia was 3.90% in Qianjiang city and the prevalence of dyslexia in boys was higher than that in girls. (2) Learning habits were significantly associated with dyslexia. (3) Home literacy environment could have impact on children's reading abilities.

Depending on the definition of dyslexia and culture differences, the prevalence rate varies. According to a previous study [14], children learning to read Chinese and Japanese suffered from the dyslexia, as well as their peers who learned English. Considering low reading ability together with average IQ, 7.5% children in Taipei met the criteria of dyslexia. If researchers applied the low achievement criteria that the child who fall behind average reading level two standard deviation was regarded as dyslexia [27], 2% of Taipei children [14] were thought to have reading disability. The difference between our study and the one in Taipei may come from the difference of two types of Chinese characters. The simplified Chinese characters are always adopted in mainland, while in Taiwan, the traditional Chinese is widely used [28]. The average number of strokes of 2000 commonly used characters is 11.2 for the traditional script used in Hong Kong and Taiwan and 9.0 for the simplified script used in Mainland China [17]. Therefore, it is harder for children to recognize the traditional characters than the simplified ones. We also noticed that the difference in the learning mechanism. Children learn to read Chinese characters via Pin-Yin (an alphabetic phonetic system) in Mainland China and Zhu-Yin-Fu-Hao (a sub-syllabic phonetic system) in Taiwan. Although both of them come from the same language origin, the difference in phonetic system may affect the prevalence of dyslexia in mainland China.

Later, a similar study was conducted in mainland China, which reported that 4.55% children were subjected to dyslexia. In our study, we also adopted the low achievement criteria. The prevalence of dyslexia in this survey was 3.9%, which was between those of above two studies. The difference may be caused by the diversity in the study subjects. In the above two studies, subjects were students in 5th grade of the primary schools, but the subjects of our study were selected from 3rd–6th. As early as 3rd grade, children have showed academic difficulties evidently. By the time whether the children suffered from dyslexia or not could be entrenched. Thus, the current results provide a better knowledge of Chinese dyslexia based on populations in the primary schools. So far, the association between prevalence rate and grade is unclear. Theoretically, the prevalence of dyslexia will be lower in lower grade, because many students may manifest the symptoms of dyslexia in higher grade. However, the prevalence of dyslexics in grade 6 was the lowest among 4 grades in this study. It may be explained by a previous study, which demonstrated that the prevalence of dyslexia in higher grade was likely to be lower than the one in lower grade, because the symptoms of some dyslexic children in higher grade would be improved through the systematic reading experience of one or two years [7]. Therefore, more studies are called to address this problem in the future.

The prevalence of Chinese dyslexia is lower than the reported prevalence rate in western countries, which were 5% to 17% [7]. The study by Siok et al. [24] provided an insight into the fundamental path physiology of dyslexia by suggesting that rather than having a universal origin, the biological abnormality of impaired reading depends on culture. Indeed, Chinese belongs to non-alphabetic languages which may result in specificity in dyslexia in contrast with alphabetic languages. The percentage of dyslexia in Chinese is lower than their peers who speak English, but the relative amount of dyslexic children is still high in China. It is necessary to employ an epidemiological investigation in China. Therefore, we need to take great effort to diagnose and treat dyslexic adolescents as early as possible.

In current study, a gender ratio was nearly 3:1 from boys to girls for dyslexic children. The logistic regression revealed that the risk of boys was 2.3 times as high as girls. A large body of studies has typically reported that there were significantly more boys than girls with dyslexia [29,30]. Our findings are coincident with previous studies. The possible reasons may be genetic difference, inherited features and development of cognition. Normand reported that a small advantage in language production for girls over boys until 36 months of age [31]. In China, boys are always expected to be proficient at science subjects, while girls are expected to be good at arts. For parents, to some extent, child's gender will influence their attitude and educational ways to child. Our study indicated that boys were more likely to be dyslexic. The gender difference in dyslexia suggested that teaching methods should be considered for boys and girls.

Our results suggested that learning habits and parents' education level were associated with dyslexia. The higher education levels the parents have, the less risk their children are suffered from. And father's higher education always relates to a better social economic status. Furthermore, education and income are the determinants of socioeconomic status which are associated with the development of children language reported by previous research [32]. Maternal characteristics such as verbal ability and personality have been shown to be related to the construction of the child's environment, therefore, influence the child's development [33]. In the previous studies, the conclusion that maternal education had been strongly associated with reading and literacy had been reported, which was confirmed by the results of current study. The traditional idea that man should work outside while woman should do housework at home has not been converted completely in China. Therefore, mother communicates with child more frequently and plays an important role in raising the child. Because of the different cognitive ability, mother with different educational level may create various reading environment. Learning habits including active learning and scheduled reading time were potential factors for dyslexia, which were seldom reported in the previous studies. Child who is active in learning behaves actively during the learning, including asking questions, discussing with teachers or classmates frequently and so on. Dyslexic children usually have difficulty in reading and the failure may decrease the motivation of learning. The interaction between active learning and dyslexia may circulate towards to worse situation. That is, those children will experience more depressed, unhappy, bored feelings to reading. In China, parents usually expect their child to achieve a higher academic goal no matter their ability, and the child endures enormous pressure. For the child with dyslexia, the pressure might be larger which cannot be assessed. The study also showed that scheduled reading time was associated with dyslexia. Motivation is important to learning because of its link to reading practice [34]. As a result, parents' guide and encouragement are crucial to children's reading. In summary, students who cannot read well and read less usually lost practice opportunities, which makes it difficult to acquire average level of reading fluency. Reading experience is the vital access to increase vocabularies, reading comprehension and related skills. Because of limited knowledge and notion, parents often ignore the importance of reading practice. Thus, it is necessary to establish reading time for children.

Home literacy environment was found to associate with dyslexia in our study. When parents tell stories to child and encourage child to read more frequently, their child has less risk of dyslexia. While the parents buy books that child is interested in, their child is less likely to be dyslexia. Fontina L. Rashid indicated that children's home literacy actives were not significantly related to any of their academic abilities, whereas parents' home literacy activities were significantly related to children's passage comprehension and spelling scores [35]. According to our results, parents' reading activities (spending more time to reading with child, more books available at home, encouraging child to read) can help to reduce the risk of dyslexia.

The difference of risk factors associated with dyslexia in low grade and high grade indicated the importance of parents. Children in high grade may face heavy pressure of entering high schools so that their parents pay more attention to their scores instead of offering a good literacy environment. Generally speaking, children in high grade process reading practice mainly in class. As a result, there were no associations between parents' relevant actives (frequency of parents tell stories, how about parents encourage the child to read book extra-curricular, frequency of parents buy the books child interested) and dyslexia. On the other hand, children in low grade will be relaxed and parents' relevant actives may be associated with dyslexia. Therefore, parents' attitude to construct what kind of literacy environment is crucial for their children.

The current study showed special culture, economy and educational system may be associated with dyslexia. Additional studies are still needed to explore issues in debate. However, there are still some shortcomings in present study. The current study was carried out in one city in China, and we could only generalize the prevalence rate to other middle-sized cities similar to Qianjiang city. More different types of cities should be sampled if we want to know the dyslexic prevalence in the whole China in the future studies. The subjects were selected from primary schools, which just reflected the prevalence rate of dyslexia among children from 9–12 years old. To a great extent, the etiology of Chinese dyslexia is still uncovered. The learning habits, home literacy environment and the other factors such as cognitive characters of children will continue to be studied in the future.

Author Contributions

Conceived and designed the experiments: ZS LZ RS. Performed the experiments: ZS LZ JZ SM. Analyzed the data: SS RZ JK XL. Contributed reagents/materials/analysis tools: JK XL. Wrote the paper: ZS LZ XM RS.

References

1. Fisher SE, Francks C, Marlow AJ, MacPhie IL, Newbury DF, et al. (2002) Independent genome-wide scans identify a chromosome 18 quantitative-trait locus influencing dyslexia. Nat Genet 30: 86–91.
2. Maughan B, Rowe R, Loeber R, Stouthamer-Loeber M (2003) Reading problems and depressed mood. J Abnorm Child Psychol 31: 219–229.
3. Willcutt EG, Pennington BF (2000) Psychiatric comorbidity in children and adolescents with reading disability. J Child Psychol Psychiatry 41: 1039–1048.
4. Casey R, Levy SE, Brown K, Brooks-Gunn J (1992) Impaired emotional health in children with mild reading disability. J Dev Behav Pediatr 13: 256–260.
5. Beitchman JH, Wilson B, Brownlie EB, Walters H, Inglis A, et al. (1996) Long-term consistency in speech/language profiles: II. Behavioral, emotional, and social outcomes. J Am Acad Child Adolesc Psychiatry 35: 815–825.
6. Heiervang E, Stevenson J, Lund A, Hugdahl K (2001) Behaviour problems in children with dyslexia. Nord J Psychiatry 55: 251–256.
7. Shaywitz SE (1998) Dyslexia. N Engl J Med 338: 307–312.
8. Katusic SK, Colligan RC, Barbaresi WJ, Schaid DJ, Jacobsen SJ (2001) Incidence of reading disability in a population-based birth cohort, 1976–1982, Rochester, Minn. Mayo Clin Proc 76: 1081–1092.
9. Rutter M, Caspi A, Fergusson D, Horwood LJ, Goodman R, et al. (2004) Sex differences in developmental reading disability: new findings from 4 epidemiological studies. JAMA 291: 2007–2012.
10. Kempe C, Gustafson S, Samuelsson S (2011) A longitudinal study of early reading difficulties and subsequent problem behaviors. Scand J Psychol 52: 242–250.
11. Shaywitz SE, Shaywitz BA, Fletcher JM, Escobar MD (1990) Prevalence of reading disability in boys and girls. Results of the Connecticut Longitudinal Study. JAMA 264: 998–1002.
12. Undheim AM, Sund AM (2008) Psychosocial factors and reading difficulties: students with reading difficulties drawn from a representative population sample. Scand J Psychol 49: 377–384.

13. Donfrancesco R, Iozzino R, Caruso B, Ferrante L, Mugnaini D, et al. (2010) Is season of birth related to developmental dyslexia? Ann Dyslexia 60: 175–182.
14. Stevenson HW, Stigler JW, Lucker GW, Lee S, Hsu C, et al. (1982) Reading disabilities: the case of Chinese, Japanese, and English. Child Dev 53: 1164–1181.
15. Ho CS, Law TP, Ng PM (2000) The phonological deficit hypothesis in Chinese developmental dyslexia. Reading and Writing 13: 57–79.
16. Ho CS, Chan DW, Tsang SM, Lee SH (2002) The cognitive profile and multiple-deficit hypothesis in Chinese developmental dyslexia. Dev Psychol 38: 543–553.
17. Ho CS, Chan DW, Lee SH, Tsang SM, Luan VH (2004) Cognitive profiling and preliminary subtyping in Chinese developmental dyslexia. Cognition 91: 43–75.
18. Ho CS, Chan DW, Chung KK, Lee SH, Tsang SM (2007) In search of subtypes of Chinese developmental dyslexia. J Exp Child Psychol 97: 61–83.
19. McBride-Chang C, Lam F, Lam C, Chan B, Fong CY, et al. (2011) Early predictors of dyslexia in Chinese children: familial history of dyslexia, language delay, and cognitive profiles. J Child Psychol Psychiatry 52: 204–211.
20. Shu H, McBride-Chang C, Wu S, Liu H (2006) Understanding chinese developmental dyslexia: Morphological awareness as a core cognitive construct. Journal of Educational Psychology 98: 122–123.
21. Shu H, Meng X, Lai A (2003) Lexical representation and processing in Chinese-speaking poor readers. In: McBride-Chang C, Chen HC, editors. Reading Development in Chinese Children. Westport: Greenwood Publishing Group. pp. 199–214.
22. Meng X, Tian X, Jian J, Zhou X (2007) Orthographic and phonological processing in Chinese dyslexic children: an ERP study on sentence reading. Brain Res 1179: 119–130.
23. Siok WT, Niu Z, Jin Z, Perfetti CA, Tan LH (2008) A structural-functional basis for dyslexia in the cortex of Chinese readers. Proc Natl Acad Sci U S A 105: 5561–5566.
24. Siok WT, Perfetti CA, Jin Z, Tan LH (2004) Biological abnormality of impaired reading is constrained by culture. Nature 431: 71–76.
25. Basic situation of Qianjiang city. Available: http//www.hbqj.gov.cn/data/2006/0825/article_15.htm. Accessed 5 November 2012.
26. National Bureau of Statistics of China (2011) China city statistical yearbook. Beijing: China Statistics Press. 23p.
27. Zhang C, Zhang J, Yin R, Zhou J, Chang S (1996) Experimental research on the reading disability of Chinese students. psychological Science 19: 222–226.
28. Jin H, He X, Mo L (2009) On the DiagnosticTests of Chinese Developmental Dyslexia. Journal of South China Normal University 5: 39–43.
29. Badian NA (1999) Reading disability defined as a discrepancy between listening and reading comprehension: a longitudinal study of stability, gender differences, and prevalence. J Learn Disabil 32: 138–148.
30. DeFries JC (1989) Gender ratios in children with reading disability and their affected relatives: a commentary. J Learn Disabil 22: 544–545.
31. Normand MT, Parisse C, Cohen H (2008) Lexical diversity and productivity in French preschooolers developmental and biosocial aspects by developmental, gender and sociocultural factors. Clin Linguist Phon 22: 47–58.
32. Nicolson RI, Fawcett AJ, Dean P (2001) Developmental dyslexia: the cerebellar deficit hypothesis. Trends Neurosci 24: 508–511.
33. Lyytinen P, Eklund K, Lyytinen H (2003) The play and language behavior of mothers with and without dyslexia and its association to their toddlers' language development. J Learn Disabil 36: 74–86.
34. Morgan PL, Fuchs D, Compton DL, Cordray DS, Fuchs LS (2008) Does early reading failure decrease children's reading motivation? J Learn Disabil 41: 387–404.
35. Rashid FL, Morris RD, Sevcik RA (2005) Relationship between home literacy environment and reading achievement in children with reading disabilities. J Learn Disabil 38: 2–11.

3

Cognitive Profile of Students Who Enter Higher Education with an Indication of Dyslexia

Maaike Callens*◔, Wim Tops◔, Marc Brysbaert

Department of Experimental Psychology, University of Ghent, Ghent, Belgium

Abstract

For languages other than English there is a lack of empirical evidence about the cognitive profile of students entering higher education with a diagnosis of dyslexia. To obtain such evidence, we compared a group of 100 Dutch-speaking students diagnosed with dyslexia with a control group of 100 students without learning disabilities. Our study showed selective deficits in reading and writing (effect sizes for accuracy between d = 1 and d = 2), arithmetic (d≈1), and phonological processing (d>0.7). Except for spelling, these deficits were larger for speed related measures than for accuracy related measures. Students with dyslexia also performed slightly inferior on the KAIT tests of crystallized intelligence, due to the retrieval of verbal information from long-term memory. No significant differences were observed in the KAIT tests of fluid intelligence. The profile we obtained agrees with a recent meta-analysis of English findings suggesting that it generalizes to all alphabetic languages. Implications for special arrangements for students with dyslexia in higher education are outlined.

Editor: Kevin Paterson, University of Leicester, United Kingdom

Funding: This research was made possible by an Odysseus research grant from the Government to Marc Brysbaert. For further details, see: http://www.fwo.be/Odysseusprogramma-huidige-detail.aspx?ID = fcdcbebe-d2a3-46c3-8393-f2e820b24664. The funders had no role in study design, data collection and analysis, decision to publish, or preparation of the manuscript.

Competing Interests: The authors have declared that no competing interests exist.

* E-mail: maaike.callens@ugent.be

◔ These authors contributed equally to this work.

Introduction

An increasing number of students with dyslexia enter higher education, most likely due to better assessment, guidance and remediation in primary and secondary education [1–2]. This creates a need for information about the characteristics of these students and the best ways to support them. Higher education differs significantly from primary and secondary school. At this age education is no longer compulsory and students have a much wider range of options (certainly compared to primary education, which in most countries is inclusive, with nearly all children given the same curriculum). Therefore, dyslexic students entering higher education can be expected to be a select group, with better than average coping skills and possibly less comorbidity (for the issue of comorbidity in dyslexia, see [3–5]).

Still, there is a need for scientific evidence about the cognitive profile of students with dyslexia in higher education, particularly for non-English speaking countries. There are a number of manuals about adult dyslexia and dyslexia in higher education (e.g. [6–8]), which contain valuable information for students with dyslexia and their counselors and tutors, but they mainly base their information and recommendations on clinical and educational practice and they focus on the state of affairs in English-speaking countries.

Because of the scarcity of scientific data, at present there are no generally-accepted guidelines, regulations, and standards for compensatory measures. Instead, the clinical experience of the local office of disability services and their considerations tend to prevail [9]. As a result, the special arrangements differ between institutes and are not appreciated by all lecturers. In the absence of theoretical and empirical evidence for the efficacy of such measures lecturers fear that reading disabled students could be beneficiaries of needless exceptions, which create extra work and may be unfair to the other students. Exceptionally, some even doubt whether students with a diagnosis of dyslexia belong in higher education, questioning their cognitive skills and work attitude. Given the current situation, these reactions are not completely without grounds. Sparks and Lovett [9–10], for instance, found that offices of disability services in American colleges often give learning disability certificates without empirical justification, and that these certificates tend to be popular when they are linked to course exemptions in colleges with foreign-language requirements.

In the present paper we first discuss what is known about the cognitive profile of students with dyslexia in American and British higher education. Then, we discuss the reasons why generalization to other countries is not straightforward, and we present the data of a new study addressing the limitation.

The Cognitive Profile of Students with Dyslexia in Higher Education: Evidence from English

A first series of studies in the 1990s [11–13] addressed the question whether individuals with dyslexia continued to have problems with reading and spelling in adulthood, or whether remediation, teaching and reading practice in primary and secondary education were able to bridge the initial gap. They had a strong focus on reading and spelling and did not take into account other functions such as memory, attention, planning, and organization. These studies all came to the conclusion that dyslexia is an enduring problem with remaining suboptimal performance for reading and writing in dyslexic university students.

A particularly interesting study was published in the UK by Hatcher, Snowling, and Griffiths [14], because it investigated a broader range of skills. The authors compared the cognitive skills of 23 university students with dyslexia and 50 controls matched on verbal and non-verbal abilities. Participants completed 17 tasks assessing literacy (reading and writing), processing skills (perceptual speed, memory span, and arithmetic), phonological skills (spoonerisms and rapid naming), verbal fluency, verbal abilities (vocabulary test), non-verbal abilities (Raven matrices), and self-reported problems in attention and organization. Surprisingly, the students with dyslexia performed worse on all but the two tasks of general cognitive abilities (Wechsler Adult Intelligence Scale Vocabulary and Raven Matrices). They showed significant deficits in reading and writing and in reading-related phonological processes. Additionally, their processing rate was overall slower and their short-term memory spans were shorter. The students with dyslexia also had poorer arithmetic performance. Dyslexic students further reported more problems with memory ("I easily forget about what has been said"), attention ("I lose track in required reading"), effort ("I do not work to my potential"), affect ("I am sensitive to criticism"), and – less so – organizing and activating ("I have difficulty getting organized and started"). Based on these results, Hatcher et al. [14] doubted about the generality of the statement that higher education students with dyslexia have compensated for their problems.

Surprisingly, Hatcher et al.'s [14] rather pessimistic conclusion was not followed by other studies of the same standards. Subsequent studies again involved small numbers of tasks and small numbers of participants, making it difficult to obtain reliable estimates of the overall cognitive profile of dyslexic students in higher education [15–16]. A further step forward was made when Swanson and Hsieh [17] published the results of a meta-analysis. By applying such an analysis, researchers can distill a coherent pattern out of a multitude of heterogeneous, small-scale studies. Swanson and Hsieh's meta-analysis was based on 52 published articles (but surprisingly without Hatcher et al. [14] and 776 comparisons of participants with reading disabilities versus participants without reading disabilities. An additional advantage of meta-analyses is that the results are communicated as effect-sizes. Swanson and Hsieh used Cohen's d statistic. This is a standardized measure with very much the same interpretation as a z-score [18]. As a rule of thumb, d-values larger than.5 have practical value and d-values larger than.8 point to a substantial difference between the groups. These effect sizes make it easy to translate research findings to the counseling practice. In contrast, individual studies have a tendency to focus on the statistical significance of their effects, often overlooking issues of power and practical importance.

Table 1 summarizes the findings reported in the meta-analysis of Swanson and Hsieh [17] as effect sizes (d) of differences between participants with reading disabilities and participants without reading disabilities. Positive values indicate poorer performance of participants with dyslexia; negative values indicate better performance of this group. For comparison purposes, we also include the data of Hatcher et al. [14] expressed as effect sizes. The convergences between both studies are clear. The top problems of adults with dyslexia are, not surprisingly: writing, reading, and phonological processing (non-word naming and spoonerisms, which involve exchanging the first sounds of two words, e.g., turning "Terry Wogan" into "Werry Togan"). The effect sizes are mostly larger than 1. In addition, reading disabled adults seem to be poorer in retrieving verbal information from long-term memory, either because this information has been processed less frequently or because of an additional weakness in individuals with dyslexia. One of the most robust findings in cognitive psychology is the (word) frequency effect, the finding that the efficiency of information processing depends on the number of times the information has been processed before (e.g. [19]). There was also poorer performance on arithmetic. This finding has recently been confirmed [20–21] and linked to the fact that arithmetic operations often depend on verbal fact retrieval, in particular for multiplication. This would explain why the difference between

Table 1. Effect sizes (d) of differences between participants with reading disabilities and participants without reading disabilities.

	S&H09	HSG02
Literacy		
Reading comprehension	1.20	
Word reading	1.37	1.14
Non-Word Reading	1.33	1.47
Word Spelling	1.57	1.31
Text Writing	0.72	1.12
Processing skills		
Perceptual speed		0.89
Short-term memory span		1.05
Phonological skills		
Phonological processing	0.87	1.32
Rapid naming	0.96	1.19
Verbal fluency		
Semantic fluency		0.46
Rhyme fluency		1.26
General intelligence		
Arithmetic	0.75	0.58
Verbal memory	0.20	
Verbal intelligence	0.63	
Vocabulary	0.71	0.10
General information	0.47	
Problem solving/reasoning	0.11	−0.01
Verbal memory	0.62	
Visuospatial memory	−0.39	
Cognitive monitoring	0.27	
Perceptual motor skills	−0.13	
Auditory perception	−0.18	
Visual perception	0.13	
Other		
Social and personal skills	0.10	
Personality	0.28	
Neuropsychological (e.g., EEG)	−0.02	
Ratings by third persons	−0.23	

Note: S&H09 = Swanson & Hsieh [17]; HSG02 = Hatcher, Snowling & Griffiths [14].

individuals with dyslexia and controls is larger for multiplication than for subtraction [20].

On the positive side, there were no differences of practical significance for general intelligence, problem solving/reasoning, cognitive monitoring, perceptuo-motor skills, auditory and visual perception, social and personal skills, personality, and neuropsychological measures (such as EEG patterns). Dyslexics slightly outperformed controls in visuo-spatial memory and tended to be rated more favorably by third persons than controls.

All in all, Swanson and Hsieh's [17] analysis paints a rather clear picture of the strengths and weaknesses of adults with dyslexia. Still, two caveats should be kept in mind. The first is that meta-analyses involve a combination of very heterogeneous studies, with varying degrees of methodological rigor. This is particularly a concern when the number of studies on which an effect size has been calculated is rather small. Then, the presence or absence of an effect could be due to a single unrepresentative study involving a less valid test or a less representative participant sample. This issue is known as the apples-and-oranges problem in meta-analyses [22]. Although the convergence between Swanson and Hsieh [17] and Hatcher et al. [14] is reassuring in this respect, one would feel more confident if the picture were confirmed in an independent series of studies given to the same groups of participants. The second caveat with respect to Swanson and Hsieh's [17] conclusions is that they are almost entirely based on English-speaking adults. Only 5% of the data were from non-English studies. Below we discuss two reasons why generalization to other languages/countries is not straightforward.

Factors that may Prevent Generalization to other Languages

A first factor that may hinder the generalization of English findings to other languages, such as Dutch, is that languages differ in the difficulty of the letter-sound mappings. This feature has been linked to the time children need for reading acquisition [23–25] and also to the prevalence of dyslexia ([26]; see also [27] and [28] for a discussion of the ways in which English differs from other languages and what impact this may have for dyslexia). Readers of languages with inconsistent mappings need more time to reach ceiling performance and also have higher chances of not succeeding. There are two types of mapping: from letters to sounds and from sounds to letters (particularly important for correct spelling but also involved in word reading; [29]). Alphabetical languages differ in the degree of complexity of these mappings [30–31] with English consistently being the most opaque for both directions, and Dutch more towards the transparent end of the continuum (the extent depending on the specific measure used).

In the absence of empirical evidence, it is not clear what to expect as a result of the language differences in letter-sound mappings. On the one hand, one could imagine that dyslexia would be less of a problem in a transparent language; on the other hand, someone with dyslexia in a transparent language may on average have a stronger deficit than someone with dyslexia in an opaque language (if indeed differences in prevalence of dyslexia because of language transparency exist).

Another factor that may limit the findings of Table 1 to English-speaking countries is the organization of the education system in different countries. In general, British-inspired education is characterized by ability-based selection at the entry together with a commitment to bring the selected candidates to a successful completion (the master-apprentice model). In many other countries, however, there are no hard entrance criteria for higher education, and selection occurs as part of the curriculum. In Belgium, for instance, everyone who has completed secondary education, is entitled to start whatever type of higher education they want (except for medicine and dentistry, where an additional entrance exam must be passed). As a result, the number of students starting higher education tends to be higher and completion rates are lower. In particular, the first year is considered as a selection year with less than half of the student succeeding. Classes in the first year, therefore, tend to be plenary lectures before large groups, and exams often are multiple choice.

Needless to say, ability-based admission criteria are likely to have implications for the cognitive profiles of the students, certainly in the first year of education. For instance, the observation that Swanson and Hsieh [17] and Hatcher et al. [14] found no differences in general intelligence or problem solving between students with and without reading problems may be a consequence of the fact that British and American universities select their students on the basis of SAT-scores (US) and A-levels (UK). Indeed, Lovett and Sparks [32] noticed that a discrepancy between general intelligence and reading skills in American university students with reading disabilities is often due to average text reading skills combined with above-average IQ. Such a pattern might be a direct consequence of the admission criteria. As these criteria are not present in Belgium, students with quite different IQ-scores can start the same degree and there is no built-in guarantee that students who present themselves with a diagnosis of dyslexia have the same abilities as students without such an assessment. On the other hand, because students with a reading disability know of the selection taking place in the first year of higher education, they may be less inclined to start a degree that is perceived as demanding, given the chances of failure.

The Cognitive Profile of Students with Dyslexia in Higher Education: Evidence from Non-English Speaking Countries

As stated before, literature on dyslexia in young adults who do not have English as mother tongue, is limited. In addition, in line with the first studies in English, they all focused on weaknesses rather than on the full pattern of strengths and weaknesses. Reid, Szczerbinski, Iskierka-Kasperek, and Hansen [33] ran a study in Polish on 15 dyslexic university students and 15 control students. As primary deficits they reported inferior word reading rate, pseudoword reading rate and text reading (both speed and accuracy). Spelling accuracy was also significantly lower. In relation to the underlying causes of dyslexia the authors observed impaired rapid automatized naming (pictures, colors, letters and digits) and phonological difficulties on a timed sound deletion task. However, group differences on spoonerism accuracy/time and sound deletion accuracy only approached significance. Similar results were found in a French study by Szenkovits and Ramus [34]. Students with dyslexia ($N = 17$) performed worse than a control group on a text reading task when a combined time and accuracy measure was reported (but see Bruyer and Brysbaert [35] for difficulties with such combined measures). Orthographic skills were also significantly lower. Moreover, a combined RAN (colors, digits and letters) score revealed impaired automatized naming and working memory. Students with dyslexia also displayed phonological deficits. Wolff [36] examined Swedish university students ($N = 40$) on a range of reading, writing and phonological skills tasks. Significant differences with large effect sizes were reported for several tasks: spoonerisms, non-word reading and writing (time and accuracy), exception word spelling, and orthographic skills (time and accuracy).

The above studies agree with the English studies showing that difficulties in reading and writing and phonological impairments persist into adulthood. However, none addressed abilities beyond reading and writing. Furthermore, they were all characterized by small sample sizes, making it dangerous to interpret the effect sizes.

A New Study

Given the limitations of the available evidence, we decided to run a new study, which would enable us to compare the American-British profile (Table 1) to the Belgian profile. In order to do things properly, we took into account the following methodological considerations.

A problem with small-scale studies for applied research is the large confidence intervals around the obtained statistics, certainly in between-groups designs involving the comparison of two samples of individuals. Only recently have researchers become sensitive to the power problem related to small-group comparisons (e.g [37–38]). The smaller the samples, the larger the difference between the groups at population level must be before it can be found reliably in an empirical study. As a rule of thumb, to assess effect sizes as small as d = .4, one requires two groups of 100 participants (Figure 1). Samples of this size also result in reasonably small confidence intervals, so that the observed effect sizes can be trusted and compared to those from the English studies (Table 1).

To further improve the relevance of our study for offices of disability studies, we ran the study on the first 100 students who were entitled to special educational support on the basis of dyslexia by a learning disability support office in the city of Ghent (Belgium) and who were willing to take part in our study. For each student we then looked for a control student matched on age, gender, and field of study. The local support office serves Ghent University as well as other colleges of higher education (including technical colleges), meaning that we could examine a wide range of students.

Methods

Participants

Two hundred first-year undergraduate students of higher education participated in the study, both students of professional bachelors (in colleges for higher education) and academic bachelors (in some colleges for higher education and in university). They all attended higher education in Ghent, one of the major cities of Flanders (the Northern, Dutch-speaking half of Belgium) and had just graduated from secondary school. The group consisted of 100 students diagnosed with dyslexia and a control group of 100 students with no known neurological or functional deficiencies. All had normal or corrected-to normal vision and were native speakers of Dutch. Students were paid for their participation. The study followed the ethical protocol of Ghent University, meaning that students gave informed consent and were

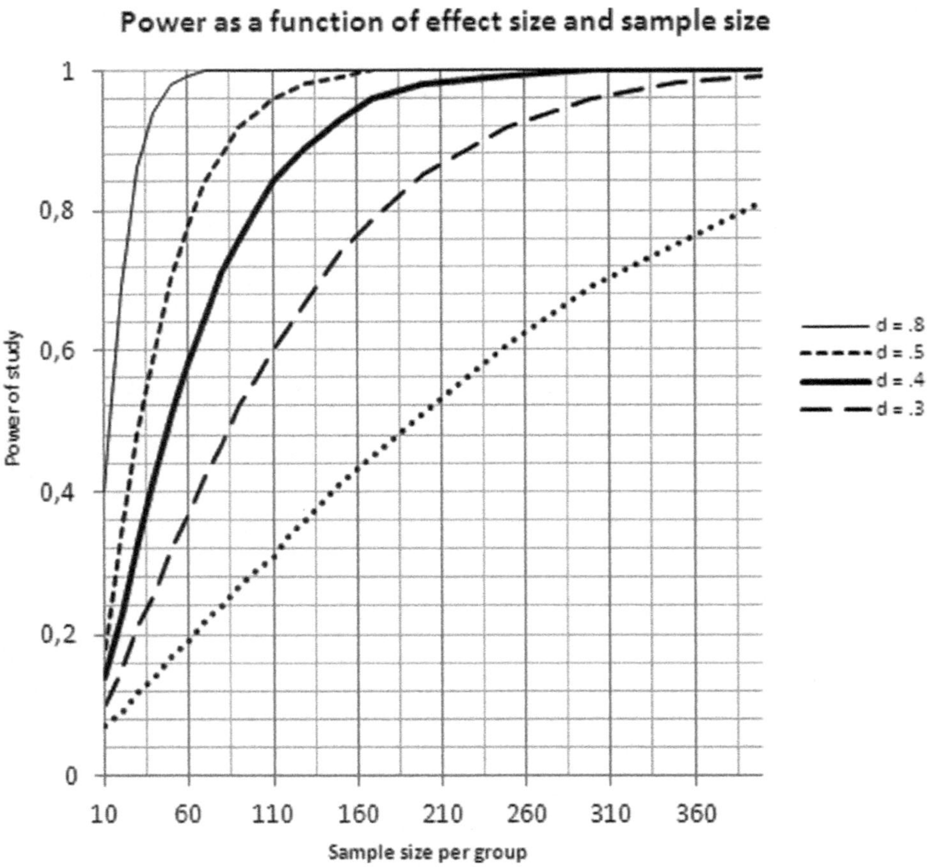

Figure 1. Power of study as a function of sample size. This figure shows the power of a study with two independent groups as a function of sample size for different levels of effect size (assuming that alpha, 2-tailed, is set at.05). For a small effect size (d = .2) we would need two samples of 393 participants to yield a power of 80%. This means that there is 80% chance of finding a significant difference between the groups, given that an effect of this size exists at the population level. For a medium effect size (d = .5) we would need two samples of 64 participants to achieve this level of power. For a large effect size (d = .8) we need 26 participants per group.

informed that they could stop at any time if they felt they were treated incorrectly.

The students with dyslexia had been diagnosed prior to our study by trained diagnosticians in accordance with the definition of SDN (Stichting Dyslexie Nederland [Foundation Dyslexia Netherlands] [39]). Because of the ongoing debate about the origin of dyslexia, the SDN uses a purely descriptive definition of dyslexia. In their guidelines dyslexia is defined as an impairment characterized by a persistent problem in learning to read and/or write words or in the automatization of reading and writing. The level of reading and/or writing has to be significantly lower than what can be expected based on the educational level and age of the individual. Finally, the resistance to instruction has to be confirmed by looking at the outcome of remedial teaching. Remedial teaching is considered adequate when it meets the requirements as stated in the "response to instruction" model [40] or the "response to intervention' model [41]. Also, the SDN definition requires ensuring that the reading and writing impairment cannot be attributed to external and/or individual factors such as socio-economic status, cultural background or intelligence. Students entering higher education in Ghent are assessed anew by the local support office (*vzw Cursief*) if their previous assessment is older than three years. All students with dyslexia had (sub) clinical scores (<pc 10) on a word reading test [42] and/or, pseudo word reading test [43] and/or word spelling test [44]. These tests are addressed further in the text. All students with dyslexia had received individual tutoring in primary or secondary education for a period of minimum 6 months by either a speech-therapist or a remedial teacher.

All students with dyslexia who applied for special facilities at the local support office in the academic year 2009–2010 were asked to participate in the study until we had a total of one hundred. To find a group of 100 participants with dyslexia who completed the full study, we had to approach an initial cohort of some 120 students. Of these 120 students a small number of students chose not to cooperate once the study was explained to them. A few more students were lost because they failed to show up at appointments.

When recruiting the subjects we tried to reflect the inflow in the first year of higher education as much as possible. Matching criteria for the control students were therefore restricted to field of study, gender and age. Because one of the goals of our project is to see how dyslexic students succeed in higher education compared to their peers and to assess the impact of their disability on their study skills we matched them on field of study. We did add age and gender as matching criteria to construct homogenous groups. To recruit the control students we used different methods. We asked the students with dyslexia for several names of fellow classmates who would be interested in participating. Amongst these names we selected someone at random. In case the dyslexic student failed to deliver any names (which was the case for about 50% of the participants), we recruited them ourselves by means of electronic platforms or the guidance counselors of the institution in question. Table 2 contains the general information on the two groups: mean age, gender, professional bachelor v. academic bachelor students, fields of study and the educational level of the parents.

The socio-economical level of the parents was not a matching criteria but no difference was found between the two groups in socio-economical level based on the educational level of the mother [$\chi^2(3) = 4.855$, $p = .183$] and father [$\chi^2(3) = 2.634$, $p = .452$]. Educational levels were: lower secondary education, higher secondary education, post secondary education either at university or a college for higher education.

Cognitive Measures and Tests Administered

In the following section, we group the tests as a function of cognitive skill. Although this is not 100% how the assessment happened (which was battery-based), it makes it easier to compare our data to those of Swanson and Hsieh [17] and Hatcher and colleagues [14]. Most cognitive skills were assessed with validated and widely used Dutch-language screening instruments. We used the Dutch version of the Kaufman Adolescent and Adult Intelligence Test [45] and an established test battery for diagnosing dyslexia in young adults [44]. We tried to obtain converging evidence from a second test designed to measure the same skill when no data about reliability and validity were available. In particular, we compared the data to the IDAA or *Interactive Dyslexia Test Amsterdam-Antwerp*, a test battery that at the time of our testing was being normed and validated [46].

The American KAIT, developed in 1993 by A.S. Kaufman and N.L. Kaufman, was translated by Dekker, Dekker, and Mulder in 2004 and norms were collected on a standardization sample in the Netherlands and Flanders. The main goal of the KAIT is to evaluate analytic intelligence in individuals from 14 to 85 years. In our study the complete version was administered. It consists of 10 subtests categorized into two types of intelligence: fluid and crystallized intelligence. The crystallized scale consists of 4 subtests: Word Definitions, Double Meanings, Auditory Comprehension, and Famous People (for more information see below). It reflects how well a person has learned concepts and knowledge that are part of one's cultural and scholar context. It is influenced by verbal conceptual development and education. The fluid intelligence scale gives an indication of the person's potential and flexibility to solve new problems, either verbal or non-verbal. The 6 subtests are Symbol Learning, Logical Reasoning, Secret Codes, Block Patterns, Delayed Auditory Memory, and Delayed Symbol Learning (for more information see below). The combination of fluid and crystallized IQ results in a total IQ-score. All three scores have a mean of 100 and a standard deviation of 15 points. Psychometric information can be found in Table 3.

We used the KAIT instead of the Wechsler Adult Intelligence Scale III [47] to avoid retest effects. Many students with dyslexia had been tested previously with the WISC or the WAIS as part of their assessment. Other reasons for choosing the KAIT were the less rigorous time constraints, which we considered an advantage for students with learning disabilities, and the inclusion of two subtests of delayed memory, namely Delayed Symbol Learning and Delayed Auditory Memory. Both subtests are considered valid measures of long term memory capacities.

We also administered the GL&SCHR, a Dutch reading and writing test battery for (young) adults [44]. This test includes many of the tasks frequently administered in dyslexia assessment (e.g. [14]). There are three tests specifically designed to evaluate reading and writing skills, namely Word Spelling, Proofreading, and Text Reading (for more information see below). Seven additional tests focus on associated language deficits such as phonological processing, rapid naming, short term memory and working memory, morphology, and vocabulary (for more information see below). Information about reliability can be found in Table 4. For different subtests different methods were used, namely KR20, Guttman split-half, and a test-retest correlation.

The IDAA or Interactive Dyslexia Test Amsterdam-Antwerp [46] is a new diagnostic instrument for the diagnosis of dyslexia in secondary school children and students in higher education. It is a test battery developed by The University of Amsterdam, Lessius College for Higher Education (Antwerp), and Muiswerk for the screening of young adults. It focuses on core skills of reading and writing such as automatized word recognition, decoding at lexical

Table 2. General information on the control group and the group with dyslexia.

	Control group		Dyslexia group	
Mean age	19 years and 11 months		19 years and 4 months	
Gender	46 male students 54 female students		46 male students 54 male students	
Degree taken	66 non university college students 34 university students		66 non university students 34 university students	
Field of study				
	Non university students	University college students	Non university students	University college students
Educational sciences	16	0	16	0
Health and behavioral sciences	21	19	21	19
Management	9	0	9	0
Sciences and Engineering	19	10	19	10
Arts and humanities	0	5	0	5
Other	1	0	1	0
Educational level father				
Lower secondary	4		7	
Higher secondary	44		36	
College	28		31	
University	16		22	
Missing	8		4	
Total	100		100	
Educational level mother				
Lower secondary	4		4	
Higher secondary	36		35	
College	45		41	
University	7		18	
Missing	8		2	
Total	100		100	

and sublexical level, and orthographic and phonological competence. The individual administration is fully computer controlled. The battery consists of six subtests. The first one is a questionnaire that assesses print exposure in Dutch and English. Next, phonological skills are evaluated with a reversal task where the participant has to state whether the second orally presented nonword is the reversal of the first (e.g. rol-lor). Then, four tests focus on orthographical skills : flash reading in Dutch, flash typing in Dutch, flash typing of nonwords in Dutch, and flash typing in English. In these tasks participants are presented with a word or nonword for 200 ms followed by a mask (###). Depending on the task the participant has to identify whether the target item was a word or nonword, or type in the word/nonword. As the names indicate, this is done both for Dutch and English. As this

Table 3. Reliability and validity indices for the different subtests of the KAIT [45].

	Internal consistency Chronbach's alpha for age groups 16–19	Test-retest reliability for age group 14–24	Content validity: correlation with WAIS –R Total IQ scores
CIQ	.92	.80	.79
Definitions	.82	.81	
Double Meanings	.81	.72	
Auditory Comprehension	.81	.71	
Famous People	.76	.87	
FIQ	.93	.84	.76
Symbol Learning	.93	.85	
Logical Reasoning	.81	.66	
Secret Codes	.80	.61	
Block Patterns	.80	.82	
Delayed Auditory Comprehension	.55	.49	
Delayed Symbol Learning	.93	.81	
TIQ	.95	.89	.84

Table 4. Reliability indices for the different subtests of the GL&SCHR [44].

	KR20	Guttman split half (γ)	test-retest
Text Reading		.77< r <.90	
Word Spelling (Word Spelling and Proofreading)		.69< r <.80	
Reading Comprehension		.61	
Morphology and Syntax		.65	
Short Term Memory		.54< r <.77	
Vocabulary	.90		
Phonological Awareness (Spoonerisms and Reversals)			.78< r <.90
Rapid naming			.62< r <.84

instrument is still in development and copyright protected, the results can only be used as validation criterion for other measures.

Finally, we also administered some standard tests for reading and calculation problems, used in the Dutch-speaking countries, such as word and nonword reading tests, and a standard arithmetic test. All in all, the following cognitive functions were assessed.

Literacy

Text comprehension. In this test from the GL&SCHR, a text is presented in printed form and at the same time read out by the computer. Afterwards, the participant has to answer questions about the text. These questions rely on either literal comprehension or deductive knowledge.

Word reading. A classic word reading test in the Dutch-speaking countries is the *EMT* [One Minute Test] [42]. Parallel-form reliability ranges from.89 to.97 in various studies, whereas test-retest reliability lies between.82 and.92. For more psychometric information about the EMT we refer to the test's manual. The list consists of 116 words of increasing difficulty printed in four columns. The participant has to read aloud as many words as possible in one minute trying to minimize reading errors. Raw scores are obtained for the total number of words read, the number of errors made, and the number of words read correctly.

English word reading. We also administered an English version of the EMT, namely the One Minute Test or OMT [48]. Validity and reliability data of the OMT have been collected by Kleijen, Steenbeek-Planting, and Verhoeven [49]. Test-retest reliability varies between 0.87 and 0.92. This test is in all aspects comparable to the Dutch EMT, except that English words are presented instead of Dutch ones.

Text reading. In this test from the GL&SCHR participants are asked to read aloud a Dutch text which becomes increasingly difficult. Substantial errors (e.g. addition/substitution/omission of letters, syllables and/or words) and time consuming errors (e.g. repeating a word/sentence, spelling a word aloud) are registered as well as the total reading time.

Silent text reading. The test that was used -"Hoe gevaarlijk is een Tekenbeet? [How Dangerous Can a Tick Be?]"- is part of a screening instrument published by Henneman, Kleijnen, and Smits [50]. It provides an indication of silent reading speed and the ability to retain information. There are no norms for Flanders. So, we made use of the raw scores. To obtain further information about the validity of the test, we looked at the correlation with the EMT word reading test in our sample. A Pearson correlation coefficient of.66 ($N = 200$) was found. The silent reading test works as follows. Participants are instructed to read a text of 1023 words in silence, taking into account that they will have to write a short summary afterwards. During reading participants have to indicate the word they just read when a signal is given after one, two, and three minutes. Afterwards, the average number of words read per minute is calculated. The written summary is evaluated based on measures of content, structure and syntax but the results of these analyses are beyond the scope of the present paper [50].

Nonword reading. The standard Dutch nonword reading test is *De Klepel* [43]. The parallel-forms correlation varies between.89 and.95. In various studies, the results of the Klepel correlate between.74 and.91 with those of the EMT. For more psychometric information about the Klepel we refer to the test's manual. The test contains 116 nonwords that follow the Dutch grapheme-phoneme correspondence rules. Administration and scoring are identical to the EMT.

Word spelling. Word spelling was measured with two tests of the GL&SCHR: *Word Spelling* and *Proofreading*. In the Word Spelling test participants write down 30 words dictated by means of an audio file with a 3 seconds interval. Afterwards they are given the opportunity to correct their answers. Half of the words follow the Dutch spelling rules; the other half are exception words (involving inconsistent sound-letter mappings that must be memorized). Participants are also asked to rate how certain they feel about each answer (certain, almost certain, uncertain). There is a score for the number of correct responses, one for the number of words written during dictation (speed of writing), and one total weighted score where the certainty per item is taken into account. When a correct answer is given and the participant is certain, the weighted item score is 5. When the word is spelled correctly but the participant is uncertain the score is only 2. The difference between the raw score and the weighted score can be considered as a measure of meta-cognitive knowledge [51–52]. In the Proofreading test participants are given 20 sentences in which they have to correct possible spelling mistakes and rate their certainty per item. Two scores are given: one for the total number of correct responses and a weighted score (see Word Spelling).

English word spelling. Given the importance of English in higher education, we also included an English word dictation test. We used a standardized English test for word spelling: the *WRAT-III English Word Dictation* [53]. The internal consistency coefficients for the English age groups 17–18 and 19–24 are both.90. For more information on validity and reliability in English we refer to the manual. Because this test has not yet been validated for bilinguals with Dutch as mother tongue, we calculated the Pearson correlation with the English flash typing test of the IDAA (r = 0.72; N = 200). The test was administered according to the guidelines in the English manual. The examiner says a word, uses it in a significant context, and repeats the word. The participant writes it down. The test consists of 42 words.

Sentence dictation. Because higher education involves academic language, we also administered an advanced spelling test (AT-GSN [General Test for Advanced Spelling in Dutch]), developed and used at the University of Leuven [54]. This test has been used in a number of scientific studies [55–56]. Further information about the validity was obtained by correlating the scores with those of the Word Spelling test of the GL&SCHR (r = .79) and with the Dutch flash typing test of the IDAA (r = .70). The test consists of 12 paragraphs with exception words and challenging spelling rules (e.g. for the verbs). The correct use of capitals and punctuation marks is also taken into account. The score is the total number of errors made.

Morphology and syntax. In this subtest of the GL&SCHR 20 sentences are presented, in which the participant has to identify the syntactical or grammatical errors. The same principles as in the Proofreading test are applied. The total score gives the number of correct answers, whereas the weighted score takes into account the certainty of the participant about the answer given.

Processing Skills

Speed of processing. To measure the participants' speed of processing, we used the CDT or Cijfer Doorstreep Test [Digit Crossing Test] [57]. This is a standardized Dutch test to detect attentional deficits and measure the speed and accuracy of processing in a task of selective attention involving task-switching. It is one of the 23 tests of the DVMH [Differential Aptitude Tests for Middle and Higher Level], a test battery published in 2003 by Dekker and De Zeeuw [58]. This test battery was developed according to Carroll's [59] Three Stratum Model in order to assess a large variety of cognitive skills such as verbal and numerical reasoning, attentional skills and language skills. The test – retest reliability scores vary between 0.79 and 0.95. The test can be administered from 14 years up to 80. There are 960 digits from 0 to 9 presented in 16 columns. Students have three minutes to underline as many fours and to cross out as many threes and sevens as possible. Scores for working pace (total numbers of items processed), concentration (total number of correct items), number of target errors, number of missed target digits and percentage of errors are obtained.

Phonological Skills

Phonological processing. Phonological awareness was tested with 2 subtests from the GL&SCHR: *Spoonerisms* and *Reversals*. In the *Spoonerisms* test the first letters of two orally presented words must be switched (e.g., Harry Potter becomes Parry Hotter). Accuracy and speed (measured with a stop-watch) are measured. In the *Reversals* test participants have to judge if two spoken words are reversals or not (e.g. rac-car). Again, accuracy and speed (measured with a stop-watch) are measured.

Rapid naming. In the RAN test of the GL&SCHR participants are asked to rapidly name letters, digits, colors, or objects presented one-by-one on a computer screen (4 tests). The participant determines the pace by pressing the Enter button. Accuracy and speed are measured.

General Intelligence

Arithmetic. We used the *Tempo Test Rekenen* (*TTR;* [60]), a Dutch standardized test for mental calculations. It is designed to examine the rate at which participants mentally perform simple mathematical operations (single and double digits). There are five lists, consisting of additions, subtractions, multiplications, divisions below 100, and a random sequence of all four operations. Participants are given one minute per list to solve as many problems as possible. The score per subtest is the number of items minus the number of errors made.

General intelligence. The scores for crystallized IQ, fluid IQ and total IQ of the KAIT give us measures of general intelligence.

Vocabulary. We used three tests to evaluate this language function: *Vocabulary* from the GL&SCHR and *Definitions* and *Double Meanings* from the KAIT. In the *Vocabulary* test participants are asked to find the low frequency word for which a definition is given (e.g., the Dutch equivalents of anonymous or simultaneous). In the *Definitions* test the participant has to find a word based on a number of letters given and a short description of the word (e.g., "A dark color :.r.n"). In the *Double Meanings* test the participant has to find a word that is in some way connected to two word pairs (e.g., the connection between biology-body and jail-lock is the target word *cell*).

General information. To obtain information about the participants' non-verbal long-term memory, we used the *Famous People* test of the KAIT. In this test pictures of famous people are shown and participants have to name the person (e.g., Ghandi).

Problem solving/reasoning. Three subtests for fluid intelligence of the KAIT [45] were used to evaluate this cognitive skill: *Symbol Learning*, *Logical Reasoning*, and *Secret codes*. In the Symbol Learning test, the participant has to remember and reproduce series of symbols in different sentence-like combinations. In the Logical Reasoning test, information is given about the relative location of a number of items (people or animals). By logical reasoning the participant has to infer the location of a target item. In the Secret Codes test three or four items are given a unique code consisting of different parts. Based on these codes the participant has to infer which codes new target items should get.

Memory

Short-term memory span. The GL&SCHR contains a short-term memory test for phonemes and non-verbal shapes (which must be drawn), and a test in which participants have to reproduce randomly presented series of letters or digits in ascending order. The participant is placed in front of a computer screen. After pressing the enter button the participant sees and hears a series of items presented one item per 2 seconds. At the end of each series the participant has to reproduce the items remembered. The number of items within a series increases steadily.

Verbal memory. The GL&SCHR contains a short-term memory test for objects. Administration is identical to the short term memory spans test of the GL&SCHR described in the previous section.

Auditory memory. The *Auditory Memory Test* of the KAIT is a delayed memory task in which questions have to be answered about a text that was read out at the beginning of the administration of the KAIT (see the Auditory Comprehension Test discussed below).

Visuo-spatial memory. Visual-spatial memory was tested with two subtests of the KAIT: *Delayed Symbol Learning*, and *Block Patterns*. The Delayed Symbol Learning test is a delayed retention task of the symbols used in the Symbol Learning test. In the Block Patterns test a yellow-black pattern has to be reproduced with cubes.

Auditory Perception

The *Auditory Comprehension* test of the KAIT comprises the presentation of short audio fragments about which the experimenter asks content questions. The participant has to provide an answer.

Procedure

The complete test protocol was administered during two sessions of about three hours each. The protocol was divided into two counterbalanced parts. The order of tests in part one and two was fixed and chosen to avoid succession of similar tests. There was a break halfway each session. If necessary, students could take additional breaks. Students with dyslexia started with part one or two according to an AB-design. Their control student always started with the same part. All tests were administered individually by three test administrators according to the manuals guidelines. The test administrators were the two first authors and a test psychologist. To standardize administration each administrator read the manuals of the tests, had a practice session, and followed three sessions of the starting administrator. Testing occurred in a quiet room with the test administrator seated in front of the student.

Results

To improve comparison with Table 1, results are given as Cohen's d effect sizes (derived from parametric or non-parametric tests, see below). In line with the English studies (Table 1), the sign of the d-values was adapted so that positive d-values represent better performance of the controls and negative values better performance of the students with dyslexia. All data were first checked on normality and equality of variance between groups (dyslexic group and control group). When the constraints for parametric statistics were satisfied, means were compared using a Student's t-test. Otherwise, the data were analyzed with the non-parametric Mann-Whitney-U test and converted into the appropriate d-value by means of the equation given in Field ([61], p. 530 on how to transform a U-value into an r-statistic) and an equation to derive the d-value from the r-statistic. Values of the t-statistics and U-statistics are not given, as these can be calculated from the d-scores. Table 5 shows performances of students with dyslexia on literacy skills in comparison with their non-dyslexic peers. For variables that were analyzed using with a t-test, confidence intervals for the effect sizes could be calculated with the use of the ESCI-CIdelta program [62]. In Table 6 the results of phonological skills and processing skills are listed. In Table 7 results on general intelligence measures are reported.

With respect to the literacy skills (Table 5), the following results stand out:

1. As in English speaking individuals, the deficiency of students with dyslexia tends to be worse in the writing tests than in the reading tests. In particular, the Word Spelling test of the GL&SCHR and the Sentence Dictation (AT-GSN) resulted in large effect sizes ($d \approx 2$).
2. Deficiencies in spelling are similar at the word level ($d = 2$) and at the sentence level ($d = 2.1$).
3. Dutch word reading ($d = 1.97$) seems to be more affected in students with dyslexia than nonword reading ($d = 1.57$), possibly because the former involved more instances of inconsistent spelling-sound mappings.
4. For our group of students in higher education deficiencies in reading and writing are not more pronounced in a second language (English) than in the first language. In English word reading the same pattern in effect sizes was found for the percentage of errors and the number of words read as in Dutch.
5. Reading deficiencies are most pronounced in speed ($1.60 < d < 1.90$). Smaller but still substantial effect sizes were found for percentage of number of errors made ($d \approx .80$).
6. Text comprehension was nearly equivalent for both groups ($d = .4$) when the text was read aloud, and better than expected on the basis of the reading scores.

Turning to the wider cognitive skills (Table 6 and 7), the following are the most important findings:

1. The differences on the IQ test are negligible and particularly caused by definitions to words ($d = .75$), although there is also a small difference for the recognition of famous persons ($d = .35$). There are no differences in fluid intelligence ($d = .1$).
2. Students with dyslexia tend to be slower than controls in processing speed as measured with the CDT($d = .6$), and a small effect size can be noted for the percentage of errors ($d = .35$).
3. Except for phonological short-term memory ($d = .71$), memory spans are quite comparable ($0.28 < d < .45$).
4. There is considerable dyslexia cost for arithmetic ($d \approx 1$), which tends to be larger for divisions ($d = 1$) and multiplications ($d = .90$) than for subtractions ($d = .61$).
5. There is a non-negligible cost ($d > 1.3$) for phonological processing. This cost again is largely due to the speed of processing, and less to the accuracy of processing.
6. Dyslexics are slower at naming letters, digits and colors, but not at naming objects ($d = .2$).

Finally, to facilitate comparison with English, Table 8 includes our results together with those of Swanson and Hsieh [17] and Hatcher et al. [14]. In particular, the correspondence with Swanson and Hsieh is impressive. The Pearson correlation between both sets is $r = .94$ ($N = 11$, $p < .001$). The correlation with Swanson and Hsieh is lower if we also include the text comprehension difference of the present study ($d = .5$) and correlate it with the reading comprehension difference reported by Swanson and Hsieh ($d = 1.2$). Then the correlations drops to $r = .74$ ($N = 12$). However, this comparison is not really justified, because in our text comprehension test the text was additionally read out by the computer. Correlation is lower with Hatcher and colleagues [14], partly because of a lack of data in that study on aspects where students with dyslexia show good performance. The correlation coefficient is.67 and reaches significance ($p < .05$).

Discussion

We designed this study to obtain an empirically based cognitive profile of students with dyslexia in higher education in a language other than English. We started from the tests we thought worthwhile, making sure those of Hatcher et al. [14] were included. Shortly after data collection began, Swanson and Hsieh [17] published their meta-analysis, providing us with an even more complete image of English-speaking students.

Despite the differences in language and educational context, our findings are remarkably similar to those in English: The pattern of strengths and weaknesses of students with reading disabilities is very much the same in Dutch as in English (Table 8). This is good news, because it means that the profile is likely to be applicable to all alphabetical languages. Also, different educational systems do not seem to play an important role in defining which students with dyslexia enter higher education.

Table 5. Performances of students with dyslexia on literacy skills in comparison with their non-dyslexic peers.

	Students with dyslexia		Students without dyslexia		Cohen's d			p
	M1	SD1	M2	SD2	d	lower CI	upper CI	
Text comprehension (GL&SCHR)								
Number correct responses	19.38	5.05	21.59	4.4	0.47[b]			**
Word reading (EMT)								
Total number read words	79.08	14.32	101.33	10.6	1.87[b]			**
Number of errors	2.05	2.10	0.91	1.12	0.67[b]			**
Correctly read words	77.03	14.21	100.42	10.58	1.97[b]			**
Percentage of errors	2.63	2.77	0.90	1.08	0.88[b]			**
English word reading (OMT)								
Total number read words	71.18	10.72	84.99	9.49	1.36[a]	1.05	1.67	**
Number of errors	3.99	2.70	2.53	2.15	0.59[b]			**
Correctly read words	66.52	10.2	82.49	10.20	1.40[a]	1.09	1.71	**
Percentage of errors	5.64	3.98	3.07	2.71	0.75[b]			**
Text reading (GL&SCHR)								
Substantial errors	15.71	10.80	7.81	5.19	0.98[b]			**
Time consuming errors	14.29	8.72	9.17	4.91	0.64[b]			**
Reading time	311.14	51.97	258.53	25.26	1.29[a]	0.98	1.59	**
Silent text reading (Tekenbeet)								
Words per minute	184.63	59.25	243.64	57.59	1.13[b]			**
Nonword reading (Klepel)								
Total number read words	46.07	9.84	63.26	12.90	1.50[b]			**
Number of errors	5.20	3.77	3.67	3.10	0.44[b]			**
Correctly read words	40.88	10.46	59.72	13.10	1.59[b]			**
Percentage of errors	11.75	9.11	6.05	5.28	0.88[b]			**
Word spelling								
Word Spelling								
Weighted score word spelling	91.59	15.87	121.40	12.84	2.28[b]			**
Correct word spelling	17.49	4.02	24.60	2.81	2.05[b]			**
Writing speed	24.89	4.01	26.50	3.40	0.43[a]	0.15	0.71	**
Proofreading	51.23	10.96	63.49	11.69	1.08[a]	0.78	1.38	**
English word spelling (WRAT)								
Correctly spelled words	16.57	4.81	24.27	5.42	1.50[a]	1.19	1.82	**
Sentence dictation (AT-GSN)								
number of errors	54.04	24.17	23.20	11.65	2.10[b]			**
Morphology and syntax (GL&SCHR)								
Weighted score	50.34	10.35	59.57	9.86	0.91[a]	0.62	1.2	**
Total score	9.06	2.64	11.24	9.06	0.87[b]			**

p<.05; **p<.01.
Note: Parametric test results are marked with a. When the data violated the constraints for a parametric test, results are marked with b.
GL&SCHR = Dutch reading and writing test battery for (young) adults; EMT = Een Minuut Test [One Minute Test]; OMT = One Minute Test;
WRAT = Wide range Achievement Test; AT-GSN = Algemene Test- Gevorderde Spelling Nederlands [General Test Advanced Spelling Dutch].

A further important conclusion from our findings is that the data agree very well with the traditional definition of dyslexia as a combination of normal intelligence with deficient reading and writing. This definition has been questioned in recent years, because it has proven difficult to find the discrepancy in all individuals. Researchers have disagreed about whether this has theoretical consequences for the relationship between reading/writing skills and other abilities, or whether it is simply a consequence of the notoriously low correlations one is bound to find for difference scores of highly correlated variables (e.g. [63]). Our data leave little doubt that, as a group, dyslexics entering higher education show exactly the profile predicted by the traditional definition of dyslexia, even though at an individual level the difference scores may show large variability. As such, our findings reinforce a similar, tentative conclusion reached by Swanson and Hsieh [17].

Table 6. Performances of students with dyslexia on phonological skills and processing skills in comparison with their non-dyslexic peers.

	Students with dyslexia		Students without dyslexia		Cohen's d			p
	M1	SD1	M2	SD2	d	lower CI	upper CI	
Processing skills								
Speed of processing (CDT)								
Working pace	421.94	84.63	467.80	79.99	0.62[b]			**
Concentration	119.25	22.85	134.29	22.03	0.51[b]			**
Number of errors	0.19	0.56	0.15	1.73	0.23[b]			
Number of missed digits	8.08	6.96	6.60	6.76	0.19[b]			
Percentage of errors/missed	2.03	1.49	1.60	1.51	0.35[b]			*
Phonological skills								
Spoonersims (GL&SCHR)								
Number correct responses	16.72	2.50	18.19	1.67	0.70[b]			**
Time	179.88	65.98	116.48	41.22	1.42[b]			**
Reversals (GL&SCHR)								
Number correct responses	15.63	2.41	17.72	2.03	1.00[b]			**
Time	106.00	33.996	76.61	16.18	1.3[b]			**
Rapid naming (GL&SCHR)								
Letters	25.72	5.85	20.62	3.99	1.02[b]			**
Digits	23.83	5.26	19.28	3.64	1.05[b]			**
Colours	32.55	6.03	28.25	4.314	0.81[b]			**
Objects	39.55	7.39	37.84	6.82	0.24[b]			

p<.05; **p<.01.
Note: Parametric test results are marked with a. When the data violated the constraints for a parametric test, results are marked with b.
CDT = Digit Crossing Test [Cijfer Doorstreep Test]. GL&SCHR = Dutch reading and writing test battery for (young) adults.

The affirmation of the traditional definition of dyslexia shows that some lecturers' doubts about the existence of isolated reading disabilities in combination with normal intelligence are unjustified. For the group we tested, we found – just like the authors before us – a pattern of results that is extremely hard to obtain on the basis of deficient general abilities, motivation, or outright malingering. Although we cannot exclude the possibility that one or two of the students who refused to take part in our study did so because they wanted to play the system, our results emphatically testify that the vast majority of students entering higher education with a diagnosis of dyslexia are the same as the other students, except for a language-related deficiency that arguably hurts them most during the school years when they have to rapidly acquire and produce a lot of new information in written form.

At the same time, it is important to keep in mind that, although the differences are not large, all test scores tended to be lower for the students with dyslexia than for the controls. When looking at the full cognitive profile of students with dyslexia, it cannot be denied that there is a quite consistent deficiency on a wide range of tasks, predominantly those involving speed of processing and retrieval of verbal information from long term memory. It would be good if students with dyslexia were properly informed about this extra challenge they are facing. The most prominent example of such a "hidden" cost is the extra time they need for mental calculations (total of operations: $d = 1$), arguably because of the extra effort to retrieve arithmetic facts from memory (see the triple code model [64]). This additional deficit was not mentioned by many students, but is likely to cause problems in courses involving the calculation of many elementary arithmetic operations (e.g., the calculation of a standard deviation in a course of statistics).

Sometimes it has been hypothesized that successful individuals with dyslexia have fully compensated for their reading and writing difficulties [65]. Hatcher et al. [14] raised doubts about this possibility, and our data confirm this to some extent, although the picture is much less pessimistic. What is encouraging is the finding that students with dyslexia tended to perform equally good on the text comprehension test, in which the text was additionally read out by the computer (see also their good scores on the auditory comprehension test). This suggests the usefulness of text-to-speech arrangements, although ideally we would have more data on this aspect, directly comparing text comprehension with and without text-to-speech assistance.

A further interesting finding of our study is that the effect sizes are not larger for tests based on sentences than for tests based on individual words (word reading $d = 1.87$, text reading $d = 1.29$; word writing $d = 2.05$, text writing $d = 2.10$). This agrees with the descriptive definition of SDN [39] arguing that the impairment in reading and spelling can be measured at the word level. Our data indicate that tests of reading and writing at the word level are enough to make a valid diagnosis. This is valuable information for diagnosticians, as it leads to a substantial time gain.

Finally, our findings have clear implications for guidelines about special arrangements. We think the following arrangements are incontestable:

Table 7. Performances of students with dyslexia on general intelligence in comparison with their non-dyslexic peers.

	Students with dyslexia		Students without dyslexia		Cohen's d			p
	M1	SD1	M2	SD2	d	lower CI	upper CI	
General Intelligence								
Arithmetic (TTR)								
Total number calculations	121.24	20.67	144.75	23.83	1.05[a]	0.76	1.35	**
Addition	30.46	3.51	33.81	3.41	0.97[a]	0.67	1.26	**
Subtraction	27.31	4.17	30.14	3.98	0.61[b]			**
Multiplication	21.74	5.02	26.78	6.19	0.90[b]			**
Division	19.73	5.82	26.29	7.27	1.00[b]			**
Mixed operations	22.93	4.45	28.33	4.98	1.12[b]			**
General Intelligence (KAIT)								
Total IQ	105.50	12.97	109.83	9.29	0.38[a]	0.1	0.66	**
Crystallized IQ	106.66	8.11	111.31	8.83	0.55[a]	0.27	0.83	**
Fluid IQ	105.36	11.04	106.78	10.83	0.13[a]	−0.14	0.41	
Vocabulary								
Vocabulary (GL&SCHR)	7.83	4.14	10.83	4.77	0.67[b]			**
Definitions (KAIT)	20.89	1.92	22.16	1.98	0.75[b]			**
Double meanings (KAIT)	14.44	3.91	16.10	3.71	0.43[b]			**
General information (KAIT)	7.26	3.14	8.41	3.25	0.35[b]			*
Problem Solving/Reasoning (KAIT)								
Symbol learning	80.45	12.64	80.93	13.14	0.07[b]			
Logical reasoning	11.32	3.48	11.78	3.18	0.12[b]			
Secret codes	26.78	5.49	27.46	4.91	−0.13[b]			
Memory								
Short term memory span (GL&SCHR)								
STM phonemes	20.11	4.7	23.23	4.56	0.71[b]			**
STM shapes	10.44	4.00	11.84	5.05	0.28[b]			*
Memory with sorting	39.34	5.03	41.54	4.34	0.45[b]			**
Verbal memory (GL&SCHR)								
STM words	35.41	5.78	37.24	5.37	0.30[a]	0.05	0.61	*
Auditory memory (KAIT)	4.99	1.40	5.54	1.50	0.37[b]			**
Visual Memory (KAIT)								
Delayed Symbol Learning	50.98	10.4	51.34	10.53	0.03[a]	−0.23	0.32	
Block Patterns	12.23	2.71	11.71	2.97	−0.17[b]			
Auditory Perception (KAIT)								
Auditory comprehension	13.26	2.96	13.60	2.80	0.09[b]			

*p<.05; **p<.01.
Note: EMT = Een Minuut Test [One Minute Test]; GL&SCHR = Dutch reading and writing test battery for (young) adults; AT-GSN = Algemene. Test- Gevorderde Spelling Nederlands [General Test Advanced Spelling Dutch]; CDT = Cijfer Doorstreep Test [Digit Crossing Test]; TTR = Tempo. Test Rekenen [Speed Test Mental Calculations], KAIT = Kaufmann Adult Intelligence Test; STM = short term memory.

1. It is clear that students with dyslexia have a specific and pervasive problem with reading and writing. This means that they are entitled to arrangements that help them with these particular deficiencies, such as text-to-speech software (also during exams) and the use of spellcheckers and word completion software when spelling errors are likely to lead to lower marks (e.g., for essay-type questions).
2. Students with dyslexia are at a disadvantage under time constraints, meaning that situations should be avoided in which they are likely to suffer more (e.g., exams and tests with strict time limits). This does not mean that students with reading disabilities should be given extended deadlines for all tasks (e.g., for the submission of essays and lab reports, which can be planned well in advance), but it does entail that they are denied a fair chance if they have to complete an exam in the same time as their peers.
3. Many students with dyslexia have a pervasive problem with mathematical tables. This should be taken into account when an exam strongly relies on them (e.g., for problem solving,

Table 8. Correspondence between the effect sizes reported in English and the effect sizes found in the current study.

	S&H09	HSG02	Dutch
Literacy			
Reading comprehension	1.2		
Word reading	1.4	1.1	2.0 (EMT correctly read)
Non-Word Reading	1.3	1.5	1.6 (Klepel correctly read)
Word Spelling	1.6	1.3	2.0 (GL&SCHR, N correct)
Text Writing	0.7	1.1	
Sentence dictation			2.0 (AT-GSN)
Processing skills			
Perceptual speed		0.9	0.6 (CDT Time)
Phonological skills			
Phonological processing	0.9	1.3	1.4 (GL&SCHR time)
Rapid naming	1.0	1.2	1.0 (GL&SCHR, without objects)
General intelligence			
Arithmetic	0.7	0.6	1.0 (TTR)
Verbal memory	0.2	1.1	0.3 (GL&SCHR, STM words)
General intelligence	0.2		0.4 (KAIT)
Vocabulary	0.7	0.1	0.6 (KAIT, GL&SCHR)
Problem solving/reasoning	0.1	−0.01	0.1 (KAIT fluid)
Auditory perception	−0.2		0.1 (KAIT, aud.compr)

Note: S&H09 = Swanson & Hsieh [17]; HSG02 = Hatcher, Snowling & Griffiths [14].EMT = Een Minuut Test [One Minute Test]; GL&SCHR = Dutch. reading and writing test battery for (young) Adults; AT-GSN = Algemene Test-Gevorderde Spelling Nederlands [General Test Advanced Spelling. Dutch]; CDT = Cijfer Doorstreep Test [Digit Crossing Test]; TTR = Tempo Test Rekenen [Speed Test Mental Calculations], KAIT = Kaufmann Adult. Intelligence Test; STM = short term memory.

where different alternatives have to be tried out). This problem can easily be solved by allowing students to use a calculator.

4. Finally, there is scope for better feedback to the students themselves. It is important for them to know of the limitations they are confronted with, so that they can prepare themselves well and insist on having the arrangements outlined above. A better knowledge of their limitations may also help them not to overestimate their abilities. One cannot deny that the average performance of the dyslexics on nearly all tests tended to be lower than that of controls. Although these differences often are too small to justify special arrangements, students with reading disability should know about these differences, so that they can better organize their studies. For instance, many institutes of higher education nowadays provide their students with ways to spread the burden (e.g., by studying part-time or distributing the exams over extra sessions). It may be an idea to discuss these options with students (and their parents), certainly when their test performances are below average, so that they can prepare themselves better in the light of the specific difficulties they will be confronted with.

The above (minimal) arrangements are easy to implement if they are part of the general organization of exams, certainly with the current availability of text-to-speech software and text writing software with built-in spellcheckers. Additionally, these measures are so specifically tailored to the proven needs of students with dyslexia that they are unlikely to be contested or misused. To our knowledge there is no evidence that text-to-speech software, spellcheckers, and a few extra hours for exams are any good in compensating for a lack of knowledge, deficient intellectual abilities, or missing achievement motivation. However, our results strongly suggest that they will make a significant difference for students with dyslexia.

Acknowledgments

The authors thank Valérie Van Hees and Charlotte De Lange from *Cursief* for their help in the study and the recruitment of participants. They also thank Joke Lauwers for her assistance in testing the participants, and Annemie Desoete for helpful suggestions.

Author Contributions

Conceived and designed the experiments: MC WT MB. Performed the experiments: MC WT. Analyzed the data: MC WT MB. Contributed reagents/materials/analysis tools: MC WT MB. Wrote the paper: MC WT MB.

References

1. Hadjikakou K, Hartas D (2008) Higher education provision for students with disabilities in Cyprus. Higher Education 55: 103–119.
2. Madriaga M, Hanson K, Heaton C, Kay H, Newitt S, et al. (2010) Confronting similar challenges? Disabled and non-disabled students' learning and assessment experiences. Studies in Higher Education 35: 647–658.
3. Landerl K, Moll K (2010) Comorbidity of learning disorders: prevalence and familial transmission. Journal of Child Psychology and Psychiatry 51: 287–294.
4. Pieters S, De Block K, Scheiris J, Eyssen M, Desoete A, et al. (2012) How common are motor problems in children with a developmental disorder: rule or exception? Child: Care, Health and Development 38: 139–145.
5. Yoshimasu K, Barbaresi WJ, Colligan RC, Killian JM, Voigt RG, et al. (2010) Gender, Attention-Deficit/Hyperactivity Disorder, and Reading Disability in a Population-Based Birth Cohort. Pediatrics 126: 788–795.
6. Du Pré EA, Gilroy DE, Miles TR (2008) Dyslexia at College. NY : Routledge.
7. Farmer M, Riddick B, Sterling CM, (2002) Dyslexia and Inclusion. Assessment and Support in Higher Education. London: Whurr Publishers Ltd.
8. Wolf LE, Schreiber HE, Wasserstein J (2008) Adult Learning Disorders: Contemporary Issues (A Neuropsychologist's Handbook). NY: Psychology Press.
9. Sparks RL, Lovett B (2009) College Students With Learning Disability Diagnoses Who Are They and How Do They Perform? Journal of Learning Disabilities 42: 494–510.
10. Sparks RL, Lovett B (2009) Objective Criteria for Classification of Post-secondary Students as Learning Disabled Effects on Prevalence Rates and Group Characteristics. Journal of Learning Disabilities 42: 230–239.
11. Everatt J, Bradshaw MF, Hibbard PB, Lages M (1997) Visual processing deficits and dyslexia. Perception 26: 1330–1330.
12. Felton RH, Naylor CE, Wood FB (1990) Neuropsychological profile of adult dyslexics. Brain and Language 39: 485–497.
13. Lefly DL, Pennington BF (1991) Spelling-errors and reading fluency in compensated adult dyslexics. Annals of Dyslexia 41: 143–162.
14. Hatcher J, Snowling MJ, Griffiths JM (2002) Cognitive assessment of dyslexic students in higher education. British Journal of Educational Psychology 72: 199–133.
15. Ransby MJ, Swanson HL (2003) Reading comprehension skills of young adults with childhood diagnoses of dyslexia. Journal of Learning Disabilities 36: 538–555.
16. Trainin G, Swanson HL (2005) Cognition, metacognition and achievement of college students with learning disabilities. Learning Disability Quarterly 28: 264–272.
17. Swanson HL, Hsieh CJ (2009) Reading Disabilities in Adults: A Selective Meta-Analysis of the Literature. Review of educational Research 79: 1362–1390.
18. Brysbaert M (2011) Basic statistics for psychologists. London: Palgrave Macmillan.
19. Keuleers E, Diependaele K, Brysbaert M (2010) Practice effects in large-scale visual word recognition studies: a lexical decision study on 14,000 Dutch mono- and disyllabic words and nonwords. Frontiers in Psychology: 1–174.

20. De Smedt B, Boets B (2010) Phonological processing and arithmetic fact retrieval: evidence from developmental dyslexia. Neuropsychologia 48: 3973–3981.
21. Göbel SM, Snowling MJ (2010) Number-processing skills in adults with dyslexia. Quarterly Journal of Experimental Psychology 63: 1361–1373.
22. Sharpe D (1997) Of Apples and Oranges, File Drawers and Garbage: Why Validity Issues in Meta-analysis Will Not Go Away. Clinical Psychology Review 17: 881–901.
23. Hanley JR, Masterson J, Spencer LH, Evans D (2004) How long do the advantages of learning to read a transparent orthography last? An investigation of the reading skills and reading impairment of Welsh children at 10 years of age. Quarterly Journal of Experimental Psychology 57: 1393–1410.
24. Seymour PHK, Aro M, Erskine JM (2003) Foundation literacy acquisition in European orthographies. British Journal of Psychology 94: 143–174.
25. Ziegler JC, Goswami U (2005) Reading acquisition, developmental dyslexia, and skilled reading across languages: A psycholinguistic grain size theory. Psychological Bulletin 131: 3–29.
26. Lindgren SD, De Renzi E, Richman LC (1985) Cross-national comparisons of developmental dyslexia in Italy and the United-States. Child Development 56: 1404–1417.
27. Landerl K, Wimmer H, Frith U (1997) The impact of orthographic consistency on dyslexia: A German-English comparison. Cognition 63: 315–334.
28. Share DL (2008) On the anglocentricities of current reading research and practice: The perils of overreliance on an "Outlier" orthography. Psychological Bulletin 134: 584–615.
29. Stone GO, Vanhoy M, VanOrden GC (1997) Perception is a two-way street: Feedforward and feedback phonology in visual word recognition. Journal of Memory and Language 36: 337–359.
30. Borgwaldt S, Hellwig F (2004) Onset entropy matters: Cross-linguistic sound-spelling analyses and empirical validation. Australian Journal of Psychology 56: 106–107.
31. Van den Bosch A, Content A, Daelemans W, De Gelder B (1994) Measuring the Complexity of Writing Systems. Journal of Quantitative Linguistics 1: 178–188.
32. Lovett BJ, Sparks RL (2010) Exploring the Diagnosis of "Gifted/LD": Characterizing Postsecondary Students With Learning Disability Diagnoses at Different IQ Levels. Journal of Psycho-educational Assessment 28: 91–101.
33. Reid AA, Szczerbinski M, Iskierka-Kasperek E, Hansen P (2006) Cognitive Profile of Adult Developmental Dyslexics: Theoretical Implications. Dyslexia 13: 1–24.
34. Szenkovits G, Ramus F (2005) Exploring dyslexics' phonological deficit I: Lexical versus sublexical and input versus output processes. Dyslexia 11: 253–268.
35. Bruyer R, Brysbaert M (2011) Combining speed and accuracy in cognitive psychology: Is the Inverse Efficiency Score (IES) a better dependent variable than the mean Reaction Time (RT) and the Percentage of Errors (PE)? Psychologica Belgica 51: 5–13.
36. Wolff U (2009) Phonological and Surface Subtypes among University Students with Dyslexia. International Journal of Disability, Development and Education 59: 73–91.
37. Campbell JID, Thompson VA (2002) More power to you: Simple power calculations for treatment effects with one degree of freedom. Behavior Research Methods, Instruments, & Computers 34: 332–337.
38. Faul F, Erdfelder E, Lang AG, Buchner A (2007) G*Power 3: A flexible statistical power analysis program for the social, behavioral, and biomedical sciences. Behavior Research Methods 39: 175–191.
39. Stichting Dyslexie Nederland (2008) Diagnose dyslexie. Brochure van de Stichting Dyslexie Nederland. Herziene versie. Bilthoven: Stichting Dyslexie Nederland.
40. Vaughn S, Fuchs LS (2003) Redefining learning disabilities as inadequate response to instruction: The promise and potential problems. Learning Disabilities Research & Practice 18: 137–146.
41. Haager D, Klinger J, Vaughn S (2007) Evidence-Based Reading Practices for Response to Intervention. Baltimore, London, Sydney: Paul H. Brookes Publishing Co.
42. Brus B, Voeten M (1991) Eén-minuut-test vorm A en B, schoolvorderingstest voor de technische leesvaardigheid bestemd voor groep 4 tot en met 8 van het basisonderwijs. Verantwoording en handleiding. Lisse: Swets & Zeitlinger.
43. van den Bos K, Spelberg H, Scheepsma A, de Vries J (1999) De klepel vorm A en B, een test voor leesvaardigheid van pseudowoorden. Verantwoording, handleiding, diagnostiek en behandeling. Lisse: Swets & Zeitlinger.
44. De Pessemier P, Andries C (2009) Test voor Gevorderd Lezen en Schrijven. Antwerpen-Apeldoorn : Garant.
45. Dekker R, Dekker PH, Mulder JL (2004) Kaufman Adolescent and Adult Intelligence Test – Nederlandstalige Versie: Handleiding. PITS: Leiden.
46. Van der Leij A, Bekebrede JI, Geudens A, Schraeyen K, Schijf GM, et al. (2012) Interactieve Dyslexietest Amsterdam- Antwerpen [Interactive Dyslexia Test Amsterdam-Antwerp] : handleiding. Uithoorn : Muiswerk Educatief. In press.
47. Wechsler Dv (2001) WAIS-III, Nederlandstalige bewerking, technische handleiding. Lisse: Swets & Zeitlinger.
48. Kleijnen R, Loerts M (2006) Protocol Dyslexie Hoger Onderwijs. Antwerpen/Apeldoorn: Garant Uitgeverij.
49. Kleijen R, Steenbeek-Planting E, Verhoeven L (2008) Toetsen en Interventies bij Dyslexie in het Voortgezet Onderwijs. Nederlands en Moderne Vreemde Talen. Antwerpen/Apeldoorn: Garant Uitgeverij.
50. Henneman K, Kleijnen R, Smits A (2004) Protocol Dyslexie Voortgezet Onderwijs : Deel 2 - Signalering, diagnose en begeleiding. KPC Groep, Expertisecentrum Nederlands, Werkverband Opleidingen Speciaal Onderwijs.
51. Tops W, Callens M, Van Cauwenberghe E, Adriaens J, Brysbaert M (2012) Beyond spelling: the writing skills of students with dyslexia in higher education. Annals of Dyslexia: In press.
52. Desoete A, Roeyers H (2002) Off-line metacognition. A domain-specific retardation in young children with learning disabilities? Learning Disability Quarterly 25: 123–139.
53. Wilkinson GS (1993) Wide Range Achievement Test. Jastak Assessment.
54. Ghesquière P (1998) Algemene toets gevorderde spelling van het Nederlands (AT-GSN) : Verantwoording en handleiding. Rapport van een specialisatiejaar: Onderzoek AT-GSN-dictee. Unpublished bachelor thesis, University Leuven, Leuven, Belgium.
55. Gauderis K, Heirman E, Vandenhoof T (2004) Normering van AT-GSN, TTR en CDR-5 bijleerlingen van het zesde jaar Algemeen Secundair Onderwijs [Standardisation of AT-GSN, TTR and CDR-5 among sixth-year students in General Secondary Education]. Unpublished bachelor thesis, University College Arteveldehogeschool, Ghent, Belgium.
56. Vanderswalmen R, Vrijders J, Desoete A (2010) Metacognition and spelling performance in college students. In A Efklides & P Misailidi (Eds.). Trends and Prospects in Metacognition Research. Springer: New York, 367–394.
57. Dekker R, Mulder JL, Dekker PH (2007) De ontwikkeling van vijf nieuwe Nederlandstalige tests. PITS: Leiden.
58. Dekker R, De Zeeuw J (2003) DVMH: Differentiële Vaardighedentests voor Midden en Hoger Niveau. PITS: Leiden.
59. Carroll JB (1993) Human Cognitive Abilities. A Survey of Factor-Analytic Studies. Cambridge: Cambridge University Press.
60. de Vos T (1992) Tempo Test Rekenen. Amsterdam: Pearson Education.
61. Field A (2005) Discovering Statistics using SPSS. London: SAGE Publications Ltd.
62. Cumming G, Finch S (2001) A primer on the understanding, use and calculation of confidence intervals based on central and noncentral distributions. Educational and Psychological Measurement 61: 530–572.
63. Cotton SM, Crewther DP, Crewther SG (2005) Measurement error: Implications for diagnosis and discrepancy models of developmental dyslexia. Dyslexia 11: 186–202.
64. Dehaene S, Piazza M, Pinel P, Cohen L (2003) Three parietal circuits for number processing. Cognitive Neuropsychology 20: 487–506.
65. Snowling MJ (2000) Dyslexia (2nd ed.). Oxford: Blackwell.

4

Grey Matter Alterations Co-Localize with Functional Abnormalities in Developmental Dyslexia

Janosch Linkersdörfer[1,2]*, Jan Lonnemann[2,3], Sven Lindberg[1,2], Marcus Hasselhorn[1,2,3], Christian J. Fiebach[1,3,4]

1 Center for Individual Development and Adaptive Education of Children at Risk, Frankfurt, Germany, **2** German Institute for International Educational Research, Frankfurt, Germany, **3** Institute for Psychology, Goethe-University Frankfurt, Germany, **4** Donders Institute for Brain, Cognition and Behaviour, Radboud University Nijmegen, The Netherlands

Abstract

The neural correlates of developmental dyslexia have been investigated intensively over the last two decades and reliable evidence for a dysfunction of left-hemispheric reading systems in dyslexic readers has been found in functional neuroimaging studies. In addition, structural imaging studies using voxel-based morphometry (VBM) demonstrated grey matter reductions in dyslexics in several brain regions. To objectively assess the consistency of these findings, we performed activation likelihood estimation (ALE) meta-analysis on nine published VBM studies reporting 62 foci of grey matter reduction in dyslexic readers. We found six significant clusters of convergence in bilateral temporo-parietal and left occipito-temporal cortical regions and in the cerebellum bilaterally. To identify possible overlaps between structural and functional deviations in dyslexic readers, we conducted additional ALE meta-analyses of imaging studies reporting functional underactivations (125 foci from 24 studies) or overactivations (95 foci from 11 studies) in dyslexics. Subsequent conjunction analyses revealed overlaps between the results of the VBM meta-analysis and the meta-analysis of functional underactivations in the fusiform and supramarginal gyri of the left hemisphere. An overlap between VBM results and the meta-analysis of functional overactivations was found in the left cerebellum. The results of our study provide evidence for consistent grey matter variations bilaterally in the dyslexic brain and substantial overlap of these structural variations with functional abnormalities in left hemispheric regions.

Editor: Bogdan Draganski, Centre Hospitalier Universitaire Vaudois Lausanne - CHUV, UNIL, Switzerland

Funding: This research was funded by the Hessian initiative for the development of scientific and economic excellence (LOEWE; http://www.hmwk.hessen.de/irj/HMWK_Internet?cid=a2396939885f8c8c0a3ba39bda517cbd). The funders had no role in study design, data collection and analysis, decision to publish, or preparation of the manuscript.

Competing Interests: The authors have declared that no competing interests exist.

* E-mail: j.linkersdoerfer@idea-frankfurt.eu

Introduction

Developmental dyslexia is a severe difficulty in learning to read accurately and fluently that affects 5–17% of all children and often persists into adulthood (e.g., [1]). The most widely accepted explanation for the origin of this disorder is an underlying deficit in the representation and processing of speech sounds [2–4]. This phonological deficit is associated with deficient grapheme-phoneme decoding skills that are crucial in the beginning stages of reading development. Early difficulties in phonological reading in turn are assumed to exert a negative impact on the establishment of orthographic representations required for fluent and effortless reading. Although phonological deficits can be found in the majority of persons with reading difficulties, dyslexia is a heterogeneous condition [5,6]. Several other sensorimotor deficits have been associated with the disorder resulting in the emergence of alternative theories describing phonological deficits as secondary consequences of basal auditory [7], visual [8], attentional [9] and/or motor problems [10].

Over the last two decades, numerous neuroimaging studies have examined functional brain abnormalities in persons with dyslexia of different ages and of different languages (for reviews see, e.g., [1,11]). Converging evidence from these studies indicates that dyslexia is associated with functional underactivations in two posterior neural systems of the left hemisphere. The first system is located dorsally in a temporo-parietal region, including the posterior part of the superior temporal gyrus and the supramarginal and angular gyri of the inferior parietal lobule, and is assumed to be involved in grapheme-phoneme decoding. The second neural system is located ventrally in an occipito-temporal region including the extrastriate fusiform and the inferior temporal gyrus. This region, often referred to as the Visual Word Form Area (VWFA; [12]; but see also [13]), is considered to gradually specialize for the fast and effortless processing of familiar visual words or frequent letter strings within words during the first years of reading experience (e.g., [1]). A common developmental interpretation is that underactivations of the ventral system, representing inferior automaticity of the reading process, are the secondary result of primary dysfunctions in the dorsal system that are associated with problems in phonological reading [1,14]. Two further areas have been proposed to exhibit differences between dyslexic and normal readers: Overactivations in bilateral inferior frontal gyri, along with other regions of the right hemisphere, have been postulated to represent compensatory processes (e.g., [11]). However, these results have been inconclusive and sometimes contradictory as other researchers reported no activation differences (e.g., [15]) or even underactivations (e.g., [16]) in the left inferior frontal gyrus in dyslexic readers. Finally, based on behavioral and brain activation differences between dyslexic and normal readers in tasks involving motor skills, the cerebellum has been proposed to play a major role in the origin of dyslexia ("cerebellar deficit hypothesis"; [10,17]).

In three recent coordinate-based meta-analyses, the results of studies showing functional differences between dyslexic and normal readers have been quantitatively analyzed. To detect topographic convergence between studies, coordinate-based meta-analyses use the reported 3D coordinates of voxels of peak statistical difference as input foci. These foci are modeled as Gaussian probability distributions centered at the given coordinates and combined to three-dimensional brain maps that represent the likelihood of activation across studies, at each voxel, and that can be tested for significance. In the first meta-analysis, Maisog et al. [18] used activation likelihood estimation (ALE; [19]) to analyze nine studies comparing adult dyslexics with control participants in reading tasks involving words, pseudowords, or letters. In addition to functional underactivations in the occipito-temporal (i.e., ventral) and temporo-parietal (i.e., dorsal) reading systems described above, they also reported maxima of underactivations in the inferior frontal gyrus, precuneus, and thalamus of the left, and the fusiform, postcentral, and superior temporal gyri of the right hemisphere. Maxima of consistent overactivations were found in the thalamus and the anterior insula of the right hemisphere. In a second ALE meta-analysis that used foci from 17 original studies examining children and adults, Richlan and colleagues [20] reported similar results regarding underactivations of the two posterior reading systems. They also found that underactivations in the inferior frontal gyrus were accompanied by overactivations in the primary motor cortex and the anterior insula of the left hemisphere and bilateral subcortical structures. The authors interpreted these results as compensatory reliance on silent articulatory access to phonological word representations. In their recent meta-analysis using signed differential mapping (SDM; [21]), Richlan et al. [22] statistically compared the results of two meta-analyses including nine studies with adult and nine studies with child participants respectively. Meta-analyses of studies with both children and adults showed underactivations in the occipito-temporal reading system suggesting an early dysfunction of this region. For adult studies, this cluster of underactivation was relatively enlarged. With respect to the temporo-parietal system, underactivations in the superior temporal gyrus were only found for adult studies, while underactivations in the inferior parietal lobule were only found for studies of children.

In addition to differences in functional activation, several studies have examined neuroanatomical variations in dyslexic readers over the last years. First evidence came from a series of post-mortem studies on the brains of diagnosed cases of developmental dyslexia [23–26]. These studies demonstrated neuronal ectopias and architectonic dysplasias mainly in perisylvian regions of the left hemisphere which were interpreted as the results of disturbed neuronal migration during the prenatal stage. Further findings were an atypical symmetry of the planum temporale and deviations in thalamic structures consisting in disorganization and smaller neurons in the magnocellular layers of the lateral geniculate nuclei bilaterally and smaller neurons in the left medial geniculate nucleus. Galaburda's case studies constitute an important step in the search for a neurophysiological basis of dyslexia. Nevertheless, the results have to be interpreted with caution as the number of analyzed brains was quite small (ranging from one to five between studies) and some of the individuals had further neurological issues.

In vivo neuroimaging studies using manual volumetric measurements that concentrated mainly on the perisylvian language regions of the left-hemisphere, especially the planum temporale, yielded inconclusive results (for reviews, see [27,28]). The advent of newly developed analysis techniques such as voxel-based morphometry (VBM; [29]) enabled an objective localization of structural differences with high spatial resolution. Furthermore, VBM studies report results in standard stereotactic space, thereby allowing for directly comparing findings from different studies as well as linking them to the results of functional imaging studies. Over the last ten years, a growing number of VBM studies has been published and structural differences in grey matter density or volume between dyslexic and normal readers have been identified in several brain regions. Locations most frequently reported to exhibit grey matter reductions in dyslexic readers include bilateral posterior temporal, temporo-parietal, and occipito-temporal regions, and the cerebellum, thereby closely resembling the above mentioned reading systems that showed functional disturbances in dyslexics. These results have been narratively reviewed in two recent publications [27,30] but up to date no quantitative meta-analysis objectively measuring convergence between the studies has been published. Furthermore, no attempt has yet been made to objectively compare the results of dyslexia studies using structural imaging to those using functional imaging.

The present study aims at closing this gap by quantitatively meta-analyzing the results of published VBM studies comparing dyslexic and control participants. A main goal was to objectively identify areas showing consistent neuroanatomical differences across the studies and to specify the broad anatomical description of grey matter abnormalities in dyslexic persons by providing results in a standard stereotaxic space. Quantitative meta-analyses of neuroimaging data allow to assess convergence between studies independently from differences regarding acquisition and analysis methods or heterogeneity of subject characteristics, which is especially important for the study of disorders as heterogenous as dyslexia. An additional goal of this study was to identify possible overlaps between structural and functional brain variations in dyslexia by quantitatively comparing the results of the meta-analysis of VBM studies to results of meta-analyses of functional imaging studies showing under- or overactivations in dyslexic readers. To this end, we conducted three ALE meta-analyses, i.e. one on VBM studies reporting grey matter reductions in dyslexic readers, including 62 foci from nine studies; a second meta-analysis of functional imaging studies reporting underactivations in dyslexics, including 125 foci from 24 studies, and a third meta-analysis of functional imaging studies reporting overactivations in dyslexics, including 95 foci from 11 studies.

Materials and Methods

Study Selection

For the VBM meta-analysis, relevant publications were identified by PubMed searches using the keywords dyslexia plus morphometry, voxel-based or voxelwise, as well as by exploration of additional publications from the reference lists of obtained articles. Studies were included in the analysis if they (1) used voxel-based morphometry, (2) reported group comparisons between dyslexic and control participants with respect to local changes in grey matter density or volume, (3) reported results in a standard reference space (Talairach or MNI) and (4) used the same threshold throughout the whole brain. Based on these criteria, nine studies were selected [16,31–38]. Together, these studies included data from 277 participants (139 dyslexics and 138 controls) and reported 62 foci of grey matter reduction in dyslexic readers. Data are current with December, 2011. Only three of the nine studies reported grey matter increases in dyslexics. Five of the nine studies examined adult and four examined child or adolescent participants. Due to the small overall number of VBM studies, we included studies with participants from all age groups into the meta-analysis (cf. [20] for a similar approach). For an overview of the main characteristics of the included VBM studies, see Table 1.

For the selection of publications to be included in the meta-analyses of functional imaging studies, we aimed at consistency with the three previously published meta-analyses. The studies analyzed in Maisog et al.'s meta-analysis [18] represent a subset of the studies analyzed in Richlan et al.'s first meta-analysis [20] which in turn represent a subset of the studies analyzed in Richlan et al.'s second meta-analysis [22], with older studies [39–41] using the same participants being replaced by more recent ones [42–44]. Therefore, we included the 17 published papers [42–58] from Richlan et al.'s second [22] and four papers from Richlan et al.'s first meta-analysis [20], which were excluded in the second study because they examined adolescent participants [33,59–60].

To identify further studies published in the meantime, we conducted a PubMed search with the same keywords (dyslexia plus imaging) as used by Richlan and colleagues and applied the same selection criteria as used by the previous meta-analyses [18,20,22]: Studies were included in the analysis if they (1) investigated reading or reading-related tasks in alphabetic languages (2) with visually presented words, pseudowords, or single letters in the participants native language, (3) reported group comparisons between dyslexic and control participants (4) in a standard stereotactic space (Talairach or MNI) and (5) used the same threshold throughout the whole brain. As we included studies with participants of all age groups in the VBM meta-analysis, we did not introduce any restrictions on the age of participants in the selection of functional imaging studies (in accordance with [20]; but in contrast to [18,22]). Following these criteria, three additional studies could be identified [62–64].

According to the approach used by Richlan et al. [20,22], if a study reported differences between dyslexic and control participants for more than one contrast (i.e., contrast of an activation condition against simple fixation or a low-level visual control task), only foci from one such contrast, typically involving the task putting highest demands on phonological processing, were included. For the 21 studies analyzed in the previously published meta-analyses, foci of under- and overactivation from the same contrasts used by Richlan and colleagues [20,22] were selected, while the three newly selected studies reported foci of functional differences only for one contrast respectively. In total, the 24 selected studies included data from 736 participants (371 dyslexics and 365 controls) and reported 125 foci of underactivations in dyslexic readers. Out of these 24 studies, 11 reported 95 foci of overactivations. The main characteristics of the included functional imaging studies are listed in Table S1.

ALE Meta-Analysis Procedure

We performed three separate ALE meta-analyses one on VBM studies reporting grey matter reductions in dyslexic readers, a second on imaging studies reporting functional underactivations in dyslexics, and a third on imaging studies reporting functional overactivations in dyslexics. As only three VBM studies reported in

Table 1. Overview of the studies included in the meta-analysis of VBM studies.

Year	First author	Native language	Dylexics		Controls		Modulated/unmodulated images	Threshold		Number of foci with	
			n	mean age	n	mean age		Voxel-level (height) p<	Cluster-level (extent) p< or no. of voxels/ mm³	grey matter decrease	grey matter increase
2011	Raschle	English	10	5.9	10	5.5	modulated	0.001 unc.	0.01 corr.	5	0
2009	Pernet	French	38	27.2	39	27.8	modulated	0.005 unc.	20 voxels	15	5
2008	Kronbichler	German	13	15.8	15	15.4	modulated	0.005 unc.	100 mm³	11	8
2008	Steinbrinck	German	7	20.1	7	23.7	modulated	0.05 corr.	650 voxels	2	0
2007	Hoeft	English	19	14.4	19	14.4	modulated	0.01 corr.	0.01 corr	6	0
2005	Eckert	English	13	11.4	13	11.3	modulated	0.00001 unc.	0.001 corr.	5	0
2005	Vinckenbosch	French	13	17–30	10	-	unmodulated	0.01 corr.	0.05 corr.	1	1
2004	Brambati	Italian	10	31.6	11	27.4	modulated	0.05 corr.	25 voxels	9	0
2001	Brown	English	16	24	14	matched	unmodulated	0.05 unc.	0.05 corr.	8	0

sum only 14 foci of grey matter increase in dyslexic participants, we did not perform an additional meta-analysis of those studies.

The meta-analyses were carried out using GingerALE software, version 2.1.1 ([65], available from http://brainmap.org/ale/). Prior to analysis, foci reported in Talairach space in the original studies were transformed into MNI space using the tal2icbm algorithm [66]. For each study, the reported foci were modeled as centers of three-dimensional Gaussian probability distributions with FWHMs determined on the basis of the number of participants in the respective study (see [67]). The probability values of all foci in a given study were then combined to a modeled activation (MA) map. To control for within-experiment effects, the MA value of each voxel was computed by taking the maximum probability associated with any one of the foci reported in the respective study [68]. Finally, voxel-wise ALE scores, representing the convergence between studies at the corresponding location, were calculated by taking the union of the individual MA maps.

In order to determine the probability of the ALE values under the null-hypothesis of spatial independence between the studies, a null-distribution was derived analytically (see [69]). Based on these probabilities, the ALE maps for the three meta-analyses were thresholded at a false discovery rate (FDR) of $p<0.05$ and a cluster threshold of 125 voxels. To examine possible overlaps between the significant clusters from the VBM meta-analysis and those from the functional meta-analyses, two formal conjunction analyses were performed by multiplying binarized versions of the thresholded ALE maps.

Results

ALE Meta-Analysis of VBM Studies

In the meta-analysis of VBM studies reporting grey matter reductions in dyslexic readers, we found six clusters of significant convergence between the studies (see Table 2; Figure 1). The largest cluster was located in the fusiform gyrus of the left hemisphere extending into the left inferior temporal gyrus. Further clusters were found bilaterally in the supramarginal gyrus and in the cerebellum. In the right hemisphere, the supramarginal cluster extended into the parietal operculum and was accompanied by an additional cluster in the posterior portion of the superior temporal gyrus.

Overlap between Structural and Functional Alterations

Expectedly, the two meta-analyses of functional imaging studies reporting over- or underactivations in dyslexic readers yielded similar clusters of convergence as the previously published meta-analyses by Maisog et al. [18] and Richlan et al. [20,22]. As the focus of the present study lies on the meta-analysis of VBM studies, these results will not be discussed in detail (see Table S2 for an overview).

The two formal conjunction analyses revealed three regional overlaps between the thresholded ALE maps from the VBM meta-analysis and those from the meta-analyses of functional imaging studies (see Table 2; Figure 1). The conjunction between the VBM meta-analysis and the meta-analysis of functional underactivations identified a large overlap of 95 voxels in the left fusiform gyrus (Figure 1, bottom row, middle panel). The supramarginal cluster from the VBM meta-analysis was located anterior and inferior, but in direct connection, to an extensive temporo-parietal cluster showing functional underactivation in dyslexics. There was a slight overlap of one voxel between the clusters in the left supramarginal gyrus (Figure 1, bottom row, left panel). The conjunction between the VBM meta-analysis and the meta-analysis of functional overactivations identified a large overlap of 99 voxels in the left cerebellum (Figure 1, bottom row, right panel).

Discussion

The present study provides the first quantitative summary of published findings on grey matter variations in dyslexic readers, by conducting an ALE meta-analysis of nine published studies reporting grey matter reductions in dyslexics. The meta-analysis revealed six clusters of topographic convergence that were located bilaterally in temporo-parietal regions and in the cerebellum, as well as in occipito-temporal regions of the left hemisphere. Subsequent conjunction analyses identified overlaps with dyslexia-related functional underactivations in the fusiform and supramarginal gyri of the left hemisphere and an overlap with functional overactivations in the left cerebellum.

Temporo-parietal Regions

The meta-analysis of VBM studies identified convergent grey matter reductions in temporo-parietal regions of both hemispheres. In the left hemisphere, one cluster with local maximum in the supramarginal gyrus was found. In the right hemisphere, a supramarginal cluster could also be identified that extended anteriorly into the parietal operculum. An additional cluster was found in the right superior temporal gyrus extending into the inferior parietal lobule.

The left parietal cluster corresponds well to the anatomical characterization of the dorsal posterior reading system which has been described by several authors [1,70,71]. This system is assumed to support the transformation of orthographic elements of visual words (graphemes) into associated phonological elements (phonemes). In the framework of the phonological theory of dyslexia, a dysfunction of this system has been proposed as the main biological basis of dyslexia [72]. Indeed, local grey matter volume in this region has been demonstrated to correlate with tasks involving phonological processing [35,36] and these correlations could not be found for dyslexic readers [35]. Structural neuroimaging studies using manual methods in temporo-parietal regions concentrated mainly on symmetry measurements of the planum temporale and the planum parietale. While some studies reported greater symmetry or rightward asymmetry of the planum temporale and greater leftward asymmetry of the planum parietale, others could not confirm those findings (for reviews, see [27,28]). Similar inconsistencies with regard to differences in asymmetry of temporo-parietal regions have been reported for other developmental disorders of speech and language, such as specific language impairment (SLI; [73,74]) or stuttering [75]. Our VBM meta-analysis found grey matter reductions in dyslexic readers in areas corresponding to the planum temporale of the right and the planum parietale of both hemispheres. While an integration of results from micro- and macrostructural methods has to be interpreted with caution, our findings of grey matter decreases in the right planum temporale are not consistent with the proposal of greater rightward asymmetry in dyslexic readers. Likewise, as grey matter reductions affected the planum parietale not only of the left, but also the right hemisphere, the presently available VBM data also fail to support the proposed leftward asymmetry of the planum parietale.

On the basis of the present data, it remains unclear whether the grey matter reductions in temporo-parietal regions of dyslexic readers can be interpreted as the underlying neurobiological cause of deficient phonological processing skills in this population or should be better understood as the result of experience-dependent structural changes occurring in the course of school or preschool

Table 2. Results of the ALE meta-analysis of VBM studies and the two conjunction analyses.

Region	MNI coordinates of local maxima			Cluster size (voxels)
	X	Y	Z	
VBM meta-analysis (Contr. >Dysl.)				
L supramarginal gyrus	−54	−34	30	156
R supramarginal gyrus	48	−40	26	143
	46	−30	24	a
R superior temporal gyrus	64	−34	18	131
L fusiform gyrus	−38	−66	−14	200
	−44	−60	−14	a
L inferior temporal gyrus	−56	−64	−10	a
L cerebellum	−26	−50	−32	158
R cerebellum	26	−54	−34	138
	18	−50	−38	a
Conjunction analyses				
VBM (Contr. >Dysl.)∩Imaging (Contr. >Dysl.)				
L supramarginal gyrus				1
L fusiform gyrus				95
VBM (Contr. >Dysl.)∩Imaging (Dysl. >Contr.)				
L cerebellum				99

a. subpeak within cluster.

education. Raschle et al. [36] found grey matter alterations in temporo-parietal regions in familial dyslexic children before the onset of formal reading instruction. These findings suggest that the structural abnormalities are not the result but the cause of later reading problems. However, an alternative interpretation could be that abnormal phonological processing, possibly due to more basal auditory deficits (e.g., [7]), leads to secondary temporo-parietal grey matter alterations in dyslexic children even before reading instruction starts. The VBM meta-analysis also identified clusters of convergence in homologous areas of the right hemisphere, which conforms to the results of post-mortem studies by Galaburda and colleagues, showing that cortical abnormalities affected mainly perisylvian areas of the left hemisphere, but were always accompanied by corresponding abnormalities in the right hemisphere (see, e.g., [76]). Thus, our findings support the notion that bilateral anatomical variations represent a pre-existing neurobiological deficit of dyslexic readers, with left hemispheric variations underlying phonological processing problems. It can be hypothesized further that the parallel development of those bilateral regions might be under genetic control. Variations in genes involved in cortical development might result in micro-structural cortical malformations through abnormal migration or maturation of neurons [77].

The left temporo-parietal cluster from the VBM meta-analysis was located directly anterior and inferior to an inferior parietal cluster from the meta-analysis of dyslexia-related functional underactivations, with an overlap of one voxel between the two clusters. The cluster of functional underactivations also included the posterior part of the supramarginal gyrus and extended into the angular gyrus and the superior parietal lobule. At its inferior border, this cluster of grey matter reductions was located in close proximity to a large occipito-temporal cluster of functional underactivations which extended into the superior temporal gyrus. In the right hemisphere, the superior temporal cluster from the VBM meta-analysis was located lateral and superior to a cluster from the meta-analysis of functional underactivations in the superior temporal gyrus.

To assess age-specific contributions to the relationship between structural and functional abnormalities, two additional meta-analyses were conducted, dividing the studies reporting functional underactivations in studies examining children and studies examining adults (for details, see Method S1; Table S3). While conjunction analyses of the results from the VBM meta-analysis with the results from both age-specific meta-analyses did not result in an overlap, the meta-analyses revealed that both child and adult studies contributed to the close connection between structural and functional deviations in left inferior parietal regions, with children's underactivations being more wide-spread and extending into the angular gyrus and the superior parietal lobule. In contrast, the proximity to superior temporal underactivations in both hemispheres was driven by adult studies (see Table S4; Figure S1, left side). Taken together, the small overlap in the temporo-parietal system does not speak for a direct correspondence between the areas showing structural and functional abnormalities in dyslexic readers. Nonetheless, as the left-hemispheric cluster from the VBM meta-analysis was located in close connection to both the temporo-parietal and the occipito-temporal cluster showing functional underactivation in dyslexics, it is tempting to speculate that the anterior part of the temporo-parietal system might serve as a connectional hub and that structural deviations in this area might secondarily cause dysfunction of occipito-temporal and temporo-parietal regions and a disruption of functional connectivity between these areas that has been demonstrated in dyslexics [78–80].

Occipito-temporal Regions

The largest cluster of dyslexia-related grey matter alteration identified by the VBM meta-analysis was located in occipito-

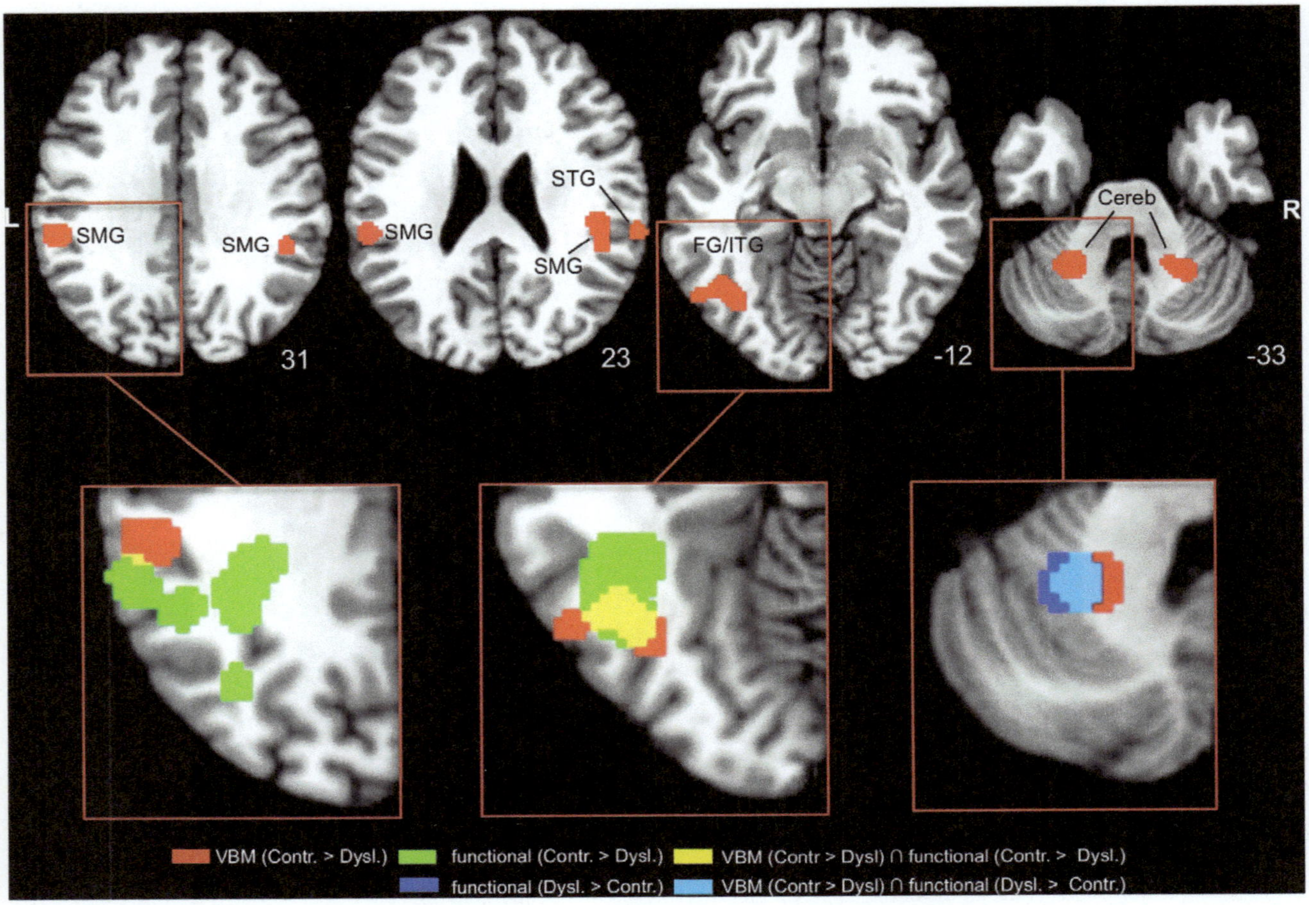

Figure 1. Results of the ALE meta-analysis of VBM studies and the conjunction analyses. Upper row–2D axial slices depicting the thresholded and binarized ALE map for the VBM meta-analysis (red) projected onto the Colin T1-template in MNI space. Images are presented in neurological convention (i.e., left = left) and MNI coordinates in the inferior-superior (Z) plane are provided with each slice. Lower row – cut-outs of the axial slices display overlaps (yellow) of the VBM meta-analysis (red) with the thresholded and binarized ALE map for the meta-analysis of functional underactivations (green) and overlaps (light blue) with the thresholded and binarized ALE map for the meta-analysis of functional overactivations (dark blue). SMG = supramarginal gyrus; STG = superior temporal gyrus; FG/ITG = fusiform gyrus/inferior temporal gyrus; Cereb = cerebellum.

temporal regions of the left hemisphere comprising mainly the fusiform gyrus and extending laterally into the inferior temporal gyrus. It thereby closely resembles the anatomical description of the ventral occipito-temporal reading system [70,71] and includes the coordinates for the visual word form area (VWFA; x = 43, y = 54; z = 12; Talairach space) reported by Cohen et al. [12]. The occipito-temporal system is assumed to underlie the fast and effortless processing of printed text in experienced readers through direct mapping of orthographic word forms onto corresponding phonological representations (e.g., [81]). This specialization is assumed to develop gradually in the course of the process of learning to read, and functional underactivations of this region in dyslexic readers have been interpreted as the result of pre-existing functional and/or structural disruptions of the temporo-parietal reading system [1,80].

As previously discussed, the results of our meta-analysis cannot answer the question whether grey matter microstructural abnormalities in dyslexics can be interpreted as the neurobiological cause of reading problems or should rather be understood as secondary, experience-dependent developmental changes. In contrast to the temporo-parietal system, where bilateral VBM effects were consistently observed, an occipito-temporal cluster of convergence between VBM studies could only be identified in the left hemisphere. If one assumes that disturbed neuronal migration should result in bilateral grey matter alterations in dyslexic readers, as suggested by the findings of post-mortem studies (cf. [76]), one might conclude that the observed structural abnormalities in left occipito-temporal regions represent the secondary result of disturbed reading and pre-reading experience. At least one VBM study, however, reported lower grey matter volume also in homologous areas of the right hemisphere [34]. Furthermore, [36] found lower grey matter volume in occipito-temporal regions of the left hemisphere in familial dyslexics in the last year before entering elementary school. As argued above, grey matter reductions might also have emerged in response to pre-school learning experiences, but it remains possible that occipito-temporal grey matter alterations may constitute a pre-existing neurobiological deficit, at least in a subgroup of dyslexics. Future, possibly longitudinal, studies examining structural abnormalities in persons suffering from or at risk for developmental dyslexia are needed to resolve this issue.

The conjunction analysis exhibited overlap between the occipito-temporal VBM cluster and an extensive occipito-temporal cluster showing reduced activation across functional imaging studies of dyslexic participants. The overlap comprised mainly the fusiform gyrus, including the above mentioned VWFA coordinates. Following the two explanatory approaches outlined above, microstructural alterations of grey matter in this region might either be the cause for a reduced functional responsiveness of the corresponding neural circuits or alternatively be the secondary result of abnormal input from and/or connectivity to temporo-parietal regions of the left hemisphere.

The age-specific meta-analyses of functional underactivations and conjunction analyses with the results from the VBM meta-analysis revealed that the occipito-temporal overlap between structural and functional deviations was driven by the studies examining adults, with an overlap of 82 voxels between the VBM meta-analysis and the meta-analysis of functional underactivations in adults. The meta-analysis of functional underactivations in children also resulted in a cluster in the fusiform gyrus, but it was located more anterior and inferior than the cluster of grey matter reduction (see Table S4; Figure S1, right side). The age-specific results highlight the increasing importance of structural and functional integrity of fusiform areas for the fast and effortless processing of words.

Cerebellum

The VBM meta-analysis identified clusters of convergence in the cerebellum bilaterally. Traditionally, the cerebellum has been exclusively considered as a motor structure, controlling the coordination of movements. Recent research, however, points to an involvement of the cerebellum in higher cognitive functions by means of cerebro-cerebellar circuits targeting non-motor cortical regions (e.g., [82]). Indeed, cerebellar activation has been found by functional imaging studies employing a variety of tasks, including spatial processing, executive functions, working memory and language [83]. In addition to numerous PET and fMRI studies [84], the importance of the cerebellum for the processing of spoken and written language has been demonstrated by clinical studies showing phonological, semantic and syntactic impairments in patients with cerebellar lesions [85]. Accordingly, the cerebellum has been proposed to play an important role in the origin of dyslexia. The cerebellar deficit theory by Nicolson and colleagues [10] states that a mild dysfunction of the cerebellum leads to deficits in motor control and skill automatization in dyslexic readers. Supporting the theory, studies using different approaches have found structural abnormalities in the cerebellum to be a valid neurobiological marker for dyslexia [86–88]. A recent longitudinal VBM study demonstrated increased grey matter volume in the right anterior cerebellum in a group of dyslexic children following an eight-week reading intervention program [89]. On the other hand, meta-analyses of functional imaging studies comparing dyslexic and control participants did not reveal any reliable evidence for underactivations in the cerebellum [18,20,22]. Furthermore, motor problems seem to be present only in a subgroup of the dyslexic population (see, e.g., [6]) and it has been suggested that they only occur in dyslexic children with comorbid attention-deficit hyperactivity disorder (ADHD; [90,91]). In their more recent work, Nicolson and colleagues [92] proposed that malfunctions in cortico-cerebellar loops might lead to procedural learning deficits which may affect both language and motor functions, either individually or in combination. An alternative explanation for morphometric alterations of cerebellar regions in dyslexic readers was raised by Ramus [93]. With reference to the work of Galaburda (for an overview see [76,77]), he suggested that a core deficit in temporo-parietal regions of the cortex following disturbed neuronal migration may, under specific conditions, cause additional dysfunctions in sub-cortical regions, resulting in optional sensorimotor symptoms in a subgroup of dyslexic readers. Our finding of reliable structural alterations in homologous regions of the cerebellum highlights the importance of cerebellar deficits in dyslexia. The bilateral clusters of grey matter reductions were located mainly in the cerebellar lobule VI. Similar clusters were also found bilaterally by a meta-analysis of PET studies investigating single-word reading in normal adult participants [19] and in the right hemisphere by a meta-analysis of verbal working memory studies [94]. The clusters from the meta-analysis of single-word reading were located medial, posterior and superior, the cluster from the working memory meta-analysis superior to the clusters reported here. In a more recent study reporting several meta-analyses of functional imaging studies with different tasks, Stoodley and Schmahmann [83] also found bilateral clusters in the cerebellar lobule VI for verbal working memory and language tasks, with clusters being located more lateral and posterior. In the same study, also for motor tasks a right lateralized cluster (but note that all the tasks were finger-tapping tasks performed with the right index finger) in similar regions was reported, that extended from the anterior lobule V. Thus, the origin and implications of the grey matter reductions in the cerebellum found in the meta-analysis of VBM studies remain unclear. Further studies are needed to explore these questions in more detail.

In the left cerebellum, a large overlap between the VBM meta-analysis and the meta-analysis of functional overactivations in dyslexic readers was identified by the conjunction analysis. Additional meta-analyses examining age-specific contributions to the overlap could not be performed in this case, due to the limited number of studies reporting functional overactivations. The overlap between structural reduction and functional overactivation seems counterintuitive as one would rather assume that structural alterations of grey matter would result in decreases of functional responsiveness in corresponding regions. We hypothesize that increased activation in cerebellar and other sub-cortical regions in dyslexic readers while processing reading-related stimuli might represent increased effort, possibly due to disorganization of cortico-cerebellar loops and/or the use of compensatory strategies involving subvocal articulation or verbal working memory.

Inferior Frontal Regions

Our meta-analysis did not find any reliable evidence for grey matter differences between dyslexic and normal readers in inferior frontal regions. The role of these regions in dyslexia has been discussed controversially — bilateral inferior frontal gyri have been found to exhibit functional overactivations in dyslexics by some researchers, while others reported no activation differences or even functional underactivations, mainly in the left inferior frontal gyrus. Some evidence for deviations in inferior frontal regions has been found in structural imaging studies: Brown et al. [31] reported grey matter reductions in dyslexic readers in the left inferior frontal gyrus. In support of this finding, some studies found grey matter density or volume in this region to be positively correlated with behavioral performance in tasks involving phonological processing [35,38,87]. In addition, neuroimaging studies using manual morphometric measurements reported rightward asymmetry of the inferior frontal gyrus [95] and a smaller left [86] and right [32,86] pars triangularis in dyslexic readers. In contrast, most published VBM studies did not identify any significant differences between dyslexic and normal readers in inferior frontal gyri, not even when applying small volume correction [34]. Thus, grey matter deviations in inferior frontal regions do not seem to play a major role in the neurobiological origin of dyslexia, but might, at least in some dyslexics, occur as a secondary consequence of deficient input from posterior reading systems or as a reflection of compensatory cognitive processes.

Limitations

Besides methodological issues associated with coordinate-based meta-analyses in general [96] and inevitable drawbacks of meta-analyses of neuroimaging data, such as differences between the analyzed studies regarding data acquisition and processing, the present meta-analysis has the following limitations: The diagnostic criteria that were applied to select dyslexic participants varied greatly between the analyzed studies. While most studies used deviation from the norm of a standardized reading test as main criterion (i.e., ranging from 0.67 to 2 SD below average between studies), often combined with an intelligence test to ensure that intelligence was in the normal range, some studies used the stronger discrepancy criterion (i.e., discrepancy between the individual test scores in a reading and an intelligence test) and yet others selected participants based on evidence for a family history of dyslexia or a childhood diagnosis. One study [36] examined participants with familial history of dyslexia in the year before entering school, at a point in time where a reliable diagnosis for dyslexia cannot be made. Thus, the symptoms and possibly also the neuroanatomy of dyslexic participants included in the analyzed studies have to be regarded as heterogeneous. A further issue concerns the variability between the analyzed studies regarding the age of participants, with mean ages ranging from 5 to 30 in the VBM meta-analysis. To determine possible developmental changes of structural differences between dyslexic and control participants in the course of formal reading instruction, a comparison between separate meta-analyses of studies examining children and those examining adults would have been of interest, but was not possible due to the small number of studies that would be available for each age group in this analysis. In addition, separate analyses of studies using unmodulated (indicating differences in concentration) and modulated images (indicating differences in volume) might have provided further information about the nature of the observed structural differences between dyslexic and normal readers, but again could not be performed at the moment due to the limited number of available studies using each method. Finally, only studies from countries with alphabetic languages were included limiting the generalizability of the results of our study to specific cultures.

Conclusion

By quantitatively integrating across individual studies, our meta analysis provides a strong empirical basis for understanding the neuroanatomical changes underlying developmental dyslexia. Clusters of topographic convergence were found exclusively in posterior brain regions, specifically in bilateral temporo-parietal and left occipito-temporal regions, and bilaterally in the cerebellum. These areas correspond well to the anatomical characterizations of neural systems that have been proposed to play a role in the origin of dyslexia by previous research. The analysis of conjunctions between the results of the VBM meta-analysis and meta-analyses of functional neuroimaging studies demonstrates that structural alterations of the reading systems in the left cerebral hemisphere co-occur with functional underactivations in these systems. Functional overactivations co-localize with grey matter reductions in the left cerebellum, possibly reflecting the compensatory use of articulatory strategies in dyslexic readers. In sum, our data suggest strong convergence between structural and functional alterations in the left hemisphere of the dyslexic brain.

Supporting Information

Figure S1 Results of the age specific conjunction analyses. Upper row — cut-outs of axial slices display the temporo-parietal and occipito-temporal overlaps (yellow) of the VBM meta-analysis (red) with the meta-analysis of functional underactivations (green) as depicted in Figure 1, bottom row. Lower row — cut outs of axial slices display the results of the conjunction of the VBM meta-analysis (red) with the meta-analyses of functional underactivations in adults (light blue) and children (dark blue) for the same regions. Overlaps between the VBM meta-analysis and the adults meta-analysis are depicted in magenta, overlaps between the age-specific meta-analyses are depicted in cyan. Images are presented in neurological convention (i.e., left = left) and MNI coordinates in the inferior-superior (Z) plane are provided.

Table S1 Overview of the studies included in the meta-analyses of functional imaging studies.

Table S2 Results of the ALE meta-analyses of functional imaging studies.

Table S3 Overview of the studies included in the age-specific meta-analyses of functional underactivation.

Table S4 Results of the age-specific ALE meta-analyses of functional underactivation and the age-specific conjunction analyses.

Method S1 Supplementary method.

Author Contributions

Conceived and designed the experiments: J. Linkersdorfer J. Lonnemann SL MH CJF. Analyzed the data: J. Linkersdorfer J. Lonnemann CJF. Wrote the paper: J. Linkersdorfer J. Lonnemann SL MH CJF.

References

1. McCandliss BD, Noble KG (2003) The development of reading impairment: a cognitive neuroscience model. Ment Retard Dev Disabil Res Rev 9: 196–204.
2. Bradley L, Bryant PE (1978) Difficulties in auditory organisation as a possible cause of reading backwardness. Nature 271: 746–7.
3. Snowling MJ (1981) Phonemic deficits in developmental dyslexia. Psychol Res 43: 219–34.
4. Vellutino FR (1979) Dyslexia: Research and theory. Cambridge, MA: MIT Press.
5. Heim S, Tschierse J, Amunts K, Wilms M, Vossel S, et al. (2008) Cognitive subtypes of dyslexia. Acta Neurobiol Exp (Wars) 68: 73–89.
6. Ramus F, Rosen S, Dakin SC, Day BL, Castellote JM, et al. (2003) Theories of developmental dyslexia: insights from a multiple case study of dyslexic adults. Brain 126: 841–65.
7. Tallal P (1980) Auditory temporal perception, phonics, and reading disabilities in children. Brain Lang 9: 182–98.
8. Stein J, Walsh V (1997) To see but not to read; the magnocellular theory of dyslexia. Trends Neurosci 20: 147–152.
9. Hari R, Renvall H (2001) Impaired processing of rapid stimulus sequences in dyslexia. Trends Cogn Sci 5: 525–532.
10. Nicolson RI, Fawcett AJ, Dean P (2001) Developmental dyslexia: the cerebellar deficit hypothesis. Trends Neurosci 24: 508–11.
11. Shaywitz SE, Shaywitz BA (2005) Dyslexia (specific reading disability). Biol Psychiatry 57: 1301–1309.
12. Cohen L, Dehaene S, Naccache L, Lehéricy S, Dehaene-Lambertz G, et al. (2000) The visual word form area: spatial and temporal characterization of an

initial stage of reading in normal subjects and posterior split-brain patients. Brain 123: 291–307.
13. Price CJ, Devlin JT (2003) The myth of the visual word form area. Neuroimage 19: 473–81.
14. Pugh KR, Mencl WE, Jenner AR, Katz L, Frost SJ, et al. (2000) Functional neuroimaging studies of reading and reading disability (developmental dyslexia). Ment Retard Dev Disabil Res Rev 6: 207–13.
15. Eden GF, Jones KM, Cappell K, Gareau L, Wood FB, et al. (2004) Neural changes following remediation in adult developmental dyslexia. Neuron 44: 411–22.
16. Brambati SM, Termine C, Ruffino M, Stella G, Fazio F, et al. (2004) Regional reductions of gray matter volume in familial dyslexia. Neurology 63: 742–5.
17. Nicolson RI, Fawcett AJ, Berry EL, Jenkins IH, Dean P, et al. (1999) Association of abnormal cerebellar activation with motor learning difficulties in dyslexic adults. Lancet 353: 1662–7.
18. Maisog JM, Einbinder ER, Flowers DL, Turkeltaub PE, Eden GF (2008) A meta-analysis of functional neuroimaging studies of dyslexia. Ann N Y Acad Sci 1145: 237–259.
19. Turkeltaub PE, Eden GF, Jones KM, Zeffiro TA (2002) Meta-analysis of the functional neuroanatomy of single-word reading: method and validation. Neuroimage 16: 765–780.
20. Richlan F, Kronbichler M, Wimmer H (2009) Functional abnormalities in the dyslexic brain: a quantitative meta-analysis of neuroimaging studies. Hum Brain Mapp 30: 3299–308.
21. Radua J, Mataix-Cols D (2009) Voxel-wise meta-analysis of grey matter changes in obsessivecompulsive disorder. Br J Psychiatry 195: 393–402.
22. Richlan F, Kronbichler M, Wimmer H (2011) Meta-analyzing brain dysfunctions in dyslexic children and adults. Neuroimage 56: 1735–42.
23. Galaburda AM, Kemper TL (1979) Cytoarchitectonic abnormalities in developmental dyslexia: a case study. Ann Neurol 6: 94–100.
24. Galaburda AM, Livingstone M (1993) Evidence for a magnocellular defect in developmental dyslexia. Ann N Y Acad Sci 682: 70–82.
25. Galaburda AM, Sherman GF, Rosen GD, Aboitiz F, Geschwind N (1985) Developmental dyslexia: four consecutive patients with cortical anomalies. Ann Neurol 18: 222–33.
26. Galaburda AM, Menard MT, Rosen GD (1994) Evidence for aberrant auditory anatomy in developmental dyslexia. Proc Natl Acad Sci U S A 91: 8010–3.
27. Eckert MA (2004) Neuroanatomical markers for dyslexia: a review of dyslexia structural imaging studies. Neuroscientist 10: 362–371.
28. Heim S, Keil A (2004) Large-scale neural correlates of developmental dyslexia. Eur Child Adolesc Psychiatry 13: 125–140.
29. Ashburner J, Friston KJ (2000) Voxel-based morphometry-the methods. Neuroimage 11: 805–21.
30. Richardson FM, Price CJ (2009) Structural mri studies of language function in the undamaged brain. Brain Struct Funct 213: 511–23.
31. Brown WE, Eliez S, Menon V, Rumsey JM, White CD, et al. (2001) Preliminary evidence of widespread morphological variations of the brain in dyslexia. Neurology 56: 781–3.
32. Eckert MA, Leonard CM, Wilke M, Eckert M, Richards T, et al. (2005) Anatomical signatures of dyslexia in children: unique information from manual and voxel based morphometry brain measures. Cortex 41: 304–15.
33. Hoeft F, Meyler A, Hernandez A, Juel C, Taylor-Hill H, et al. (2007) Functional and morphometric brain dissociation between dyslexia and reading ability. Proc Natl Acad Sci U S A 104: 4234–9.
34. Kronbichler M, Wimmer H, Staffen W, Hutzler F, Mair A, et al. (2008) Developmental dyslexia: Gray matter abnormalities in the occipitotemporal cortex. Hum Brain Mapp 29: 613–625.
35. Pernet CR, Andersson J, Paulesu E, Demonet JF (2009)When all hypotheses are right: a multifocal account of dyslexia. Hum Brain Mapp 30: 2278–92.
36. Raschle NM, Chang M, Gaab N (2011) Structural brain alterations associated with dyslexia predate reading onset. Neuroimage 57: 742–9.
37. Steinbrink C, Vogt K, Kastrup A, Müller HP, Juengling FD, et al. (2008) The contribution of white and gray matter differences to developmental dyslexia: insights from dti and vbm at 3.0 t. Neuropsychologia 46: 3170–8.
38. Vinckenbosch E, Robichon F, Eliez S (2005) Graymatter alteration in dyslexia: converging evidence from volumetric and voxel-by-voxel mri analyses. Neuropsychologia 43: 324–31.
39. Brunswick N, McCrory E, Price CJ, Frith CD, Frith U (1999) Explicit and implicit processing of words and pseudowords by adult developmental dyslexics: A search for wernicke's wortschatz? Brain 122: 1901–17.
40. Meyler A, Keller TA, Cherkassky VL, Lee D, Hoeft F, et al. (2007) Brain activation during sentence comprehension among good and poor readers. Cereb Cortex 17: 2780–7.
41. Schulz E, Maurer U, van der Mark S, Bucher K, Brem S, et al. (2008) Impaired semantic processing during sentence reading in children with dyslexia: Combined fmri and erp evidence. Neuroimage 41: 153–168.
42. Meyler A, Keller TA, Cherkassky VL, Gabrieli JDE, Just MA (2008) Modifying the brain activation of poor readers during sentence comprehension with extended remedial instruction: a longitudinal study of neuroplasticity. Neuropsychologia 46: 2580–92.
43. Paulesu E, Démonet JF, Fazio F, McCrory E, Chanoine V, et al. (2001) Dyslexia: cultural diversity and biological unity. Science 291: 2165–7.
44. Schulz E, Maurer U, van der Mark S, Bucher K, Brem S, et al. (2009) Reading for meaning in dyslexic and young children: distinct neural pathways but common endpoints. Neuropsychologia 47: 2544–57.
45. Blau V, van Atteveldt N, Ekkebus M, Goebel R, Blomert L (2009) Reduced neural integration of letters and speech sounds links phonological and reading deficits in adult dyslexia. Curr Biol 19: 503–8.
46. Blau V, Reithler J, van Atteveldt N, Seitz J, Gerretsen P, et al. (2010) Deviant processing of letters and speech sounds as proximate cause of reading failure: a functional magnetic resonance imaging study of dyslexic children. Brain 133: 868–79.
47. Booth JR, Bebko G, Burman DD, Bitan T (2007) Children with reading disorder show modality independent brain abnormalities during semantic tasks. Neuropsychologia 45: 775–783.
48. Brambati SM, Termine C, Ruffino M, Danna M, Lanzi G, et al. (2006) Neuropsychological deficits and neural dysfunction in familial dyslexia. Brain Res 1113: 174–85.
49. Cao F, Bitan T, Chou TL, Burman DD, Booth JR (2006) Deficient orthographic and phonological representations in children with dyslexia revealed by brain activation patterns. J Child Psychol Psychiatry 47: 1041–1050.
50. Hoeft F, Hernandez A, McMillon G, Taylor-Hill H, Martindale JL, et al. (2006) Neural basis of dyslexia: a comparison between dyslexic and nondyslexic children equated for reading ability. J Neurosci 26: 10700–10708.
51. Ingvar M, af Trampe P, Greitz T, Eriksson L, Stone-Elander S, et al. (2002) Residual differences in language processing in compensated dyslexics revealed in simple word reading tasks. Brain Lang 83: 249–67.
52. van der Mark S, Bucher K, Maurer U, Schulz E, Brem S, et al. (2009) Children with dyslexia lack multiple specializations along the visual word-form (vwf) system. Neuroimage 47: 1940–9.
53. McCrory EJ, Mechelli A, Frith U, Price CJ (2005) More than words: a common neural basis for reading and naming deficits in developmental dyslexia? Brain 128: 261–7.
54. Paulesu E, Frith U, Snowling M, Gallagher A, Morton J, et al. (1996) Is developmental dyslexia a disconnection syndrome? evidence from pet scanning. Brain 119 (Pt 1): 143–57.
55. Richlan F, Sturm D, Schurz M, Kronbichler M, Ladurner G, et al. (2010) A common left occipitotemporal dysfunction in developmental dyslexia and acquired letter-by-letter reading? PLoS One 5.
56. Rumsey JM, Nace K, Donohue B, Wise D, Maisog JM, et al. (1997) A positron emission tomographic study of impaired word recognition and phonological processing in dyslexic men. Arch Neurol 54: 562–73.
57. Temple E, Poldrack RA, Salidis J, Deutsch GK, Tallal P, et al. (2001) Disrupted neural responses to phonological and orthographic processing in dyslexic children: an fmri study. Neuroreport 12: 299–307.
58. Wimmer H, Schurz M, Sturm D, Richlan F, Klackl J, et al. (2010) A dual-route perspective on poor reading in a regular orthography: an fmri study. Cortex 46: 1284–98.
59. Georgiewa P, Rzanny R, Hopf JM, Knab R, Glauche V, et al. (1999) fmri during word processing in dyslexic and normal reading children. Neuroreport 10: 3459–65.
60. Grünling C, Ligges M, Huonker R, Klingert M, Mentzel HJ, et al. (2004) Dyslexia: the possible benefit of multimodal integration of fmri- and eeg-data. J Neural Transm 111: 951–69.
61. Kronbichler M, Hutzler F, Staffen W, Mair A, Ladurner G, et al. (2006) Evidence for a dysfunction of left posterior reading areas in german dyslexic readers. Neuropsychologia 44: 1822–1832.
62. Hu W, Lee HL, Zhang Q, Liu T, Geng LB, et al. (2010) Developmental dyslexia in chinese and english populations: dissociating the effect of dyslexia from language differences. Brain 133: 1694–706.
63. Maurer U, Schulz E, Brem S, der Mark Sv, Bucher K, et al. (2011) The development of print tuning in children with dyslexia: evidence from longitudinal erp data supported by fmri. Neuroimage 57: 714–22.
64. Pecini C, Biagi L, Brizzolara D, Cipriani P, Di Lieto MC, et al. (2011) How many functional brains in developmental dyslexia? when the history of language delay makes the difference. Cogn Behav Neurol 24: 85–92.
65. Laird AR, Fox PM, Price CJ, Glahn DC, Uecker AM, et al. (2005) Ale meta-analysis: controlling the false discovery rate and performing statistical contrasts. Hum Brain Mapp 25: 155–64.
66. Lancaster JL, Tordesillas-Gutiérrez D, Martinez M, Salinas F, Evans A, et al. (2007) Bias between mni and talairach coordinates analyzed using the icbm-152 brain template. Hum Brain Mapp 28: 1194–205.
67. Eickhoff SB, Laird AR, Grefkes C, Wang LE, Zilles K, et al. (2009) Coordinate-based activation likelihood estimation meta-analysis of neuroimaging data: a random-effects approach based on empirical estimates of spatial uncertainty. Hum Brain Mapp 30: 2907–26.
68. Turkeltaub PE, Eickhoff SB, Laird AR, Fox M, Wiener M, et al. (2011) Minimizing withinexperiment and within-group effects in activation likelihood estimation meta-analyses. Hum Brain Mapp.
69. Eickhoff SB, Bzdok D, Laird AR, Kurth F, Fox PT (2011) Activation likelihood estimation metaanalysis revisited. Neuroimage.
70. Démonet JF, Taylor MJ, Chaix Y (2004) Developmental dyslexia. Lancet 363: 1451–1460.
71. Sandak R, Mencl WE, Frost SJ, Pugh KR (2004) The neurobiological basis of skilled and impaired reading: Recent findings and new directions. Scientific Studies of Reading 8: 273–292.

72. Shaywitz SE, Morris R, Shaywitz BA (2008) The education of dyslexic children from childhood to young adulthood. Annu Rev Psychol 59: 451–475.
73. Webster RI, Shevell MI (2004) Neurobiology of specific language impairment. J Child Neurol 19: 471–81.
74. Herbert MR, Kenet T (2007) Brain abnormalities in language disorders and in autism. Pediatr Clin North Am 54: 563–83, vii.
75. Cykowski MD, Kochunov PV, Ingham RJ, Ingham JC, Mangin JF, et al. (2008) Perisylvian sulcal morphology and cerebral asymmetry patterns in adults who stutter. Cereb Cortex 18: 571–83.
76. Galaburda AM (2005) Dyslexia-a molecular disorder of neuronal migration: the 2004 norman geschwind memorial lecture. Ann Dyslexia 55: 151–65.
77. Galaburda AM, LoTurco J, Ramus F, Fitch RH, Rosen GD (2006) From genes to behavior in developmental dyslexia. Nat Neurosci 9: 1213–7.
78. Horwitz B, Rumsey JM, Donohue BC (1998) Functional connectivity of the angular gyrus in normal reading and dyslexia. Proc Natl Acad Sci U S A 95: 8939–8944.
79. van der Mark S, Klaver P, Bucher K, Maurer U, Schulz E, et al. (2011) The left occipitotemporal system in reading: disruption of focal fmri connectivity to left inferior frontal and inferior parietal language areas in children with dyslexia. Neuroimage 54: 2426–36.
80. Pugh KR, Mencl WE, Shaywitz BA, Shaywitz SE, Fulbright RK, et al. (2000) The angular gyrus in developmental dyslexia: task-specific differences in functional connectivity within posterior cortex. Psychol Sci 11: 51–6.
81. Schlaggar BL, McCandliss BD (2007) Development of neural systems for reading. Annu Rev Neurosci 30: 475–503.
82. Strick PL, Dum RP, Fiez JA (2009) Cerebellum and nonmotor function. Annu Rev Neurosci 32: 413–34.
83. Stoodley CJ, Schmahmann JD (2009) Functional topography in the human cerebellum: a metaanalysis of neuroimaging studies. Neuroimage 44: 489–501.
84. Price CJ (in press) A review and synthesis of the first 20 years of pet and fmri studies of heard speech, spoken language and reading. Neuroimage.
85. Murdoch BE (2010) The cerebellum and language: historical perspective and review. Cortex 46: 858–68.
86. Eckert MA, Leonard CM, Richards TL, Aylward EH, Thomson J, et al. (2003) Anatomical correlates of dyslexia: frontal and cerebellar findings. Brain 126: 482–94.
87. Pernet CR, Poline JB, Demonet JF, Rousselet GA (2009) Brain classification reveals the right cerebellum as the best biomarker of dyslexia. BMC Neurosci 10: 67.
88. Rae C, Lee MA, Dixon RM, Blamire AM, Thompson CH, et al. (1998) Metabolic abnormalities in developmental dyslexia detected by 1h magnetic resonance spectroscopy. Lancet 351: 1849–52.
89. Krafnick AJ, Flowers DL, Napoliello EM, Eden GF (2011) Gray matter volume changes following reading intervention in dyslexic children. Neuroimage 57: 733–41.
90. Raberger T, Wimmer H (2003) On the automaticity/cerebellar deficit hypothesis of dyslexia: balancing and continuous rapid naming in dyslexic and adhd children. Neuropsychologia 41: 1493–7.
91. Wimmer H, Mayringer H, Raberger T (1999) Reading and dual-task balancing: evidence against the automatization deficit explanation of developmental dyslexia. J Learn Disabil 32: 473–8.
92. Nicolson RI, Fawcett AJ (2007) Procedural learning difficulties: reuniting the developmental disorders? Trends Neurosci 30: 135–41.
93. Ramus F (2004) Neurobiology of dyslexia: a reinterpretation of the data. Trends Neurosci 27: 720–6.
94. Chein JM, Fissell K, Jacobs S, Fiez JA (2002) Functional heterogeneity within broca's area during verbal working memory. Physiol Behav 77: 635–9.
95. Robichon F, Levrier O, Farnarier P, Habib M (2000) Developmental dyslexia: atypical cortical asymmetries and functional significance. Eur J Neurol 7: 35–46.
96. Salimi-Khorshidi G, Smith SM, Keltner JR, Wager TD, Nichols TE (2009) Meta-analysis of neuroimaging data: a comparison of image-based and coordinate-based pooling of studies. Neuroimage 45: 810–23.

Subtle Increases in Interletter Spacing Facilitate the Encoding of Words during Normal Reading

Manuel Perea[1]*, Pablo Gomez[2]

1 ERI-Lectura and Departament de Metodologia, Universitat de València, Valencia, Spain, 2 Psychology Department, DePaul University, Chicago, Illinois, United States of America

Abstract

Background: Several recent studies have revealed that words presented with a small increase in interletter spacing are identified faster than words presented with the default interletter spacing (i.e., w a t e r faster than water). Modeling work has shown that this advantage occurs at an early encoding level. Given the implications of this finding for the ease of reading in the new digital era, here we examined whether the beneficial effect of small increases in interletter spacing can be generalized to a normal reading situation.

Methodology: We conducted an experiment in which the participant's eyes were monitored when reading sentences varying in interletter spacing: i) sentences were presented with the default (0.0) interletter spacing; ii) sentences presented with a +1.0 interletter spacing; and iii) sentences presented with a +1.5 interletter spacing.

Principal Findings: Results showed shorter fixation duration times as an inverse function of interletter spacing (i.e., fixation durations were briefest with +1.5 spacing and slowest with the default spacing).

Conclusions: Subtle increases in interletter spacing facilitate the encoding of the fixated word during normal reading. Thus, interletter spacing is a parameter that may affect the ease of reading, and it could be adjustable in future implementations of e-book readers.

Editor: Kevin Paterson, University of Leicester, United Kingdom

Funding: The research reported in this article has been supported by Grant PSI2011-26924 from the Spanish Ministry of Science and Innovation. No additional external funding was received for this study. The funders had no role in study design, data collection and analysis, decision to publish, or preparation of the manuscript.

Competing Interests: The authors have declared that no competing interests exist.

* E-mail: mperea@valencia.edu

Introduction

The study of the perceptual factors that may facilitate the ease of reading have a long history (see [1,2] for review; see also [3,4] for recent evidence on the role of visual factors during web browsing and normal reading). One of these potentially relevant factors is interletter spacing. This is a feature that can be easily adjustable in current word-processing software and it applies to all characters (including spaces): compare New York vs. N e w Y o r k (default vs. +1.5 interletter spacing). A +1.5 interletter spacing refers to an expanded 1.5 inter-character spacing in MS-Word (via points to default, where a point is approximately 0.35 millimeters; see Table 1 for illustration). Importantly, three recently published studies ([5,6,7]), using a word identification task ("is the letter string a word?"; see [8], for a review of the lexical decision task) revealed that response times to individual words are shorter when the interletter spacing is slightly wider than the default settings (around +1.2 versus the default 0.0; e.g., w a t e r faster than water). This beneficial effect occurs not only with adult skilled readers ([5,6,7]), but also with young readers and with developmental dyslexics ([7,9]).

What is the alleged locus of the beneficial effect of small increases of interletter spacing during word processing? Perea and Gomez [6] showed, using fits from Ratcliff's [10] diffusion model, that this effect occurs at an early encoding stage. According to their modeling work, interletter spacing affects the parameter related to stimulus encoding in the diffusion model (see [11] for the initial application of the diffusion model to the lexical decision task). Perea and Gomez [6] argued that this encoding advantage was due to two non-exclusive explanations: i) small increases in interletter spacing led to less lateral masking from the neighboring letters (i.e., less "crowding" effects), and ii) small increases in interletter spacing produced less letter position uncertainty in the letter string (see [12,13], for two input-coding schemes which assume some position uncertainty). Unsurprisingly, when interletter spacing exceeds some critical point (e.g., as in the sequence a v o i d t o o m u c h i n t e r l e t t e r s p a c i n g), the process of word-identification – and reading speed – would be slowed down (see [14,15]).

The goal of the present study is to examine whether subtle increases in interletter spacing also influence the eye movement pattern in normal silent reading (i.e., whether the beneficial effect of small increases in interletter spacing obtained with isolated words can be generalized to normal reading). This is important for theoretical and applied reasons. On the theoretical side, it is important to examine how small increases in interletter spacing – a

Table 1. Illustration of the interletter spacing conditions in the experiment.

Interletter spacing (points to default)	Example
Default (0.0)	My cousin has bought an aquarium for her new home
Expanded (+1.0)	My cousin has bought an aquarium for her new home
Expanded (+1.5)	My cousin has bought an aquarium for her new home

Note: The original sentence in Spanish was "Mi prima ha comprado una pecera para su nueva casa".

factor which has been found to benefit early encoding in visual-word recognition experiments – affect eye movement control during sentence reading. On the applied side, if reading times during normal reading are faster in those sentences with small increases of interletter spacing than with the sentences with the default settings, this would suggest that current word-processing software may not employ the optimal settings. Keep in mind that the default settings in the current publishing companies and e-book applications have been set without a clear empirical basis [16], and hence it may not be optimal –note that unlike word-processing software, current e-book readers do not allow changes in the default interletter spacing settings.

Previous eye movement research on normal silent reading has generally replicated the effects previously obtained in visual-word identification experiments ([17]; see also [18,19] among others). If a small increase in interletter spacing produces a more efficient encoding stage on the fixated word during normal silent reading because of a decrease in "visual crowding", this may lead to shorter fixation durations. Nonetheless, the generalization to normal reading may not be straightforward as with other phenomena. Small increases in interletter spacing can also have a deleterious effect during sentence reading because the non-fixated words will be more distant from the fixation than when the interletter spacing is smaller. This may lead to a decline in acuity when processing the words in the parafovea which may lead to a larger number of (re)fixations, thus producing slower (total) reading times (i.e., "visual acuity" explanation). In this respect, neither of the two most influential models of reading – the E-Z Reader model [20] and the SWIFT model [21] – makes direct predictions because perceptual factors such as interletter spacing are beyond the scope of their current implementations.

In the present experiment, one-line sentences were presented with the default interletter settings or with small increases of interletter spacing while the participants' eye movements were monitored. It was conducted on a CRT screen –note that using an e-reader would not have allowed for precise eye-tracking. To our knowledge, no published studies have systematically examined the effect of small increases of interletter spacing during normal silent reading while the participants' eye movements are monitored. Nonetheless, we should note that, in a recent experiment, Paterson and Jordan [15] examined the combined effect of increases in interletter and interword spacing in normal reading. Specifically, in one of the key conditions, they added an extra space between all letters of a word in a proportional font (Courier), as in t h e T h a i r e s t a u r a n t. This added space interfered with the normal process of reading, relative to the default condition (i.e., the Thai restaurant) in average fixation durations and total reading times, among other variables. Leaving aside that the interletter spacing manipulation was rather large (around +7.0) – which could have hindered the words' integrity – the increases to interletter spacing in that condition also decreased the saliency of interword spaces. Indeed, the reading cost relative to the default condition was smaller when an extra space as added between words (e.g., t h e T h a i r e s t a u r a n t). In fairness to Paterson and Jordan [15], we should indicate that the focus of their experiment was not to examine the beneficial effects of increases of interletter spacing, but rather the examination of the inter-play between inter-letter and inter-word spacing.

The participants' eyes were monitored when reading sentences varying in interletter spacing (see Table 1 for illustration): i) sentences were presented with the default (0.0) interletter spacing; ii) sentences presented with a +1.0 interletter spacing; and iii) sentences presented with a +1.5 interletter spacing. These three values of interletter spacing were chosen on the basis of the lexical decision experiment of Perea and Gomez ([6]; see also [5,7]). Perea and Gomez found a linear decrement of word identification times when presenting words with −0.5, 0.0, +0.5, +1.0, and +1.5 interletter spacings. As in the lexical decision experiments of Perea and cols, sentences were presented in a widely used font (14-pt Times New Roman).

To examine the role of interletter spacing during normal reading, we recorded global measures on each sentence such as reading times, average fixation durations, and number of fixations. In addition, to explore in greater detail the pattern of eye movements when interletter spacing is manipulated, local measures of a target word embedded in the sentences were also analyzed. In particular, we examined the duration of the initial fixation (first fixation duration), the duration of all fixations before leaving the target word (gaze duration), the total time (the sum of all fixations on the target word; i.e., including regressive saccades), and the initial landing position on the target word. Importantly, we also manipulated the frequency of a target word embedded in the sentence (low-frequency vs. high-frequency). Word-frequency is a well-studied predictor of the ease of word-identification in visual-word recognition and reading. If the effect of interletter spacing occurs in an early encoding process (see [6]), the effects of word-frequency and interletter spacing should not interact (see also [5], for evidence of additive effects in lexical decision).

Results

EyeDoctor software (http://www.psych.umass.edu/eyelab/software/) was employed to process the raw eye-tracking data. All fixations shorter than 80 ms that were within one letter of the next/previous saccade were combined into that fixation, and subsequently, all fixations with individual fixations shorter than 80 ms or longer than 800 ms were excluded (less than 4%). The statistical analyses were conducted over participants (F_1) and items (F_2). List (list 1, list 2, list 3) was included as a dummy factor in the analyses to partial out the variability due to the counterbalancing lists [22]. The average eye movement data for the global and local analyses are displayed in Tables 2 and 3, respectively.

Table 2. Global measures for each of the conditions in the experiment (means and standard deviations): total sentence reading time (in ms), progressive saccade length (in number of characters), forward/backward fixation duration (in ms), and number of forward/backward fixations.

	Total reading time		Saccade length		Fixation duration				Number of fixations			
					Forward		Backward		Forward		Backward	
Interletter spacing	M	SD	M	SD	M	SD	M	SD	M	SD	M	SD
Default (0.0)	2119	406	7.6	0.8	228	22	216	29	7.4	1.1	2.1	0.8
Expanded (+1.0)	2068	398	7.5	0.8	221	20	205	21	7.4	0.9	2.1	0.8
Expanded (+1.5)	2103	408	7.3	0.9	216	20	205	31	7.7	1.0	2.2	0.9

Global Measures

Total reading time. The Analyses of Variance (ANOVAs) on total reading time revealed a significant effect of interletter spacing only in the participant analysis, $F_1(2, 42) = 3.85$, $MSE = 5679.4$, $\eta^2 = .16$, $p = .03$; $F_2(2, 234) = 1.80$, $MSE = 28820.3$, $\eta^2 = .02$, $p = .16$. Pairwise comparisons revealed that there were no signs of a difference between the default condition and the +1.5 condition, $F_1(1, 21) = 1.11$, $p = .30$; $F_2(1, 117) < 1$, $p = .95$. More important, reading times were shorter in the +1.0 spacing condition than in the default condition in the participant analysis (2068 vs. 2119 ms, respectively), $F_1(1, 21) = 6.31$, $MSE = 6747.4$, $\eta^2 = .23$, $p = .02$; $F_2(1, 117) = 2.32$, $MSE = 32003.8$, $\eta^2 = .02$, $p = .13$, and the +1.5 spacing condition in the item analysis (2068 vs. 2103 ms, respectively), $F_1(1, 21) = 3.28$, $MSE = 5307.0$, $\eta^2 = .14$, $p = .08$; $F_2(1, 117) = 3.93$, $MSE = 20541.5$, $\eta^2 = .03$, $p = .050$.

Average fixation duration (progressive saccades). The ANOVA on the average fixation durations following progressive saccades revealed a significant effect of interletter spacing, $F_1(2, 42) = 31.05$, $MSE = 25.8$, $\eta^2 = .60$, $p < .001$; $F_2(2, 234) = 25.23$, $MSE = 88.7$, $\eta^2 = .18$, $p < .001$: fixation durations were shorter in the +1.5 spacing condition than in the +1.0 spacing condition (216 vs. 221 ms, respectively), $F_1(1, 21) = 10.33$, $MSE = 25.5$, $\eta^2 = .33$, $p = .004$; $F_2(1, 117) = 12.38$, $MSE = 72.2$, $\eta^2 = .10$, $p = .001$, and in turn, fixation durations were shorter in the +1.0 spacing condition than in the default condition (221 vs. 228 ms, respectively), $F_1(1, 21) = 24.43$, $MSE = 22.8$, $\eta^2 = .54$, $p < .001$; $F2(1, 117) = 14.43$, $MSE = 94.7$, $\eta^2 = .11$, $p < .001$.

Average fixation duration (regressive saccades). The ANOVA on the fixation durations following regressive saccades also revealed a significant effect of interletter spacing, $F_1(2, 42) = 5.45$, $MSE = 200.8$, $\eta^2 = .21$, $p = .008$; $F_2(2, 234) = 5.00$, $MSE = 810.2$, $\eta^2 = .04$, $p = .007$. This reflected shorter fixation durations in the +1.5 condition than in the default condition (205 vs. 216 ms, respectively), $F_1(1, 21) = 9.09$, $MSE = 185.0$, $\eta^2 = .30$, $p = .007$; $F_2(1, 117) = 5.36$, $MSE = 1019.7$, $\eta^2 = .04$, $p = .02$, and briefer fixation durations in the +1.0 expanded condition than in the default condition (205 vs. 216 ms, respectively), $F_1(1, 21) = 8.20$, $MSE = 195.3$, $\eta^2 = .28$, $p = .009$; $F_2(1, 117) = 10.67$, $MSE = 620.6$, $\eta^2 = .06$, $p = .001$. There were virtually no differences in the average fixation duration of regressive saccades between the +1.5 and +1.0 conditions, both $Fs < 1$, both ps $> .79$.

Number of (progressive) saccades. The ANOVA on the number of progressive saccades revealed an effect of interletter spacing, $F_1(2, 42) = 15.37$, $MSE = 0.045$, $\eta^2 = .42$, $p < .001$; $F_2(2, 234) = 9.29$, $MSE = 0.28$, $\eta^2 = .07$, $p < .001$. This reflected that there were more progressive fixations in the +1.5 condition than in the +1.0 condition (7.69 vs. 7.41, respectively), $F_1(1, 21) = 17.79$, $MSE = 0.052$, $\eta^2 = .46$, $p < .001$; $F_2(1, 117) = 18.31$, $MSE = 0.19$, $\eta^2 = .14$, $p < .001$, and in the default condition (7.69 vs. 7.36, respectively), $F_1(1, 21) = 38.22$, $MSE = 0.029$, $\eta^2 = .65$, $p < .001$; $F_2(1, 117) = 12.37$, $MSE = 0.35$, $\eta^2 = .10$, $p = .001$. The number of fixations was similar in the +1.0 and the default conditions, both $Fs < 1$ and both $ps > .67$.

Progressive saccade length (defined as the actual number of characters). The ANOVA on the length of progressive saccades revealed an effect of interletter spacing, $F_1(2, 42) = 14.91$, $MSE = 0.039$, $\eta^2 = .42$, $p < .001$; $F_2(2, 234) = 5.15$, $MSE = 0.38$, $\eta^2 = .04$, $p = .006$. (Progressive saccade length was smaller in the +1.5 condition than in the +1.0 condition (7.27 vs. 7.52, respectively), $F_1(1, 21) = 10.99$, $MSE = 0.062$, $\eta^2 = .34$, $p = .003$; $F_2(1, 117) = 5.53$, $MSE = 0.47$, $\eta^2 = .05$, $p = .02$, and in the default condition (7.27 vs. 7.58, respectively), $F_1(1, 21) = 39.98$, $MSE = 0.026$, $\eta^2 = .66$, $p < .001$; $F_2(1, 117) = 15.07$, $MSE = 0.22$, $\eta^2 = .11$, $p < .001$. The saccade length in the default condition and in the +1.0 condition did not differ significantly (7.58 vs. 7.52, respectively), $F_1(1, 21) = 1.21$, $p = .28$; $F_2(1, 117) < 1$, $p = .79$.

Number of (regressive) saccades. The ANOVA on the number of regressive fixations did not reveal any significant effects, both $Fs < 1$, both $ps > .47$.

Local Measures

First fixation duration. The ANOVA on the first fixation durations revealed a significant effect of interletter spacing, $F_1(2, 42) = 5.83$, $MSE = 596.1$, $\eta^2 = .22$, $p = .006$; $F_2(2, 224) = 5.54$, $MSE = 723.6$, $\eta^2 = .05$, $p = .004$. This reflected shorter fixation durations in the +1.5 condition than in the default condition (215 vs. 227 ms, respectively), $F_1(1, 21) = 8.89$, $MSE = 649.9$, $\eta^2 = .30$, $p = .007$; $F_2(1, 112) = 10.17$, $MSE = 734.5$, $\eta^2 = .08$, $p = .002$, and the +1.0 expanded condition (215 vs. 225 ms), $F_1(1, 21) = 10.23$, $MSE = 447.6$, $\eta^2 = .33$, $p = .004$; $F_2(1, 112) = 6.95$, $MSE = 580.0$, $\eta^2 = .06$, $p = .01$. There were no differences between the default and the +1.0 conditions, both $Fs < 1$, both $ps > .30$. First-fixation durations were, on average, 5 ms faster for high-frequency words than for low-frequency words, but this difference was not statistically significant, $F_1(1, 21) = 2.80$, $MSE = 520.9$, $\eta^2 = .12$, $p = .11$; $F_2(1, 112) = 1.53$, $MSE = 1224.4$, $\eta^2 = .01$, $p = .21$. Finally, there were no signs of an interaction between the two factors, both $Fs < 1$, both $ps > .56$.

Skipping rate. The ANOVA on the percentage of skipping rate revealed that high-frequency words were skipped more often than low-frequency words, $F_1(1, 21) = 6.77$, $MSE = 54.0$, $\eta^2 = .24$, $p = .02$; $F_2(1, 112) = 6.42$, $MSE = 176.3$, $\eta^2 = .05$, $p = .01$. (Thus, the lack of reliable effect of word-frequency in first-fixation durations was not due to some shallow processing of the target

Table 3. Local measures (target word) for the different experimental conditions in the experiment (mean and standard deviation): First fixation duration (in ms), Gaze duration (in ms), Total time (in ms), Initial Landing Position (range 0–5), and Skipping rate (in %).

	First fixation duration				Gaze duration				Total time				Landing position				Skipping rate			
	Low-frequency		High-frequency		Low-frequency		High-frequency		Low-frequency		High-frequency		Low-frequency		High-frequency		Low-frequency		High-frequency	
Interletter spacing	M	SD	M	SD	M	SD	M	SD	M	SD	M	SD	M	SD	M	SD	M	SD	M	SD
Default (0.0)	227	24	227	34	284	45	256	44	366	77	310	61	2.0	0.5	2.1	0.5	12.9	12.3	9.2	10.7
Expanded (+1.0)	227	25	222	30	295	35	264	40	359	69	306	50	1.8	0.4	1.7	0.6	10.1	11.4	8.3	6.7
Expanded (+1.5)	219	22	212	24	291	51	264	38	352	80	328	73	1.8	0.5	1.6	0.4	10.6	9.0	6.9	7.6

words; indeed, as indicated below, there was a robust effect of word-frequency for gaze durations.) Target words in the default condition were skipped more often (11.0%) than in +1.0 or +1.5 conditions (9.2 and 8.8%, respectively), but the main effect of inter-letter spacing was not significant, $F_1<1$, $p=.46$; $F_2(2, 224)=1.00$, $p=.36$. The interaction between the two factors was not significant either, both Fs <1, both ps >.40.

Gaze durations. The ANOVA on the gaze durations only revealed an effect of word-frequency (261 vs. 290 ms, for high- and low-frequency words, respectively), $F_1(1, 21)=21.52$, $MSE=2681.9$, $\eta^2=.51$, $p<.001$; $F_2(1, 112)=13.09$, $MSE=5421.4$, $\eta^2=.11$, $p<.001$. Neither the effect of interletter spacing ($F_1(2, 42)=2.13$, $MSE=606.8$, $\eta^2=.09$, $p=.13$; $F_2(2, 224)<1$, $p>.41$) nor the interaction between the two factors (both Fs <; both ps>.57) approached significance.

Total time. The ANOVA on the total times only revealed an effect of word-frequency (315 vs. 359 ms, for high- and low-frequency words, respectively), $F_1(1, 21)=25.93$, $MSE=5171.8$, $\eta^2=.55$, $p<.001$; $F_2(1, 112)=10.75$, $MSE=15220.0$, $\eta^2=.09$, $p=.001$. The effect of interletter spacing was not significant (both Fs <1, both ps >.50). Finally, the interaction between the two factors was significant in the analyses by items, $F_1(2, 42)=1.97$, $MSE=2084.4$, $\eta^2=.19$, $p=.15$; $F_2(2, 224)=3.28$, $MSE=4349.6$, $\eta^2=.03$, $p=.04$. This reflected some reading cost for high-frequency words in the +1.5 spacing condition (see Table 3).

Initial landing position. The number of letters of the target words in the experiment varied between six and nine. For that reason, before conducted the analyses of initial landing position, each word was divided into five fixation areas of the same size (see [23,24] for similar analyses).The ANOVA on the landing position only revealed a significant effect of interletter spacing, $F_1(2, 42)=10.20$, $MSE=0.41$, $\eta^2=.33$, $p<.001$; $F_2(2, 234)=14.17$, $MSE=0.41$, $\eta^2=.11$, $p<.001$. This reflected that initial landing position on the target word in the default condition was closer to the middle of the target word than in the +1.0 condition (2.1 vs. 1.8, respectively), $F_1(1, 21)=7.48$, $MSE=0.59$, $\eta^2=.26$, $p=.012$; $F_2(1, 117)=14.85$, $MSE=0.46$, $\eta^2=.12$, $p<.001$, or the +1.5 condition (2.1 vs. 1.7, respectively), $F_1(1, 21)=16.11$, $MSE=0.47$, $\eta^2=.43$, $p<.001$; $F_2(1, 117)=21.08$, $MSE=0.50$, $\eta^2=.16$, $p<.001$. There were no differences between the +1.0 and the +1.5 conditions (1.8 vs. 1.7, respectively) $F_1(1, 21)=2.66$, $MSE=0.15$, $\eta^2=.11$, $p=.11$; $F_2(1, 117)=1.40$, $MSE=0.26$, $\eta^2=.01$, $p>.20$. Neither the effect of frequency ($F_1(1, 21)=1.30$, $MSE=0.072$, $\eta^2=.06$, $p=.27$; $F_2<1$, $p=.40$) nor the interaction between the frequency and spacing ($F_1(2, 42)=1.85$, $MSE=0.129$, $\eta^2=.08$, $p=.17$; $F_2<1$, $p=.63$) approached significance.

Discussion

The present experiment examined how small increases in interletter spacing affected eye movement control during normal silent reading relative to the default settings. We found shorter average fixation durations for the sentences with small increases in interletter spacing, both at the local level and the global level – thus providing a replication of the lexical decision experiments of Perea and cols. ([5,6,7]) using a more ecologically valid procedure.

Consistent with the experiments using isolated words (see [5,6,7]), there is an early encoding advantage on the fixated word when there is a slight increase in interletter spacing - note that 22 out of 24 participants showed an advantage of small increases in interletter spacing. At the local level, this beneficial effect of small increases in interletter spacing occurred in the first fixation durations on the target words, whereas it disappeared in gaze durations and total times. The effect of interletter spacing did not interact with word-frequency. If one applies the additive-factor logic (see [5,15,23,24] for a similar reasoning), this suggests that the facilitative effect of interletter spacing on the fixated word appears to occur at an early stage of processing (see also Perea et al. [5], for a similar finding in a visual-word recognition task). This interpretation is consistent with the claim that interletter spacing affects the encoding of letters in words within the context of accumulation of evidence models that assume an encoding process that extracts information to be used in the decision making process during the process of lexical access (see [6] for modeling work on the diffusion model). We should note that, unlike the present experiment, Paterson and Jordan [15] found an interaction between interletter spacing and word-frequency in the local measures for gaze durations, with less frequent words being hindered by large increases in interletter spacing than more frequent words. However, as discussed by Perea et al. [5], the interaction occurred mainly because of the condition in which there were no obvious boundary cues between (as in `t h e T h a i r e s t a u r a n t`), which affected substantially more the low-frequency than the high-frequency words. In the present experiment, the manipulation of the interletter spacing occurred for all characters, including spaces (see Table 1) so that between-word boundaries were well-defined.

The data from the average fixation durations might be taken to suggest that there would be a beneficial effect of small increases in interletter spacing in total reading times, consistent with the processing advantage at encoding the fixated words. However, the story is more complex. Increases in interletter spacing were also accompanied by more fixations and shorter saccade lengths (in number of characters), especially in the +1.5 condition. This deleterious effect of interletter spacing is probably related to the fact that the initial landing position in the target word in the increased interletter spacing conditions was closer to the beginning to the word than to the optimal viewing position (i.e., the position in the word –just before the word center– in which performance is superior in word recognition tasks; see [25]). This may have led to more (re)fixations, thus cancelling the initial advantage of the small increases in interletter spacing during a very early encoding stage – note that the presence of a shorter average fixation duration when the fixation is to the left of the optimal viewing position (i.e., an inverted optimal viewing position effect) is not new (e.g., see [26]), and it reflects the interplay between lexical and oculomotor factors during normal reading. The detrimental effect of increases of interletter spacing is also consistent with the decrease in acuity of the neighboring words (e.g., parafoveal preview benefits), especially in the +1.5 interletter spacing condition, in which the saccade length was shorter than in the other conditions. Although the lack of a significant difference for the skipping data suggests that there was no effect of the spacing manipulation on parafoveal preview benefit, the skipping rate was slightly lower for the +1.5 interletter spacing condition than for the default condition (8.8 vs. 11.0%, respectively). Thus, the benefits to gaze durations and total times may not have emerged because the benefits of easier encoding (which are reflected in the average fixation durations) were outweighed by difficulties in integrating the word as a whole when the spacing was somewhat large –in particular in the +1.5 spacing condition. As an anonymous reviewer indicated, a similar dissociation has been made when examining the role of inserting spaces in normally concatenated German compounds: Inhoff, Radach, and Heller ([27]) found initial benefits of the spaced compounds (e.g., initial fixation duration) but later costs –Inhoff and cols attributed to difficulties in understanding the compound as a whole.

In the present experiment, total reading times were slightly faster when the letters within a word were slightly more separated (+1.0 interletter spacing condition) than with the default settings. Nonetheless, we are cautious in making strong inferences from the total reading data because: i) the observed effect was numerically small in magnitude; ii) only two-thirds of the participants showed this advantage in total reading times; and iii) the effect did not reach the significance level in the item-analysis –note that the effect was barely significant ($p = .029$) when using a linear mixed model analysis for this comparison; and iv) the effect did not occur for total reading times or gaze durations at the local (word) level. Clearly, a question for further research is the role of the individual differences in the choice of the optimal interletter spacing during normal reading using paragraphs (rather than single-text sentences) and a psychophysical approach. In order to increase the applicability of the present findings, we applied the interletter manipulation to all characters (i.e., as current word processors do). Nonetheless, it may be of interest to examine experimentally how subtle increases in interletter spacing interact with interword spacing, thus extending the work of Paterson and Jordan [15].

What are the implications of the present findings? At the theoretical level, the present experiment has revealed that eye movement control is sensitive to a rather subtle manipulation of interletter spacing. This was clearly so on the decision of <u>when</u> to move the eyes (i.e., average fixation durations): small increases in interletter spacing appear to facilitate the encoding the target word. This is consistent with the "visual crowding" account stated in the Introduction –i.e., interletter spacing would affect the earliest stages of letter processing in the EZ Reader or SWIFT models. Importantly, the fact that the effect of interletter spacing did not appear in gaze durations at the local level does suggest that some effort was required in the conditions with an increased interletter spacing which cancelled out the initial encoding benefit. Indeed, the interletter spacing manipulation affected the decision of <u>where</u> to move the eyes: the initial landing position was closer to the beginning of the word for the words with increases interletter spacing. As an anonymous reviewer suggested, landing position differences could be the result of readers failing to accommodate their oculomotor behavior to account for the increased distance between words in the conditions with increased interletter spacing –in particular in the +1.5 interletter spacing condition in which the saccade length was smaller than in the other two conditions.

At the practical level, the present data suggest that the choice of the default interletter spacing made by publishing/software companies may not be the optimal settings. Further research should be conducted to examine the potential benefits of small increases of interletter spacing across a variety of devices not just with adult skilled readers, but also in other populations. In a recent study, Perea et al. [7] found a clear advantage of interletter spacing with a group of individuals with developmental dyslexia, both in the lexical decision times and in the total reading times of a continuous reading task. (The eye movements were not monitored in that study, though.) Importantly, when the parallel experiments were conducted with a group of control children, the benefit of interletter spacing only occurred in the lexical decision times, but not in the total reading times of the continuous reading task ([7]; see also [9] for similar evidence in Italian and French). This suggest that the potential benefits of interletter spacing in the early stages of processing for readers with dyslexia overcome the potential disadvantage of increasing interletter spacing at the parafoveal level – probably because the deleterious effects of crowding are typically greater for readers with dyslexia than for an age-control group (e.g., see [28]). Additional caution is required if one wants to generalize the obtained findings to many of the devices used for reading e-books (e.g., Kindle, iPad). These devices have some differences (besides portability) with the CRT screen typically used in eye-tracking experiments like the present one: the resolution is better, which leads to less anti-aliasing, which might alter fixation patterns (see [4]). In addition, we only employed one font, Times New Roman (i.e., the same employed in our previous experiments on this issue, see [5,6,7]). Different fonts may have a different interletter spacing by default, and Times New Roman is a more narrowly spaced font (e.g., compare finding vs. finding; Times New Roman vs. Calibri). Clearly, the choice of font may qualify the optimal interletter settings – note that fonts may also differ in a number of other aspects (e.g., x-height, absence/presence of serifs, etc; see [4] for an analysis of the effects of fonts during normal reading).

In sum, the present experiment has revealed that eye movement control in adult skilled readers is affected by subtle increases in interletter spacing. In particular, fixation durations on the fixated word are shorter when there is a small increase in interletter spacing. This suggests that interletter spacing is a relevant parameter when processing text, and implementations of e-book applications should include an option to modify interletter spacing –as is currently the case in most word-processing applications. More research should be committed to examine in greater depth how interletter spacing affects eye movement control during normal reading with other populations (e.g., young children learning to read, readers with dyslexia, see [7,9]).

Materials and Methods

Ethics Statement

All participants gave informed consent in writing – the experiment was conducted with the approval of the "Comité Ético de Investigación en Humanos de la Comisión de Ética en Investigación Experimental de la Universitat de València" (Ethics Committee for Human Research at the University of Valencia).

Participants

Twenty-four students (average age: 20 years) from the University of Valencia participated in the experiment. They received a small monetary compensation (3 €). They were native speakers of Spanish, had normal (or corrected-to-normal) vision, and were naïve as to the purpose of the experiment.

Apparatus

The participants' eye movements were recorded using an Eyelink II eyetracker (SR Research Ltd, Canada). This is a video-based eye tracking device with cameras that sample pupil location at a 500-Hz rate. Viewing was binocular, but only the data from the right eye were registered. The average gaze position error is less than 0.5°. The sentences were presented on a 22-inch ViewSonic Professional series P225f CRT monitor. The participant's situation with respect to the monitor was controlled by a head-tracking camera that served for compensating possible head motion. Participants were seated 70 cm from the screen. At this distance, the number of letters in 14-pt Times New Roman font in 1° of visual angle was approximately 3.71 for the default spacing, 3.47 for the +1.0 interletter spacing, and 3.05 for the +1.5 interletter spacing –note that Times New Roman is not a monospaced font so that different letters may correspond to different angles.

Materials and Design

We employed the 120 sentences created by Perea and Acha [24]. For each sentence, there was a target word which could be of low-frequency (average frequency: 4.5 per million in the B-Pal database [29]) or of high-frequency (average frequency: 87.3 per million) of the same length, as in "Mi prima ha comprado una pecera/alarma para su nueva casa" and "El vendedor ha colocado una pecera/alarma en el escaparate"; "pecera" [fishbowl] is a low-frequency word, and alarma [alarm] is a high-frequency word). The average number of letters of the target words was 7.3 (range: 6–9). Two counterbalanced sets of stimuli were created so that participants read the 120 target words in one of the two sentence frames (e.g., for a given participant, the sentence "Mi prima ha comprado una pecera para su nueva casa" [the low-frequency word pecera is the target word], would be accompanied by the sentence "El vendedor ha colocado una alarma en el escaparate", in which high-frequency word would appear in the other sentence frame). All sentences were easily comprehensible in Spanish (as deduced from the results of a norming task), and all target words had a low predictability (less than 5% in a "cloze" task; see [24] for additional details). The list of sentences is available at [24]. For each participant, forty sentences were presented with the default interletter spacing (i.e., 0.0 interletter spacing; twenty with a low-frequency target word, and twenty with a high-frequency target word), forty sentences with a +1.0 interletter spacing (twenty with a low-frequency target word, and twenty with a high-frequency target word), and forty sentences with a +1.5 interletter spacing (twenty with a low-frequency target word, and twenty with a high-frequency target word) (see Table 1). Interletter spacing was counterbalanced across three lists for each sentence frame. The order of the sentences was randomized for each participant.

Statistical Analyses

Two types of analyses were carried out. For the three interletter spacing conditions (0.0, +1.0, +1.5), we examined six global measures: reading time (in ms), average fixation duration [for both progressive and regressive saccades], saccade length (in number of characters), and number of saccades [for both progressive and regressive saccades]). For the local measures on the target word, we examined the first fixation duration (i.e., the duration of the initial fixation on the target word), skipping rate (i.e., the percentage of skipping the target word), the gaze duration (i.e., the sum of all fixations on the target word before leaving it), the total time (i.e., the sum of all fixations on the target word, including regressive saccades), and the initial landing position as a function of interletter spacing (0.0, +1.0, +1.5) and word-frequency (low, high).

Procedure

Each participant sat in front of the computer monitor in a quiet, dimly lit room. Participants were instructed to read the sentences silently for comprehension, as they would normally do. They were also asked to press a button in a game-pad when they finished reading each sentence. Before proceeding with the experiment, each participant was instructed to follow several dots on the computer monitor to calibrate the eye tracker. Then, each sentence was displayed on a single line of text. Eight practice trials were employed to familiarize the participants with the procedure, and this was followed by the 120 experimental sentences. Before the presentation of each sentence, the eye tracker was checked –it was recalibrated when necessary. The sequence in each trial was the following. A black square appeared on the left-hand side of the monitor. Once the participant looked at that square, the sentence appeared. The location of the square corresponded with the initial letter of the sentence. To ascertain that participants were actually reading the sentences for comprehension, yes/no questions were asked after 20% of the sentences. Participants had no difficulty responding to these questions (error rates were less than 4% and similarly distributed across conditions). Sentences were presented in a different random order for each participant.

Author Contributions

Conceived and designed the experiments: MP PG. Performed the experiments: MP. Analyzed the data: MP. Wrote the paper: MP PG.

References

1. Morrison RE, Inhoff AW (1981) Visual factors and eye movements in reading. Visible Lang 15: 129–146.
2. Tinker MA (1963) Legibility of print. Iowa: Iowa State University Press.
3. Simola J, Kuisma J, Öörni A, Uusitalo L, Hyönä J (2011) The impact of salient advertisements on reading and attention on web pages. J Exp Psychol-Appl 17: 174–190. doi:10.1037/a0024042.
4. Slattery TJ, Rayner K (2010) Eye movements and text legibility. Appl Cognitive Psych 24: 1129–1148. doi: 10.1002/acp.1623.
5. Perea M, Moret-Tatay C, Gomez P (2011) The effects of interletter spacing in visual-word recognition. Acta Psychol 137: 345–351. doi: 10.1016/j.actpsy.2011.04.003.
6. Perea M, Gomez P (2012) Increasing interletter spacing facilitates encoding of words. Psychon Bull Rev 19: 332–338. doi: 10.3758/s13423-011-0214-6.
7. Perea M, Panadero V, Moret-Tatay C, Gomez P (2012) The effects of interletter spacing in visual-word recognition: Evidence with young normal readers and developmental dyslexics. Learn Instr 22: 420–430. doi: 10.1016/j.learninstruc.2012.04.001.
8. Dufau S, Duñabeitia JA, Moret-Tatay C, McGonigal A, Peeters D, et al (2011) Smart phone, smart science: How the use of smartphones can revolutionize research in cognitive science. PLoS ONE 6(9): e24974. doi:10.1371/journal.pone.0024974.
9. McCandliss B (2012) Helping dyslexic children attend to letters within visual word forms. Proc Natl Acad Sci 109: 11064–11065 doi: 10.1073/pnas.1209921109.
10. Ratcliff R (1978) A theory of memory retrieval. Psychol Review 85: 59–108. doi: 10.1037/0033-295X.85.2.59.
11. Ratcliff R, Gomez P, McKoon G (2004) A diffusion model account of the lexical decision task. Psychol Rev 111: 159–182. doi: 10.1037/0033-295X.111.1.159.
12. Davis CJ (2010) The spatial coding model of visual word identification. Psychol Rev 117: 713–758. doi: 10.1037/a0019738.
13. Gomez P, Ratcliff R, Perea M (2008) The overlap model: A model of letter position coding. Psychol Rev 115: 577–601. doi: 10.1037/a0012667.
14. Chung STL (2002) The effect of letter spacing on reading speed in central and peripheral vision. Invest Ophth Vis Sci 43: 1270–1276.
15. Paterson KB, Jordan TR (2010) Effects of increased letter spacing on word identification and eye guidance during reading. Mem Cognition 38: 502–512. doi:10.3758/MC.38.4.502.
16. McLeish E (2007) A study of the effect of letter spacing on the reading speed of young readers with low vision. Brit J Vis Impair 25: 133–143.
17. Rayner K (1998) Eye movements in reading and information processing: 20 years of research. Psychol Bull 124: 372–422. doi:10.1037/0033-2909.124.3.372.
18. Davis CJ, Perea M, Acha J (2009) Re(de)fining the orthographic neighbourhood: The role of addition and deletion neighbours in lexical decision and reading. J Exp Psychol Human 35: 1550–1570. doi: 10.1037/a0014253.
19. Johnson RL, Perea M, Rayner K (2007) Transposed-letter effects in reading: Evidence from eye movements and parafoveal preview. J Exp Psychol Human 33: 209–229. doi: 10.1037/0096-1523.33.1.209.
20. Reichle ED, Pollatsek A, Fisher DL, Rayner K (1998) Towards a model of eye movement control in reading. Psychol Rev 105: 125–157. doi: 10.1037/0033-295X.105.1.125.
21. Engbert R, Nuthmann A, Richter E, Kliegl R (2005) SWIFT: A dynamical model of saccade generation during reading. Psychol Rev 112: 777–813. doi: 10.1037/0033-295X.112.4.777.
22. Pollatsek A, Well AD (1995) On the use of counterbalanced designs in cognitive research: A suggestion for a better and more powerful analysis. J Exp Psychol Learn 21: 785–794. doi:10.1037//0278-7393.21.3.785.
23. Rayner K, Fischer MH (1996) Mindless reading revisited: Eye movements during reading and scanning are different. Percept Psychophys 58, 734–747. doi: doi:10.3758/BF03213106.
24. Perea M, Acha J (2009) Space information is important for reading. Vision Res 49: 1994–2000. doi: 10.1016/j.visres.2009.05.009.
25. O'Regan JK, Lévy-Schoen A, Pynte J, Brugaillere B (1984) Convenient fixation location within isolated words of different length and structure. J. Exp. Psychol. Hum. Percept. Perform 10: 250–257. doi:10.1037//0096-1523.10.2.250.
26. Vitu F, McConkie GW, Kerr P, O'Regan JK (2001) Fixation location effects on fixation durations during reading: an inverted optimal viewing position effect. Vision Res 41: 3513–3533. doi: 10.1016/S0042-6989(01)00166-3.
27. Inhoff AW, Radach R, Heller D (2000) Complex compounds in German: Interword spaces facilitate segmentation but hinder assignment of meaning. J Mem Lang 42: 23–50. doi:10.1006/jmla.1999.2666.
28. Spinelli D, de Luca M, Judica A, Zoccolotti P (2002) Crowding effects on word identification in developmental dyslexia. Cortex 8: 179–200. doi: 10.1016/S0010-9452(08)70649-X.
29. Davis CJ, Perea M (2005) BuscaPalabras: A program for deriving orthographic and phonological neighborhood statistics and other psycholinguistic indices in Spanish. Behav Res Meth 37: 665–671. doi: 10.3758/BF03192738.

6

New Insights on Developmental Dyslexia Subtypes: Heterogeneity of Mixed Reading Profiles

Rachel Zoubrinetzky[1,2]*, Frédérique Bielle[1], Sylviane Valdois[1,2]

1 Centre Référent de Diagnostic des Troubles du Langage et des Apprentissages, Pôle Couple-Enfant, Centre Hospitalier Universitaire, Grenoble, France, **2** Laboratoire de Psychologie et NeuroCognition, CNRS, UMR 5105, Université Grenoble Alpes, Grenoble, France

Abstract

We examined whether classifications based on reading performance are relevant to identify cognitively homogeneous subgroups of dyslexic children. Each of the 71 dyslexic participants was selected to have a mixed reading profile, i.e. poor irregular word and pseudo-word reading performance (accuracy and speed). Despite their homogeneous reading profile, the participants were found to split into four distinct cognitive subgroups, characterized by a single phonological disorder, a single visual attention span disorder, a double deficit or none of these disorders. The two subgroups characterized by single and contrasted cognitive disorders were found to exhibit a very similar reading pattern but more contrasted spelling performance (quantitative analysis). A qualitative analysis of the error types produced in reading and spelling provided some cues about the participants' underlying cognitive deficit. The overall findings disqualify subtyping based on reading profiles as a classification method to identify cognitively homogeneous subgroups of dyslexic children. They rather show an opaque relationship between the cognitive underpinnings of developmental dyslexia and their behavioral manifestations in reading and spelling. Future neuroimaging and genetic studies should take this issue into account since synthesizing over cognitively heterogeneous children would entail potential pitfalls.

Editor: Evelyn Kroesbergen, Utrecht University, Netherlands

Funding: This work was supported by ANR Blanc ORTHOLEARN: ANR-12-BSH2-0013-01. The funders had no role in study design, data collection and analysis, decision to publish, or preparation of the manuscript.

Competing Interests: The authors have declared that no competing interests exist.

* E-mail: rachel.zoubri@gmail.com

Introduction

Developmental dyslexia is a specific learning disability characterized by an unexpected difficulty in learning to read in children who have at least average intelligence, who do not have general learning difficulties, and whose reading problems are not due to extraneous factors that might interfere with learning to read, such as sensory acuity deficits, severe emotional problems, acquired brain damage or inadequate educational opportunity [1]. The dyslexic population is highly heterogeneous so that different dyslexic children may exhibit different reading profiles and their poor reading performance can be associated with different cognitive impairments and different brain dysfunctions [2–5]. Classification systems have been proposed to reduce this heterogeneity and identify more homogeneous subgroups [6,7]. A very popular subtyping approach is based on the recognition of different reading profiles as a way to distinguish cognitively distinct subtypes of developmental dyslexia.

Individual differences in developmental dyslexia have been conceptualized using dual route models [8,9]. The case study approach revealed the existence of two distinct reading profiles of developmental phonological and surface dyslexia. Prototypical cases of developmental phonological dyslexia show selective difficulties in pseudo-word reading but relatively preserved irregular word reading [10–15]. This reading profile is viewed as resulting from the inability of dyslexic children to acquire grapheme-phoneme conversion rules due to a phonological disorder. The converse reading pattern characterizes developmental surface dyslexia in which pseudo-word reading is preserved but irregular word reading is selectively impaired [15–21]. Within the dual route framework, this profile is viewed as following from the selective impairment of the lexical pathway due to a specific orthographic processing disorder.

Through group studies, subtypes of reading disability have been identified based on the relative imbalances on the tasks of irregular word and pseudo-word reading. Regression techniques were then used to identify dyslexics with larger than expected discrepancies between irregular word and pseudo-word reading, based on the linear relationship between irregular words and pseudo-words in the control group. Using this procedure, two groups of phonological and surface dyslexic children have been identified as compared to age-matched controls. However, only about a third of the children exhibited strict discrepancies between irregular word and pseudo-word reading (i.e., poor performance on one type of items but not the other); most were impaired on both types of items, thus showing a pattern of mixed dyslexia. The preponderance of mixed reading profiles in the dyslexic population was estimated from 53% to 76% depending on the studies [8,22–26] (see [27] for a cross-language review).

Although classifications based on reading patterns were initially proposed to identify cognitively homogeneous subgroups of developmental dyslexia, there is no strong evidence for such a direct relationship. To the contrary, comparative studies of the phonological-like and surface-like groups as defined through regression analyses failed to show contrasted cognitive profiles.

In fact, a phonological disorder was reported not only in the phonological dyslexia subtype but also in the group of children identified through regression methods as having a surface-like profile [28,24,26]. Moreover, most studies focused on the phonological and surface dyslexia profiles; none explored what cognitive disorders were associated with the most frequent mixed dyslexia subtype and none provided a straightforward account of why this pattern predominates in the dyslexic population. The main purpose of the present study was to investigate the cognitive underpinnings of the dyslexic group characterized by a mixed reading pattern. We focused on the mixed reading pattern because of its prevalence in the dyslexic population and because of the difficulty of theoretical models to account for its overrepresentation. We will show that mixed dyslexia is associated with a variety of distinct cognitive disorders, against the hypothesis of a one-to-one mapping between reading patterns and cognitive disorders. To explore more in-depth the relationship between cognitive disorders and their behavioral manifestations, we will then focus on the two subsets of dyslexic children with a single but contrasted cognitive disorder to explore whether contrasted cognitive impairments differently modulated reading and spelling performance. More generally, the present study will address the issue of the relationship between cognitive disorders and their behavioral manifestations. We will provide new insights on the relevance of dyslexia subtypes while questioning the validity of classifications based on reading patterns.

1. Classical accounts of mixed reading patterns

Typically, dual route models interpret mixed dyslexia as cumulating the disorders of phonological and surface dyslexia, thus showing dysfunctions of both the analytic and lexical reading pathways [22]. However, dual route models do not provide any straightforward account of the higher probability for a double deficit rather than a single in the dyslexic population. The preponderance of double deficits seems rather implausible statistically and should be cognitively and neurologically explained if observed. The high incidence of mixed reading patterns is thus challenging for dual route models.

Subsequent theoretical advances led to the new hypothesis that mixed dyslexia might follow from a single phonological disorder. Indeed, Share's self-teaching hypothesis postulates that the development of orthographic knowledge mainly relies on phonological processing abilities [29–31]. The child who encounters a word he never read before will decode it by applying grapheme-phoneme conversion rules. Each successful decoding will provide the opportunity to gradually strengthen word orthographic knowledge in long-term memory, thus leading to acquire the large sight vocabulary required for rapid recognition of words and fluent reading. The self-teaching hypothesis suggests that dyslexic children who show a phonological disorder should exhibit a pseudo-word reading disorder as a direct consequence of their poor decoding skills but they should further show a (regular and irregular) word reading problem due to the impact of their poor decoding on the self-teaching device. Theoretical evidence for a central role of phonological processing in the building up of the two (analytic and lexical) reading pathways is well in line with the hypothesis that developmental dyslexia follows from a core phonological disorder [32,33]. This hypothesis is further supported by behavioral and modeling data. At the behavioral level, phonological and decoding skills appear as key agents of learning to read [34] and strong predictors of successful orthographic learning [31]. Within the framework of PDP connectionist models, Harm & Seidenberg [35] showed through simulations that a mild phonological disorder primarily impacted pseudo-word reading while additional word reading problems occurred following a more severe phonological disorder (also [22,23]). Thus, both the self-teaching hypothesis and modeling data from PDP connectionist networks support the hypothesis that mixed dyslexia could follow from a single phonological disorder. However, PDP connectionist models as dual route models cannot straightforwardly account for the prevalence of mixed reading profiles, unless explaining why phonological problems should be more often severe rather than moderate or mild in the dyslexic population.

2. The multitrace memory (MTM) model account of mixed reading profiles

The MTM model [36] postulates that developmental dyslexia can result from two distinct disorders, either a phonological or a visual attention (VA) span disorder, or both. The phonological disorder would primarily impact pseudo-word reading and further prevent normal acquisition of orthographic knowledge, as postulated by the self-teaching account, so that a single phonological disorder can result in a mixed dyslexia profile. However, the most innovative prediction of the model is that a VA span reduction should also result in developmental dyslexia, and sometimes in a mixed reading profile.

Within this framework, the VA span corresponds to the amount of orthographic information that can be simultaneously processed when reading [2]. In delineating the number of letters that are simultaneously processed at each step of the reading process, the VA span is involved in the processing of all relevant multi-letter orthographic units from graphemes to whole words [37]. Accurate reading of irregular words and rapid recognition of regular words require a large VA span that encompasses all the letters of the word sequence. A VA span reduction that prevents the entire word letter string to be simultaneously processed may thus result in poor accuracy performance on irregular words and slowed reading speed on words, thus generating a reading profile of surface dyslexia [37]. In line with this hypothesis, a VA span reduction was reported in some prototypical cases of surface dyslexia [38,39,15,5]. Regardless of dyslexia subtypes, group studies further revealed that the VA span disorder contributed to the poor reading outcome of dyslexic children independently of their phoneme awareness skills [2]. A VA span disorder was reported in dyslexic children who demonstrated no phonological problems [2,5,39–42], while other dyslexic participants showed a phonological disorder but preserved VA span [2,12]. Both the MTM model and behavioral data suggest that the VA span acts as a second core disorder in developmental dyslexia and is a key agent of reading acquisition. Indeed, a study carried out on a large sample of typically developing children from first, third and fifth grades showed that the VA span predicts variations in learning to read at all grades, independently of the influence of phoneme awareness [43]. Moreover, this study revealed that VA span abilities contributed not only to word reading but also to pseudo-word reading performance (see also [2]). Indeed, pseudo-word reading requires the VA span to be large enough to process in parallel all the letters of relevant sublexical units (as multi-letter graphemes or syllables). A reduced VA span could thus result in poor performance in both word and pseudo-word reading, thus leading to a mixed reading profile.

This prediction was first assessed through the case study of Martial, a 9 year-old child with a severe mixed dyslexia [42]. Martial was found to have remarkably preserved phonological abilities (i.e., good oral language, good phoneme awareness and good verbal short-term memory skills) but a severely reduced VA span. When asked to report as many letters as possible from a briefly presented 5-consonant letter string, he could only identify two letters out of 5 at the expected level. When asked to process briefly presented words of different length (from 3 to 9 letters long), he could only report 3 letters accurately on average whatever word length. Thus, Martial's case study exemplifies the MTM model's prediction that mixed dyslexia can follow from a single VA span disorder. Simulations carried out within the connectionist network that implemented the MTM model confirmed that a selective VA span reduction could affect both real word and pseudo-word reading [36].

In fact, the MTM model provides a multifactorial account of mixed reading patterns in developmental dyslexia. The model posits that a single phonological disorder can result in a mixed reading profile if further impacting the self-teaching device. It further emphasizes the importance of the VA span as a second key component of learning to read and predicts that a mixed reading profile can follow from a single VA span disorder but preserved phonological skills. Of course, a double deficit of phonological processing and VA span would further result in a mixed reading profile. The MTM model thus predicts that the mixed reading pattern in developmental dyslexia may follow from three distinct cognitive dysfunctions: a single phonological disorder, a single VA span disorder or a double deficit. Evidence for different cognitive disorders in mixed dyslexia is a very important issue that may provide a straightforward account of the prevalence of this reading profile in the dyslexic population.

3. Overview of the current study

The current study was carried out by reference to the MTM model of reading, thus discarding the potential influence of other mechanisms (as rapid automatized naming) not involved in the model. Our aim was to assess whether each of a single phonological disorder or a single VA span disorder or both disorders may result in a mixed reading profile. Overall, our working hypothesis will be that mixed dyslexia is characterized by a causal heterogeneity, i.e. a many-to-one mapping across the cognitive and behavioral levels [44]. Within this framework, each phonological and VA span disorder is viewed as necessary and sufficient to result in a mixed dyslexia profile. Note that the phonological and VA span processes are components of the reading system that play an independent role in reading acquisition [2,43,37]. As expected within interactive frameworks, simulations already showed that mixed reading profiles can follow from a single phonological disorder [35] or a single VA span disorder [36]. We therefore expected each of these cognitive disorders to characterize subsets of children with a mixed dyslexia profile, whatever the associated symptoms (comorbidity) they might otherwise exhibit.

For this purpose, the current study focused on a group of dyslexic children chosen to have a mixed reading profile at the individual level - i.e., poor (regular and irregular) word and pseudo-word reading performance (accuracy and speed) - and for whom phoneme awareness and VA span abilities were investigated. The first section of the paper (Part 1) will focus on the whole population to explore whether this mixed reading profile dyslexic population falls into distinct cognitive subgroups characterized by either a single phonological disorder, or a single VA span disorder, or both disorders. The methodology we used is very close to that of Bosse et al. [2]. In this previous paper however, the issue of multiple cognitive disorders was explored in a dyslexic population that was not a priori selected to have a specific reading profile. Accordingly, this study provided no insight on the relationship between cognitive disorders and reading profiles, which is specifically addressed in the current study. Contrary to Bosse et al's results [2], the classical view of mixed dyslexia (based on dual route models) would predict a large predominance of double deficits (poor phoneme awareness AND reduced VA span) in our sample of dyslexic individuals. The causal heterogeneity hypothesis does not make such a strong prediction within the framework of interactive models and reading acquisition. In this framework, a single deficit may be detrimental for the building up of the whole reading system whether it selectively affects phonological processing or the VA span. Evidence for distinct cognitive disorders in a population characterized by a homogeneous reading profile of mixed dyslexia will be taken as first evidence that subtyping based on reading profiles is not relevant to identify cognitively homogeneous subtypes of developmental dyslexia.

In a second section (Part 2), we will focus on two groups of dyslexic children selected from the whole population to have a single phonological or a single VA span disorder but similar chronological age and reading level. We will first compare their VA span and phoneme awareness performance to that of two control groups matched for chronological age and reading age. Our main purpose will be to show that the group with a pure VA span disorder remains impaired when compared to younger children of the same reading level (similar findings are further expected with respect to phoneme awareness). We will then conduct quantitative and qualitative analyses to explore to what extent these cognitively distinct subgroups differ at the behavioral level. The quantitative analysis will focus on performance in reading and spelling that were both expected to suffer from either a VA span disorder or a phonological disorder [45,15,42]. In particular, we will investigate whether a pure phonological disorder yields poorer performance in pseudo-word reading than a pure VA span disorder, as poor pseudo-word reading is typically viewed as reflecting poor phonological skills. In the same way, a phonological disorder was expected to prevent accurate pseudo-word spelling which should be mainly preserved following a VA span disorder. In contrast, similar reading and spelling performance in the two groups of dyslexic children with distinct cognitive disorders would be strong evidence that cognitively distinct subtypes of developmental dyslexia do not necessarily yield distinct reading/spelling profiles. We will lastly conduct a qualitative analysis to explore whether contrastive cognitive disorders result in distinct error patterns. Phonological errors are expected in the context of a phonological disorder while regularization errors in reading and phonologically plausible errors in spelling should predominate in cases of dyslexia related to a VA span deficit but preserved phonological skills. In line with previous evidence from a single case study [42], we will further expect visual errors to predominate in the group with a single VA span disorder; parsing errors due to partial decoding of the whole letter-string that forms complex graphemes (e.g., "AIN" read "A"-"IN" instead of "AIN" /ɛ̃/) will be in particular expected following limited visual attention resources.

Overall, there is substantial evidence that the dyslexic population is cognitively and neurophysiologically heterogeneous. We will here explore whether reading profile subtyping is relevant or not to select homogeneous groups of dyslexic children from which meaningful conclusions at the cognitive, neurobiological, genetic, and therapeutic level can be made.

Part 1: Whole population investigation

1. Method

1.1. Participants. One hundred and forty-two French native speakers took part in this experiment: 71 dyslexic children with mixed dyslexia and 71 control children. The research was approved by the local ethic committee of the Université de

Grenoble. All children and their parents or guardians have provided their written informed consent to participate in this study. Dyslexic participants were recruited at the center for learning disabilities of Grenoble University Hospital where they received a complete medical, psychological and cognitive assessment. All participants had normal IQ (exclusion if Progressive Matrices <25° percentile or if VCI and PRI <85 on the Wechsler Intelligence Scale for Children IV); they attended school regularly and none of them had any history of neurological illness or brain damage. Dyslexic children were excluded from the study if their reading disorder was associated with a specific language impairment or an attention disorder with or without hyperactivity. Each selected dyslexic child showed poor performance (at least 1.6 SD below the norm) in both irregular word and pseudo-word reading (accuracy or speed) at the individual level (median SD below the norm of the selected SDs, on accuracy score or speed, for irregular word = −4.4 SD, for pseudo-words = −3.8 SD). As a group, dyslexic children achieved a mean reading age of 7 years and 6 months on the Alouette Reading Test [46], corresponding to a reading delay of more than three years on average. Normally developing children were monolingual French speakers recruited from schools of the Grenoble urban area. They reported no history of oral language or reading disorder. None had repeated a grade. The two groups of dyslexic participants (mean age = 10 years 5 months, SD = 22 months) and normally developing control children (mean age = 10 years 5 months, SD = 14 months) were matched on chronological age (t (141) = −0.33, $p = .74$) but they differed in reading age (10 years and 5 months, SD = 22 months for control children, 7 years and 3 months, SD = 6 months for dyslexics children, t (141) = 13.8, $p < .0001$). Descriptive data of the groups is provided on Table 1.

1.2. Material and procedure. The test session included three reading tasks, three phoneme awareness tasks and two visual attention span tasks, plus a control single letter identification task. The dyslexic children were tested individually at the center for Learning Disabilities of Grenoble University Hospital. The control children were tested individually in one or two sessions in a quiet room of their school. The phonological, visual attention span and reading tests were presented in a random order that varied from one child to the other.

Reading skills were assessed using tasks of isolated word and pseudo-word reading, taken from the ODEDYS neuropsychological battery [47]. Participants were administered six lists of 20 items each for a total of 40 regular and 40 irregular words of high and low frequency (HF and LF), and 40 pseudo-words. The regular and irregular word lists were matched for letter and syllable length, grammatical class and frequency. The 40 pseudo-words were legal pseudo-words without lexical neighbors. The participants were instructed to read aloud each of the six lists of 20 items as quickly and as accurately as possible. Both accuracy and reading speed were taken into account. A composite score was created from performance on the two lists of pseudo-words and the two HF and LF lists for the regular and irregular words to obtain an average reading accuracy (maximal = 20) and an average reading speed performance.

The phoneme awareness was assessed using a phoneme deletion task and a phoneme segmentation task which were taken from [43], and an acronyms task from the BELEC battery [48]. For each task, the participants were given a set of practice items for which they received feedback. No feedback was provided on the experimental items. The dependent variable was the percentage of correct responses.

In the phoneme deletion task, the participants had to delete the first sound of a spoken word and produce the resulting pseudo-word (e.g., "outil" /uti/: /ti/; "placard" /plakaR/: /lakaR/). Twenty experimental words were presented: 7 began with a vocalic phoneme corresponding to a multiple letter grapheme so that the omission of the first letter (instead of the first phoneme) yielded incorrect responses, 9 began with a consonantal cluster, 4 with a singleton.

In the phoneme segmentation task, the participants had to successively sound out each phoneme of a spoken word (e.g. /kado/ 'cadeau' gift: /k/- /a/- /d/- /o/). Fifteen words were

Table 1. Descriptive data.

	CA controls		Dyslexics			
	Mean (SD)	Range	Mean (SD)	Range	t (140)	*p*
Age (months)	125,1 (13,7)	99–146	125,9 (16,4)	98–175	−0,33	*0,744*
Reading Age (months)	125,2 (22,4)	88–171	87,4 (5,6)	78–102	13,80	*<0,001*
RW score (/20)	19,3 (0,8)	17–20	15,6 (2,7)	6–20	10,94	*<0,001*
RW time (sec)	16,1 (4,9)	8–30	49,2 (20,6)	18–159	−13,15	*<0,001*
IW score (/20)	17 (2,5)	10–20	9,8 (3,5)	1–20	14,08	*<0,001*
IW time (sec)	18 (6,9)	7–41	60,5 (29,2)	18–229	−11,92	*<0,001*
PW score (/20)	17,8 (1,4)	14–20	11,5 (3,2)	3–18	15,12	*<0,001*
PW time (sec)	22 (6,3)	11–43	57,7 (20,4)	19–192	−14,09	*<0,001*
Deletion (%)	84,4 (16,8)	40–100	69,4 (21,2)	30–100	4,69	*<0,001*
Segmentation (%)	57,3 (27,5)	6–100	53,1 (28,7)	0–100	0,88	*0,383*
Acronyms (%)	84,5 (15)	50–100	66,3 (24,3)	0–100	5,36	*<0,001*
Letter identification (/50)	44,4 (6,3)	26–50	39,2 (7,5)	17–50	4,51	*<0,001*
Whole report (%)	83,9 (9,6)	63–100	70 (11,6)	46–90	7,81	*<0,001*
Partial report (%)	87,9 (8,1)	64–100	75 (13,1)	38–100	7,00	*<0,001*

Mean scores, standard deviation (SD) and ranges of regular word (RW), irregular word (IW), and pseudo-word (PW) reading, phonological and visual attention span tasks for the dyslexic and chronological age matched (CA) control participant.

presented that were made up of 4 phonemes on average (range 3–5).

In the acronyms task, two words were successively pronounced (one word per second). The children were asked to extract the first phoneme of each word and blend them to produce a new syllable (e.g. "photo" "artistique" /foto/-/aRtistik/ says /fa/). The test comprised 10 series of two words made up of 4.4 phonemes on average (range 2–8). Seven words began with a phoneme corresponding to a digraph so that an erroneous word was generated if the first letter was extracted instead of the first phoneme (response /pa/ instead of /fa/ if orthographically biased in the above example).

Two tasks of global and partial letter report were used to assess VA span abilities. A task of single letter identification threshold was further administered to control for single letter processing. Although they involve a verbal response and use verbal stimuli, there is strong evidence that the letter report tasks primarily address visual attention span abilities. Indeed, performance on these tasks is not sensitive to verbal memory load [40] and not affected by concurrent articulation [49]. Dyslexic children with poor letter report performance are similarly impaired when using non-verbal tasks and non-verbal material [50]. Lastly, the VA span involves attentional but not phonological brain regions [51,41,5,52]. Moreover, similar brain activations are observed regardless of the verbal or non-verbal nature of the stimuli to be processed [53]. The letter report tasks were displayed on a PC computer using E-prime software (E-prime Psychology Software Tools Inc., Pittsburgh, USA).

For the global and partial letter report tasks, random five letter-strings (e.g., RHSDM; angular size = 5.4°) were built up from 10 consonants (B, P, T, F, L, M, D, S, R, H). The strings contained no repeated letters. The 5-consonant strings never matched the skeleton of a real word (e.g.: FLMBR for FLAMBER "burn"). Two subsequent letters never corresponded to a French grapheme (e.g. PH, TH) or a frequent bigram in French (e.g. TR, PL, BR). The letters were presented in upper case (Arial, 7 millimeters high) in black on a white background. The distance between adjacent letters was of 0.57° in order to minimize crowding. Twenty 5-letter strings were displayed in Global Report. Each letter was used ten times and appeared twice in each position. Fifty random 5-letter strings were used in Partial Report. Each letter occurred 25 times (5 times in each position). At the beginning of each trial, a central fixation point was presented for 1000 ms followed by a blank screen for 50 ms. Then, a letter-string was displayed at the center of the screen for 200 ms, a duration which corresponds to the mean duration of fixations in reading, long enough for an extended glimpse, yet too short for a useful eye movement. In the Global report condition, children had to report verbally as many letters as possible immediately after the string disappeared. In Partial Report, a vertical bar indicating the letter to be reported was displayed 1.1° below the target letter, at the offset of the letter-string. Each letter was used as target once in each position. Participants were asked to report the cued letter only. In both tasks, the experimenter pressed a button to start the next trial after the participant's oral response. The experimental trials were preceded of 10 training trials for which participants received feedback. No feedback was given during the experimental trials. The dependent measure was the percentage of letters accurately reported (identity not location) across the 20 trials in Global report or across the 50 trials in Partial report.

In the letter identification control task, each of the 10 letters used in the report tasks were randomly presented (5 times each) with the same physical characteristics as in the experimental tasks, at 5 different presentation durations (33, 50, 67, 84 and 101 ms). At the offset of the letter, a mask (13 mm high, 37 mm wide) was displayed for 150 ms. Participants were asked to name each letter immediately after its presentation. The test trials were preceded of 10 practice trials (2 for each presentation time) for which participants received feedback. Children were excluded when the maximal score of 10 good responses was not reached at the maximal presentation duration of 101 ms. The total score was the sum of scores at each display duration.

1.3. Design and analyses. A correlation analysis was first conducted on the measures of Age, Reading, Phonological Awareness and Visual Attention Span, for the whole population of dyslexic and control children (Bonferroni correction: $p<0.05/(14*14)$). When required, data were log-transformed to meet normality assumption. Second, to reduce the data set before exploring the concurrent predictors of reading skills among mixed dyslexic and normally developing children, we conducted a principal components analysis with varimax rotation on the data from the 3 phonological tasks and the 2 visual scores. All factor loadings greater than /0.70/ were used for interpretation. A hierarchical regression analysis from the factor scores derived on the basis of the principal components analysis was used to explore the contribution of each factor to reading skills. We then studied the participant's repartition according to their factorial coefficients and we distinguished cognitively based subgroups among the mixed dyslexia population.

2. Results

2.1. Overview of the participants' performance. Performance of the dyslexic and control participants on each task of the assessment battery is provided in Table 1. The dyslexic group shows poorer performance than the control group on all the reading and VA span tasks. The dyslexic participants further show lower performance on two of the phoneme awareness tasks, namely deletion and acronyms but not in phoneme segmentation. On average, they also identified fewer briefly presented single letters than normal readers.

2.2. Correlation analyses. Results of correlation analyses carried out on the measures of reading, phonological skills and VA span - with and without controlling for age (CA) and letter identification skills (Letter Id.) - are provided in Table S1. Strong correlations were found between the measures thought to reflect the same cognitive processes. However as typically found, performance on the phonological and VA span tasks was mainly unrelated, suggesting that these tasks tap different cognitive processes. In line with our previous findings, both phonological and reading skills on one hand and VA span and reading skills on the other hand correlated significantly.

2.3. Principal components analyses. To reduce the data set before exploring the concurrent predictors of reading skills among mixed dyslexic and control children, we computed a principal components analysis with varimax rotation on the two VA span and the three phonological tasks. The analysis revealed a two-factor solution. The first factor accounted for 30.8% of the variance and received high loadings from the deletion, segmentation and acronyms tasks (from 0.76 to 0.80 - called phonological factor hereafter). The second factor with high loadings from the global and partial report tasks (0.91 and 0.92 - called VA span factor here after) accounted for a further 31.4% of the variance.

The individual phonological and VA span factorial coefficients were then used as potential predictors of reading subskills. Two different sets of hierarchical regressions were carried out. In all cases, chronological age and letter identification were entered as control tasks at step 1. We then forced the entry of either the phonological factor or the VA span factor at step 2 to assess the

Table 2. Results of hierarchical regressions.

	R^2 Change					
Factor	**RW score**	**RW time**	**IW score**	**IW time**	**PW score**	**PW time**
1. Control	.073**	.108***	.142***	.127***	.064**	.103***
2. Phonological	.204***	.065**	.220***	.066***	.156***	.031*
3. VA span	.186***	.302***	.262***	.261***	.277***	.292***
2. VA span	.188***	.303***	.264***	.262***	.279***	.293***
3. Phonological	.203***	.063***	.218***	.065***	.155***	.030**
Total	.465***	.475***	.624***	.454***	.497***	.427***

Contribution of each of the phonological and VA span factors to regular word (RW), irregular word (IW) and pseudo-word (PW) reading, accuracy and speed. The First Step corresponds to the forced entry of the two control variables (CA and letter identification).
*** p<.001 ** p<.01 *p<.05.

unique contribution of each factor to the different reading measures at step 3. Results of these analyses are shown in Table 2.

The whole model accounted for more than 40% of the variance in each reading task (from 42.7% to 62.4%). The phonological factor and the VA span factor both independently contributed to accuracy (from 15.5% to 27.7%), and speed performance (from 3% to 30.2%) on all reading sub-skills. In line with the self-teaching account, phonological skills independently contributed to irregular word reading (22% accuracy, 6% speed). Interestingly, the VA span factor was found to account for 28% of unique variance in pseudo-word reading accuracy (29% for speed), suggesting a non-trivial contribution of this "visual" factor to pseudo-word reading.

2.4. Identification of cognitively based dyslexic subtypes. In the above analyses, two distinct cognitive processes have been identified that independently contribute to the reading performance of dyslexic and control children. The next step is to explore whether different cognitive subgroups can be identified within this homogeneous population with regard to the reading profile. For this purpose, we analyzed the distribution of the individual VA span and phonological factor coefficients derived from the principal components analysis. The dyslexic children whose score on one or the other factor fell below the 10th percentile of the control group factorial coefficients were considered as having a cognitive impairment, either a VA span (−0.43 for the VA span factor) or a phoneme awareness disorder (−0.60 for the phonological factor). Figure 1 shows the scatterplot of the participants, dyslexic and control children, based on their VA span and phonological factorial coefficients. Despite their homogeneous reading profile, our group of dyslexic children splits into four cognitively-distinct subgroups. Indeed, 23 dyslexic children (32%) show a single phonological disorder, 24 (34%) show a single VA span deficit and 12 (17%) a double disorder characterized by poor phonological and VA span abilities. A remaining 17% shows none of these two cognitive deficits.

Part 2: Focusing on subgroups with a single cognitive disorder

In Part 1, we provided evidence that a group of dyslexic children selected to have a homogeneous mixed reading profile nevertheless show a variety of cognitive disorders. This finding suggests a rather weak relationship between reading profiles and cognitive disorders. In the second part of the investigation, we will address this issue by directly comparing reading and spelling performance in the two groups of dyslexic children previously identified as having either a pure phonological disorder or a pure VA span disorder. The two groups were first matched for chronological age, reading age and single letter identification skills. We further ensured that their phonological and VA span disorder remained when compared to a younger group of control children of the same reading level. Our purpose was to compare two groups with contrasted cognitive disorders that were otherwise matched. We then focused on these two contrasted groups and carried out a quantitative and a qualitative analysis of their performance. The analysis of performance of cognitively-distinct subgroups of dyslexic children was expected to provide additional insights on the degree of transparency/opacity of the relationship between reading profiles and cognitive disorders. In particular, we were interested in potential imbalances with poorer pseudo-word than irregular word reading abilities in the group with a single phonological disorder and a reverse pattern in the group with a single VA span disorder.

1. Characteristics of the participants in the two contrasted subgroups

Nine children of the phonological group and 10 VA span impaired children who did not match for chronological age, reading age or single letter identification were excluded from the analysis. Fourteen children from the VA span group and fourteen matched children from the phonological group were retained together with, fourteen CA matched control children. An additional reading-age-matched control group of fourteen children was further included to establish whether the phonological and VA span deficits highlighted through comparison with children of the same chronological age further remained when compared to younger children of the same reading level. The four groups' characteristics are presented in Table 3.

An ANOVA was carried out with Group as a between-subject factor (Phonological impaired group, VA span impaired group, CA controls and RA controls). A composite phonological score was computed from performance on the three phonological tasks, and a composite VA span score from the two global and partial report tasks. As shown in Table 3, the phonological disorder that characterized the phonological group in the comparison with CA controls [$F(1,52) = 26.79$; $p < 0.001$] remained when compared to

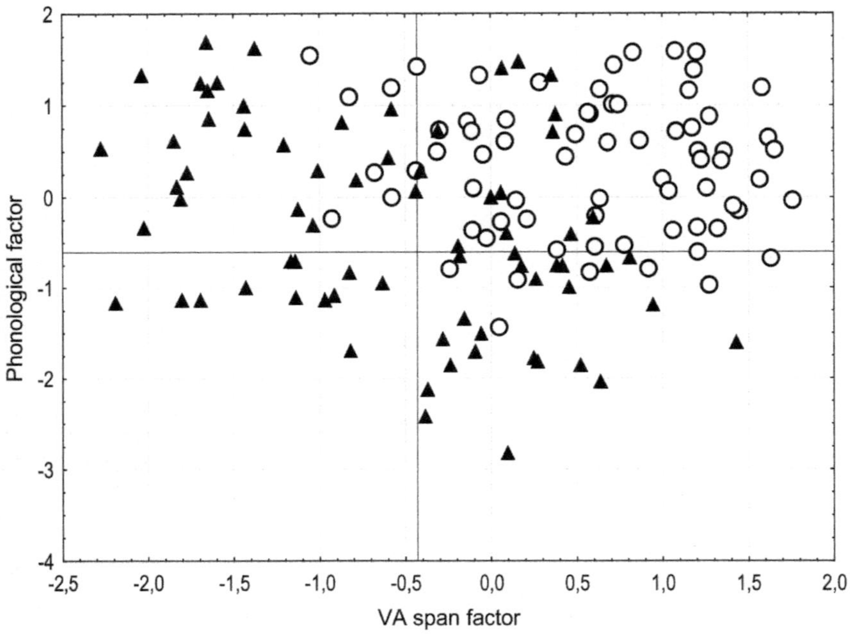

Figure 1. Scatterplot of the participants according to their factorial coefficients. Scatterplot of the dyslexic (triangle) and control participants (empty circle) according to their visual attention (VA) span and phonological factorial coefficients.

RA matched controls [F(1,52) = 9.11; *p* = *0.004*]. By construction, the VA span group performed as CA controls on phoneme awareness tasks [F(1,52) = 1.18; *p* = *0.282*] and slightly better than RA matched children [F(1,52) = 10.53; *p* = *0.002*]. The VA span dyslexic group performed significantly lower than both CA controls [F(1,52) = 39.77; *p*<*0.001*] and RA controls in the VA span tasks [F(1,52) = 12.09; *p* = *0.001*]. By construction, the phonological dyslexic group performed as CA controls [F(1,52) = 0.004; *p* = *0.949*] and better than RA controls on the VA span tasks [F(1,52) = 7.64; *p* = *0.008*]. The phonological dyslexic group and the VA span group were as efficient as CA controls in single letter processing [respectively F(1,52) = 0.003; *p* = *0.957* and F(1,52) = −0.63; *p* = *0.432*] and showed better performance than RA matched children [respectively F(1,52) = 19.53; *p*<*0.001* and F(1,52) = 12.77; *p*<*0.001*]. Note that lower ability of the younger RA matched control group to identify single letters might account for their relatively low VA span performance, whereas poor VA span performance in the VA span dyslexic group was found despite very good single letter processing skills. Overall these findings attest the existence of a selective phonological disorder in one dyslexic group and a selective VA span disorder in the other group. These cognitive disorders remain in the comparison with younger children of the

Table 3. Scores and comparisons of the two dyslexic groups, and the two control groups.

Age and Tasks	Dyslexics VA (a) Mean (SD) Range	Dyslexics P (b) Mean (SD) Range	Controls CA (c) Mean (SD) Range	Controls RA (d) Mean (SD) Range
CA	120,4 (14,2)*d*	122,4 (10,8)*d*	118,6 (13,1)*d*	84,3 (3,9)*abc*
	98–146	102–142	101–141	77–88
RA	86,5 (4,2)*c*	88,1 (6,9)*c*	111,2 (15,5)*abd*	87,6 (5,6)*c*
	79–94	78–99	88–134	79–101
Phonological score	76,4 (9,4)*bd*	43,5 (12,8)*acd*	70,7 (12,9)*bd*	59,4 (18,9)*abc*
	64,4–92,8	17,8–59,4	51,1–94,4	17,8–91,7
Letter Identification	39,4 (5,3)*d*	41,6 (6,5)*d*	41,5 (6,3)*d*	30,1 (9)*abc*
	30–49	21–47	28–49	18–44
VA span score	63,4 (7,3)*bcd*	80,6 (4,3)*ad*	80,8 (7,3)*ad*	73,0 (9,3)abc
	52,5–73	74,5–88,5	70,5–93,5	59,5–95

Mean and standard deviation (SD), range and comparisons (significant differences at p<.05 indicated by the group letter in italics) of the two dyslexic group, with phonological deficit (P) and with VA span deficit (VA)s, the CA matched control group and the RA matched control group on the phonological composite score, the VA composite score, and control (age and letter identification) tasks.

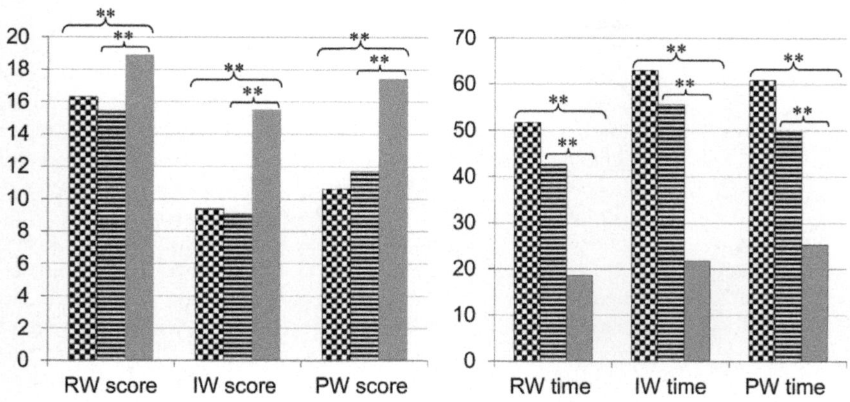

Figure 2. Performances of the dyslexic and control groups on reading tasks. Number of correct responses (max = 20) and reading times (in seconds) on reading tasks for dyslexics with a VA span deficit (checker board) or a phonological deficit (lines), and chronological age (CA) controls (grey) on regular words (RW), irregular words (IW) and pseudo-words (PW). **p<0,001 between CA controls and both dyslexics groups.

same reading age, thus leading to exclude any interpretation in terms of reading delay.

2. Quantitative analysis

2.1. Material and predictions. Performance of the two phonologically impaired and VA span impaired dyslexic groups and CA controls was compared for the regular word, irregular word and pseudo-word reading tasks previously described in Part 1. Two additional tasks of single word and pseudo-word spelling were administered. Children were asked to spell a list of 66 words [53]. The list included 22 regular words that could be spelled correctly by application of the most frequent phoneme-grapheme conversion rules, 22 irregular words including an inconsistent phoneme associated to a relatively infrequent grapheme and 22 exception words including an orthographic particularity or a rare grapheme which could not be inferred from the phonemic analysis of the oral input. The three types of words were matched in length and frequency. Regular, irregular and exception word frequency was 126, 131 and 134 per million respectively (from MANULEX, a database from French elementary school-readers [55]. The 66 words were randomly mixed, then dictated in a fixed order. Pseudo-word spelling was assessed using two lists of 10 bi-syllable and 10 tri-syllable pseudo-words from the ODEDYS battery [46]. The items were legal pseudo-words with no lexical neighbors.

We reasoned that if reading profiles were relevant to distinguish cognitively distinct subgroups, the two groups of children with contrasted cognitive disorders should differ in reading. Indeed, although the dyslexic participants were a priori selected to show both poor irregular word and poor pseudo-word reading performance, opposite word/pseudo-word imbalances were expected in the two contrasted subgroups of children. Lower pseudo-word reading performance was expected in the phonologically impaired group than in the VA span impaired group whereas VA span impaired dyslexic children might show lower scores in irregular word reading as compared to their phonologically impaired peers. We further extended the comparison to spelling performance. Indeed, if theoretical models of reading predict that performance in both pseudo-word and irregular word reading should be affected by either a phonological disorder or a VA span disorder, predictions slightly differ in spelling. Indeed, whereas both disorders should affect irregular word spelling, pseudo-word spelling might be differently affected as far as it mainly relies on phonological skills (i.e., the ability to identify the pseudo-word constitutive phonemes and knowledge of phoneme-grapheme mappings).

2.2. Results of the quantitative analysis. An ANOVA with group as the between-subject factor was carried out to compare the two dyslexic groups and each dyslexic group with the CA control group. Results are presented in Figure 2 and Figure 3 (see also Table S2 for more details). With respect to reading, the two dyslexic groups differ from CA controls by lower reading accuracy performance and longer reading times. However, the two dyslexic groups show very similar performance in word reading (accuracy and speed). In particular, they do not differ in irregular word reading and show very impaired performance on these items whatever the associated phonological or VA span disorder. Surprisingly, VA span impaired dyslexic children show the same low pseudo-word (accuracy and speed) reading performance as phonologically impaired children. For spelling, as previously for reading, the two groups do not differ in word spelling performance. In particular, the VA span group does not show lower performance on the irregular or exception words. However, the two dyslexic groups do differ in pseudo-word spelling with lower performance for the group with an associated phonological disorder. Interestingly, comparison with the control group revealed that pseudo-word spelling was preserved in the dyslexic group with a VA span disorder but impaired in the phonological group.

3. Qualitative analysis

3.1. Material and Predictions. We analyzed reading and spelling errors to explore whether contrasted cognitive disorders resulted in distinct error patterns. The errors were divided into seven mutually exclusive categories in reading, six in spelling. The different categories of errors are presented in Table 4.

Phonological errors (i.e., voice-voiceless substitutions) in both reading and spelling were expected in the context of a phonological disorder while regularization errors in reading and phonologically plausible errors in spelling should predominate when dyslexia relates to a single VA span deficit but preserved phonological skills. Based on previous findings from Martial's case study [42], we further expected a dysfunction in the allocation of attention to the letter string of the whole word or pseudo-word orthographic units to yield specific errors in reading. A difficulty to simultaneously process all the letters of multi-letter graphemes should yield grapheme parsing errors due to splitting these units' letter-string into shorter graphemes. A VA span reduction should

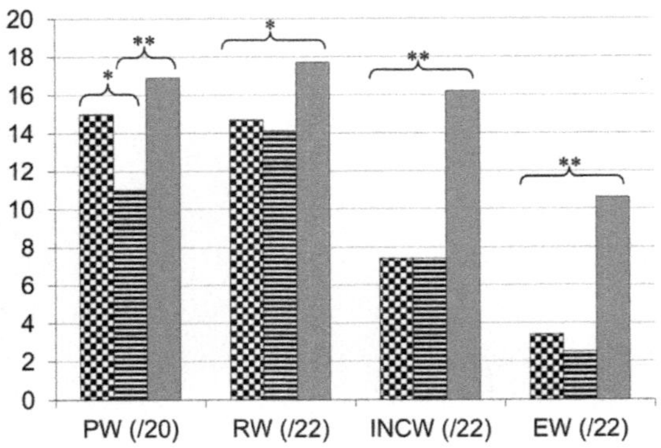

Figure 3. Performance of the dyslexic and control groups on the spelling tasks. Correct responses for dyslexics with visual attention span deficit (checker board), dyslexics with phonological deficit (lines), and chronological age (CA) controls (grey) on pseudo-word (PW), regular word (RW), inconsistent words (INCW) and exception words (EW) stimuli for spelling tasks. *p<0,01; **p<0,001 between CA controls and both dyslexics groups.

also limit processing of the graphemes' surrounding context thus leading to errors on contextual sensitive graphemes (s/z errors were excluded because such errors could follow from voiced-voiceless confusions as well). Partial decoding of the letter string could further result in letter omissions and a difficulty to code letter order within strings. However while graphemic parsing errors should be relatively specific, the other error types (i.e., omissions, letters order and contextual errors) are more ambiguous and could follow from a phonological disorder as well. We further hypothesized that partial decoding and poor letter order processing might result in a tendency for reporting the target word as another visually similar and more frequent real word as previously reported in some cases of visual attention dyslexia [56].

Specific errors were also expected in spelling. If a VA span reduction prevents normal development of orthographic knowledge (see [45] for supporting evidence), then the disorder should prevent normal extraction of orthographic statistical regularities then leading to higher probability for the production of illegal sequences as first described in [54] and poor knowledge of purely orthographic constraints which control for the final schwa adjunction in French. Contextual errors were further expected in spelling as in reading, assuming that normal acquisition of contextually sensitive relationships between orthographic and phonological units requires a VA span large enough to process the contextual grapheme and its surrounding context simultaneously. However as for reading, contextual errors may also reflect a phonological disorder and poor knowledge of more complex grapheme-phoneme relationships. Letter order errors in spelling were expected to primarily result from poor phonological skills.

The rate of phonologically plausible errors (PPE) in spelling was further documented using either a strict or a lax criterion. According to the strict criterion, an error was classified as phonologically plausible whenever the written word sounded as the dictated word when applying strict grapheme-phoneme conversion rules. Following this criterion, the phoneme /s/ had to be converted into "SS" between two vowels and "TE" was expected to translate the phoneme /t/ at the end of French words. According to the lax criterion, graphemes that could be pronounced as the dictated phonemes without consideration for mapping frequencies or orthographic context were considered as phonologically plausible (/s/ written "S" was then considered as phonologically plausible even in the two vowel context, and "T" was considered as plausible to translate the final phoneme /t/). We reasoned that these two categories of phonologically plausible errors both reflect good phonological processing skills. Indeed, even expanded phonologically plausible errors (lax criterion) require good ability to segment spoken words into phonemes but without consideration for the conventional orthographic rules.

3.2. Results of the qualitative analysis. The error analysis was restricted to those words and pseudo-words that included a single error type, all other errors were considered as complex. The proportion of errors in each category is shown for each group in Table 5 and Figure 4. Chi-square tests were used to compare

Table 4. Example of the error types considered in reading and spelling.

Error types	Examples
In Reading	
Voice-voiceless substitutions (f/v, t/d, p/b, k/g, ch/j, s/z)	JALOUX read /chalou/ not /jalou/
Regularizations	FEMME read /fèm/ not /fam/
Omissions	ESCROC read /esco/ not /escro/
Letter order errors	SOIF read /fois/ not /soif/
Parsing errors	AVANIE read /avan-ni/ not /avani/
Contextual errors	CARGO read /carjo/ not/cargo/
Paralexias	CARGO "cargo" read /escargo/ "snail"
In Spelling	
Voice-voiceless substitutions (f/v, t/d, p/b, k/g, ch/j, s/z)	/carp/ written GARPE not CARPE
Phonologically plausible errors	/fam/ written FAME not FEMME
Final schwa additions	/mirwar/ written MIROIRE not MIROIR
Final schwa omissions	/verb/ written VERB not VERBE
Contextual errors	/jenti/ written GANTI (/genti/) not GENTIL
Illegal sequences	/mirwar/ written MIROIRR not MIROIR
Letter order errors	/frit/ written FIRTE not FRITE

reading and spelling error rates between the phonological and the VA span dyslexic group. In reading tasks, results show that confusions between voiced/voiceless consonants are more frequent in phonologically impaired dyslexic children and quite rare in the VA span impaired group. Conversely, the dyslexic children with a VA span deficit produced more grapheme parsing errors, than the dyslexic children with a phonological deficit. Omissions, letter order errors, and contextual errors occurred in similar proportions in the two dyslexic groups. Likewise, the proportion of formal paralexias and regularization errors on irregular words was similar in the VA span impaired and phonologically impaired groups. In spelling as in reading, voiced/voiceless confusion errors were more frequent in phonologically impaired dyslexic children than in the group with a VA span deficit. However, more illegal sequences and more omissions of the final schwa were found on words for the VA span group as compared to the phonological group. Results further showed that PPE and expanded PPE were more frequent in the group of children with a VA span deficit than in children with a phonological deficit. The two groups did not differ in the rate of final additions, contextual errors, or letter order errors.

Discussion

The well-recognized heterogeneity of the dyslexic population led researchers to propose classifications based on reading profiles [8,57,22,58,24]. Different reading profiles were thought to distinguish subsets of dyslexic children with different cognitive disorders. However, the classification based on reading profiles yielded a relatively poor description of the dyslexic population [59]. Indeed, a deficiency in phoneme awareness and phonological processing tasks was reported not only in phonological but also in surface profiles [28,24,60,26]. Moreover, reading-based subtypes did not show stability over time thus suggesting they did not reliably characterize cognitively distinct subgroups [61]. Accordingly, the existence of developmental subtypes was denied and the tendency was to treat developmental dyslexia as a unitary syndrome with a phonological deficit as the proximal cause [33,62,24,32,63].

Evidence for a failure of reading profile subtypes to account for the heterogeneity of developmental dyslexia was interpreted as evidence against dyslexia subtypes. However, such a failure might reflect the irrelevance of the reading-profile-based subtypes rather than being strong evidence against cognitively-based subtypes. Recent evidence that some children with developmental dyslexia exhibit a visual attention span disorder that typically dissociates from phonological problems [2] and taps attentional brain regions while leaving preserved those associated with phonological processing [53,41,5] put the subtype issue back on the front row.

In this paper, we focused on mixed developmental dyslexia, a condition characterized by poor pseudo-word and poor regular and irregular word reading. Despite its severity and its high incidence in the dyslexic population (two third of cases), very few studies investigated this form of developmental dyslexia (see however [42]). The 71 dyslexic children who participated showed very poor performance on all types of items (regular or irregular words and pseudo-words) either considering reading accuracy or reading speed. This is potentially an important issue as reading latency may be more prone than accuracy measures to reflect a reading disorder, at least in more transparent languages than English [24,27]. This group of children was very severely impaired since demonstrating a 38 months delay in reading for an average chronological age of 10 years 5 months. They were administered tasks of phoneme awareness and global/partial letter report to respectively assess their phonological and visual attention span skills, two independent cognitive skills involved in reading acquisition [2,43,37]. Our purpose was to focus on the cognitive underpinnings of developmental dyslexia as defined within the framework of the multi-trace memory model [36] and for this reason, only the phonological and VA span mechanisms which are basic mechanisms of the reading system were taken into account.

We first assessed whether children of this group - which was homogeneous with respect to reading profile - showed the same cognitive disorder or whether the group was cognitively heterogeneous. We then explored whether distinct and unrelated cognitive disorders translated in different reading and spelling patterns.

1. One reading profile, multiple cognitive disorders

Although our dyslexic participants exhibited poor phoneme awareness skills and poor VA span abilities as a group, only a few participants (12%) showed a double deficit. In fact, a majority of children exhibited either a single phonological disorder (32%), or a single VA span disorder (34%), two independent cognitive factors which were further found to independently contribute to all reading measures. These findings are clear evidence that children with a similar mixed reading profile do not form a homogeneous population with respect to the associated cognitive disorder.

Surprisingly, the current findings largely replicate those reported by [2] whereas the later study was conducted on an unselected population of French dyslexic children who did exhibit a variety of reading profiles. Not only is our population of mixed dyslexic children heterogeneous at the cognitive level but further, incidence of a double deficit in this population is not higher than in previous studies conducted on unselected groups of either French or English dyslexic participants [2]. This finding undermines the classical explanation of mixed dyslexia [22] according to which this condition would follow from two independent disorders, one involved in the build-up of the phonological procedure (responsible for phonological dyslexia), the other one preventing normal orthographic knowledge acquisition (as seen in surface dyslexia). Such a view would have predicted a majority of double deficits in the mixed dyslexia population, cumulating the phonological disorder typically described in children with poor pseudo-word reading [10,12,14] and the VA span disorder reported in cases with poor orthographic knowledge [39,15].

Our results show to the contrary that even severely impaired children with mixed dyslexia suffer, for more than 60% of them, from an isolated cognitive disorder: a phonological deficit or a VA span deficit. The self-teaching theory provides a straightforward account of the impact of a single phonological disorder on the building-up of the reading system [29–31,64]. This theory assumes that the ability to translate unfamiliar printed words into their spoken equivalents is the main way by which orthographic knowledge is acquired [65–68]. The self-teaching theory thus predicts that poor phonological skills preventing normal acquisition of letter-sound mapping would disturb phonological recoding of unfamiliar words, thus leading to poor pseudo-word reading. In turn, poor phonological decoding would compromise normal development of word-specific orthographic knowledge, alter irregular word reading and thus lead to the mixed dyslexia profile.

However, a main finding of the current study is to show that a mixed reading profile can be associated with a single VA span disorder (see [42], for similar findings in a single case study). The MTM model [36] provides a straightforward account of this finding. Indeed within this framework, a VA span disorder that hampers the entire letter sequence of most words to be processed in a single step would primarily affect irregular word reading [37]. However, analytic processing requires the VA span to be large

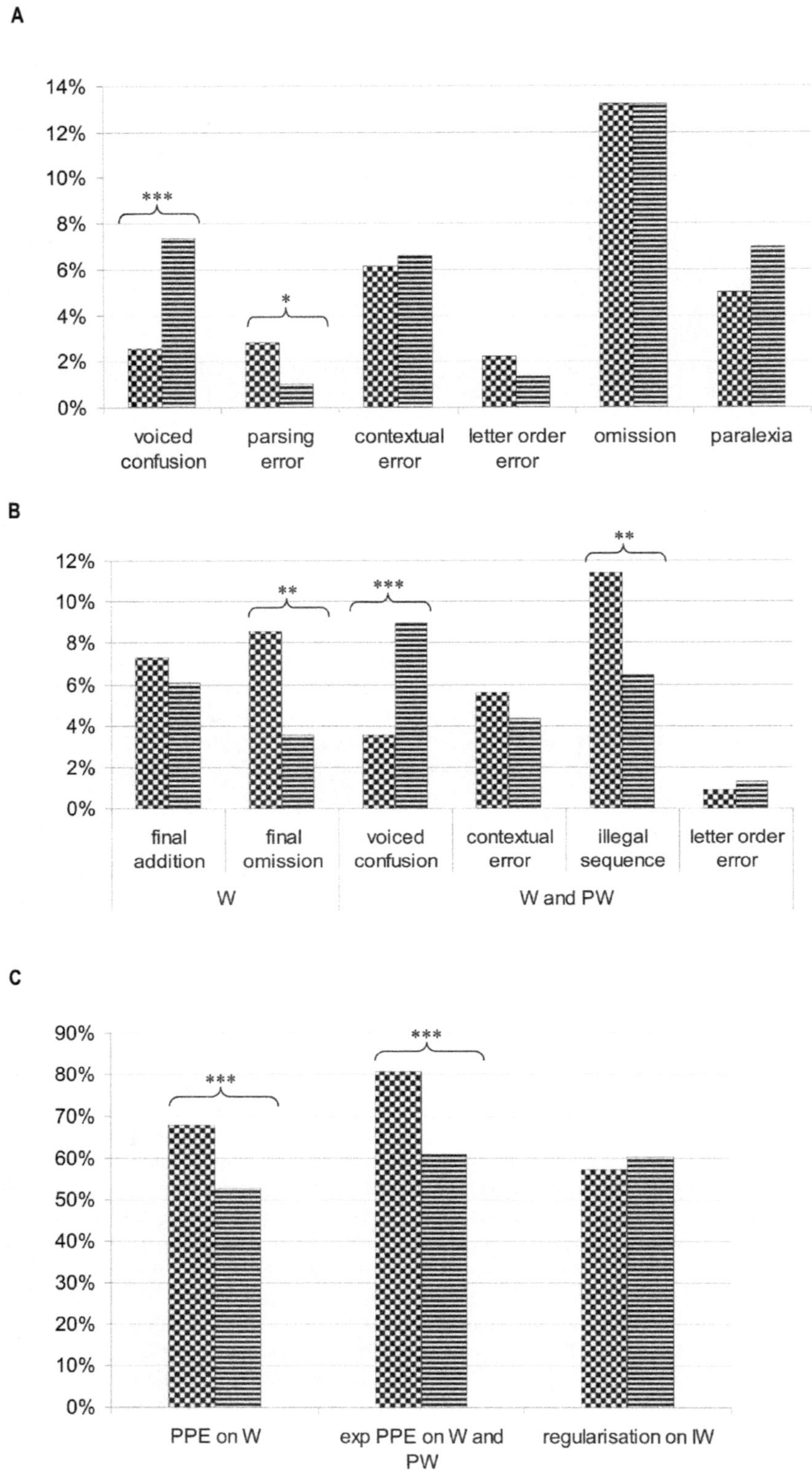

Figure 4. Percentage of each type of errors for both dyslexic groups. Percentage of each type of errors for dyslexics with visual attention span deficit (checker board) and dyslexics with phonological deficit (lines), on reading tasks (A), on spelling tasks (B) and phonologically plausible errors on spelling tasks (PPE and expanded PPE) and on irregular word reading task (C). *p<0,05; **p<0,01; ***p<0,001.

enough to process in parallel all the letters of relevant orthographic units (such as multi-letter graphemes or syllables). It follows that a VA span impairment can result not only in difficulties for processing words globally but it will further prevent normal processing of multi-letter orthographic units, thus leading to the word and pseudo-word reading difficulties that characterize mixed

Table 5. Comparison of the two dyslexic groups on error types.

Error type	Dys VAS		Dys P		Chi2 (1)
Reading					
Voice-voiceless confusions	17/665	2,6%	49/665	7,4%	16,33***
Parsing errors	19/665	2,9%	7/665	1,1%	5,65*
Contextual errors	41/665	6,2%	44/665	6,6%	0,11
Letter order errors	15/665	2,3%	9/665	1,4%	1,53
Omissions	88/665	13,2%	88/665	13,2%	0,00
Visual paralexias on words	21/403	5,2%	28/432	6,5%	0,61
Regularizations on IW	171/298	57,4%	183/304	60,2%	0,49
Spelling					
Final schwa additions on words	34/466	7,3%	29/477	6,1%	0,56
Final schwa omissions on words	40/466	8,6%	17/477	3,6%	10,46**
Voice-voiceless confusions	19/536	3,5%	54/603	9,0%	13,85***
Contextual errors	30/536	5,6%	26/603	4,3%	1,00
Illegal sequences	61/536	11,4%	39/603	6,5%	8,55**
Letter order errors	5/536	0,9%	8/603	1,3%	0,39
PPE on words	316/466	67,8%	252/477	52,8%	22,09***
Expanded PPE on words	418/466	89,7%	361/477	75,7%	32,24***
Expended PPE on PWs	14/70	20,0%	7/126	5,6%	9,81*

Comparisons of the two dyslexic groups, with phonological deficit (P) and with visual attention span deficit (VA), on the rate of each error types in reading and spelling tasks.
*** $p<.001$ ** $p<.01$ *$p<.05$.

dyslexia. The MTM model thus predicts a causal relationship between VA span deficit and dyslexia, as evidenced through simulations showing that a VA span reduction impacts reading performance independently of the model's phonological processing [36]. Further support for a causal relationship comes from evidence that intensive VA span-based intervention results in higher VA span abilities, increased reading performance and specific brain activity modulations [69].

Another main finding of the current study is to provide a straightforward account of the high incidence of mixed reading profiles in the dyslexic population. We indeed show here that mixed reading profiles can be associated with either a single phonological disorder, or a single VA span disorder or a double deficit, and potentially some other, not yet identified, cognitive disorder able to account for the group of children with none of the phonological or VA span disorder (it is worth noting that the double deficit group does not differ from the single deficit groups in reading delay). This suggests that the mixed reading profile may have different causes, which would in turn yield higher prevalence in the dyslexic population. More generally, the current findings confirm the prevalence of isolated cognitive deficits in the dyslexic population and the cognitive heterogeneity of developmental dyslexia [2].

2. Different cognitive disorders, subtle reading and spelling differences

In the second part of this paper, we focused on the two groups of dyslexic children previously identified as having a single phonological or VA span disorder. The two groups were matched on chronological age and reading age, to ensure that any observed difference could not be attributed to differences in print exposure or neural maturation. We further compared the phonological and VA span performance of the two groups with that of a new reading age-matched control group to demonstrate that their underlying cognitive disorder was not just the consequence of their poor reading skills [70]. The phonological dyslexic group showed a selective phonological processing disorder relative to the two control groups. This finding is well in agreement with previous evidence that phonological awareness scores in developmental dyslexia typically lag behind those of younger but typical children matched for reading age [25,22]. This also emerged from the comparison of the VA span dyslexic group and the reading age control group. Indeed, results clearly showed that VA span impaired dyslexic children had a more reduced VA span than younger controls of the same reading level. Lower performance than reading age-matched controls excludes any effect of the level of reading attained by our dyslexic participants and may rather suggest a causal relationship between VA span abilities and reading performance. Previous studies have already suggested that VA span abilities are not just the consequence of the children's poor reading performance [15,71].

We reasoned that comparison of the reading and spelling performance patterns of the two dyslexic groups would provide insights on the consequences of each of the phonological and VA span disorder on the establishment of the reading system. In particular, based on the fact that the difficulties experienced by dyslexic individuals in reading pseudo-words are generally explained in terms of their poor phonological skills (especially in phoneme awareness), we expected children from the phonological group to show lower pseudo-word reading and spelling performance relative to the VA span impaired dyslexic group.

Against the view that different cognitive disorders would yield imbalances in irregular word and pseudo-word reading, our two groups of dyslexic children despite contrasted cognitive disorders were found to only very slightly differ in reading and spelling. It is first noteworthy that their accuracy performance on words (in particular for the irregular, inconsistent and exception words) was very similarly low in both reading and spelling. The two groups did not differ either in regular and irregular word reading latency. This result suggests that poor phonological skills or poor VA span abilities similarly impact orthographic knowledge acquisition. Although the role of phonology in orthographic learning is well documented [72,73,31], the potential role of VA span has received little attention. As indirect evidence, Bosse et al. [45] showed that the orthographic form of new words is better memorized in a self-teaching paradigm when the entire word orthographic information is available for visual processing at once than when the word sublexical units are discovered in turn one at a time. In line with this result, the current findings suggest that beyond phonological skills and decoding abilities, VA span abilities may play an important role in word orthographic learning.

Another unexpected finding concerns pseudo-word processing. The two groups show very low pseudo-word reading accuracy and speed performance and no relative imbalance in favor of the VA span group. First, these findings reveal an asymmetric relation between phonological disorders and pseudo-word reading. While a phonological disorder results in poor pseudo-word reading accuracy and slow pseudo-word reading speed, poor pseudo-word performance (accuracy and speed) does not necessarily reflect a phonological disorder. This is a very important issue as there is a very strong tradition in the literature that considers a disorder in pseudo-word reading as the hallmark of a phonological deficit [74–76,62]. Second, our results suggest that a VA span disorder can affect pseudo-word reading as a phonological disorder does. In line with this finding, VA span abilities in typical readers have been shown to contribute to pseudo-word reading performance independently of children's phonological skills [43]. Furthermore, some studies have reported cases of surface or mixed reading profiles which were associated with slow pseudo-word reading but preserved phonological skills [42,17,15,77], suggesting that a non-phonological disorder might affect pseudo-word reading speed. It is clear from the current study (see also [2]–[43]) that a single VA span disorder contributes to poor pseudo-word reading (accuracy and speed). This is quite compatible with the MTM prediction [36] that VA span allows grapheme identification within the pseudo-word letter string. Reduced VA span abilities yield dyslexic children to process shorter sub lexical units than their non-dyslexic peers, with direct incidence on pseudo-word reading speed. The overall data thus suggests that phonological and VA span problems both compromise normal acquisition and use of alphabetic knowledge.

Another important finding is the strong pseudo-word spelling impairment in the phonological group whereas the VA span group performs as CA matched non dyslexic children. In the absence of strong behavioral differences in reading between our two cognitively contrasted dyslexic groups, we focused on the participants' spelling performance which is typically viewed as another marker of dyslexia. As pseudo-word spelling relies on the ability to accurately parse the pseudo-word phonological string into phonemes, a phonological disorder is expected to have strong impact on pseudo-word spelling, which was found. In contrast, a VA span disorder was expected to prevent normal processing of the visual input in reading but should have no detrimental effect in spelling which primarily relies on the phonological analysis of the spoken input. In line with these expectations, pseudo-word spelling was less accurate when developmental dyslexia was associated with a phonological disorder, but the children with a VA span disorder showed normal pseudo-word spelling abilities, as expected given their preserved phonological skills.

3. Different error types depending on the underlying cognitive disorder

Interestingly, the qualitative analysis of reading and spelling performance provided some insights on the two groups' cognitive underpinnings. A first important issue is that confusions between voiced/voiceless consonants in either reading or spelling were more frequently observed in the phonologically impaired group but quite rare in the VA span group. Such errors may suggest a difficulty to discriminate between phonologically similar phonemes or identify phonemes appropriately, in line with the well-documented categorical perception deficit in developmental dyslexia [78,79].

Evidence for a higher incidence of phonologically plausible errors (PPE) or expanded PPE in spelling in the VA span group provides further evidence for reliance on phonological recoding skills, well in line with the VA span group's good phonological abilities. In contrast the VA span group was more prone to produce grapheme parsing errors in reading, as expected if children cannot simultaneously process the whole grapheme letter strings due to their poor VA span abilities. It has been hypothesized that an inability to process the whole word letter string during reading would result in poor orthographic knowledge acquisition [56]. Accordingly, we found that VA span impaired children produced more illegal sequences in spelling and a higher rate of final schwa omission errors due to a disrupted analysis of orthographic statistical regularities and poor knowledge of orthographic constraints.

As a matter of fact, the main difference between the two dyslexic groups highlighted from the quantitative analysis is first that phonological skills and pseudo-word spelling are associated and second, that pseudo-word spelling performance is not impaired in the VA span group of dyslexic children. There is indeed strong evidence that pseudo-word spelling primarily relies on the ability to identify and isolate each of the spoken pseudo-word constitutive phonemes in order to activate their corresponding graphemes and provide a phonologically plausible translation of the dictated pseudo-word. In contrast, the VA span hypothesis would predict good pseudo-word spelling skills in the group of children with a single VA span disorder, which is observed.

Conclusion

The current study questioned the relevance of reading profiles to identify cognitively homogeneous subgroups of dyslexic children. We first showed that dyslexic children selected to have the same reading profile nevertheless split into distinct cognitive subgroups. We further showed that the two subgroups characterized by distinct and independent cognitive disorders nevertheless exhibited very similar reading and spelling performance. The overall findings question the validity of reading profile subtypes as a classification method to reduce heterogeneity in the dyslexic population and define cognitively homogenous subgroups.

More and more evidence is accumulating that VA span abilities contribute to reading performance in both skilled and dyslexic readers, independently of their phonological skills. The VA span involves parietal regions known for their role in visual attention, not phonology [53,41]. The analysis of two contrasted cases of developmental dyslexia with either a single phonological disorder or a single VA span disorder, further established that these cognitively distinct subtypes further dissociated at the neural level [5]. Available data thus supports the existence of distinct cognitively based subgroups but suggests an opaque relationship between these cognitive subgroups and their reading profiles. Future neuroimaging and genetic studies should take this issue into account since synthesizing over cognitively heterogeneous children would entail potential pitfalls.

Lastly, the present findings have important implications from a clinical perspective. Although reading profiles provide valuable information on the development of the reading system, our results clearly indicate that they provide no reliable information on the cognitive disorders involved in the reading disorder. Even if some cues about the underlying cognitive deficit can be found in reading and spelling performance, the clinician has to conduct additional investigations more directly targeted towards the identification of the associated cognitive disorders. Assessment of the child phonological skills is absolutely necessary, all the more that our results indicate that poor pseudo-word reading is not a sufficient clue to conclude that an underlying phonological disorder is at play. Investigation of the child VA span abilities is further required as more and more evidence suggests a specific contribution of this component to normal and atypical reading and spelling [2,43,45,80]. Assessment of the phonological and VA span abilities of dyslexic children is a very important issue in clinical practice. This step is indeed crucial to identify which remediation program is more appropriate to improve the child's reading performance.

Supporting Information

Table S1 Correlations. Correlations among Chronological Age (CA), Letter Identification (Letter Id.), Deletion, Segmentation (Segment.), Acronyms, Whole report, Partial report, Reading Age (RA), Regular word (RW) reading score and time, Irregular word (IW) reading score and time, Pseudo-word (PW) reading score and time, and partial correlations (controlling for chronological age and letter identification) below the diagonal (N = 142). * p<.00025 (Bonferroni correction).

Table S2 Scores and comparisons of the two dyslexic groups and the two control groups. Scores and comparisons of the two dyslexic groups and the chronological age (CA) matched control group in word reading (accuracy and speed), and spelling of regular words (RW), irregular words (IW), pseudo-words (PW), inconsistent words (INCW) and exception words (EW).

Acknowledgments

Thanks to Estelle Gillet-Perret, Delphine Lassus-Sangosse, Camille Durel and Marie-Ange Nguyen-Morel from the "Centre Référent des Troubles du Langage et des Apprentissages" (CHU de Grenoble, France) for their help in the participants' recruitment.

Author Contributions

Conceived and designed the experiments: RZ FB SV. Performed the experiments: RZ FB. Analyzed the data: RZ FB SV. Contributed reagents/materials/analysis tools: RZ FB SV. Wrote the paper: RZ FB SV.

References

1. Valdois S (2010) Dyslexia (developmental). In: Koob GF, Le Moal M, Thompson RF, editors. Encyclopedia of behavioral neuroscience.Elsevier. pp. 454–460.
2. Bosse ML, Tainturier MJ, Valdois S (2007) Developmental dyslexia: The visual attention span deficit hypothesis. Cognition 104: 198–230.
3. Hadzibeganovic T, Van den Noort MWML, Bosch MPC, Prec M, Van Kralingen R, et al. (2010) Cross-linguistic neuroimaging and dyslexia: A critical view. Cortex 46: 1312–1316.
4. Lallier M, Thierry G, Tainturier MJ (2013) On the importance of considering individual profiles when investigating the role of auditory sequential deficits in developmental dyslexia. Cognition 126: 121–127.
5. Peyrin C, Lallier M, Démonet JF, Baciu M, Le Bas JF, et al. (2012) Neural dissociation of phonological and visual attentional span disorders in developmental dyslexia: fMRI evidence from two case reports. Brain Lang 120(3): 381–394.
6. King WM, Giess SA, Lombardino LJ (2007) Subtyping of children with developmental dyslexia via bootstrap aggregated clustering and the gap statistic: Comparison with the double deficit hypothesis. Int J Lang Commun Disord42: 77–95.
7. Heim S, Tschierse J, Amunts K, Wilms M, Vossel S, et al. (2008) Cognitive subtypes of dyslexia. Acta Neurobiol Exp68: 73–89.
8. Castles A, Coltheart M (1993) Varieties of developmental dyslexia. Cognition 47: 149–180.
9. Coltheart M, Rastle K, Perry C, Langdon R, Ziegler J (2001) DRC: A dual route cascaded model of visual word recognition and reading aloud. Psychol Rev108: 204–256.
10. Campbell R, Butterwoth B (1985) Phonological dyslexia and dysgraphia in a highly literate subject: A developmental case with associated deficits of phonemic processing and awareness. Q J Exp Psychol A 37: 435–475.
11. Howard D, Best W (1996) Developmental phonological dyslexia: Real word reading can be completely normal. Cogn Neuropsychol 13: 887–934.
12. Lallier M, Donnadieu S, Berger C, Valdois S (2010) A case study of developmental phonological dyslexia: Is the attentional deficit in the perception of rapid stimuli sequences amodal? Cortex 46: 231–241.
13. Snowling MJ, Hulme C (1989) A longitudinal case study of developmental phonological dyslexia. Cogn Neuropsychol 6: 379–403.
14. Temple CM, Marshall JC (1983) A case study of developmental phonological dyslexia. Br J Psychol 74: 517–533.
15. Valdois S, Bosse ML, Ans B, Carbonnel S, Zorman M, et al. (2003) Phonological and visual processing deficits can dissociate in developmental dyslexia: Evidence from two case studies. Read Writ 16: 541–572.
16. Brunsdon R, Coltheart M, Nickels L (2005) Treatment of irregular word spelling in developmental surface dysgraphia. Cogn Neuropsychol 22: 213–251
17. Castles A, Coltheart M (1996) Cognitive correlates of developmental surface dyslexia: A single case study. Cogn Neuropsychol 13: 25–50.
18. Dubois M, De Micheaux PL, Noel MP, Valdois S (2007) Preorthographical constraints on visual word recognition: Evidence from a case study of developmental surface dyslexia. Cogn Neuropsychol 24: 623–660.
19. Hanley JR, Gard F (1995) A dissociation between developmental surface and phonological dyslexia in two undergraduate students. Neuropsychologia 33: 909–914.
20. Goulandris NK, Snowling M (1991) Visual memory deficits: a plausible cause of developmental dyslexia? Evidence from a single case study. Cogn Neuropsychol 8: 127–154.
21. Romani C, Stringer M (1994) Developmental dyslexia: A problem acquiring orthographic/phonological information in the face of good visual memory and good short-term memory. Brain Lang 47: 482–485.
22. Manis FR, Seidenberg MS, Doi LM, McBride-Chang C, Peterson A (1996) On the bases of two subtypes of developmental dyslexia. Cognition 58: 157–195.
23. Peterson RL, Pennington BF, Olson RK (2013) Subtypes of developmental dyslexia: Testing the predictions of the dual-route and connectionist frameworks. Cognition 126(1): 20–38.
24. Sprenger-Charolles L, Colé P, Lacert P, Serniclaes W (2000) On subtypes of developmental dyslexia: Evidence from processing time and accuracy scores. Can J Psychol 54: 87–103.
25. Stanovich KE, Siegel LS, Gottardo A (1997) Progress in the search for dyslexia subtypes. In: Hulme C, Snowling M, editors. Dyslexia: Biology, Cognition and Intervention.London: Whurr Publishers. pp. 108–130.
26. Ziegler JC, Castel C, Pech-Georgel C, George F, Alario FX, et al. (2008) Developmental dyslexia and the dual route model of reading: Simulating individual differences and subtypes. Cognition 107: 151–178.
27. Sprenger-Charolles L, Siegel LS, Jiménez JE, Ziegler JC (2011) Prevalence and reliability of phonological, surface, and mixed profiles in dyslexia: A review of studies conducted in languages varying in orthographic depth. Sci Stud Read 15: 498–521.
28. Jimenez JE, Rodríguez C, Ramírez G (2009) Spanish developmental dyslexia: Prevalence, cognitive profile and home literacy experiences. J Exp Child Psychol 103: 167–185.
29. Cunningham AE, Perry KE, Stanovich KE, Share DL (2002) Orthographic learning during reading: examining the role of self-teaching. J Exp Child Psychol 82: 185–199.
30. Share DL (1995) Phonological recoding and self-teaching: Sine qua non of reading acquisition. Cognition 55: 151–218.
31. Share DL (1999) Phonological recoding and orthographic learning: A direct test of the self-teaching hypothesis. J Exp Child Psychol 72: 95–129.
32. Vellutino FR, Fletcher JM, Snowling MJ, Scanlon DM (2004) Specific reading disability (dyslexia). What have we learned in the past four decades? J Child Psychol Psychiatry 45: 2–40.
33. Ramus F, Rosen S, Dakin SC, Day BL, Castellote JM, et al. (2003) Theories of developmental dyslexia: Insights from a multiple case study of dyslexic adults. Brain 126: 841–865.

34. Castles A, Coltheart M (2004) Is there a causal link from phonological awareness to success in learning to read? Cognition 91(1): 77–111.
35. Harm MW, Seidenberg MS (1999) Phonology, reading acquisition and dyslexia: Insights from connectionist models. Psychol Rev106: 491–528.
36. Ans B, Carbonnel S, Valdois S (1998) A connectionist multi-trace memory model of polysyllabic word reading. Psychol Rev105: 678–723.
37. Valdois S, Bosse ML, Tainturier MJ (2004) Cognitive correlates of developmental dyslexia: Review of evidence for a selective visual attentional deficit. Dyslexia 10: 1–25.
38. Bouvier-Chaverot M, Peiffer E, Nguyen-Morel MA, Valdois S (2012) Un cas de dyslexie développementale avec trouble isolé de l'empan visuo-attentionnel (A case study of developmental dyslexia with a selective visual-attention span disorder). Revue de Neuropsychologie 4: 24–35.
39. Dubois M, Kyllingsbaek S, Prado C, Musca SC, Peiffer E, et al. (2010) Fractionating the multi-character processing deficit in developmental dyslexia: Evidence from two case studies. Cortex 46: 717–738.
40. Lassus-Sangosse D, Nguyen-Morel MA, Valdois S (2008) Sequential or simultaneous visual processing deficit in developmental dyslexia. Vision Res 48: 979–988.
41. Peyrin C, Démonet JF, Baciu M, Le Bas JF, Valdois S (2011) Superior parietal lobe dysfunction in a homogeneous group of dyslexic children with a single visual attention span disorder.Brain Lang 118: 128–138.
42. Valdois S, Bidet-Ildei C, Lassus-Sangosse D, Reilhac C, N'Guyen MA, et al. (2011) A visual processing but no phonological disorder in a child with mixed dyslexia. Cortex 47: 1197–1218.
43. Bosse ML, Valdois S (2009) Influence of the visual attention span on child reading performance: a cross-sectional study. J Res Read 32: 230–253.
44. Pennington BF (2006) From single to multiple-deficit models of developmental disorders. Cognition 10(2): 385–413.
45. Bosse ML, Chaves N, Largy P, Valdois S (2014) Orthographic learning during reading: The role of whole word visual processing. J Res Read. In press.
46. Lefavrais P (1965) Test de l'Alouette (The "Alouette" Reading Test). Paris: Editions du Centre de Psychologie Appliquée.
47. Jacquier-Roux M, Valdois S, Zorman M (2002) l'Odédys, un outil de dépistage des dyslexies. Grenoble: Laboratoire cogni-sciences, IUFM de Grenoble.
48. Mousty P, Leybaert J, Alegria J, Content A, Morais J (1994) BELEC. Batterie d'évaluation du langage écrit et de ces troubles. In Grégoire J, Piérart B, editors. Evaluer les troubles de la lecture. Les nouveaux modèles théoriques et leurs implications diagnostiques. Bruxelles: De Boeck. pp. 127–145.
49. Valdois S, Lassus-Sangosse D, Lobier M (2012) Poor letter string processing in developmental dyslexia: What visual-to-phonological code mapping disorder. Dyslexia 18: 77–93.
50. Lobier M, Zoubrinetzky R, Valdois S (2012) The VA span deficit in developmental dyslexia is visual not verbal. Cortex 48(6): 768–773.
51. Peyrin C, Lallier M, Valdois S (2008) Visual attention span brain mechanisms in normal and dyslexic readers. In: Baciu M, editors. Neuropsychology and Cognition of language: Behavioural, neuropsychological and neuroimaging studies of spoken and written language. Trivandrum: Research Signpost. pp. 22–40.
52. Reilhac C, Peyrin C, Démonet JF, Valdois S (2013) Role of the superior parietal lobules in letter-identity processing within strings: fMRI evidence from skilled and dyslexic readers. Neuropsychologia 51(4): 601–612.
53. Lobier M, Peyrin C, Le Bas JF, Valdois S (2012) Pre-orthographic character string processing and parietal cortex: A role for visual attention in reading? Neuropsychologia 50:195–204.
54. Martinet C, Valdois S (1999) L'apprentissage de l'orthographe et ses troubles dans la dyslexie développementale de surface. L'Année Psychologique 99: 577–622.
55. Lété B, Sprenger-Charolles L, Colé P (2004) MANULEX: A lexical database from French readers. Behavioral Research Methods, Instruments and Computers 36: 156–166.
56. Valdois S, Gerard C, Vaneau P, Dugas M (1995) Developmental dyslexia: A visual attentional account? Cogn Neuropsychol 12: 31–67.
57. Douklias S, Masterson J, Hanley JR (2009) Surface and phonological developmental dyslexia in Greek.Cogn Neuropsychol 26: 705–723.
58. Marshall JC (1984) Toward a rational taxonomy of the developmental dyslexia. In: Malatesha RN, Whitaker HA, editors. Dyslexia: a global issue. The Hague: Martinus Nijhoff. pp. 45–58.
59. Griffiths YM, Snowling MJ (2002) Predictors of exception word and nonword reading in dyslexic children: The severity hypothesis. J Educ Psychol 94: 34–43.
60. Zabell C, Everatt J (2002) Surface and phonological subtypes of adult developmental dyslexia. Dyslexia 8: 160–177.
61. Manis FR, Bailey CE (2008) Exploring heterogeneity in developmental dyslexia: A longitudinal investigation. In: Reid G, Fawcett A, Manis F, Siegel L, editors. The SAGE handbook of dyslexia.London: SAGE Publications ltd. pp. 149–173.
62. Snowling MJ (2000) Dyslexia (2nd ed.). Oxford: Blackwell.
63. Ziegler JC, Goswami U (2005) Reading acquisition, developmental dyslexia, and skilled reading across languages: A psycholinguistic grain size theory. Psychol Bull 131: 3–29.
64. Share DL (2004) Orthographic learning at a glance: On the time course and developmental onset of self-teaching. J Exp Child Psychol 87: 267–298.
65. Bowey JA, Muller D (2005) Phonological recoding and rapid orthographic learning in third-grade children's silent reading: a critical test of the self-teaching hypothesis. J Exp Child Psychol 92: 203–219.
66. Cunningham AE (2006) Accounting for children's orthographic learning while reading text: Do children self-teach? J Exp Child Psychol 96: 56–77.
67. De Jong PF, Share DL (2007) Orthographic learning during oral and silent reading. Sci Stud Read 11: 55–71.
68. Kyte CS, Johnson CJ (2006) The role of phonological recoding in orthographic learning. J Exp Child Psychol 93: 166–185.
69. Valdois S, Peyrin C, Lassus-Sangosse D, Lallier M, Démonet JF, et al. (2014). Dyslexia in a French-Spanish bilingual girl: Behavioral and neural modulations following a specific visual-attention span intervention program. Cortex. In press. doi: 10.1016/j.cortex.2013.11.006
70. Goswami U (2003) Development and developmental disorders: The case of dyslexia. Trends Cogn Sci 7: 534–540.
71. Bosse ML, Valdois S (2003). Patterns of developmental dyslexia according to a multi-trace memory model of reading. Curr Psychol Lett 1: 10. Available: http://cpl.revues.org/document
72. Castles A, Nation K (2006) How does orthographic learning happen? In: Andrews S, editors. From ink marks to ideas: Challenges and controversies about word recognition and reading.London: Psychology Press. pp. 151–179.
73. Castles A, Nation K (2008) Orthographic Processes in Reading. Special issue of the J Res Read. Oxford: Blackwell Publishing.
74. Bradley L, Bryant P (1983) Categorising sounds and learning to read – a causal connection. Nature 301: 419–421.
75. Hulme C, Hatcher PJ, Nation K, Brown A, Adams J, et al. (2002) Phoneme awareness is a better predictor of early reading skill than onset-rime awareness. J Exp Child Psychol 82: 2–28.
76. Wimmer H, Landerl K, Linortner R, Hummer P (1991) The relationship of phonemic awareness to reading acquisition: More consequence than precondition but still important. Cognition 40: 219–249.
77. Tree JJ, Kay J (2006) Phonological dyslexia and phonological impairment: An exception to the rule? Neuropsychologia 44: 2861–2873.
78. Bogliotti C, Serniclaes W, Messaoud-Galusi S, Sprenger-Charolles L (2008) Discrimination of speech sounds by children with dyslexia: Comparisons with chronological age and reading level controls. J Exp Child Psychol 101: 137–155.
79. Serniclaes W, Sprenger-Charolles L, Carré R, Démonet JF (2001) Perceptual discrimination of speech sounds in developmental dyslexia. J Speech Lang Hear Res 44 (2): 384–399.
80. Lobier M, Dubois M, Valdois S (2013) The role of visual processing speed in reading speed development. Plos One 8(4): e58097. doi: 10.1371/journal.pone.0058097

7

The Zebrafish Orthologue of the Dyslexia Candidate Gene *DYX1C1* Is Essential for Cilia Growth and Function

Gayathri Chandrasekar[1], Liselotte Vesterlund[1], Kjell Hultenby[2], Isabel Tapia-Páez[1], Juha Kere[1,3,4]*

1 Center for Biosciences, Department of Biosciences and Nutrition, Karolinska Institutet, Huddinge, Sweden, **2** Clinical Research Center, Department of Laboratory Medicine, Karolinska Institutet, Stockholm, Sweden, **3** Folkhälsan Institute of Genetics, Helsinki and Molecular Neurology Program, Research Programs Unit, University of Helsinki, Helsinki, Finland, **4** Science for Life Laboratory, Karolinska Institutet, Stockholm, Sweden

Abstract

DYX1C1, a susceptibility gene for dyslexia, encodes a tetratricopeptide repeat domain containing protein that has been implicated in neuronal migration in rodent models. The developmental role of this gene remains unexplored. To understand the biological function(s) of zebrafish *dyx1c1* during embryonic development, we cloned the zebrafish *dyx1c1* and used morpholino-based knockdown strategy. Quantitative real-time PCR analysis revealed the presence of *dyx1c1* transcripts in embryos, early larval stages and in a wide range of adult tissues. Using mRNA in situ hybridization, we show here that *dyx1c1* is expressed in many ciliated tissues in zebrafish. Inhibition of *dyx1c1* produced pleiotropic phenotypes characteristically associated with cilia defects such as body curvature, hydrocephalus, situs inversus and kidney cysts. We also demonstrate that in *dyx1c1* morphants, cilia length is reduced in several organs including Kupffer's vesicle, pronephros, spinal canal and olfactory placode. Furthermore, electron microscopic analysis of cilia in *dyx1c1* morphants revealed loss of both outer (ODA) and inner dynein arms (IDA) that have been shown to be required for cilia motility. Considering all these results, we propose an essential role for *dyx1c1* in cilia growth and function.

Editor: Sheng-Ping Lucinda Hwang, Institute of Cellular and Organismic Biology, Taiwan

Funding: This work was supported by Swedish Research Council (www.vr.se); Swedish Royal Bank Tercentennial Foundation, Swedish Brain Foundation (Hjärnfonden)(www.hjarnfonden.se); Knut and Alice Wallenberg Foundation (www.wallenberg.com); Center for Biosciences and Sigrid Jusélius Foundation(www.sigridjuselius.fi). The funders had no role in study design, data collection and analysis, decision to publish, or preparation of the manuscript.

Competing Interests: The authors have declared that no competing interests exist.

* E-mail: juha.kere@ki.se

Introduction

Dyslexia is the most common learning disability affecting approximately 5–10% of school children worldwide. The dyslexia susceptibility 1 candidate gene 1 (*DYX1C1*) is the first gene implicated as a candidate gene for dyslexia [1]. Although mixed replication results for *DYX1C1* in dyslexia were first reported, several independent studies that followed later have confirmed its association to dyslexia, verbal short term memory and orthographic skills in many populations [2,3,4,5,6,7,8,9,10].

Subtle malformations in the cerebral cortex have been associated with dyslexia [11,12]. Consistent with the impairments seen in dyslectic brains, inhibition of *Dyx1c1* in rats by in utero RNAi was shown to affect neuronal migration in the neocortex resulting not only in similar cortical and hippocampal heterotopias but also impairments in the auditory processing, spatial learning and spatial working memory [13,14,15,16].

Genetic studies in humans have led to the identification of several other candidate genes for dyslexia, among which *DCDC2*, *KIAA0319* and *ROBO1* have been strongly implicated in either neuronal migration in the developing cortex or axon and dendritic guidance [17,18,19,20,21]. In addition, analyses of brain structure and the SNPs in *DYX1C1*, *KIAA0319* and *DCDC2* in children and young adults have suggested a neuronal basis for reading abilities involving the white matter volume in the left temporo-parietal regions of the brain [22]. Despite the growing evidence that implicates defective cortical neuron migration in dyslexia, the precise cellular and molecular mechanisms are still not clearly understood. The DYX1C1 protein was recently implicated in regulating estrogen signalling [23].

The dyslexia candidate gene *DCDC2* was recently shown to localize to neuronal cilia upon overexpression and regulate cilia length and signalling [24]. The primary cilium, an organelle extending from the surface of the cell is present in almost all cells in vertebrates and is important for normal development and for various biological processes. Cilia are bound to the cell surface through the basal body and consist of a microtubule framework, termed the ciliary axoneme. The primary cilia or non-motile cilia have 9+0 axoneme, 9 outer microtubule doublets, no central microtubule and no ODA and IDA and mainly function as chemosensors or mechanosensors or osmosensors. Cilia on the epithelial cells of mammalian lungs and oviduct are motile and possess a 9+2 axoneme with two central microtubules and dynein arms [25]. Monocilia of mouse embryonic node are motile and generate a unidirectional fluid flow inside the node that is crucial for the initiation of organ left-right asymmetry [26,27]. The importance of cilia in brain development and function has been recognized recently [28,29]. Defects in cilia are associated with a broad range of human diseases categorized as ciliopathies, which share overlapping symptoms including neurological symptoms [30].

In this study we have used zebrafish as a model to study the biological function of *DYX1C1* through its orthologous gene *dyx1c1*. Here, we show that the zebrafish ortholog is expressed in ciliated organs including Kupffer's vesicle (KV), otic vesicle, pronephros, spinal canal and olfactory placode. We performed a knockdown of *dyx1c1* using antisense morpholino oligonucleotides (MO) which resulted in pleiotropic phenotypes similar to those previously observed in zebrafish mutants with defective cilia [31]. Our results also show defects of cilia structure and length in various organs in *dyx1c1* morphants. Disruption of *dyx1c1* results in loss of ODA and IDA, thus disrupting cilia motility. Our results provide the first evidence that *dyx1c1* is essential for vertebrate ciliogenesis and function.

Materials and Methods

Ethics Statement

All experiments were carried out in accordance with ethical permits approved by the relevant ethical committee (Stockholm North Experimental Animal Committee Dnr N29-12). Dissection on adult fish was performed under tricaine treatment to ameliorate animal suffering.

Zebrafish Maintenance

Zebrafish (Danio rerio) were reared and maintained according to standard procedures [32]. Wild-type embryos were obtained from AB strain fish by natural spawnings and raised at 28°C. Embryos were staged to hours post fertilization (hpf) and days post fertilization (dpf). To prevent pigmentation in embryos older than 24 hpf, phenylthiourea was used as described previously [32].

Cloning of the *dyx1c1* mRNA

RNA was extracted from 50 zebrafish embryos at 50% epiboly stage using trireagent (Sigma Aldrich, St Lois, MO, USA). One microgram of total RNA was used for cDNA synthesis according to the Superscript III protocol (Invitrogen, Inc, CA). A proofreading polymerase Accuprime Pfx, (Invitrogen, Inc, CA) was used to amplify the coding region of zebrafish *dyx1c1* transcript. In short, one microliter of the cDNA synthesis reaction was used as template in a touchdown PCR ranging in annealing temperatures from 60°C to 56°C. Primers used were 5′-CGCTGAGGAGAGTCAGAGATG-3′ (forward) and 5′-AAAG-GATGCGGTGTCATTAT-3′ (reverse). The PCR assay was run on a 1% agarose gel from which a PCR product of approximately 1300 bp was sliced and extracted (Qiagen, The Netherlands) and subsequently cloned into the pCR-II-Blunt TOPO vector (Invitrogen, Inc, CA). The zebrafish *dyx1c1* clone was then validated using Sanger sequencing (Eurofin MWG Operon).

Quantitative Real Time PCR (qPCR)

Tissues including eyes, brain, heart, gill, swimbladder, liver, kidney, ovary, and testis were isolated from adult (1 year old, AB strain) male and female zebrafish and pooled by tissue type for RNA extraction. Embryos of different stages of development including <3 and 10 hpf and 1–5 dpf were collected for RNA extraction. RNA extraction, cDNA synthesis and real-time PCR assays were performed as described previously [33]. For measuring the transcript levels of *dyx1c1*, F- 5′-CACCGCGCTCAGA-GAGTC-3′ and R-5′TCCGCCTGCTTCTTCAAC-3′ were used as forward and reverse primers respectively. β-actin was used as the internal reference control to normalize the expression levels of *dyx1c1*. RNA from the stage before zygotic transcription (<3 hpf) and eye were used as calibrators in qPCR analysis in embryos and adult tissues. Each PCR assay was performed on two independent sets of cDNA samples in triplicates.

Whole-mount in situ Hybridization

Whole-mount in situ hybridization was carried out using digoxigenin-labeled riboprobes as previously described [34]. Antisense RNA probe for zebrafish *dyx1c1* was in vitro synthesized by T7 polymerase after linearising the template with SpeI. Riboprobes for the laterality markers, *otx5* [35], *foxa3* [36] and *lov* [37] were generated as described previously. Images of the stained embryos were obtained using a Nikon digital camera.

Morpholino Based Knockdown and Rescue Experiments

Morpholinos targeting the ATG translation start site (ATGMO; 5′- GTGATCTCTCACTATCAGCGGCATC-3′), exon 2-intron 2 splice site (SPMO; 5′-TGACAGTCAACATGTCTTACC-GATG-3′), a 5 bp mismatch control MOs (misATGMO; 5′-GTCATGTCTCAGTATCACCCGCATC-3′, misSPMO; 5′-TGACACTGAACATCTCTTAGCCATG-3′), a standard control MO (5′-CCTCTTACCTCAGTTACAATTTATA-3′) and a p53MO (5′-GCGCCATTGCTTTGCAAGAATTG-3′) were purchased from Genetools, (Genetools Inc, OR, USA). MOs dissolved in 1× Danieau buffer were injected into zebrafish embryos at 1–2 cell stages at varying concentrations of 50, 100, 150, 200 and 250 μM. To test the off-target effects of MOs, 200 μM concentration of p53MO was injected alone or together with 100 μM each of ATGMO+SPMO. To confirm the specificity of the *dyx1c1* MOs (ATGMO and SPMO), a 5′ capped mRNA of *dyx1c1* was synthesized using mMessage Machine kit (Ambion, TX, USA) and coinjected along with the *dyx1c1* MOs. Splice morpholino specificity was confirmed by RT-PCR using primers spanning exon 2 (F- 5′-GAGATGAAATGTGGGAGCAG-3′) and exon 5 (R-5′-ACTCGTGGAGTGAAGCTGAT-3′) of *dyx1c1* gene. PCR was carried out using the amplification program that consists of 4 min of initial denaturation at 95°C, 40 cycles of 30 s at 95°C, 30 s at 57°C for *dyx1c1* and 58°C for *β-actin*, 60 s at 72°C followed by 10 min of final extension at 72°C.

Acridine Orange Staining

Apoptotic cell death was detected by acridine orange staining following the protocol described previously [38]. All fluorescent images were accquired with Leica camera mounted on a Leica stereomicroscope.

Histology

Zebrafish embryos (2 dpf and 3 dpf) were fixed in 4%PFA overnight at 4°C. The fixed specimens were then serially dehydrated in 70%, 80%, 95% and 100% ethanol for 5 min each, treated with xylene twice for 10 min and embedded in paraffin. Paraffin blocks were then sectioned using a microtome at 3 μm thickness and the sections were stained with Hematoxylin and Eosin.

Immunohistochemistry

Embryos were fixed in 4% PFA overnight at 4°C. Fixed embryos were rinsed four times in PBS and permeabilized in cold acetone for 20 min at −20°C. Embryos were then washed in PBS and blocked for 2 h at RT in blocking solution (1× PBS, pH 7.4, 1% DMSO, 0.5% Tween20, 1% BSA, 10% normal goat serum). Following blocking, embryos were incubated with anti-acetylated tubulin antibody (1:1000, Sigma-Aldrich, St Lois, MO) at 4°C overnight. Goat anti-mouse Alexa 488 was used as the secondary antibody (1:500, Invitrogen, Inc, CA, USA). For nuclear staining of KV cells, 14 hpf embryos were first immunostained with anti-acetylated tubulin antibody as mentioned above and subsequently stained with DAPI (5 mg/ml, Molecular Probes) at 1:50 dilution in dark for 10 min at RT. The confocal images were obtained with Andor spinning disk confocal microscope using a 60× water objective.

Transmission Electron Microscopy

Three days old embryos were fixed in 2% glutaraldehyde solution containing 1% PFA in 0.1 M phosphate buffer (PB), pH 7.4 at RT and stored at 4°C until use. Specimens were rinsed in 0.1M PB, pH 7.4 and then post-fixed with 2% osmium tetroxide in 0.1M PB, pH 7.4 at 4°C for 2 h, dehydrated in ethanol followed by acetone and then embedded in LX-112 (Ladd, Burlington, Vermont, USA). Semithin sections were cut and stained with toluidine blue O and used for light microscopic analysis. Ultrathin sections of approximately 40–50 nm were cut by a Leica EM UC 6 (Leica, Wien, Austria) and stained with uranyl acetate followed by lead citrate and examined in a Tecnai 10 transmission electron microscope (FEI Company, Eindhoven, The Netherlands) at 100 kV. Images were acquired using a Veleta camera (Olympus Soft Imaging Solutions, GmbH, Münster, Germany).

Results

Identification, Cloning and Sequence Analysis of *dyx1c1* Gene in Zebrafish

By searching the zebrafish genome database, we identified the zebrafish ortholog of *dyx1c1* (ENSDARG00000007792). The zebrafish *dyx1c1* is located on chromosome 13 and is predicted to encode a protein of 420 amino acids. Comparison of the zebrafish Dyx1c1 protein sequence with that of human and mouse revealed 54% and 53% sequence identity, respectively (Fig. 1A, B). In addition, we found a high degree of conservation in the intron-exon architecture of zebrafish *dyx1c1* with its mammalian counterparts (Fig. 1C). The protein coding region comprised 9 exons separated by 8 introns. Although the length of the introns varied between the three species, their positions were conserved. The exons also displayed high similarity in the number of amino acids they coded for; exons 1, 2 and 8 coded for the same number of amino acids in all the species, whereas exons 3 and 5 coded for the same number of amino acids in human and mouse but not in zebrafish. The total number of amino acids coded by exons 6 and 7 were the same in human and zebrafish but not in mouse. Exon 4 and 9 of the protein coding region showed the most variability among the three species analyzed. The DYX and TPR domains were highly conserved between the three species, whereas the zebrafish p23 domain was less conserved with respect to the mamalian p23 domain. However, the three domains spanned across the same exons in all the species (Fig. 1C). Analyses of the genomic region near *dyx1c1* revealed synteny between zebrafish and humans both including genes coding for ccpg1, pygo1 and prtg (data not shown).

Using qPCR, the coding region of *dyx1c1* was amplified from embryos at 50% epiboly stage. The amplified fragment was then purified and cloned into a TOPO vector.

Expression of *dyx1c1* in Developing Embryos and Adult Organs

Using qPCR, we measured the mRNA levels of *dyx1c1* in developing embryos and in early larval stages. Zebrafish *dyx1c1* was maternally expressed as seen at <3 hpf, a stage before mid-blastula transition (MBT) and its expression levels increased until 1 dpf. The mRNA levels of *dyx1c1* dropped down by 2 dpf and remained at low levels during larval stages (Fig. 2A). To further analyze the spatial expression of *dyx1c1*, we performed whole-mount *in situ* hybridization on developing embryos. At 10 hpf, a weak expression of *dyx1c1* was detected in KV (Fig. 2C). At 15 somites stage, *dyx1c1* expression was localized in the otic vesicle, pronephros and neural tube (Fig. 2D). By 26 hpf, *dyx1c1* expression was evident in several regions of the brain including telencephalon, midbrain, and tegmentum and was persistently expressed in the otic vesicle, spinal canal and pronephros (Fig. 2E–G). However the expression of *dyx1c1* was reduced by 49 hpf and was detected strongly only in the olfactory placode (Fig. 2H). It is evident from RNA *in situ* hybridization that *dyx1c1* is expressed in ciliated tissues suggesting that it might have a role in cilia development and/or function.

The relative mRNA levels of *dyx1c1* in different pooled tissues of adult male and female zebrafish were measured by qPCR. Highest expression of *dyx1c1* was seen in the testis. *dyx1c1* was also detected in other organs including brain, swimbladder, liver, kidney and ovary (Fig. 2B). Our results are consistent with the expression analysis of *DYX1C1* in human tissues [1].

Knockdown of *dyx1c1* Leads to Body Curvature, Hydrocephalus and Kidney Cysts

To investigate the biological role of *dyx1c1* during embryonic development in zebrafish we used MOs to knockdown the protein expression of Dyx1c1. Both translation start-site MO (ATGMO) and splice-site MO (SPMO) targeting the splice junction of exon 2 and intron 2, were injected alone into 1-cell embryos at varying concentrations of 50, 100, 150, 200 and 250 μM. The efficiency of the MOs was dose dependent; at 50 μM dose no visible morphological defects were observed whereas at higher concentrations, both the MOs resulted in similar phenotypes as described below (Fig. 3A, S1). At the highest concentration, the MOs increased the percentage of mortality in the morphants to more than 70%.

The effects of the loss-of-function of *dyx1c1* were observed in higher percentage (>90%) of morphants at 200 μM for both the MOs. The knockdown efficiency of SPMO was strong at 1 dpf but decreased at 2 dpf. As both ATGMO and SPMO resulted in identical phenotypes we used a combined dose of 100 μM each to get a total of 200 μM for all experiments unless otherwise specified. For all experiments, a total concentration of about 8 ng of ATGMO or SPMO or combination of both (4 ng each) was injected per embryo. The 5 bp mismatch control MO (misATGMO and misSPMO) that were tested at the same concentration range had no effects at 50 and 100 μM but produced a phenotype identical to that seen with ATGMO or SPMO in 10% of the injected embryos at 200 μM. Microjection of a standard control MO (cMO) had no effects at the same concentration range and the injected embryos appeared normal like the wild-type uninjected embryos. Wild-type (WT) embryos were used as controls in all experiments.

The specificity of the SPMO was confirmed by RT-PCR which revealed aberrant splicing events in 1 and 2 dpf morphants. Sequencing of the misspliced transcript revealed the inclusion of 32 bp from intron 2 which might encode nonfunctional truncated Dyx1c1 protein in the splice morphants (Fig. 3B). However at 3.5 dpf the efficiency of SPMO was reduced in embryos showing weak phenotype (Fig. S1). We therefore used only morphants showing prominent body curvature, hydrocephalus and kidney cysts for all our experiments. Coinjection of 5′capped mRNA of zebrafish *dyx1c1* along with 200 μM of ATGMO or SPMO or combination of both, rescued the curved body axis phenotype to normal WT phenotype (Fig. 3G).

Wild-type embryos injected with ATGMO and SPMO either alone or together developed numerous morphological changes

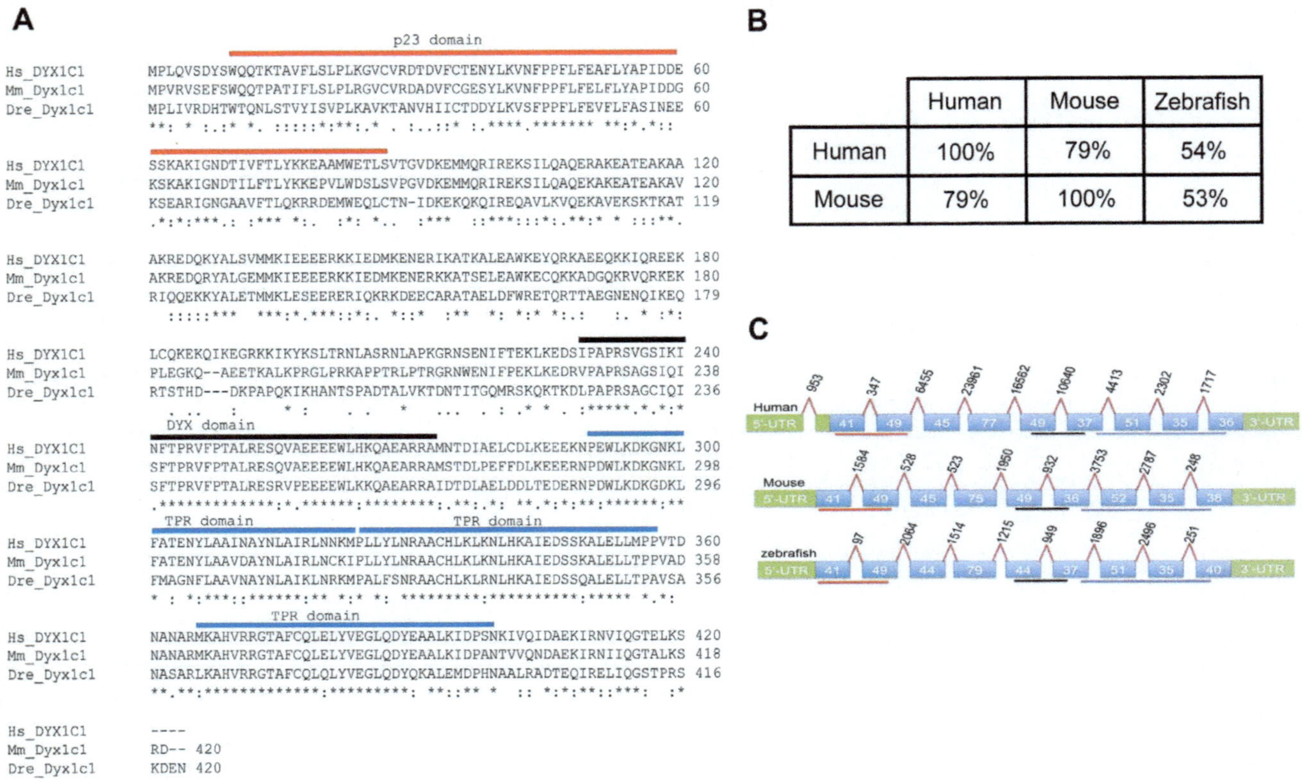

	Human	Mouse	Zebrafish
Human	100%	79%	54%
Mouse	79%	100%	53%

Figure 1. Sequence alignment and genomic structure of the vertebrate *DYX1C1/Dyx1c1/dyx1c1* genes and proteins. Sequence comparison of zebrafish (*Danio rerio*; Dre) Dyx1c1 protein with that of Human (*Homo sapiens*; Hs) and mouse (*Mus musculus*; Ms) protein sequences (A). The p23, DYX and TPR domains are denoted by red, black and blue lines respectively. Protein sequence identity shown in percentage for the three species (B). The comparison of *dyx1c1* cDNAs from Human, mouse and zebrafish reveals 9 exons intercepted by 8 introns (C). Human cDNA sequence shows the presence of an additional intron in the 5'untranslated region (UTR). The UTRs are denoted by green boxes, exons by blue boxes with the number of amino acids they code and introns are represented by slanting lines connecting the exons with the number of nucleotides (nt) on top. The conserved domains are denoted by red (for p23 domain), black (for DYX domain) and blue (for TPR domain) lines below the cDNA structure for each species.

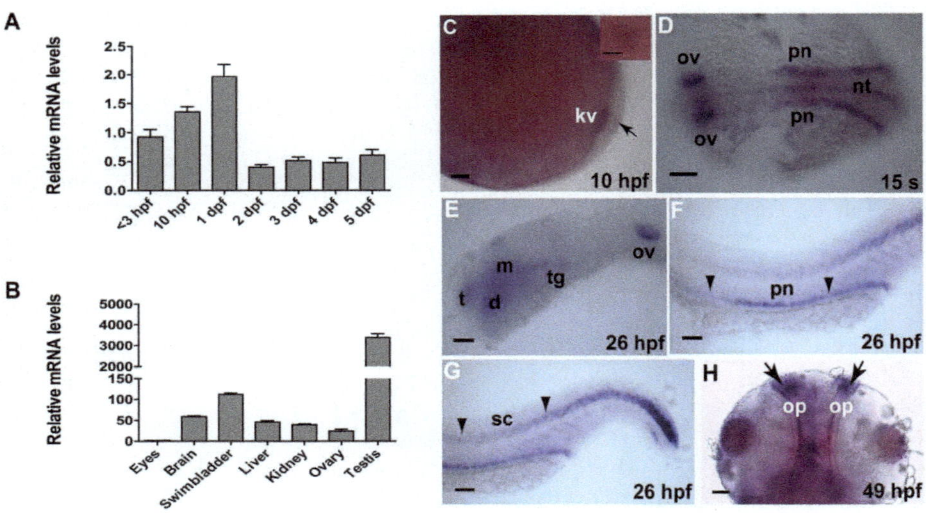

Figure 2. Expression of *dyx1c1* mRNA during embryonic development and in adult tissues. qPCR analysis of the transcript levels of *dyx1c1* during embryonic development (A) and in adult tissues (B). Whole-mount *in situ* hybridization showed that *dyx1c1* is expressed in KV at 10 hpf (C). Inset in C is a close-up view of KV. At 15-somites, *dyx1c1* was expressed specifically in the otic vesicle, pronephros and neural tube (D). At 26 hpf *dyx1c1* was detected in the brain and is still maintained in otic vesicle, pronephros and spinal canal (E–G). Later at 49 hpf, *dyx1c1* was visible in the olfactory placode (H). Panels E–G show lateral views of embryos. Panels D and H show dorsal and ventral views of embryos, respectively. Scale bars indicate 100 μm. Abbreviations: KV, Kupffer's vesicle: nt, neural tube: pn, pronephros: t, telencephalon: d, diencephalon: m, midbrain: tg, tegmentum: ov, otic vesicle: sc, spinal canal: op, olfactory placode.

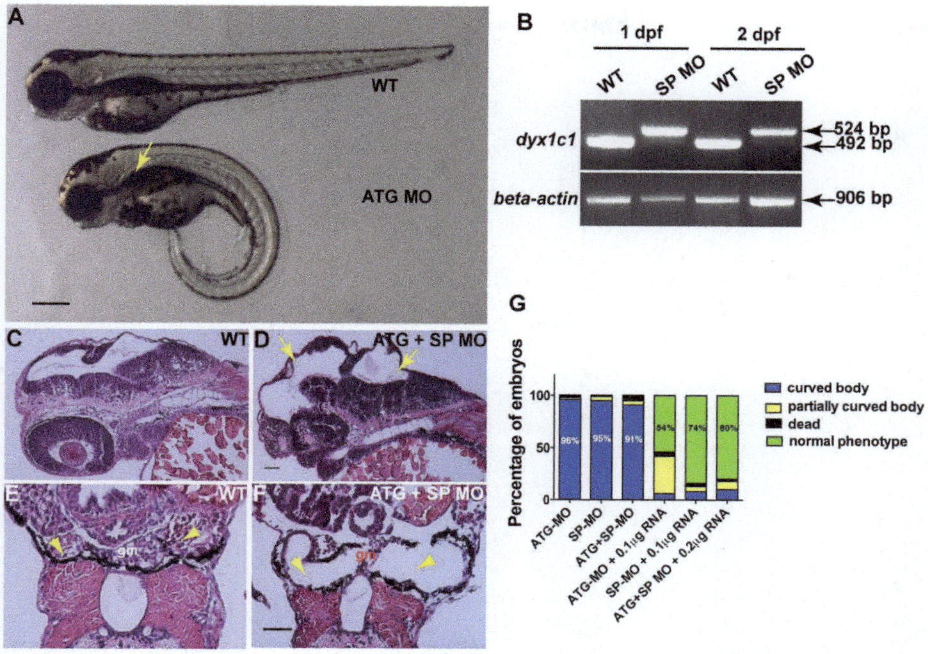

Figure 3. Knockdown of *dyx1c1* showed typical cilia phenotypes. Injection of ATGMO or SPMO at 200 μM concentration produced ventrally curved body axis, hydrocephalus and kidney cysts (A). Arrow in panel A denotes kidney cyst in ATG morphant. RT-PCR showed aberrant splice transcripts in SPMO injected embryos at 1 and 2 dpf (B). Histological sections of 2 day old embryos injected with both ATGMO and SPMO (100 μM each) showed hydrocephalus (D; yellow arrows) compared to normal size brain ventricles in WT (C). Transverse histological sections across the pronephros at 3.5 dpf showed normal pronephros in WT embryos (E). Section of *dyx1c1* morphant (ATGMO+SPMO) showed severe pronephric distention and a thin glomerulus in the center (F). Yellow arrowheads in panel E and F point out normal pronephros in WT and dilated pronephros in morphant embryo, respectively. Quantitative analysis of the rescue of *dyx1c1* morphant phenotype to WT phenotype with different combinations of MOs and *dyx1c1* mRNA (G). Scale bars indicate 100 μm. Abbreviation: gm, glomerulus.

that were visible from 1 dpf onward. *dyx1c1* morphants developed ventrally curved body axis, hydrocephalus and pronephric cysts which became visible only at 3 dpf (Fig. 3A). Additionally, upon mechanical stimulus the morphants exhibited abnormal circular swimming behaviour. Histological analysis of transverse sections of WT and *dyx1c1* morphant clearly showed hydrocephalus in 2 days old morphant embryos and dilated pronephric tubules in 3.5 dpf morphant embryos (Fig. 3C–F).

One of the major off-target effects caused by MOs is p53 mediated cell death [38]. Thus, to further confirm that the MOs are specifically targeting *dyx1c1,* we performed acridine orange staining on wild-type, *p53* morphants, *dyx1c1* morphants and p53MO coinjected embryos to visualize apoptosis. Our results show that coinjection with p53MO does not produce any phenotypic changes in *dyx1c1* morphants, thus confirming that the phenotypes are caused by true loss-of-function of *dyx1c1* (Fig. S2).

Loss-of-function of *dyx1c1* in Zebrafish Leads to *situs inversus* in Different Organs

Zebrafish cilia mutants display phenotypes including curvature of the body axis, hydrocephalus and kidney cysts similar to that of *dyx1c1* morphant embryos suggesting a potential role for *dyx1c1* in cilia formation and/or function [31]. As cilia have been implicated in the specification of left-right (LR) asymmetry of the body plan, we sought to analyze the left-right patterning in asymmetrically placed organs such as the heart, epithalamus and visceral organs. The percentage of morphant embryos showing randomization in LR asymmetry in different organs is shown in Table 1. To assess brain asymmetry, the expression of markers for parapineal (*otx5*) and habenular nuclei (*lov*) were analyzed by *in situ* hybridization on two days old embryos [35,37]. In WT control embryos, the normal position of the parapineal organ is on the left side, whereas in 41% of the *dyx1c1* morphant embryos it was reversed (Fig. 4A, B). The expression of *lov* was stronger on the left habenula in WT control embryos but 42% of the *dyx1c1* morphants showed stronger expression of *lov* on the right habenula and in 5% of the morphants *lov* was symmetrically expressed (Fig. 4C–E). Using *cardiac myosin light chain 2* (*cmlc2*) gene expression as marker, we determined the heart looping in WT and *dyx1c1* morphant embryos [39]. Normal heart looping, with left placement of the ventricle and right placement of the atrium was observed in 98% of wild-type embryos, whereas, in 26% of the *dyx1c*1 morphants the looping was inverted and in 24% of morphant embryos the heart failed looping at all (Fig. 4F–H). Assessment of the positioning of the visceral organs in WT embryos and morphants using the endodermal marker *foxa3* revealed that the position of the gut, liver and pancreas was irregular in the morphants [36]. About 52% of the *dyx1c1* morphants showed situs inversus and 5% showed heterotaxia with respect to the positioning of the liver (Fig. 4I–K).

Loss-of-function of *dyx1c1* Affects Cilia Length in Multiple Organs

The KV in zebrafish is a transient ciliated organ which is essential for specifying organ laterality [40]. To test whether the L–R asymmetry defects observed in *dyx1c1* morphants were due to impaired ciliogenesis, we performed immunolabelling with an antibody against acetylated tubulin to visualize cilia in KV. Measurement of cilia number in KV of 10-somite stage WT and

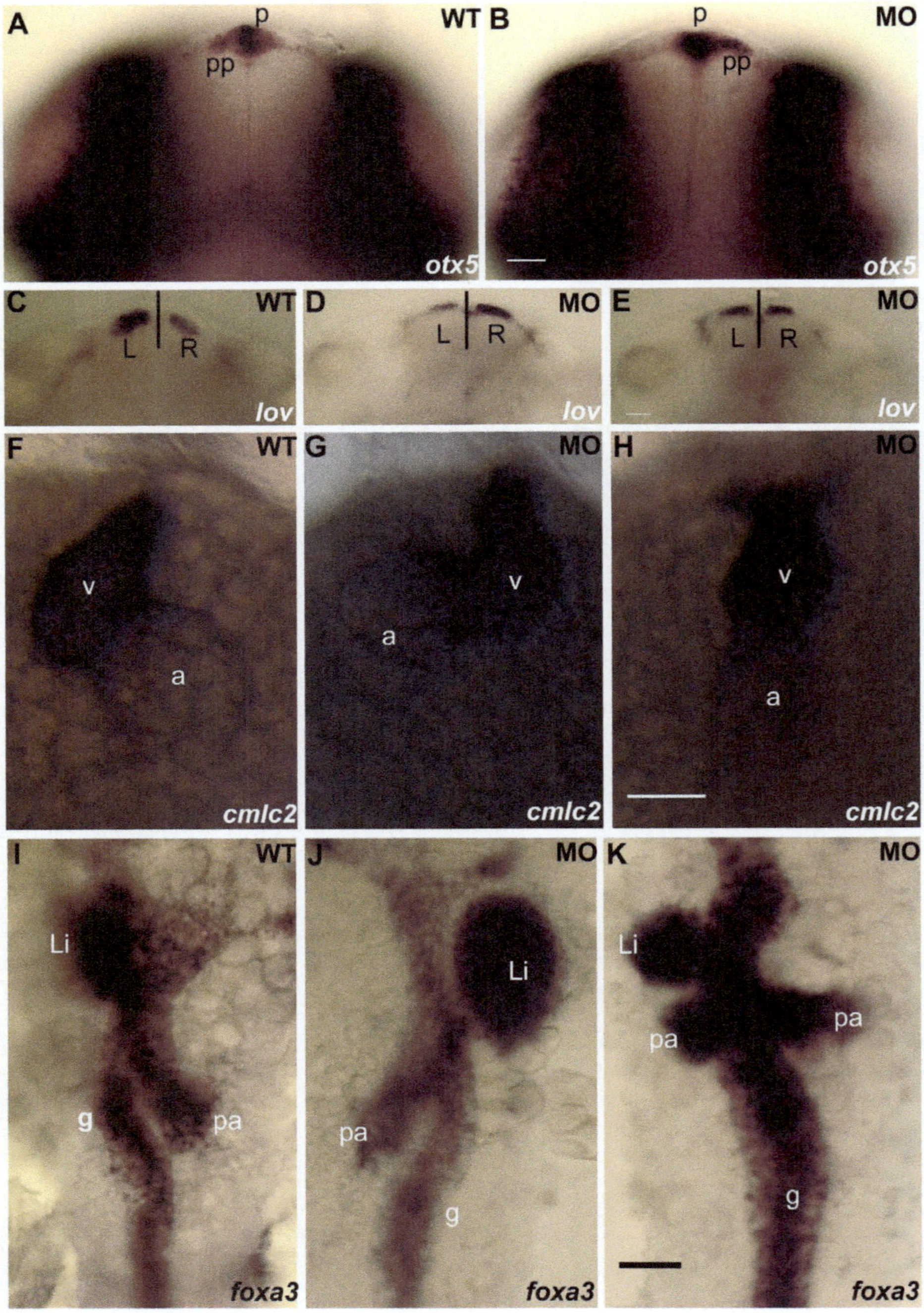

Figure 4. Loss-of-function of *dyx1c1* caused L–R assymetry defects in zebrafish. Whole-mount in situ hybridization showing the expression of laterality markers in WT and *dyx1c1* morphants (ATGMO+SPMO) at 2 dpf. The position of the asymmetrically placed organs was irregular in at least 50% of the embryos injected with *dyx1c1* MO. *otx5* expression showing the left sided placement of the parapineal organ in WT (A). In *dyx1c1* morphant, the parapineal position was reversed (B). *lov* was strongly expressed in the left habenular in WT (C). In *dyx1c1* morphant *lov* expression was stronger in the right or expressed symmetrically (D & E). Knockdown of *dyx1c1* altered heart looping. Ventral views of embryos at 2 dpf (F–H). *cmlc2* expression showed normal heart looping in WT (F). Cardiac looping was reversed (G) or absent in *dyx1c1* morphant embryos (H). Expression of *foxa3* revealing the position of the gut, liver and pancreas in WT embryo (I). The positions of the liver, gut and pancreas were irregular in *dyx1c1* morphants (J & K). Panels A, B, C, D, E, I, J and K are dorsal views with anterior to the top. Frontal views are shown in panels F–G. Scale bars indicate 50 μm. Abbreviations: p, pineal organ: pp, parapineal organ: v, ventricle: a, atrium: li, liver: pa, pancreas: g, gut.

morphant embryos revealed that cilia number was significantly reduced in *dyx1c1* morphants when compared to those of the WT embryos (Fig. 5A, B, I). Examination of DAPI stained KV cell nuclei showed no difference in the total number of cells in KV between WT and morphant embryos suggesting that reduction in cilia number in morphant embryos is not produced by loss of ciliated cells (Fig. 5J–L). We also found slight reduction in cilia length in KV of *dyx1c1* morphants (Fig. 5A, B).

The expression of *dyx1c1* in many ciliated organs such as the pronephros, spinal canal, otic vesicle and olfactory placode

Table 1. Percentage of embryos showing normal or altered organ laterality in WT and *dyx1c1* morphants.

Markers		Normal	Reversed	Bilateral	Absent
otx5	WT (n = 94)	97%	3%	–	–
	MO (n = 120)	**58%**	**41%**	–	–
lov	WT (n = 81)	98%	2%	–	–
	MO (n = 81)	**53%**	**42%**	**5%**	–
cmlc2	WT (n = 131)	97%	3%	–	–
	MO (n = 152)	**48%**	**26%**	–	**24%**
foxa3	WT (n = 87)	98%	2%	1%	–
	MO (n = 101)	**47%**	**52%**	**5%**	–

Asymmetry of the parapineal organ and habenular nuclei was detected by *otx5* and *lov* expression. Bilateral expression of *lov* in morphants refers to equal expression of *lov* on both left and right habenula. Heart looping in WT and morphant was detected using *cmcl2*. About 24% of morphant embryos showed no looping which is denoted as absent in the table. Randomization of the liver position is quantified with *foxa3* expression.

prompted us to examine cilia in these organs. In zebrafish, cilia in the pronephros and spinal canal are motile and are essential for driving fluid flow within these organs. Disruption of cilia structure or motility in the pronephros and spinal canal leads to fluid accumulation and organ distention subsequently resulting in kidney cysts and hydrocephalus respectively [41]. As expected the proximal region of WT zebrafish pronephros was densely populated with cilia that were long and extended into the lumen of the kidney tubule. Interestingly, the pronephric cilia of *dyx1c1* morphants were less dense and were severely shortened in length (Fig. 5E, F). Likewise, spinal canal cilia of *dyx1c1* morphants were dramatically reduced in length in contrast to that seen in WT embryos (Fig. 5G, H). We next visualized cilia in the olfactory placode of 2 dpf WT and morphant embryos. We found in the WT embryos numerous cilia projecting from the epithelial cells of the olfactory placode. Strikingly, we detected very few olfactory cilia in the *dyx1c1* morphants and those present were severely shortened in length (Fig. 5C, D). Together, these data suggest that *dyx1c1* might have a central role in regulating cilia length in many organs in zebrafish.

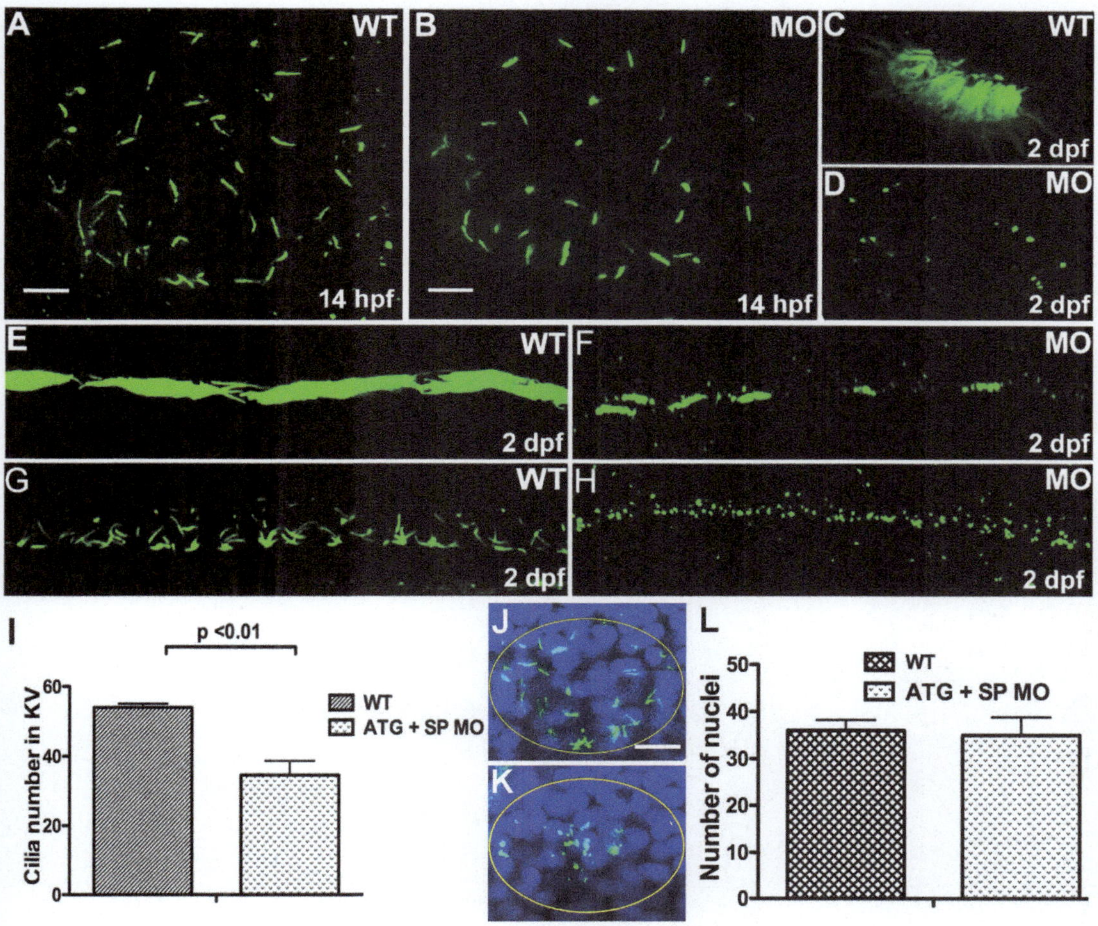

Figure 5. Knockdown of *dyx1c1* reduced cilia length and number in different organs. Immunolabelling of KV cilia with anti-acetylated tubulin in WT (A) and *dyx1c1* morphants (B) at 14 hpf showed reduction in cilia length in morphant embryos. Compared to WT control (C), morphant embryo (D) revealed fewer and shortened cilia in the olfactory placode. At 2 dpf, cilia in *dyx1c1* morphants were shortened in pronephros and spinal canal (F, H) compared to WT (E, G). Measurement of cilia number in WT and morphants (I). Confocal images of KV in WT and morphant embryos at 14 hpf stained with anti-acetylated tubulin and DAPI (J, K). Graphical representation of total number of nuclei/KV in WT and morphant embryos (L). Panel C, D, E, F, G and H are lateral views with anterior to the left in E, F, G and H. Scale bars indicate 10 μm.

Zebrafish *dyx1c1* is Needed for Dynein Arm Assembly

Transmission electron microscopy was used to examine the ultrastructural defects in cilia to better understand the functional role of *dyx1c1* in ciliogenesis. The cilium consists of 9 microtubule doublets (A and B subunits) arranged in the border and two central tubules. Each outer A subunit has a set of arms attached, IDA and ODA. Lack of dynein arms have been shown to render cilia immobile [42]. We analyzed ultrathin sections of the pronephros because zebrafish pronephros is a multiciliated tissue providing easy access to examine motile cilia, and secondly, because kidney cysts, a manifestation of defective cilia motility, were apparent in *dyx1c1* morphants from 3 dpf onward. In WT embryos staged at 3.5 dpf, a dense brush border of apical microvilli projecting from the epithelial cells and numerous cilia were evident in the pronephric duct (Fig. 6A). However in the morphant embryos the pronephric duct was dilated and the epithelia completely lacked microvilli (Fig. 6B). Furthermore, we observed abnormal cilia axoneme structure in the morphants. In most of the *dyx1c1* morphants, both ODA and IDA were absent as compared to WT controls (Fig. 6C, D). Ocassionally, in some morphants remnants of ODA were noticeable but the IDA were still missing (data not shown). As in the pronephros, dynein arms were also missing in the olfactory placode cilia (Fig. S3).

dyx1c1 mRNA Rescues Cilia Defects in *dyx1c1* Morphants

To confirm that the cilia defects observed were due to true loss-of-function of *dyx1c1*, we performed rescue experiments by coinjecting *dyx1c1* mRNA with ATGMO+SPMO. The laterality defects caused by suppression of *dyx1c1* was greatly reduced by *dyx1c1* mRNA injection (Fig. S4). Also, the dramatic reduction of cilia length in the pronephros was rescued by coinjection of *dyx1c1* mRNA (Fig. S4). Ultrastructural analyses revealed that the loss of dynein arms caused by knockdown of *dyx1c1* was rescued efficiently in the pronephric cilia as well as in the olfactory placode cilia by coinjection of *dyx1c1* mRNA with ATG-MO+SPMO (Fig. 6E, Fig. S3).

Discussion

In the present study, we show that the ortholog of the dyslexia candidate gene *dyx1c1* is essential for cilia growth and motility in zebrafish. Cilia are membrane-bound organelles that are crucial for vertebrate development, organ morphogenesis and differentiation of sensory cells. Ciliary dysfunction has been described in a dozen of human ciliopathies such as primary ciliary dyskinesia (PCD), Autosomal Dominant Polycystic Kidney Disease (ADPKD), Nephronophthisis (NPHP), Bardet Biedl Syndrome (BBS) and Jouberts syndrome (JBTS) and the list continues to expand as more ciliary proteins are being identified [43,44,45,46]. Zebrafish has been used extensively to study cilia structure, function and signalling and several cilia mutants have been generated. Interestingly, the ciliary mutants and morphants with defects in diverse ciliary genes display defects including body curvature, hydrocephalus, kidney cysts and left-right asymmetry [47,48,49,50]. Here, we demonstrate that zebrafish *dyx1c1* is specifically expressed in ciliated tissues and its inhibition results in ciliopathy-related phenotypes consistent with those seen in zebrafish cilia mutants [31,49,51].

Beating of the motile ependymal cilia in the brain propels cerebrospinal fluid (CSF) flow in brain ventricles and impairment of ependymal cilia has been linked to the formation of hydrocephalus in different animal models [52,53,54]. In humans, hydrocephalus has been noticed in some patients with PCD [55]. The presence of renal cysts in patients of cystic kidney diseases has been suggested to result from the functional failure of renal primary cilia, possibly through abnormal cilia-mediated Ca^{2+} signalling as suggested by *in vitro* studies [56,57]. Spinal cord cilia and renal cilia in zebrafish are motile and their beating is essential to move fluid within these organs [41]. Our observation of

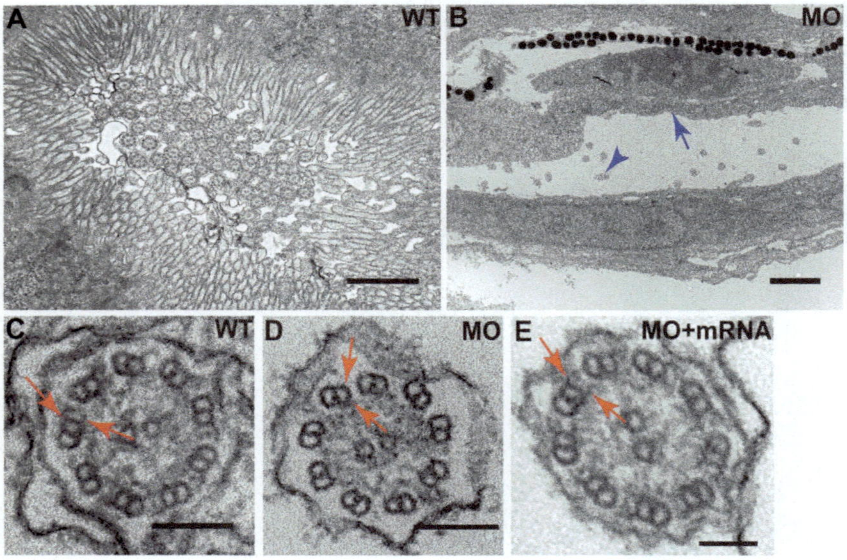

Figure 6. Disruption of *dyx1c1* leads to pronephric brush border defects and loss of cilia dynein arms. Ultrastructure of WT (3.5 dpf) pronephric duct showed dense brush border of apical microvilli extending from the epithelial cells and the presence of numerous cilia in the lumen (A). Apical microvilli were absent in *dyx1c1* morphants (ATGMO+SPMO) at 3.5 dpf (B). Arrow in blue denotes missing brush border and blue arrowhead denotes cilia. Electron micrography of pronephric cilia axoneme in *dyx1c1* morphant embryo at 3.5 dpf showed the absence of both ODA and IDA on the outer microtubules (D) whereas the dynein arms were present in WT embryos (C). Coinjection of *dyx1c1* mRNA with MO rescued both ODA and IDA (E). Arrows in red indicate ODA and IDA in WT, morphant and rescued embryo. Scale bars in panels A and B indicate 1 μm and 2 μm respectively. Scale bars in panels C and D are 100 nm and 200 nm in E.

hydrocephalus and pronephric cysts in *dyx1c1* morphants strongly suggested that cilia motility might be compromised in these organs.

We report randomization of LR asymmetry of different organs in *dyx1c1* morphant embryos (Fig. 4) and cilia in many organs including the spinal canal, pronephros and olfactory placode appeared greatly stunted (Fig. 5). Significant reduction in cilia number was also detected in the KV and olfactory placode. It is important to note that among all tissues examined, KV cilia was least affected which could possibly be due to the incomplete suppression of maternally supplied mRNA not affected by SPMO. Interestingly, laterality defects have been observed in PCD patients and also in mice carrying mutation in genes implicated in cilia function [58,59]. The unique motile cilia of zebrafish KV, an organ homologous to mouse node function to set up left-right asymmetry of organs in zebrafish [40]. We suggest that the fewer number of short cilia in KV of *dyx1c1* morphants may not be able to generate a clockwise fluid flow within this organ, which is required for specifying LR organ asymmetry. Supporting our hypothesis, cilia length has been shown previously to play a crucial role in regulating speed and direction of fluid flow inside KV [60]. Previous work has shown that zebrafish mutants showing ciliary length defects also exhibit kidney cysts and hydrocephalus [31,48,49,51]. Taken together, these results suggest that *dyx1c1* could be important for controlling cilia length in different organs in zebrafish.

Structural abnormalties of cilia have been previously shown to affect cilia motility [61,62]. Human PCD subjects with mutations in the *DNAAF3* gene lack ODA and IDA in their cilia, a phenotype which could also be reproduced in zebrafish by morpholino knockdown of *dnaaf3* [63]. Thus, absence of dynein arms in *dyx1c1* morphants suggests that *dyx1c1* might be required for cilia movement through maintenance of the assembly of ODA and IDA. Interestingly, some zebrafish mutants and morphants that lack both ODA and IDA do not have short cilia whereas mutations in ciliary genes in *chlamydomonas* that show defects in outer or inner dynein arms do cause a reduction in the average length of the flagella [63,64,65,66]. Elongation and maintenance of cilia axoneme is dependent on the bidirectional intraflagellar transport (IFT) of IFT protein complex. Chlamydomonas ODA16 is an IFT associated protein that is needed for the proper assembly of outer dynein arm proteins. Short cilia observed in *dyx1c1* morphants could possibly result from the disruption of IFT and perhaps *dyx1c1* functions in zebrafish to transport specific components of outer and inner dynein arms to the ciliary axoneme [66,67]. Molecular chaperones such as HSP90, HSP70 and TCP1 are known to modulate the assembly of cytoskeletal proteins [68]. Similar to other family of TPR domain containing proteins, DYX1C1 has been shown to act as a co-chaperone for HSP70 and HSP90 [69]. Interestingly, the DYX1C1 protein interactome in SH-SY5Y cells by Tammimies et al., reveals that DYX1C1 interacts with several microtubule and cytoskeletal proteins [70]. Based on the accumulated evidence and our *in vivo* data, we hypothesize that DYX1C1 might function to deliver structural and functional components of the axoneme from the cytoplasm to the axoneme by interacting with proteins essential for IFT. Further studies are needed to test this hypothesis.

A role for cilia in dyslexia has not been shown until recently. DCDC2 was the first dyslexia protein shown to regulate ciliary signalling [24]. A recent report using a large-scale gene coexpression analysis of microarray data sets from human ciliated tissues suggest that *DYX1C1, KIAA0319* and *DCDC2* have a role in ciliary functions [71]. Also, an earlier comparative genomic screen identified DYX1C1 as one of the proteins involved in ciliary and basal body biogenesis [72]. A recent study on the transcriptional profiling of multiciliated mouse tracheal epithelial cells showed that Dyx1c1 is localized to centrosome and cilia and upregulated during ciliogenesis [73]. Our results in zebrafish provide direct evidence for the role of the *dyx1c1* in the biology and function of cilia suggesting a similar function for DYX1C1. Disruption of *DYX1C1, DCDC2* and *KIAA0319* individually results in neuronal migration abnormalities in rat neocortex. Whether the neuronal phenotype observed in animal models and in human dyslectic brains is a consequence of defects in neuronal cilia structure and function remains unknown. However, the significance of primary cilium in brain patterning including cortical morphogenesis has been implicated previously [28,74]. Cognitive impairments are often observed in ciliopathy syndromes such as Joubert Syndrome, Bardet-Biedl Syndrome and Alström Syndrome and it is possible that these symptoms are manifestations of defects in neuronal cilia [75]. Until now it was not clear whether migrating neurons possess cilia, but a recent study in mouse suggests that cilia growth occurs only after the completion of neuronal migration in the cortex [76]. Thus, the function of primary cilia in migration of neurons still remains poorly characterized and further studies with respect to cilia biology in the CNS are required.

Centrosome positioning is considered as a crucial factor for proper migration of neurons in the cortex. In our previous work we have shown that DYX1C1 localizes to the centrosome and also interacts with Lissencephaly 1 (LIS1), another centrosomal protein. Mutations in LIS1 lead to a severe neuronal migration disorder lissencephaly in humans [70,77]. However, it remains to be determined if this interaction regulates centrosomal orientation during the migration of neurons.

The zebrafish is a very powerful model to study ciliopathies. In this work we show for the first time the involvement of *dyx1c1* in ciliary function in an animal model. With direct evidence implicating now DYX1C1 and DCDC2 in ciliary functions and the bioinformatic suggestion of a role for KIAA0319 as well, we propose that dyslexia should become considered as a new type of ciliopathy.

Supporting Information

Figure S1 Morphological phenotypes induced by ATGMO and SPMO. Both ATGMO and SPMO when injected alone produced identical phenotypes. Hydrocephalus and kidney cysts were clearly visible in the morphants at 2 dpf (B & C) and 3 dpf (E & F) respectively as compared to the nomal phenotype in wild-type (A & D). Arrows denote hydrocephalus and kidney cysts are denoted by arrowheads. RT-PCR showing the efficiency of SPMO at 3.5 dpf in embryos showing strong and weak phenotypes (G). Scale bars indicate 100 μm.

Figure S2 Morpholino specificity confirmed by coinjection with p53. Analysis of apoptotic cell death in WT (A–D), p53 morphants (E–H), *dyx1c1* morphants (ATGMO+SPMO; I–L) and *dyx1c1+ p53* morphants (M–P). Bright field (A,E,I,M) and fluorescent images of wild-type and morphants (B–D, F–H, J–L, N–P) at 1 dpf. Fluorescent signal in *dyx1c1* morphants appeared similar to that seen in WT. *dyx1c1* morphant phenotype was not affected by p53 coknockdown. Scale bars indicate 100 μm.

Figure S3 Dynein arms of olfactory cilia affected in *dyx1c1* morphants. Ultrastructure of olfactory cilia at 3 dpf showed loss of ODA and IDA in *dyx1c1* morphants (B) as compared to WT (A). Coinjection with *dyx1c1* mRNA rescued both the dynein arms (C). Arrows denote ODA and IDA. Scale bars indicate 200 nm.

Figure S4 ***dyx1c1*** **mRNA rescues cilia defects in** ***dyx1c1*** **morphants.** Anti-acetylated tubulin staining of cilia in the pronephros of wild-type (A), *dyx1c1* morphant (B) and mRNA coinjected embryo (C). Percentage of embryos showing left-side (normal), right-side (situs inversus) placement of liver and heterotaxia in wild-type, *dyx1c1* morphants and mRNA injected embryos (D). Scale bar indicate 10 μm.

Acknowledgments

The authors are thankful to the zebrafish core facility, Karolinska Institutet for providing embryos and adult fish. We thank Eva Blomen for the EM work at the electron microscopy unit, Department of Laboratory Medicin, Karolinska Institutet. We are also thankful to Dr. Satish Srinivas Kitambi for the generous gift of *cmlc2* riboprobe. This study was in part performed at the Live Cell Imaging unit, Department of Biosciences and Nutrition, Karolinska Institutet, Huddinge.

Author Contributions

Conceived and designed the experiments: GC LV ITP JK. Performed the experiments: GC LV KH. Analyzed the data: GC KH. Contributed reagents/materials/analysis tools: GC LV ITP KH JK. Wrote the paper: GC ITP LV JK.

References

1. Taipale M, Kaminen N, Nopola-Hemmi J, Haltia T, Myllyluoma B, et al. (2003) A candidate gene for developmental dyslexia encodes a nuclear tetratricopeptide repeat domain protein dynamically regulated in brain. Proc Natl Acad Sci U S A 100: 11553–11558.
2. Lim CK, Ho CS, Chou CH, Waye MM (2011) Association of the rs3743205 variant of DYX1C1 with dyslexia in Chinese children. Behav Brain Funct 7: 16.
3. Meng H, Hager K, Held M, Page GP, Olson RK, et al. (2005) TDT-association analysis of EKN1 and dyslexia in a Colorado twin cohort. Hum Genet 118: 87–90.
4. Marino C, Citterio A, Giorda R, Facoetti A, Menozzi G, et al. (2007) Association of short-term memory with a variant within DYX1C1 in developmental dyslexia. Genes Brain Behav 6: 640–646.
5. Dahdouh F, Anthoni H, Tapia-Paez I, Peyrard-Janvid M, Schulte-Korne G, et al. (2009) Further evidence for DYX1C1 as a susceptibility factor for dyslexia. Psychiatr Genet 19: 59–63.
6. Scerri TS, Fisher SE, Francks C, MacPhie IL, Paracchini S, et al. (2004) Putative functional alleles of DYX1C1 are not associated with dyslexia susceptibility in a large sample of sibling pairs from the UK. J Med Genet 41: 853–857.
7. Marino C, Giorda R, Luisa Lorusso M, Vanzin L, Salandi N, et al. (2005) A family-based association study does not support DYX1C1 on 15q21.3 as a candidate gene in developmental dyslexia. Eur J Hum Genet 13: 491–499.
8. Bellini G, Bravaccio C, Calamoneri F, Donatella Cocuzza M, Fiorillo P, et al. (2005) No evidence for association between dyslexia and DYX1C1 functional variants in a group of children and adolescents from Southern Italy. J Mol Neurosci 27: 311–314.
9. Cope NA, Hill G, van den Bree M, Harold D, Moskvina V, et al. (2005) No support for association between dyslexia susceptibility 1 candidate 1 and developmental dyslexia. Mol Psychiatry 10: 237–238.
10. Venkatesh SK, Siddaiah A, Padakannaya P, Ramachandra NB (2011) An examination of candidate gene SNPs for dyslexia in an Indian sample. Behav Genet 41: 105–109.
11. Galaburda AM, Sherman GF, Rosen GD, Aboitiz F, Geschwind N (1985) Developmental dyslexia: four consecutive patients with cortical anomalies. Ann Neurol 18: 222–233.
12. Humphreys P, Kaufmann WE, Galaburda AM (1990) Developmental dyslexia in women: neuropathological findings in three patients. Ann Neurol 28: 727–738.
13. Wang Y, Paramasivam M, Thomas A, Bai J, Kaminen-Ahola N, et al. (2006) DYX1C1 functions in neuronal migration in developing neocortex. Neuroscience 143: 515–522.
14. Rosen GD, Bai J, Wang Y, Fiondella CG, Threlkeld SW, et al. (2007) Disruption of neuronal migration by RNAi of Dyx1c1 results in neocortical and hippocampal malformations. Cereb Cortex 17: 2562–2572.
15. Threlkeld SW, McClure MM, Bai J, Wang Y, LoTurco JJ, et al. (2007) Developmental disruptions and behavioral impairments in rats following in utero RNAi of Dyx1c1. Brain Res Bull 71: 508–514.
16. Szalkowski CE, Hinman JR, Threlkeld SW, Wang Y, LePack A, et al. (2011) Persistent spatial working memory deficits in rats following in utero RNAi of Dyx1c1. Genes Brain Behav 10: 244–252.
17. Meng H, Smith SD, Hager K, Held M, Liu J, et al. (2005) DCDC2 is associated with reading disability and modulates neuronal development in the brain. Proc Natl Acad Sci U S A 102: 17053–17058.
18. Burbridge TJ, Wang Y, Volz AJ, Peschansky VJ, Lisann L, et al. (2008) Postnatal analysis of the effect of embryonic knockdown and overexpression of candidate dyslexia susceptibility gene homolog Dcdc2 in the rat. Neuroscience 152: 723–733.
19. Paracchini S, Thomas A, Castro S, Lai C, Paramasivam M, et al. (2006) The chromosome 6p22 haplotype associated with dyslexia reduces the expression of KIAA0319, a novel gene involved in neuronal migration. Hum Mol Genet 15: 1659–1666.
20. Hannula-Jouppi K, Kaminen-Ahola N, Taipale M, Eklund R, Nopola-Hemmi J, et al. (2005) The axon guidance receptor gene ROBO1 is a candidate gene for developmental dyslexia. PLoS Genet 1: e50.
21. Andrews W, Liapi A, Plachez C, Camurri L, Zhang J, et al. (2006) Robo1 regulates the development of major axon tracts and interneuron migration in the forebrain. Development 133: 2243–2252.
22. Darki F, Peyrard-Janvid M, Matsson H, Kere J, Klingberg T (2012) Three Dyslexia Susceptibility Genes, DYX1C1, DCDC2, and KIAA0319, Affect Temporo-Parietal White Matter Structure. Biol Psychiatry 72: 671–676.
23. Massinen S, Tammimies K, Tapia-Paez I, Matsson H, Hokkanen ME, et al. (2009) Functional interaction of DYX1C1 with estrogen receptors suggests involvement of hormonal pathways in dyslexia. Hum Mol Genet 18: 2802–2812.
24. Massinen S, Hokkanen ME, Matsson H, Tammimies K, Tapia-Paez I, et al. (2011) Increased expression of the dyslexia candidate gene DCDC2 affects length and signaling of primary cilia in neurons. PLoS One 6: e20580.
25. Ibanez-Tallon I, Heintz N, Omran H (2003) To beat or not to beat: roles of cilia in development and disease. Hum Mol Genet 12: R27–35.
26. McGrath J, Somlo S, Makova S, Tian X, Brueckner M (2003) Two populations of node monocilia initiate left-right asymmetry in the mouse. Cell 114: 61–73.
27. Nonaka S, Tanaka Y, Okada Y, Takeda S, Harada A, et al. (1998) Randomization of left-right asymmetry due to loss of nodal cilia generating leftward flow of extraembryonic fluid in mice lacking KIF3B motor protein. Cell 95: 829–837.
28. Willaredt MA, Hasenpusch-Theil K, Gardner HA, Kitanovic I, Hirschfeld-Warneken VC, et al. (2008) A crucial role for primary cilia in cortical morphogenesis. J Neurosci 28: 12887–12900.
29. Breunig JJ, Arellano JI, Rakic P (2010) Cilia in the brain: going with the flow. Nat Neurosci 13: 654–655.
30. Badano JL, Mitsuma N, Beales PL, Katsanis N (2006) The ciliopathies: an emerging class of human genetic disorders. Annu Rev Genomics Hum Genet 7: 125–148.
31. Zhao C, Malicki J (2007) Genetic defects of pronephric cilia in zebrafish. Mech Dev 124: 605–616.
32. Westerfield M (1995) The Zebrafish Book: A guide for laboratory use of zebrafish (*Danio rerio*). Eugene: University of Oregon Press. 385 p.
33. Chandrasekar G, Archer A, Gustafsson JA, Andersson Lendahl M (2010) Levels of 17beta-estradiol receptors expressed in embryonic and adult zebrafish following in vivo treatment of natural or synthetic ligands. PLoS One 5: e9678.
34. Thisse B, Heyer V, Lux A, Alunni V, Degrave A, et al. (2004) Spatial and temporal expression of the zebrafish genome by large-scale in situ hybridization screening. Methods Cell Biol 77: 505–519.
35. Gamse JT, Shen YC, Thisse C, Thisse B, Raymond PA, et al. (2002) Otx5 regulates genes that show circadian expression in the zebrafish pineal complex. Nat Genet 30: 117–121.
36. Odenthal J, Nusslein-Volhard C (1998) fork head domain genes in zebrafish. Dev Genes Evol 208: 245–258.
37. Gamse JT, Kuan YS, Macurak M, Brosamle C, Thisse B, et al. (2005) Directional asymmetry of the zebrafish epithalamus guides dorsoventral innervation of the midbrain target. Development 132: 4869–4881.
38. Robu ME, Larson JD, Nasevicius A, Beiraghi S, Brenner C, et al. (2007) p53 activation by knockdown technologies. PLoS Genet 3: e78.
39. Yelon D, Horne SA, Stainier DY (1999) Restricted expression of cardiac myosin genes reveals regulated aspects of heart tube assembly in zebrafish. Dev Biol 214: 23–37.
40. Essner JJ, Amack JD, Nyholm MK, Harris EB, Yost HJ (2005) Kupffer's vesicle is a ciliated organ of asymmetry in the zebrafish embryo that initiates left-right development of the brain, heart and gut. Development 132: 1247–1260.
41. Kramer-Zucker AG, Olale F, Haycraft CJ, Yoder BK, Schier AF, et al. (2005) Cilia-driven fluid flow in the zebrafish pronephros, brain and Kupffer's vesicle is required for normal organogenesis. Development 132: 1907–1921.
42. Schidlow DV (1994) Primary ciliary dyskinesia (the immotile cilia syndrome). Ann Allergy 73: 457–468; quiz 468–470.

43. Blacque OE, Leroux MR (2006) Bardet-Biedl syndrome: an emerging pathomechanism of intracellular transport. Cell Mol Life Sci 63: 2145–2161.
44. Torres VE, Harris PC, Pirson Y (2007) Autosomal dominant polycystic kidney disease. Lancet 369: 1287–1301.
45. Hildebrandt F, Zhou W (2007) Nephronophthisis-associated ciliopathies. J Am Soc Nephrol 18: 1855–1871.
46. Cantagrel V, Silhavy JL, Bielas SL, Swistun D, Marsh SE, et al. (2008) Mutations in the cilia gene ARL13B lead to the classical form of Joubert syndrome. Am J Hum Genet 83: 170–179.
47. Drummond IA, Majumdar A, Hentschel H, Elger M, Solnica-Krezel L, et al. (1998) Early development of the zebrafish pronephros and analysis of mutations affecting pronephric function. Development 125: 4655–4667.
48. Sun Z, Amsterdam A, Pazour GJ, Cole DG, Miller MS, et al. (2004) A genetic screen in zebrafish identifies cilia genes as a principal cause of cystic kidney. Development 131: 4085–4093.
49. Pathak N, Obara T, Mangos S, Liu Y, Drummond IA (2007) The zebrafish fleer gene encodes an essential regulator of cilia tubulin polyglutamylation. Mol Biol Cell 18: 4353–4364.
50. Omori Y, Zhao C, Saras A, Mukhopadhyay S, Kim W, et al. (2008) Elipsa is an early determinant of ciliogenesis that links the IFT particle to membrane-associated small GTPase Rab8. Nat Cell Biol 10: 437–444.
51. Sullivan-Brown J, Schottenfeld J, Okabe N, Hostetter CL, Serluca FC, et al. (2008) Zebrafish mutations affecting cilia motility share similar cystic phenotypes and suggest a mechanism of cyst formation that differs from pkd2 morphants. Dev Biol 314: 261–275.
52. Torikata C, Kijimoto C, Koto M (1991) Ultrastructure of respiratory cilia of WIC-Hyd male rats. An animal model for human immotile cilia syndrome. Am J Pathol 138: 341–347.
53. Ibanez-Tallon I, Pagenstecher A, Fliegauf M, Olbrich H, Kispert A, et al. (2004) Dysfunction of axonemal dynein heavy chain Mdnah5 inhibits ependymal flow and reveals a novel mechanism for hydrocephalus formation. Hum Mol Genet 13: 2133–2141.
54. Obara T, Mangos S, Liu Y, Zhao J, Wiessner S, et al. (2006) Polycystin-2 immunolocalization and function in zebrafish. J Am Soc Nephrol 17: 2706–2718.
55. Greenstone MA, Jones RW, Dewar A, Neville BG, Cole PJ (1984) Hydrocephalus and primary ciliary dyskinesia. Arch Dis Child 59: 481–482.
56. Balci S, Bostanoglu S, Altinok G, Ozaltin F (1999) Sibs diagnosed prenatally with situs inversus totalis, renal and pancreatic dysplasia, and cysts: a new syndrome? Am J Med Genet 82: 166–169.
57. Praetorius HA, Spring KR (2001) Bending the MDCK cell primary cilium increases intracellular calcium. J Membr Biol 184: 71–79.
58. Supp DM, Witte DP, Potter SS, Brueckner M (1997) Mutation of an axonemal dynein affects left-right asymmetry in inversus viscerum mice. Nature 389: 963–966.
59. Kennedy MP, Omran H, Leigh MW, Dell S, Morgan L, et al. (2007) Congenital heart disease and other heterotaxic defects in a large cohort of patients with primary ciliary dyskinesia. Circulation 115: 2814–2821.
60. Lopes SS, Lourenco R, Pacheco L, Moreno N, Kreiling J, et al. (2010) Notch signalling regulates left-right asymmetry through ciliary length control. Development 137: 3625–3632.
61. Merveille AC, Davis EE, Becker-Heck A, Legendre M, Amirav I, et al. (2011) CCDC39 is required for assembly of inner dynein arms and the dynein regulatory complex and for normal ciliary motility in humans and dogs. Nat Genet 43: 72–78.
62. Lee JE, Silhavy JL, Zaki MS, Schroth J, Bielas SL, et al. (2012) CEP41 is mutated in Joubert syndrome and is required for tubulin glutamylation at the cilium. Nat Genet 44: 193–199.
63. Mitchison HM, Schmidts M, Loges NT, Freshour J, Dritsoula A, et al. (2012) Mutations in axonemal dynein assembly factor DNAAF3 cause primary ciliary dyskinesia. Nat Genet 44: 381–389, S381–382.
64. Panizzi JR, Becker-Heck A, Castleman VH, Al-Mutairi DA, Liu Y, et al. (2012) CCDC103 mutations cause primary ciliary dyskinesia by disrupting assembly of ciliary dynein arms. Nat Genet 44: 714–719.
65. Gao C, Wang G, Amack JD, Mitchell DR (2010) Oda16/Wdr69 is essential for axonemal dynein assembly and ciliary motility during zebrafish embryogenesis. Dev Dyn 239: 2190–2197.
66. Ahmed NT, Mitchell DR (2005) ODA16p, a Chlamydomonas flagellar protein needed for dynein assembly. Mol Biol Cell 16: 5004–5012.
67. Ahmed NT, Gao C, Lucker BF, Cole DG, Mitchell DR (2008) ODA16 aids axonemal outer row dynein assembly through an interaction with the intraflagellar transport machinery. J Cell Biol 183: 313–322.
68. Liang P, MacRae TH (1997) Molecular chaperones and the cytoskeleton. J Cell Sci 110: 1431–1440.
69. Chen Y, Zhao M, Wang S, Chen J, Wang Y, et al. (2009) A novel role for DYX1C1, a chaperone protein for both Hsp70 and Hsp90, in breast cancer. J Cancer Res Clin Oncol 135: 1265–1276.
70. Tammimies K, Vitezic M, Matsson H, Le Guyader S, Burglin TR, et al. (2013) Molecular networks of DYX1C1 gene show connection to neuronal migration genes and cytoskeletal proteins. Biol Psychiatry 73: 583–590.
71. Ivliev AE, t Hoen PA, van Roon-Mom WM, Peters DJ, Sergeeva MG (2012) Exploring the transcriptome of ciliated cells using in silico dissection of human tissues. PLoS One 7: e35618.
72. Li JB, Gerdes JM, Haycraft CJ, Fan Y, Teslovich TM, et al. (2004) Comparative genomics identifies a flagellar and basal body proteome that includes the BBS5 human disease gene. Cell 117: 541–552.
73. Hoh RA, Stowe TR, Turk E, Stearns T (2012) Transcriptional program of ciliated epithelial cells reveals new cilium and centrosome components and links to human disease. PLoS One 7: e52166.
74. Gorivodsky M, Mukhopadhyay M, Wilsch-Braeuninger M, Phillips M, Teufel A, et al. (2009) Intraflagellar transport protein 172 is essential for primary cilia formation and plays a vital role in patterning the mammalian brain. Dev Biol 325: 24–32.
75. Louvi A, Grove EA (2011) Cilia in the CNS: the quiet organelle claims center stage. Neuron 69: 1046–1060.
76. Arellano JI, Guadiana SM, Breunig JJ, Rakic P, Sarkisian MR (2012) Development and distribution of neuronal cilia in mouse neocortex. J Comp Neurol 520: 848–873.
77. Wynshaw-Boris A, Gambello MJ (2001) LIS1 and dynein motor function in neuronal migration and development. Genes Dev 15: 639–651.

8

Dyslexia Impairs Speech Recognition but Can Spare Phonological Competence

Iris Berent[1]*, Vered Vaknin-Nusbaum[2], Evan Balaban[3], Albert M. Galaburda[4]

1 Department of Psychology, Northeastern University, Boston, Massachusetts, United States of America, **2** Western Galilee College, Akko & Univeristy of Haifa, Haifa, Israel, **3** Department of Psychology, McGill University, Montreal, Canada, **4** Department of Neurology, Division of Cognitive Neurology, Harvard Medical School, Beth Israel Deaconess Medical Center, Boston, Massachusetts, United States of America

Abstract

Dyslexia is associated with numerous deficits to speech processing. Accordingly, a large literature asserts that dyslexics manifest a phonological deficit. Few studies, however, have assessed the phonological grammar of dyslexics, and none has distinguished a phonological deficit from a phonetic impairment. Here, we show that these two sources can be dissociated. Three experiments demonstrate that a group of adult dyslexics studied here is impaired in phonetic discrimination (e.g., *ba* vs. *pa*), and their deficit compromises even the basic ability to identify acoustic stimuli as human speech. Remarkably, the ability of these individuals to generalize grammatical phonological rules is intact. Like typical readers, these Hebrew-speaking dyslexics identified ill-formed AAB stems (e.g., *titug*) as less wordlike than well-formed ABB controls (e.g., *gitut*), and both groups automatically extended this rule to nonspeech stimuli, irrespective of reading ability. The contrast between the phonetic and phonological capacities of these individuals demonstrates that the algebraic engine that generates phonological patterns is distinct from the phonetic interface that implements them. While dyslexia compromises the phonetic system, certain core aspects of the phonological grammar can be spared.

Editor: Kevin Paterson, University of Leicester, United Kingdom

Funding: This research was supported by National Institute on Deafness and Other Communication Disorders grant R01DC003277 to IB, Canadian Fund for Innovation 9908 to EB and National Insitutes of Health grant HD057853 to AMG. The funders had no role in study design, data collection and analysis, decision to publish, or preparation of the manuscript.

Competing Interests: The authors have declared that no competing interests exist.

* E-mail: i.berent@neu.edu

Introduction

Developmental dyslexia is a reading disability, defined as a difficulty in acquiring reading skill that is unexplained by intellectual, emotional or social factors [1]. Although dyslexia is first and foremost a reading impairment, it is frequently associated with difficulties in spoken language processing [1–3], including subtle abnormalities in the recognition of spoken words (e.g., contrasting *bin* and *pin* [4–14], their maintenance in memory [15], their discrimination from nonspeech [16], and the gaining of conscious awareness of word internal structure (e.g., the initial sound in *pin* [17,18]). Moreover, these impairments already manifest themselves in early development, well before reading difficulties are evident [19–21].

In view of these widely documented difficulties in processing the sound structure of language–both printed [22,23] and spoken [4–6,15,16]–many researchers have asserted that dyslexics manifest a deficit that compromises the core of the phonological system [1,5,15,16,24–28]. The support for this hypothesis, however, has been rather mixed. This is by no means due to a paucity of evidence. Hundreds of studies have attempted to gauge the phonological competence of dyslexic individuals by exploring their capacity to process speech. To date, however, no aspect of speech processing has been found to be impaired in all dyslexic individuals [29]. The divergence among studies undoubtedly results from multiple sources, including methodological factors (e.g., different task demands on attention, working memory, meta-linguistic skills, [30]). Here, however, we would like to explore the possibility that the divergence might originate from the definition of the phonological system itself.

Many researchers identify phonology with speech processing. For example, a recent review paper by Ramus and Ahissar ([29], p. 3) defines phonology as "the mental representation and processing of speech sounds, both in perception and in production". Similarly, Perrachione and colleagues [16] view phonology as the system that allows people to distinguish between the voices of different talkers. Accordingly, any deficit to the processing of speech sounds would indicate a phonological deficit, and such deficits could potentially encompass a vast gamut, ranging from the formation of phonetic categories to the extraction of phonological regularities–either statistical knowledge of language-particular phonotactic, or universal grammatical constraints.

But the equation of phonology with speech processing is theoretically unmotivated. Most linguistic accounts assume that the patterning of speech sounds engages at least two linguistic systems: the phonological grammar and the phonetic interface [31–33]. The phonological grammar is a system of productive algebraic rules that compute the structure of discrete meaningless linguistic primitives (e.g., phonemes, syllables [34–36]). While, in hearing communities, phonology is typically externalized as speech, phonological structure is an amodal pattern of meaningless linguistic elements, rather than speech sounds, specifically. And indeed, sign languages manifest phonological organization akin to the structure of spoken languages [37] and recent research has shown that phonological structure can even emerge spontaneously in nascent sign languages [38,39].

The human capacity to form comparable phonological patterns across modalities is explained by the abstract algebraic nature of phonological rules. Like syntactic rules, phonological generalizations demonstrably extend across the board, to novel phonological elements [40]. For example, consider voicing agreement in English. English requires that the suffix agrees with the stem's final consonant on the voicing feature: stems ending with a voiceless consonant (e.g., ***cat***) take a voiceless suffix/kæts/; elsewhere, the suffix is voiced (e.g.,/dogz/; [41]). Crucially, English speakers extend this restriction not only to novel words (e.g.,/zɛgz/vs./zɛps/) but even to novel phonemes (e.g., Bachs/bɑxs/, not/bɑxz/, [42]). While languages differ in the specific phonological structures that they manifest–English, for example, allows *blogs*, not *lbogs* whereas Russian tolerates both–modern linguistic theory has shown that the phonological grammars of different language share common representational primitives and constraints [34,43], and these conclusions are borne out by experimental evidence. For example, across languages, syllables like *blog* are preferred to *lbog*, and experimental studies have shown that speakers of different languages converge on the same preferences even when both types of syllables are unattested in their own language [44]. The universality of phonological knowledge, its spontaneous regenesis, early developmental onset and its role in shaping reading and writing are all consistent with the view of the phonological grammar as a biological system of core knowledge [36].

While the phonological grammar computes abstract, algebraic representations, the phonetic system is an interface dedicated to the mapping of those abstract patterns onto a specific sensorimotor modality–either speech sounds (in spoken language) or manual gestures (for signs). Unlike the discrete and algebraic phonological representations, phonetic representations are analog and continuous [32,45]. For example, the English phonological system distinguishes *big* from *pig* by a binary contrast in the voicing feature (*big* is voiced, *pig* is not), whereas the phonetic system encodes the specific voice onset time (VOT) that characterizes specific *pig* tokens (e.g., a VOT of 60 ms. vs. 155 ms., [33,46]) and registers subtle variations in the implementation of this contrast across talkers and utterances [47,48].

In view of this analysis, it is clear that the speech-processing deficit in dyslexia might have multiple linguistic origins (as well as nonlinguistic ones). To probe for a phonological deficit, it is therefore necessary to rule out the phonetic system as the source of the observed impairment. Doing so presents formidable empirical challenges, as the phonological and phonetic systems are clearly interdependent. The extraction of phonological patterns hinges on phonetic analysis, whereas a deficit in the phonological system can be partly compensated for by retrieving stored phonetic tokens of familiar words. Nonetheless, one could dissociate the phonological and phonetic systems by exploiting their distinct computational properties. While intact algebraic phonological knowledge should allow participants to extend the relevant generalizations across the board–to novel words and novel phonological elements, intact phonetic knowledge would support the extraction of detailed variation within phonetic categories. Conversely, a congenital phonological deficit should compromise the generalization of phonological principles, especially principles that are putatively universal, whereas a phonetic deficit should impair fine distinctions between phonetic exemplars. Armed with this yardstick, we can now proceed to determine whether the difficulties of dyslexics in spoken language processing are due to the phonological grammar, the phonetic system, or both.

Surprisingly, only a handful of studies have specifically addressed the phonological grammar in dyslexia [49–52]. While some of these reports note differences between dyslexics and controls [49,50], these studies did not systematically gauge the phonetic abilities of participants. Accordingly, one cannot determine whether the observed deficits result from the phonological grammar or from a phonetic impairment. Only one previous study has systematically examined both phonological and phonetic abilities [8]. The results indicated that Dutch dyslexic children overly relied on word context in extracting phonetic speech categories, but their sensitivity to the phonological process of place assimilation was intact (e.g., *tui**n**bank*→*tui**m**bank*, 'garden chair'). The findings of this pioneering study hint at the possibility that phonological and phonetic systems might dissociate in dyslexia. Unfortunately, however, the assessment of the phonological grammar was based on responses to a single pair of familiar words. The hallmark of grammatical phonological knowledge, however, is productivity–the ability to extend linguistic regularities to novel items [32]. No previous study has systematically examined the capacity of dyslexic individuals to productively generalize their phonological knowledge and dissociate it from phonetic sensitivity.

The present research seeks to clarify the origins of the speech-processing deficit in dyslexia. To this end, we systematically evaluate the state of the phonological grammar in dyslexia and dissociate it from the phonetic interface. Our investigation of grammatical phonological generalizations targets a fundamental phonological principle that restricts the occurrence of identical phonological elements. Identity restrictions have been documented in many human languages–both spoken [53–59] and signed [60]- and they manifest themselves in a host of phonological phenomena, ranging from the above-mentioned case of voicing agreement (cf., dogz/vs./kæts/) to sonority restrictions [61]. Their precursors are evident practically at birth [62,63]. In view of its early onset and generality across languages and modalities, the restriction on identical phonological elements is likely to reflect a universal grammatical principle that is central to the phonological system [36]. Here, we ask whether this broad phonological rule is spared in dyslexia, and whether it is dissociable from a phonetic impairment.

As a specific case study, we gauge the restriction on identical consonants in Hebrew. Like other Semitic languages, Hebrew systematically restricts the location of identical consonants in the stem. It allows identical consonants to occur at the right edge of the stem (ABB, e.g., *simum*), but bans them at the left edge [64] (AAB, e.g., *sisum*). Although Hebrew speakers are not consciously aware of this regularity [65], they nonetheless freely generalize this tacit restriction to novel stems, including stems with novel phonemes [40,65–69]. Moreover, computational simulations demonstrate that such generalizations are unattainable by various computational mechanisms that lack algebraic rules [70,71]. Together, these findings suggest that the restrictions on identical stem consonants are encoded by an algebraic rule (e.g., *AAB, where * indicates a ban, and A and B stand for any phoneme) that is core to the phonological grammar. Of interest is whether this rule is intact in the phonological grammar of dyslexics.

Experiments 1–2 address this question using a simple discrimination task. Participants in Experiment 1 were presented with spoken words–either existing Hebrew words (e.g., *tipul*, treatment), or novel words, matched to the words with respect to their vowel pattern (e.g., *titug*), and they were asked to quickly indicate whether each stimulus was a real word (i.e., a lexical-decision task). In Experiment 2, the same nonword stimuli were mixed with nonspeech analogs, generated by electronically manipulating those speech inputs, and participants made a simple forced choice as to whether the stimulus was speech or non-speech. Our main phonological manipulation concerns the structure of nonword stimuli. Nonwords were composed of three types–either ill-formed AAB stems (e.g., *titug*), or well-formed ABB and ABC controls (e.g., *gitut* and *gitul*). We reasoned that, if dyslexics accurately encode the algebraic ban on *AAB forms, then this knowledge should be evident in their responses to nonwords. AAB nonwords should be rendered ill-formed, hence, they should be identified as nonwords more quickly and more accurately than well-formed controls.

Finding that dyslexics can freely generalize the phonological restrictions on stem structure would suggest that any speech-processing deficits exhibited by these participants originate from impairments to the phonetic interface, not the phonological grammar. Our experiments probe for this possibility in multiple ways. Experiments 1–2 test the gross phonetic capacities of these individuals by evaluating their ability to discriminate spoken linguistic stimuli–either the discrimination of words from non-words (in Experiment 1) or speech from nonspeech (in Experiment 2). Experiment 3 directly probes for a phonetic impairment by gauging the structure of their phonetic categories. Here, participants were presented with four speech-continua that progressively varied between two syllables that contrasted by a single phoneme–either a consonant (e.g., *ba-pa*; *da-ta*) or a vowel (e.g., *a-e*, *o-u*) and they were tested for their ability to identify these phonetic stimuli and discriminate between them. Of interest is whether dyslexic participants are impaired in phonetic identification and discrimination despite their demonstrably full sensitivity to the relevant phonological rules. To the extent that the phonological and phonetic systems dissociate, this would introduce the novel notion that dyslexia impairs the phonetic interface but spares at least some important aspects of the phonological system of core algebraic rules.

Results

Reading Tests

Before we consider the phonological grammar of our dyslexic participants, we first gauged their reading ability by examining their capacity to decode phonological structure from print. To this end, we administered participants three Hebrew reading tests that assess phonological decoding, and their errors and speed were recorded. A series of independent samples t-tests (see Table 1) demonstrated that performance of dyslexics was reliably impaired on all tests. These results converge with many past findings to indicate that dyslexics manifest difficulties in decoding the phonological structure of printed words [1,22,23].

Experiment 1 (Lexical Decision)

In view of the difficulties of dyslexic participants in decoding phonological structure from print, we next moved to examine whether their deficits originate from impairment to the grammatical phonological encoding of spoken language.

A comparison of the ability of dyslexic individuals and controls to discriminate spoken words and nonwords showed that dyslexics are indeed impaired in processing spoken language. Compared to controls, dyslexic participants exhibited an attenuated discrimination (d′, $t1(40) = 2.88$, $p < .007$, see Figure 1a; for individual subject data, see Figure S1). Our main interest concerns the source of this impairment–whether it results from a deficit in the phonological grammar, or deficits to subsidiary phonetic or auditory processing.

To gauge the grammatical competence of dyslexics, we compared the sensitivity of dyslexic and skilled readers to the grammatical structure of novel Hebrew stems (nonwords). A grammatical deficit should decrease the ability of dyslexic individuals to distinguish novel, ill-formed AAB stems from well-formed ABB and ABC controls.

To address this possibility, we submitted the response time and error data (arcsine transformed, see Table 2) to nonwords to 3 stem type (AAB/ABB/ABC)×2 group (dyslexic vs. controls) ANOVAs, conducted using both participants and items as random effects (stem type was manipulated within participants and items; group was manipulated between participants and within items; for individual subject data, see Figure S2). These analyses yielded a significant main effect of stem-type on response time ($F1(2, 80) = 37.96$, $p < .0001$; $F(2, 54) = 10.01$, $p < .0002$; for errors: $F1(2, 80) = 4.63$, $p < .02$; $F(2, 54) = 1.25$, $p > .30$). Planned comparisons showed that AAB nonwords elicited faster responses than well-formed control nonwords with ABB ($t1(42) = 2.12$, $p < .04$, $t2(80) = 1.99$, $p < .06$) or ABC stems ($t1(42) = 8.38$, $p < .0001$, $t2(80) = 4.48$, $p < .0001$, Figure 1b). In addition, ABB stems elicited faster responses than ABC controls ($t1(42) = 6.26$, $p < .0001$, $t2(80) = 2.49$, $p < .02$). The same ANOVAs also yielded a main effect of group (In errors: $F(1, 40) = 5.66$, $p < .03$; $F2(1, 27) = 46.93$, $p < .0001$; In response time: $F1 < 1$; $F2(1, 27) = 1.07$, $p > .31$) due to the higher error rate of dyslexic individuals. These effects, however, did not interact, indicating that stem-structure affects both dyslexic individuals and controls, irrespective of reading ability (for the interaction, all $F < 1.16$, $p > .32$ in both response time and errors).

The results of Experiment 1 offer initial evidence that dyslexic participants are sensitive to phonological rules. Like skilled readers, dyslexics were faster to classify ill-formed AAB stems as nonwords relative to well-formed controls–either AAB or ABC. These two contrasts–the AAB-ABB and AAB-ABC could conceivably result from different sources, so their interpretation requires some caution. Because our word stimuli were mostly ABC stems (see Methods), reduplication can be used to predict the status of the stimulus as nonword. Accordingly, dyslexics' full sensitivity to the AAB-ABC contrast only suggests their intact ability to encode phonological representations, but it does not necessarily reflect grammatical constraints on their structure. However, participants in our experiments were sensitive not only to the presence of reduplication, but crucially, they further constrained its location: they were faster to respond to ill-formed AAB nonwords than to well-formed ABB controls. Unlike the across-the-board effect of reduplication, this productive restriction on its location can only be informed by linguistic rules. Our results thus suggest that grammatical phonological knowledge of stem structure appears to be preserved in dyslexics despite their difficulties in phonological decoding from print and in gross aspects of speech processing.

Experiment 2 (Speech/Nonspeech Discrimination)

The intact sensitivity of dyslexics to phonological rules suggests that their difficulties with spoken word recognition might originate from a phonetic source, rather than from a grammatical phonological deficit. Experiment 2 further tested this possibility by gauging the ability of dyslexics to recognize human speech (the same nonwords used in Experiment 1) from their matched nonspeech analogs, generated from these same speech stimuli. Our analyses first assess the capacity of the two groups to discriminate speech from nonspeech, followed by separate analysis of their sensitivity to the structure of speech and nonspeech stimuli.

Speech-nonspeech discrimination. A comparison of the sensitivity (d′) of participants to the status of our stimuli (speech/nonspeech) showed that dyslexics were impaired in speech/nonspeech discrimination (d′) compared to skilled readers ($t1(34) = 2.18$, $p < .04$; $t2(29) = 4.07$, $p < .0004$, see Figure 2A; the two groups did

Table 1. Reading scores of dyslexic and control participants in Experiments 1–3.

Experiment	Population	N	Gender (# of females)	Task							
				Pseudoword reading		Homophone reading		Text 1 (without diacritics)		Text 2 (with diacritics)	
				Response time (minutes)	Error	Response time (minutes)	Error	Response time (minutes)	Error	Response time (minutes)	Error
1	Skilled	21	13	1.09	0.90	2.38	0.24	0.53	0.38	0.53	0.29
	Dyslexic	21	16	1.40	7.33	2.75	3.29	0.78	1.43	0.67	1.57
	t(40)			2.53	9.97	1.46	3.63	3.28	3.23	1.88	5.69
	p			0.0155	0.0000	0.1527	0.0008	0.0022	0.0025	0.0681	0.0000
2	Skilled	18	15	1.08	0.67	2.49	0.33	0.52	0.22	0.49	0.06
	Dyslexics	18	13	1.43	7.11	2.80	3.61	0.80	1.56	0.70	1.50
	t(34)			2.59	9.34	1.16	3.47	3.36	4.03	2.58	7.47
	p			0.0140	0.0000	0.2549	0.0014	0.0020	0.0003	0.0144	0.0000
3	Skilled	19	12	1.12	1.63	2.31	0.68	0.57	0.37	0.58	0.37
	Dyslexics	21	14	1.46	7.19	2.91	2.76	0.79	1.57	0.67	1.52
	t(38)			2.35	8.12	2.08	3.52	2.51	3.33	1.02	4.62
	p			0.0242	0.0000	0.0440	0.0011	0.0165	0.0020	0.3122	0.0000

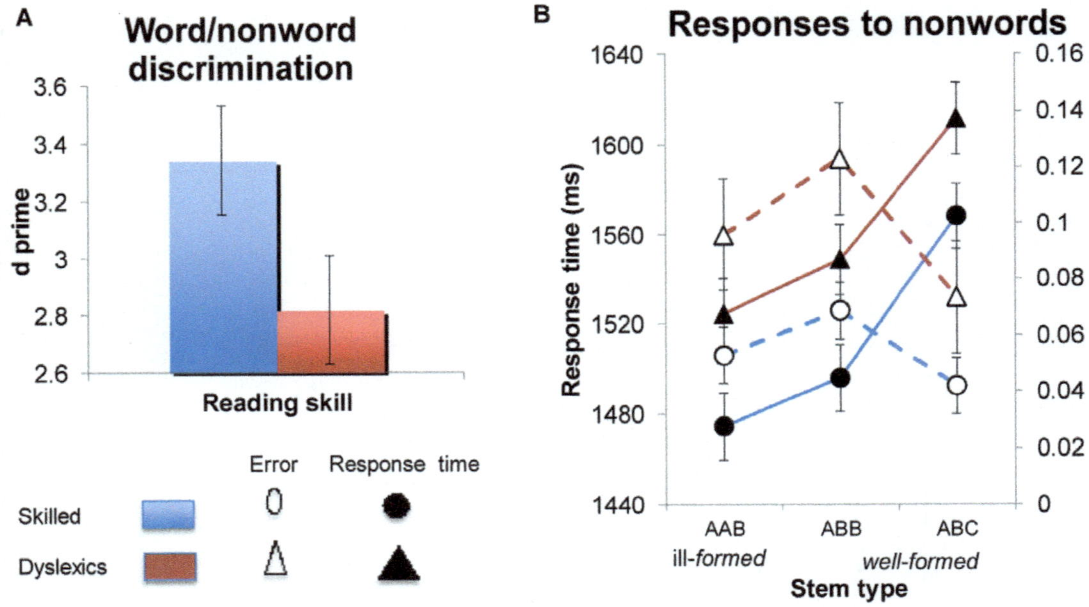

Figure 1. Word/nonword discrimination. (A) Discrimination (d′) by dyslexics and skilled readers (controls). (B) The sensitivity of dyslexics and controls to the phonological structure of Hebrew stems in the discrimination of auditory nonwords from words (Error bars are confidence intervals for the difference between the means).

not differ reliably on response time to either speech ($t1(34)<1$, $t2(29)=8.24$, $p<.0001$) or (nonspeech $t1(34)=1.24$, $p>.22$, $t2(29)=12.47$, $p<.0001$; for individual subject data, see Figure S3). Remarkably, however, this basic deficit in speech discrimination does not taint the phonological grammar. The evidence, once again, comes from the effect of stem-structure.

We reasoned that ill-formed stimuli (speech and nonspeech) should be easier to ignore, and consequently, an intact grammar should process the speech-status of ill-formed AAB stimuli more rapidly than well-formed controls–a prediction borne out by past research with typical readers [72]. Our question here is whether dyslexics automatically apply this phonological rule despite its irrelevance to the experimental task–speech recognition–and even when the auditory stimuli are not identified as human speech.

To examine this question, we submitted the speech-nonspeech discrimination (d′) and response time data to 2 group x 3 stem-type ANOVAs. As in Experiment 1, group was manipulated between participants and within items; stem-type was varied within participants and items. The 2 group×3 stem-type ANOVAs on speech-nonspeech discrimination (d′) again yielded no interaction ($F<1$; the error means are provided in Table 3)[a]. The same interaction also did not approach significance when response times to speech stimuli were analyzed separately (all $F<1$), nor was the main effect of group significant across participants ($F1<1$; $F2(1, 29)=67.96$, $p<.0001$). To directly assess the sensitivity of dyslexic and control subjects to the grammatical restriction on stem structure, we next turned to analyze their response times to speech and nonspeech stimuli.

Response time to speech stimuli. The 2 group×3 stem type ANOVAs on response time to speech stimuli yielded marginally significant main effects of stem-type ($F1(2,68)=4.64$, $p<.02$, $F2(2, 29)=2.20$, $p<.13$). This effect of stem type was not further modulated by group (both $F<1$) nor was the main effect of group reliable across participants ($F1(1, 34)<1$; $F2(1, 29)<67.96$, $p<.0001$). Planned comparisons showed that dyslexics and controls both identified ill-formed AAB speech stimuli more rapidly than well-formed ABC controls ($t1(68)=2.96$, $p<.005$; $t2(58)=2.05$, $p<.05$; Figure 2B; for individual subject data, see Figure S4).

Response time to nonspeech stimuli. To determine whether dyslexics (and skilled readers) are sensitive to the phonological structure of nonspeech stimuli, we next submitted the response times to nonspeech stimuli to 2 group×3 stem-type ANOVAs. The main effect of group was not significant across participants ($F1(1, 34)=1.55$, $p<.23$; $F2(1, 29)=155.50$, $p<.0001$). However, the main effect of stem type was significant ($F1(2, 34)=6.00$, $p<.005$; $F2(2, 58)=3.18$, $p<.05$), and its interaction with group was likewise marginally significant ($F1(2, 68)=2.80$, $p<.07$; $F2(2, 58)=3.27$, $p<.05$).

To determine the source of this interaction, we next proceeded to gauge the sensitivity of the two groups to well-formedness (the AAB vs. ABB contrast) and the structure of well-formed stems (the ABB vs. ABC contrast) by testing for these simple interactions (2 group x 2 stem-type) separately.

Reading skill did not modulate the effect of well-formedness (both $F<1$, for the 2 (AAB/ABB)×group interaction), and the main effect of reading skill was not reliable across participants ($F1(1, 34)=1.17$, $p>.29$; $F2(1, 29)=155.5$, $p<.0001$). Thus, both groups identified AAB nonspeech stimuli more readily than ABB counterparts ($F1(1, 34)=13.34$, $p<.001$; $F2(1, 29)=5.72$, $p<.03$).

Table 2. Accuracy (proportion errors) of skilled and dyslexic participants in word/nonword discrimination (Experiment 1).

		Skilled readers	Dyslexics
Words		0.0574	0.0965
Nonwords	AAB	0.0528	0.0959
	ABB	0.0685	0.123
	ABC	0.0419	0.0734

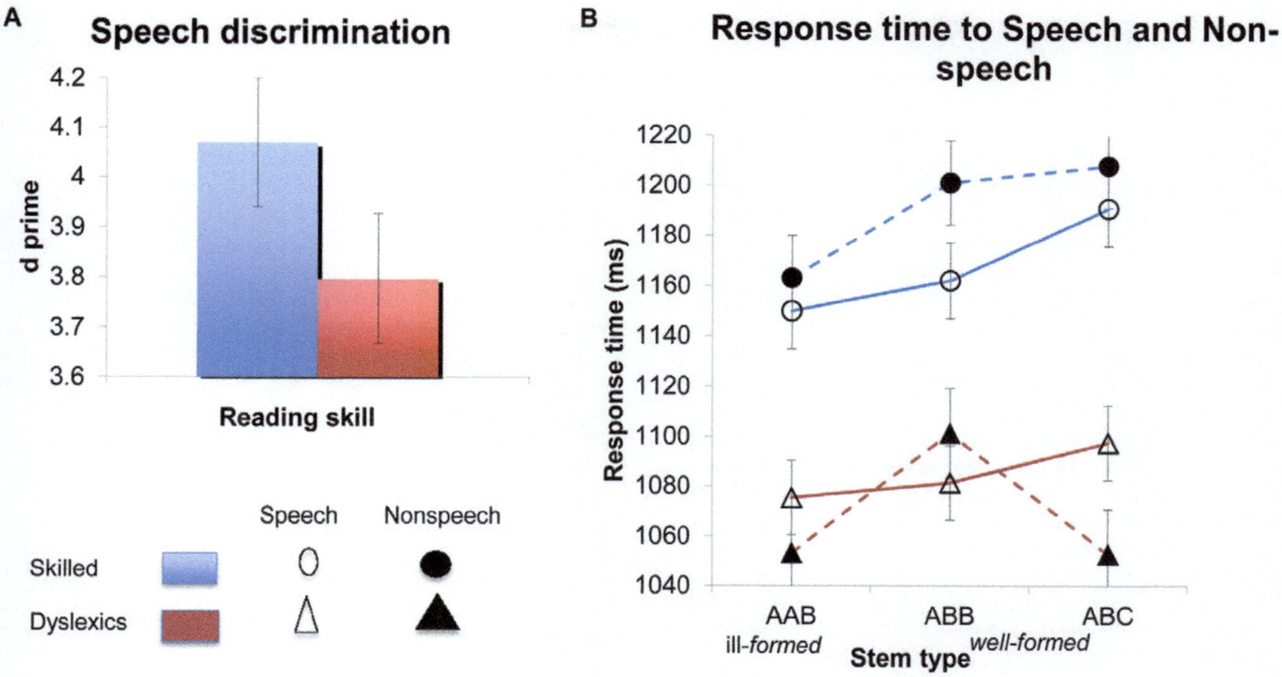

Figure 2. Speech-nonspeech discrimination. (A) Discrimination (d') by dyslexics and skilled readers (controls). (B) The sensitivity of dyslexics and controls to the phonological structure of Hebrew stems in a speech discrimination task (Error bars are confidence intervals for the difference between the means).

The easier identification of AAB stems–speech and nonspeech–suggests that phonological ill-formedness indeed renders these stimuli easier to ignore. Dyslexics' sensitivity to ill-formedness is remarkable because it implies that, like typical readers, their grammar automatically computes phonological structure even when it is irrelevant to the task, and even when the inputs are not consciously identified as human speech. Nonetheless, dyslexics were less sensitive to the structure of well-formed nonspeech stimuli.

A 2 group×2 (ABB/ABC) ANOVA on the responses to nonspeech stimuli yielded a reliable interaction ($F1(1, 34) = 4.47$, $p < .05$; $F2(1, 29) = 5.20$, $p < .04$). Because both ABB and ABC structures are well-formed, the enhanced sensitivity of dyslexics to their structure is unlikely to result from a deficit to their phonological grammar. Instead, this effect probably originates from the structure of their lexicon. Unlike ABB structures, whose well-formedness can be discerned from grammatical rules [40], the resemblance of ABC nonwords to Hebrew words must rely on lexical analogy (akin to analogizing *pake* to the English *bake*). For skilled readers, grammatical and lexical constraints were both operative, as responses to ABB and ABC nonspeech stimuli did not differ ($t < 1$). Dyslexics, however, classified ABC nonspeech stimuli more readily than ABB nonspeech controls ($t1(34) = 2.62$, $p < .02$; $t2(29) = 2.78$, $p < .01$), suggesting an attenuation in lexical analogy–a result consistent with the lexical discrimination deficit found in Experiment 1.

Table 3. Accuracy (proportion errors) of skilled and dyslexic participants in speech/nonspeech discrimination (Experiment 2).

		Stem type	Skilled readers	Dyslexics
Errors	*Speech*	AAB	0.0019	0.015
		ABB	0.0037	0.0167
		ABC	0.0056	0.0186
	Nonspeech	AAB	0.026	0.0432
		ABB	0.0316	0.0582
		ABC	0.0093	0.0261
d prime		AAB	4.08	3.82
		ABB	4.01	3.7
		ABC	4.12	3.88

Experiment 3 (Phonetic Discrimination/Identification)

Why are dyslexics impaired in speech discrimination and lexical access? While lexical access might be independently impaired in dyslexia, and the results of Experiment 2 provide some support for this possibility, lexical deficits alone cannot explain why dyslexic participants were impaired in speech/nonspeech discrimination. Since our results yielded no evidence for a grammatical phonological impairment, and our manipulations imposed only minimal demands on memory and attention, the persistent difficulties in both word/nonword and speech/nonspeech discrimination are likewise not due to resource limitations (e.g., in memory and attention). Our results, however, can be readily explained by the hypothesis that dyslexic participants manifest an impairment that affects the phonetic system. Indeed, a deficit in the formation of phonetic categories (e.g., *b* vs. *p*) will blur the recognition of speech and may impair lexical access. These two deficits might further interact, and such an interaction would explain why dyslexics showed attenuation in lexical analogy (gauged by the ABB/ABC contrast) with the phonetically-challenging nonspeech stimuli (in Experiment 2), but not with natural speech (in Experiment 1).

To probe for a phonetic deficit, we next presented our participants with two standard phonetic tasks. These tasks featured four 10-step speech continua. Each continuum varied progressively between two syllables that differed by a single phoneme– either a consonant (*ba-pa* and *da-ta*) or a vowel (*o-u* and *a-e*). In the identification task, participants were presented with a single step along the continuum, and they were asked to identify it (e.g., did you hear *ba* or *pa*?). In the discrimination task (ABX), participants were presented with two syllables (A & B) followed by a third syllable X, and they were asked to determine whether X was identical to A or B. If the speech processing deficit in dyslexia originates from a phonetic impairment, then, despite their full grammatical sensitivity, these same dyslexic individuals will manifest abnormalities in the identification of phonetic categories and their discrimination.

a. Identification results. Figure 3 plots the identification functions of dyslexic and control participants for our four continua (for individual subject data, see Figures S5, S6, S7, S8). An inspection of the means suggests that participants generally categorized the continua endpoints as intended (e.g., as *ba* vs. *pa*), and their identification varied systematically along the continua-steps. Of interest is whether the identification functions of dyslexic and skilled readers differed.

To address this question, we compared the performance of dyslexic and skilled readers for each of the four continua using separate mixed effects logit models, with group and continuum step as fixed effects (sum-coded), and participant as a random effect. We evaluated the group x continuum-step interaction by testing whether the interaction term improved the model's fit relative to a model in which these two factors were additive[b]. These tests indicated that the interaction was not reliable for either the *ba-pa* ($\chi(9)^2 = 8.81$, $p>.45$, n.s.) or *a-e* continua ($\chi(9)^2 = 8.88$, $p>.45$). For the *o-u* continuum, however, the test of the interaction was significant ($\chi(9)^2 = 25.07$, $p<.003$).

An inspection of the means suggested that dyslexics were less likely to identify the *u* endpoint as such, and they were also less likely to identify the *o* endpoint as intended. Pair-wise comparisons of dyslexic and skilled readers found that these differences were significant in step 8 ($\beta = 1.10$, $Z = 2.01$, $p<.05$) and step 9 ($\beta = 1.45$, $Z = 2.18$, $p<.03$), and marginally so in step 1 ($\beta = -1.01$, $Z = -1.83$, $p<.07$). We were unable to test for the interaction for the *da-ta* continuum, as two of the steps did not yield any variance. However, pairwise tests found that the group difference was marginally significant at step 5 ($\beta = -0.627$, $Z = -1.95$, $p<.06$). In addition, the two groups also differed at step 3, as all skilled readers identified step 3 as *da* (no variance) whereas dyslexics did not.

The identification results suggest that dyslexics differed from skilled readers in their ability to identify clearly presented speech sounds. While these differences were not found in all continua, their presence is nonetheless remarkable given that the task imposes minimal attention and memory demands, and that the speech stimuli are not masked by noise. To the extent these individuals exhibit a phonetic impairment, we expect such a deficit to also impair ABX discrimination.

b. Discrimination results. An inspection of the discrimination results (see Figure 4; for individual subject data, see Figure S9, S10, S11, S12) suggests that dyslexics were overall less accurate than skilled readers. To test for the group differences, we submitted the results of the four continua to four separate mixed effects logit models, with group and continuum step as sum-coded fixed effects, and participants as a random effect. The group factor did not reliably modulate responses to the *ba-pa* continuum ($\beta = -0.13$, $Z = -1.21$, $p<0.23$, n.s.), but it was reliable or marginally so in all other cases. Specifically, dyslexics were reliably less accurate than skilled readers with the *da-ta* ($\beta = -0.34$, $Z = -3.33$, $p<0.0009$) and *o-u* continua ($\beta = -0.269$, $Z = -2.65$, $p<0.009$), and they were marginally less accurate with the *a-e* continuum ($\beta = -0.191$, $Z = -1.76$, $p<0.08$). These group differences were not further modulated by step continuum, as the group x step interaction term did not reliably improve the model's fit (for *da-ta*: $\chi(7)^2 = 8.57$, $p>.28$, n.s., for *ba-pa*: $\chi(7)^2 = 3.20$, $p>.87$, n.s for *o-u*: $\chi^2\ (7)^2 = 12.03$, $p>.10$, n.s.; for the *a-e* continuum: $\chi(7)^2 = 3.06$, $p>.88$, n.s.)[c].

The findings from the discrimination task converge with the identification results to suggest that dyslexic participants are impaired in their ability to extract phonetic categories. Across experiments, this phonetic deficit was rather subtle, and it did not emerge in all continua. Whether these occasional failures to detect group differences are due to systematic properties of these specific continua, or difficulties with the detection of an underlying subtle deficit is a question we cannot presently address. Remarkably, however, this deficit in extracting phonetic categories associates with the capacity to identify human speech, and it is dissociable from productive grammatical phonological rules.

Discussion

Much research has argued that dyslexia is associated with a phonological impairment, but the evidence for this hypothesis is rather scant. Most of the support for the phonological deficit hypothesis has come from speech processing. Speech processing, however, relies on multiple types of linguistic knowledge, including both phonological and phonetic principles. Accordingly, a speech-processing deficit could result from either a deficit to the phonological grammar or to the analog phonetic interface.

To distinguish between these possibilities, the present research included distinct manipulations that systematically dissociated productive grammatical principles from the phonetic interface. Grammatical phonological knowledge was gauged by the capacity of dyslexic individuals (speakers of Hebrew) to extend the restriction on identical consonants to novel forms. Phonetic processing, in turn, was examined by evaluating both the global capacity of the same individuals to process spoken stimuli (distinguish words from nonwords, and speech from nonspeech) as well as their capacity to extract the detailed structure of phonetic categories.

The results from Experiments 1–2 converged to show that the sample of dyslexics tested here were fully able to generalize a grammatical phonological rule. Like their typical counterparts, dyslexics judged ill-formed stems as less acceptable than well-formed controls, and they could compute grammatical well-formedness automatically, even for stimuli that were not consciously identified as speech. But despite their full grammatical sensitivity, the same individuals manifested systematic difficulties with speech perception. Compared to skilled readers, dyslexic participants in Experiment 1 manifested difficulties in word/nonword discrimination, and, in Experiment 2, they were even impaired in the identification of auditory stimuli as human speech.

The intact grammatical competence of these dyslexic individuals cannot be explained away by the choice of our control baseline–if anything, the phonological competence of our good-reading controls overestimated the general population of skilled readers, and as such, they provided a stringent baseline for detecting a grammatical phonological impairment. Conversely, detection of speech processing deficits in the same

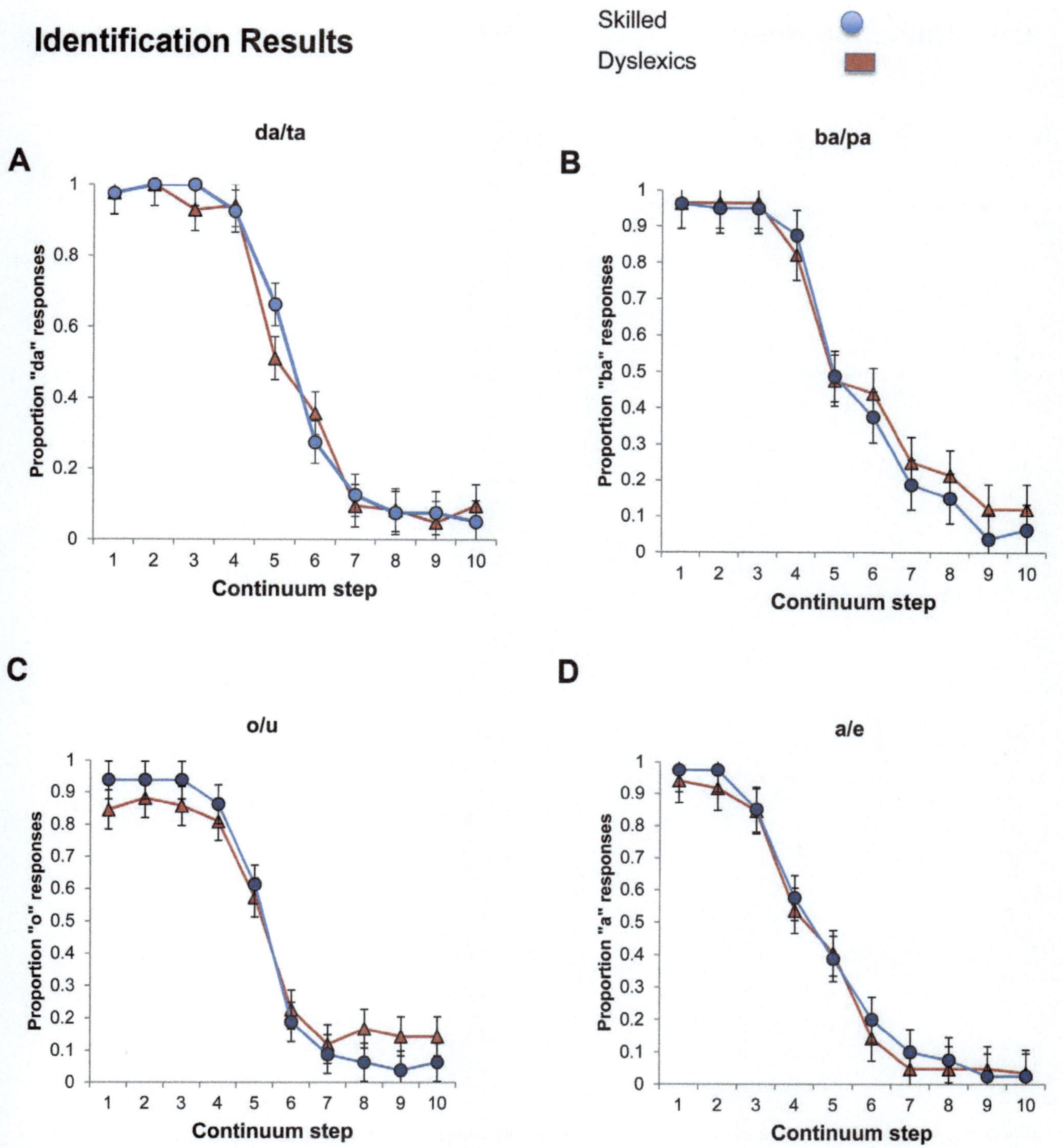

Figure 3. Phonetic identification of consonants and vowels by skilled readers and dyslexics along a 10-step continuum. Step continuum denotes the target stimulus. Error bars reflect confidence intervals for the difference between the group means.

individuals using the same tasks challenges plausible non-linguistic explanations (task demands, lapses in attention or working memory limitations) as the source of the speech impairment. Had the speech perception impairment of our dyslexic participants originated from such nonlinguistic sources, one would have expected to see similar impairments in our phonological manipulations. The selectivity of the group differences to speech perception counters this explanation. Together, these results implicate a phonetic origin that is dissociable from the phonological grammar. The findings of Experiment 3 directly support the phonetic-deficit hypothesis by demonstrating that these same dyslexic individuals are impaired in standard phonetic-categorization tasks for both consonants and vowels.

Taken as a whole, these results demonstrate that dyslexics manifest a basic phonetic deficit that impairs the identification of

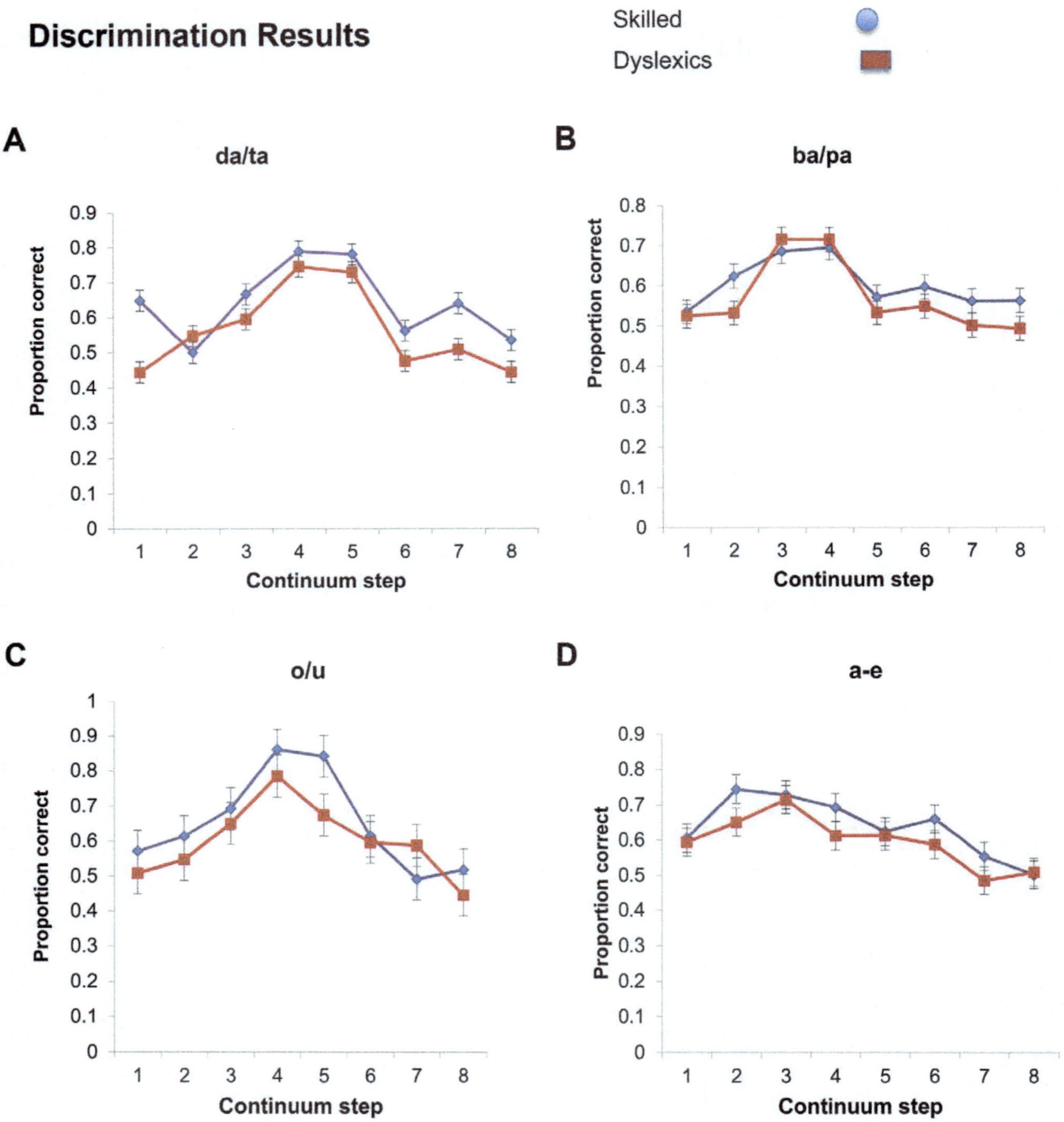

Figure 4. Phonetic discrimination of consonants and vowels by skilled readers and dyslexics along a 10-step continuum. Step continuum denotes the midpoint between the two stimuli (A and B) presented for discrimination. Error bars reflect confidence intervals for the difference between the group means.

conspecific vocalizations. These findings converge with past research showing that dyslexics individuals are impaired in the recognition of spoken words [73–77], voice recognition and phonetic categorization [5,7–14], and their impairment extends to the decoding of phonological structure from print. Our results, however, demonstrate for the first time that this phonetic deficit does not necessarily compromise the phonological grammar. These conclusions converge with findings from other languages [8,51,52], showing that other aspects of the grammatical phonological grammar are conserved in dyslexia. Our results, however, establish that the (intact) phonological competence of dyslexics concerns productive grammatical rules, and it dissociates from their (impaired) phonetic processing. Such dissociation of the phonological grammar from the phonetic interface is indeed consistent with linguistic evidence [31–33,78], neuroimaging data [79,80], neurological disorders [80,81].

The fact that both control and dyslexic participants successfully extracted the grammatical structure of the input regardless of its speech status–speech or nonspeech–also carries some methodological implications. Much research on dyslexia has used nonspeech analogs to adjudicate between auditory vs. language-specific origins for the speech-processing impairment [4,11,18,82–84]. Underlying this approach is the assumption that the processing of nonspeech analogs does not engage the language system. Our present results challenge this assumption. Replicating past research [72,85,86], we found that the language system can extract the linguistic structure even when the input is not consciously identified as speech. And indeed, previous research has shown that, when presented with our experimental stimuli, English speakers manifest quite a different pattern of responses than Hebrew speakers [72]. Similar effects of linguistic competence on the processing of nonspeech analogs were also reported with English and Russian speakers [86]. These conclusions caution against the common practice of using nonspeech stimuli as a selective test of auditory, nonlinguistic processing.

These findings nonetheless leave several open questions. One question concerns the generality of the phonetic deficit [29]. Although phonetic deficits are widely documented in dyslexia [5,7–14], the scope of these deficits is limited–they do not obtain in all groups [18,87–89], they are not found in every dyslexic individual [11,14,18,90,91], nor do they correlate with measures of reading and phonemic awareness [14,92]. We do not believe these limitations are inconsistent with a phonetic deficit hypothesis. Phonetic categorization and phonemic awareness tasks tap onto different representations and elicit different processing demands, so in view of the subtle nature of the phonetic deficit itself, it is not surprising that the correlation between these tasks is rather fragile. The present dissociation of the phonetic impairment from the phonological grammar further underscores the specificity of this deficit.

Our present results also cannot fully determine the status of the phonological grammar in dyslexia. Although our sample of adult participants showed no evidence of a grammatical phonological impairment, we cannot rule out the possibility that transient phonological deficits might have existed earlier in life and may have ameliorated with time [93–95]; nor can we rule out the possibility that some dyslexic individuals may show both phonological and phonetic impairments. The present evaluation of the phonological grammar based on a single phonological rule further limits our conclusions. We should note, however, that much linguistic and experimental evidence suggests that identity restrictions tap into a universal grammatical constraint that is at the core of the phonological grammar [53,55,62,63], and as such, they are likely to extend to other phonological systems. However, even if the phonological grammar were intact, dyslexics could still experience difficulties with other grammatical phonological distinctions because lower-level phonetic/auditory deficits [96,97] might prevent them from applying intact rules in on-line language processing.

In view of these limitations, we cannot presently determine whether the phonological grammar is generally spared in all dyslexic individuals, nor can we gauge the scope of the phonetic impairment. Clearly, however, the resolution of these questions requires an accurate characterization of the phonological and phonetic components. Our present demonstration that these two components can be dissociated underscores the urgent need for a more precise definition of the phonological- and phonetic-deficit hypotheses. We hope these conclusions foster further research into these questions.

Methods

Participants in Experiments 1–3

Dyslexic and control participants were native Hebrew speakers, students at the University of Haifa. Dyslexics were sampled from a group of 24 individuals who presented a documented diagnosis of dyslexia, issued by a certified clinician. Since all students at the University of Haifa must attain a minimum score of 450 points on a standardized psychometric test (the Israeli SAT, M = 540, SD = 70, range: 200–800), and since SAT scores are known to correlate with IQ [98,99], our participants likely fell within the normal IQ range. To assure that control participants were skilled readers, we first administered a battery of reading tests to two larger groups of about 50 participants each, and we next selected the top-performing individuals for inclusion in Experiments 1–2, matched to the number of dyslexic participants. We were unable to apply these same selection criteria to Experiment 3, but in each experiment, control participants' reading scores were significantly better than those of dyslexics (see Table 1).

Experiments 1–3 each included two groups of dyslexic participants and controls (N = 21, N = 18, N = 21 per group). Two additional dyslexic participants who took part in Experiment 2 were excluded–one due to a computer error, and another because his/her mean response accuracy to nonspeech stimuli was 32% (nearly 4SD below the group's mean). One additional control participant was excluded from Experiment 2 because his/her mean accuracy with nonspeech stimuli was 72%, (nearly 4SD below the group's mean). The data of two control participants from Experiment 3 were lost due to a computer error.

Reading tests. Reading ability was assessed by means of three tests. In the nonword naming task (from [100]), participants read aloud a list of 37 nonwords (printed with orthographic diacritics, to indicate all vowels). In the homophone detection task (from [101]), participants were presented with a list of 104 pseudohomophones (printed with vowel diacritics) and they were asked to mark the ones that spell out words of a given conceptual category. To use an English illustration, people were asked to detect food items from a list including *kat, bred,* and *roze.* Finally, in the text reading task (developed by M. Shani, A Biemiller & I. Ben-Dror) people were presented with two short passages consisting of 100 words each (one printed with vowel diacritics and one without them) and asked to read them aloud.

Task order. Participants took part in Experiments 1–3 in three sessions. Experiments 1–2 were administered in counter-balanced order in two sessions separated by approximately one week. Experiments 3a–3b (discrimination/identification) were likewise administered in counter-balanced order, approximately two weeks after the completion of the two previous experiments.

Experiment 1

Materials. The experimental materials consisted of 90 Hebrew words and 90 nonwords. Nonwords were of three types. One type (AAB) had identical consonants at the left edge of the stem (e.g., *titug*)–a structure that is illicit in Hebrew. The two other structures were well formed: one had identical consonants at the right edge of the stem (ABB, e.g., *gitut*) whereas the other had no identical consonants (ABC, e.g., *gitul*). These nonwords stimuli were arranged in 30 triplets, matched for the reduplicated consonants. The two well-formed members (ABB and ABC) were further matched for the frequency of their consonant-co-occurrence in Hebrew roots. Participants were presented with all 30 nonword triplets, but responses from two of these nonword triplets were excluded because they were identified as words in over 50% of the trials. Words (e.g., *tiupl,* 'treatment') were matched to the nonwords (e.g., *titug*) for their word pattern ($C_1iC_2uC_3$) and most words (89/90) comprised of three distinct consonants. All materials were recorded by the same Hebrew-speaking female (for details, see [69], Experiment 6). A list of all words and nonwords is provided in Appendix S1.

Procedure. Participants wore headphones, and sat in front of a computer. They initiated each trial by pressing the spacebar. Their response triggered the presentation of a fixation point (+, for 500 ms) followed by an auditory stimulus. Participants were asked to make a rapid forced choice as to whether the auditory stimulus was a real Hebrew word (1 = word, 2 = nonword). Slow (RT >3500 ms) and inaccurate responses triggered a warning message. Prior to the experiment, participants received a short practice session with similar items that did not reappear in the experimental session.

Experiment 2

Materials. Experiment 2 used the same 90 auditory nonwords from Experiment 1, along with 90 nonspeech stimuli synthesized from the waveforms of the speech stimuli.

The nonspeech materials were synthesized from their speech counterparts as detailed in [72]. Briefly, we produced the first, low-frequency component by lowpass filtering the stimulus waveforms at 400 Hz (slope of −85 dB per octave), and deriving its spectral contour from spectrograms of the filtered speech stimuli (256 point DFT, 0.5 ms time increment, Hanning window) using a peak-picking algorithm, which also extracted the corresponding amplitude values to produce an amplitude contour. We next shifted up the low-frequency spectral contour by multiplying it by 1.47, and resynthesized it into a sound component using a voltage-controlled oscillator modulated by the amplitude contour. The second, intermediate-frequency sound component was produced by bandpass filtering the original stimulus waveforms between 2000 and 4000 Hz (slope of −85 dB per octave), and deriving a single spectral contour of the frequency values in this intermediate range from spectrograms of the filtered speech stimuli (256 point DFT, 0.5 ms time increment, Hanning window) using a peak-picking algorithm–a procedure that also extracted the corresponding amplitude values to produce an amplitude contour. This intermediate spectral contour was next shifted down in frequency by multiplying it by 0.79 and resynthesized into a sound component using a voltage-controlled oscillator modulated by the amplitude contour. The third, high-frequency sound component was produced by bandpass filtering the original stimulus waveforms between 4000 and 6000 Hz (slope of −85 dB per octave), and deriving a single spectral contour of the frequency values in this high range from spectrograms of the filtered speech stimuli (256 point DFT, 0.5 ms time increment, Hanning window) using a peak-picking algorithm, which also extracted the corresponding amplitude values to produce an amplitude contour. Finally, we summed these three components together with relative amplitude ratios of 1.0:0.05: 2.0 (low-frequency component: intermediate-frequency component : high-frequency component) to produce the nonspeech version of each stimulus. The structure of these nonspeech stimuli and their natural speech counterparts is illustrated in Figure 5 (a sample of the materials is available at http://www.northeastern.edu/berentlab/gtt-material/).

Procedure. The procedure was the same as in Experiment 1, except that participants were now asked to quickly determine whether the auditory stimulus was speech or nonspeech (1 = speech; 2 = nonspeech), and the onset of the "slow responses" warning was set to 1000 ms.

Experiment 3a: Phonetic Identification

Materials. The materials were four 10-step continua generated from recordings made by a native Hebrew speaking female. Each such continuum varied progressively between two syllables that contrasted by a single phoneme–/ba/−/pa/,/da/−/ta/,/o/ −/u/ and /a/−/e/. In each trial, participants were presented a single continuum step and they were asked to quickly indicate their percept (e.g., *ba* or *pa*?).

The four continua were presented in separate blocks. Each block was preceded by a display, announcing the following continuum and the appropriate response keys. Each such block repeated the 10 continuum-steps four times (a total of 40 trials), and each such block was repeated four times (a total of 160 experimental trials). Prior to each block, participants were presented with 8 practice trials, and provided feedback on their accuracy. The order of the four blocks was counter-balanced across participants; within each block, trials were randomized.

The preparation of the consonant continua. The original syllables were recorded from a native Hebrew-speaking female (44,100 Hz sampling rate, 16-bit encoding). For the *ba-pa* continuum, the first six steps of the continuum were created by successively deleting ~30-msec portions out of the (initially) 180-msec long, initial-voiced part of the *ba* syllable. These deletions preserved the shape of the waveform, which is why they were not all exactly 30 msec long. The next 3 steps in the continuum were created by taking the initial 25 msec of the noise burst from the beginning of the pa syllable (normalized to have the same total root-mean-square amplitude as the *ba*), and adding an incrementally-amplified version of this to the beginning of the result from step 6 of the series, at a position in time corresponding to the position where the original *ba* syllable had started (amplification factors of 0.05, 0.1, and 0.3, respectively). The final step of the series was the original *pa*-syllable itself. For the *da-ta* continuum, a "hybrid" *da*-syllable was created from a *ta*-syllable with the initial noise burst removed, onto which the initial 150-msec prevoiced part of the *da*-syllable was grafted, preserving the waveform shape at the transition. The first 5 steps in the continuum were made by successively removing ~30 msec portions of the prevoiced part as above. For the next 4 steps of the continuum, the initial 30–msec of the *ta* noise burst were added to the beginning of result from step 5, in the same way as above (with amplification factors of 0.1, 0.2, 0.35, and 0.65, respectively). The final step of the series was the original *ta*-syllable itself. All stimuli were normalized to have the same root-mean-square amplitude. All of these manipulations were carried out using the SIGNAL Digital Sound Analysis System (Engineering Design, Berkeley, CA).

The preparation of the vowel continua. Ten-step vowel continua were made using the Praat computer program (3), based on a script written by Holger Mitterer, of the Max Planck Institute, Nijmegen, made freely available (4). The script made continua between two voiced speech sounds by first using the pitch-synchronous overlap and add (PSOLA) technique to equate their durations and pitch contours, and then by interpolating between the two sounds in steps of 0.1 to produce 10-step continua.

Procedure. Participants wore headphones, and sat in front of a computer. Each trial began with a message indicating the trial number and a fixation point (*), which remained visible throughout the trial. Participants initiated each trial by pressing the spacebar. They were asked to quickly categorize their percept using two computer keys (*ba* = 1, *pa* = 2; *da* = 1, *ta* = 2; o = a, u = 2, a = 1, e = 2), and their response triggered the presentation of an auditory stimulus. Slow responses (RT >2500 ms) triggered a computer warning (there was no accuracy feedback).

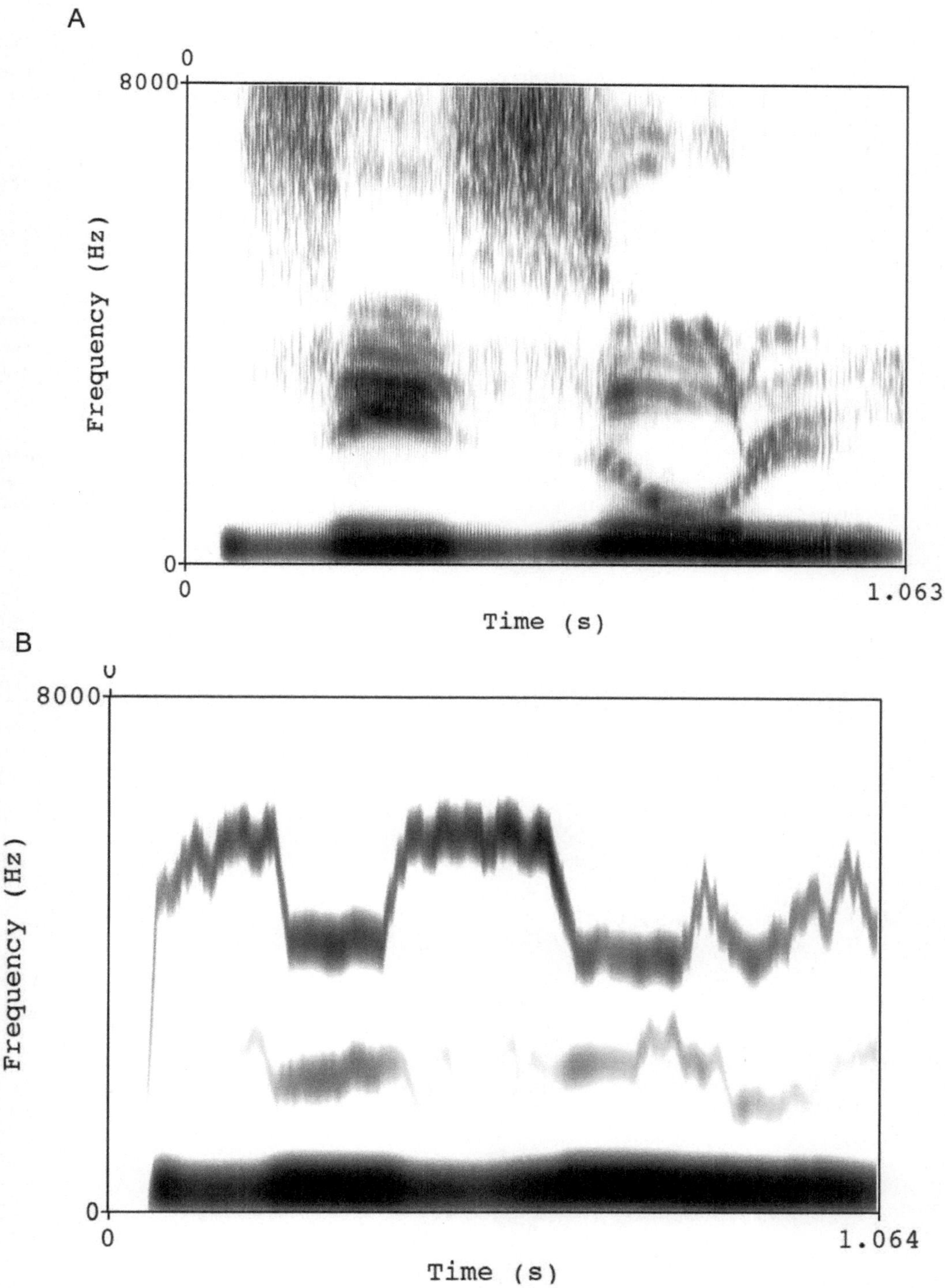

Figure 5. Spectrograms of a natural speech stimulus *zizul* (A) and its nonspeech counterpart (B).

Experiment 3b: Phonetic Discrimination

Materials and procedure. The materials corresponded to the same four continua used in Experiment 3a. In each trial, participants were presented with two step-members (A and B) followed by a third stimulus X, the probe, which was identical to either A or B. Stimulus A corresponded to steps 1–8, whereas stimulus B was always two steps higher than A (i.e., 1–3, 2–4, 3–5, etc.), a total of 8 combinations. Each of these 8 combinations was repeated twice–in half the trials, the probe X corresponded to A, in the other half, it corresponded to B, and the entire 16-trial sequence was repeated 4 times. Thus, each continuum (*ba-pa, da-ga, o-u, a-e*) gave rise to a block of 48 trials. Prior to each such block, participants were presented with 6 practice trials, comprising the naturally produced Likewise, the identification and discrimination tasks were administered in a counter-balanced order endpoints of the relevant continuum. The order of the four continua was counter-balanced; within each block, trials were randomized.

Each trial began with a message indicating the trial number and a fixation point (*), which remained visible throughout the trial. Participants initiated each trial by pressing the spacebar, and their response triggered the presentation of three auditory stimuli. Stimulus A was presented for 700 ms, followed (ISI = 500 ms) by stimulus B (displayed for 700 ms), and succeeded (ISI = 800 ms) by the probe X. Participants were asked to quickly indicate whether X was identical to A or B. Slow responses (RT>2500 ms) triggered a warning message (there was no accuracy feedback).

Supporting Information

Figure S1 The effect of reading skill on the discrimination of words from nonwords (in Experiment 1). Note: Box plots mark one SE above and below the mean. Each whisker bar marks 2 SD. Individual data plots are indicated by triangles.

Figure S2 Response time and response accuracy to nonwords as a function of reading skill and stem type (in Experiment 1). Note: Box plots mark two SE above and below the mean. Each whisker bar marks two SD.

Figure S3 The effect of reading skill on the discrimination of speech from nonspeech (in Experiment 2). Note: Box plots mark one SE above and below the mean. Each whisker bar marks two SD. Individual data plots are indicated by triangles.

Figure S4 Response of type time to speech and nonspeech as a function of reading skill and stem type (in Experiment 2). Note: Box plots mark one SE above and below the mean. Each whisker bar marks two SD. Individual data plots are indicated by triangles.

Figure S5 Identification of the da-ta continuum by dyslexic and skilled readers. Regression lines were fit to each individual's response data across step (treated as a continuous variable) using logistic regression.

Figure S6 Identification of the *ba-pa* continuum by dyslexic and skilled readers. Regression lines were fit to each individual's response data across step (treated as a continuous variable) using logistic regression.

Figure S7 Identification of the *o-u* continuum by dyslexic and skilled readers. Regression lines were fit to each individual's response data across step (treated as a continuous variable) using logistic regression.

Figure S8 Identification of the *a-e* continuum by dyslexic and skilled readers. Regression lines were fit to each individual's response data across step (treated as a continuous variable) using logistic regression.

Figure S9 Discrimination in the *da-ta* continuum by dyslexic and skilled readers. Regression lines were fit to each individual's accuracy data across step using logistic regression with a natural cubic spline (df = 2).

Figure S10 Discrimination in the *ba-pa* continuum by dyslexic and skilled readers. Regression lines were fit to each individual's accuracy data across step using logistic regression with a natural cubic spline (df = 2).

Figure S11 Discrimination in the *o-u* continuum by dyslexic and skilled readers. Regression lines were fit to each individual's accuracy data across step using logistic regression with a natural cubic spline (df = 2).

Figure S12 Discrimination in the *a-e* continuum by dyslexic and skilled readers. Regression lines were fit to each individual's accuracy data across step using logistic regression with a natural cubic spline (df = 2).

Appendix S1

Acknowledgments

We wish to thank Monica Bennett for her technical assistance and Maureen Gillespie, for statistical advice.

Author Contributions

Conceived and designed the experiments: IB. Performed the experiments: VVN. Analyzed the data: IB. Contributed reagents/materials/analysis tools: EB. Wrote the paper: IB EB AMG.

References

1. Shaywitz S (1998) Dyslexia. The New England journal of medicine 338: 307–312.
2. Dehaene S (2009) Reading and the brain: The science and evolution of a human invention. New-York: Viking.
3. Gabrieli JDE (2009) Dyslexia: a new synergy between education and cognitive neuroscience. Science (New York, NY) 325: 280–283.
4. Serniclaes W, Sprenger-Charolles L, Carré R, Demonet JF (2001) Perceptual discrimination of speech sounds in developmental dyslexia. Journal Of Speech, Language, And Hearing Research: JSLHR 44: 384–399.
5. Mody M, Studdert-Kennedy M, Brady S (1997) Speech perception deficits in poor readers: auditory processing or phonological coding? Journal of experimental child psychology 64: 199–231.
6. Ziegler JC, Pech-Georgel C, George F, Lorenzi C (2009) Speech-perception-in-noise deficits in dyslexia. Developmental Science 12: 732–745.
7. Godfrey JJ, Syrdal-Lasky AK, Millay KK, Knox CM (1981) Performance of dyslexic children on speech perception tests. Journal of Experimental Child Psychology 32: 401–424.
8. Blomert L, Mitterer H, Paffen C (2004) In search of the auditory, phonetic, and/or phonological problems in dyslexia: context effects in speech perception. Journal Of Speech, Language, And Hearing Research: JSLHR 47: 1030–1047.
9. Chiappe P, Chiappe DL, Siegel LS (2001) Speech perception, lexicality, and reading skill. Journal of Experimental Child Psychology 80: 58–74.
10. Brandt J, Rosen JJ (1980) Auditory phonemic perception in dyslexia: categorical identification and discrimination of stop consonants. Brain and Language 9: 324–337.
11. Rosen S, Manganari E (2001) Is there a relationship between speech and nonspeech auditory processing in children with dyslexia? Journal Of Speech, Language, And Hearing Research: JSLHR 44: 720–736.
12. Werker JF, Tees RC (1987) Speech perception in severely disabled and average reading children. Canadian Journal of Psychology 41: 48–61.
13. Serniclaes W, Van Heghe S, Mousty P, Carré R, Sprenger-Charolles L (2004) Allophonic mode of speech perception in dyslexia. Journal of Experimental Child Psychology 87: 336–361.
14. Paul I, Bott C, Heim S, Wienbruch C, Elbert TR (2006) Phonological but not auditory discrimination is impaired in dyslexia. The European Journal Of Neuroscience 24: 2945–2953.
15. Paulesu E, Demonet JF, Fazio F, McCrory E, Chanoine V, et al. (2001) Dyslexia: Cultural diversity and biological unity. Science 291: 2165–2167.
16. Perrachione TK, Del Tufo SN, Gabrieli JDE (2011) Human voice recognition depends on language ability. Science 333: 595–595.

17. Bradley L, Bryant PE (1978) Difficulties in auditory organisation as a possible cause of reading backwardness. Nature 271: 746–747.
18. Ramus F, Rosen S, Dakin SC, Day BL, Castellote JM, et al. (2003) Theories of developmental dyslexia: insights from a multiple case study of dyslexic adults. Brain 126: 841–865.
19. Lalain M, Joly-Pottuz B, Nguyen N, Habib M (2003) Dyslexia: The articulatory hypothesis revisited. Brain And Cognition 53: 253–256.
20. van Herten M, Pasman J, van Leeuwen TH, Been PH, van der Leij A, et al. (2008) Differences in AERP responses and atypical hemispheric specialization in 17-month-old children at risk of dyslexia. Brain Research 1201: 100–105.
21. Leppänen PHT, Richardson U, Pihko E, Eklund KM, Guttorm TK, et al. (2002) Brain responses to changes in speech sound durations differ between infants with and without familial risk for dyslexia. Developmental Neuropsychology 22: 407–422.
22. Olson R, Wise B, Conners F, Rack J (1990) Organization, heritability, and remediation of component word recognition skills in disabled readers. In: Carr TH, Levy BA, editors. Reading and its development: Component skills approach. New-York: Academic Press. 261–322.
23. Rack JP, Snowling MJ, Olson RK (1992) The nonword reading deficit in developmental dyslexia: A review. Reading Research Quarterly 27: 28–53.
24. Pugh KR, Mencl WE, Shaywitz BA, Shaywitz SE, Fulbright RK, et al. (2000) The angular gyrus in developmental dyslexia: task-specific differences in functional connectivity within posterior cortex. Psychological Science 11: 51–56.
25. Olson RK (2002) Dyslexia: nature and nurture. Dyslexia (Chichester, England) 8: 143–159.
26. Savill NJ, Thierry G (2011) Reading for sound with dyslexia: evidence for early orthographic and late phonological integration deficits. Brain Research 1385: 192–205.
27. Tanaka H, Black JM, Hulme C, Stanley LM, Kesler SR, et al. (2011) The brain basis of the phonological deficit in dyslexia is independent of IQ. Psychological Science 22: 1442–1451.
28. Shankweiler D (2012) Reading and phonological processing. In: Ramachandran VS, editor. Encyclopedia of human behavior: Academic press. 249–256.
29. Ramus F, Ahissar M (2012) Developmental dyslexia: The difficulties of interpreting poor performance, and the importance of normal performance. Cogn Neuropsychol.: doi 10.1080/02643294.2012.677420.
30. Ramus F, Szenkovits G (2006) What phonological deficit? Quarterly Journal Of Experimental Psychology 61: 129–141.
31. Hayes BP (1999) Phonetically driven phonology: The role of Optimality Theory and inductive grounding. In: M. Danell EAM, F Newmeyer, M Noonan & K. W Wheatley, editor. Formalism and functionalism in linguistics. Amsterdam: Benjamins. 243–285.
32. Chomsky N, Halle M (1968) The sound pattern of English. New York: Harper & Row.
33. Keating PA (1984) Phonetic and Phonological Representation of Stop Consonant Voicing. Language 60: 286–319.
34. Prince A, Smolensky P (1993/2004) Optimality theory: Constraint interaction in generative grammar. Malden, MA: Blackwell Pub.
35. de Lacy P (2004) Markedness conflation in Optimality Theory. Phonology 21: 145–188.
36. Berent I (2012) The phonological mind. Cambridge: Cambridge University Press.
37. Sandler W, Aronoff M, Meir I, Padden C (2011) The gradual emergence of phonological form in a new language. Natural Language and Linguistic Theory 29: 505–543.
38. Sandler W, Lillo-Martin DC (2006) Sign language and linguistic universals. Cambridge: Cambridge University Press.
39. Brentari D, Coppola M, Mazzoni L, Goldin-Meadow S (2012) When does a system become phonological? Handshape production in gestures, signers and homesigners. Natural Language & Linguistic Theory 30.
40. Berent I, Marcus GF, Shimron J, Gafos AI (2002) The scope of linguistic generalizations: evidence from Hebrew word formation. Cognition 83: 113–139.
41. Mester A, R., Ito J (1989) Feature predictability and underspecification: palatal prosody in Japanese mimetis. Language 65: 258–293.
42. Pinker S, Prince A (1988) On language and connectionism: Analysis of a parallel distributed processing model of language acquisition. Cognition 28: 73–193.
43. McCarthy JJ, Prince A (1995) Prosodic morphology. In: Goldsmith JA, editor. Phonological theory. Oxford: Basil Blackwell. 318–366.
44. Berent I, Lennertz T, Jun J, Moreno MA, Smolensky P (2008) Language universals in human brains. Proceedings of the National Academy of Sciences 105: 5321–5325.
45. Abler WL (1989) On the particulate principle of self-diversifying systems. Journal of Social and Biological Systems 12: 1–13.
46. Lisker L, Abramson A (1964) A cross-language study of voicing in initial stops: Acoustical measurements. Word 20: 384–422.
47. Theodore RM, Miller JL (2010) Characteristics of listener sensitivity to talker-specific phonetic detail. Journal of the Acoustical Society of America 128: 2090–2099.
48. Theodore RM, Miller JL, DeSteno D (2009) Individual talker differences in voice-onset-time: Contextual influences. Journal of the Acoustical Society of America 125: 3974–3982.
49. Marshall CR, Van Der Lely HKJ (2009) Effects of word position and stress on onset cluster production: evidence from typical development, specific language impairment, and dyslexia. Language 85: 39–57.
50. Soroli E, Szenkovits G, Ramus F (2010) Exploring dyslexics' phonological deficit III: Foreign speech perception and production. Dyslexia: An International Journal of Research and Practice 16: 318–340.
51. Maionchi-Pino N (2012) Phonological Restriction Knowledge in Dyslexia: Universal or Language-Specific? In: Wydell T, editor. A Comprehensive and International Approach.
52. Marshall CR, Ramus F, van der Lely H (2010) Do children with dyslexia and/or specific language impairment compensate for place assimilation? Insight into phonological grammar and representations. Cognitive Neuropsychology 27: 563–586.
53. Suzuki K (1998) A typological investigation of dissimilation. Tucson, AZ: University of Arizona.
54. McCarthy JJ (1981) A prosodic theory of nonconcatenative morphology. Linguistic Inquiry 12: 373–418.
55. McCarthy JJ (1986) OCP effects: Gemination and antigemination. Linguistic Inquiry 17: 207–263.
56. McCarthy JJ. (1989) Linear order in phonological representation. Linguistic Inquiry 20: 71–99.
57. Yip M (1988) The Obligatory Contour Principle and phonological rules: A loss of identity. Linguistic Inquiry 19: 65–100.
58. Bat-El O (2006) Consonant identity and consonant copy: the segmental and prosodic structure of Hebrew reduplication. Linguistic Inquiry 37: 179–210.
59. Rose S, Walker R (2004) A typology of consonant agreement as correspondence. Language 80: 475–531.
60. Brentari D (1998) A prosodic model of sign language phonology. Cambridge, Mass.: MIT Press.
61. Smolensky P (2006) Optimality in Phonology II: Harmonic completeness, local constraint conjunction, and feature domain markedness. In: Smolensky P, Legendre G, editors. The harmonic mind: From neural computation to Optimality-theoretic grammar. Cambridge, MA: MIT Press. 27–160.
62. Gervain J, Macagno F, Cogoi S, Peña M, Mehler J (2008) The neonate brain detects speech structure. Proc Natl Acad Sci U S A 105: 14222–14227.
63. Gervain J, Berent I, Werker J (2012) Binding at birth: Newborns detect identity relations and sequential position in speech. Journal of Cognitive Neuroscience 24: 564–574.
64. Greenberg J, H. (1950) The patterning of morphemes in Semitic. Word 6: 162–181.
65. Berent I, Shimron J (1997) The representation of Hebrew words: Evidence from the Obligatory Contour Principle. Cognition 64: 39–72.
66. Berent I, Everett DL, Shimron J (2001) Do phonological representations specify variables? Evidence from the obligatory contour principle. Cognitive Psychology 42: 1–60.
67. Berent I, Shimron J, Vaknin V (2001) Phonological constraints on reading: Evidence from the Obligatory Contour Principle. Journal of Memory and Language 44: 644–665.
68. Berent I, Bibi U, Tzelgov J (2006) The autonomous computation of linguistic structure in reading: Evidence from the Stroop task. The Mental Lexicon 1: 201–230.
69. Berent I, Vaknin V, Marcus G (2007) Roots, stems, and the universality of lexical representations: Evidence from Hebrew. Cognition 104: 254–286.
70. Berent I, Wilson C, Marcus G, Bemis D (2012) On the role of variables in phonology: Remarks on Hayes and Wilson. Linguistic Inquiry 43: 97–119.
71. Marcus G (2001) The algebraic mind: Integrating connectionism and cognitive science. Cambridge: MIT press.
72. Berent I, Balaban E, Vaknin-Nusbaum V (2011) How linguistic chickens help spot spoken-eggs: phonological constraints on speech identification. Frontier in Language Sciences 2: doi: 10.3389/fpsyg.2011.00182.
73. Janse E, de Bree E, Brouwer S (2010) Decreased sensitivity to phonemic mismatch in spoken word processing in adult developmental dyslexia. Journal of Psycholinguistic Research 39: 523–539.
74. Zeguers MHT, Snellings P, Tijms J, Weeda WD, Tamboer P, et al. (2011) Specifying theories of developmental dyslexia: a diffusion model analysis of word recognition. Developmental Science 14: 1340–1354.
75. Szenkovits G, Ramus F (2005) Exploring dyslexics' phonological deficit I: Lexical vs sub-lexical and input vs output processes. Dyslexia: An International Journal of Research and Practice 11: 253–268.
76. Poulsen M (2011) Do dyslexics have auditory input processing difficulties? Applied Psycholinguistics 32: 245–261.
77. Corina DP, Richards TL, Serafini S, Richards AL, Steury K, et al. (2001) fMRI auditory language differences between dyslexic and able reading children. NeuroReport: For Rapid Communication of Neuroscience Research 12: 1195–1201.
78. Zsiga EC (2000) Phonetic alignment constraints: consonant overlap and palatalization in English and Russian. Journal of Phonetics 28: 69–102.
79. Phillips C, Pellathy T, Marantz A, Yellin E, Wexler K, et al. (2000) Auditory cortex accesses phonological categories: an MEG mismatch study. Journal Of Cognitive Neuroscience 12: 1038–1055.
80. Wolmetz M, Poeppel D, Rapp B (2011) What does the right hemisphere know about phoneme categories? Journal Of Cognitive Neuroscience 23: 552–569.

81. Buchwald AB, Rapp B, Stone M (2007) Insertion of discrete phonological units: An articulatory and acoustic investigation of aphasic speech. Language and Cognitive Processes 22: 910–948.
82. Helenius Pi, Salmelin R, Richardson U, Leinonen S, Lyytinen H (2002) Abnormal auditory cortical activation in dyslexia 100 msec after speech onset. Journal of Cognitive Neuroscience 14: 603–617.
83. Parviainen T, Helenius Pi, Salmelin R (2005) Cortical differentiation of speech and nonspeech sounds at 100 ms: implications for dyslexia. Cerebral Cortex (New York, NY: 1991) 15: 1054–1063.
84. Vandermosten M, Boets B, Luts H, Poelmans H, Golestani N, et al. (2010) Adults with dyslexia are impaired in categorizing speech and nonspeech sounds on the basis of temporal cues. Proceedings of the National Academy of Sciences of the United States of America 107: 10389–10394.
85. Azadpour M, Balaban E (2008) Phonological Representations Are Unconsciously Used when Processing Complex, Non-Speech Signals. PLoS ONE 3: e1966.
86. Berent I, Balaban E, Lennertz T, Vaknin-Nusbaum V (2010) Phonological universals constrain the processing of nonspeech. Journal of Experimental Psychology: General 139: 418–435.
87. Maassen B, Groenen P, Crul T, Assman-Hulsmans C, Gabreëls F (2001) Identification and discrimination of voicing and place-of-articulation in developmental dyslexia. Clinical Linguistics & Phonetics 15: 319–339.
88. Hazan V, Messaoud-Galusi S, Rosen S, Nouwens S, Shakespeare B (2009) Speech perception abilities of adults with dyslexia: is there any evidence for a true deficit? Journal Of Speech, Language, And Hearing Research: JSLHR 52: 1510–1529.
89. Robertson EK, Joanisse MF, Desroches AS, Ng S (2009) Categorical speech perception deficits distinguish language and reading impairments in children. Developmental Science 12: 753–767.
90. Adlard A, Hazan V (1998) Speech perception in children with specific reading difficulties (dyslexia). The Quarterly Journal Of Experimental Psychology 51: 153–177.
91. McArthur G, Atkinson C, Ellis D (2009) Atypical brain responses to sounds in children with specific language and reading impairments. Developmental Science 12: 768–783.
92. Messaoud-Galusi S, Hazan V, Rosen S (2011) Investigating speech perception in children with dyslexia: is there evidence of a consistent deficit in individuals? Journal Of Speech, Language, And Hearing Research: JSLHR 54: 1682–1701.
93. Temple E, Deutsch GK, Poldrack RA, Miller SL, Tallal P, et al. (2003) Neural deficits in children with dyslexia ameliorated by behavioral remediation: evidence from functional MRI. Proceedings of the National Academy of Science 100: 2860–2865.
94. Galaburda AM, LoTurco J, Ramus F, Fitch RH, Rosen GD (2006) From genes to behavior in developmental dyslexia. Nat Neurosci 9: 1213–1217.
95. White S, Milne E, Rosen S, Hansen P, Swettenham J, et al. (2006) The role of sensorimotor impairments in dyslexia: a multiple case study of dyslexic children. Developmental Science 9: 237–255.
96. Lehongre K, Ramus F, Villiermet N, Schwartz D, Giraud A-L (2011) Altered low-gamma sampling in auditory cortex accounts for the three main facets of dyslexia. Neuron 72: 1080–1090.
97. Ouimet T, Balaban E (2009) Auditory stream biasing in children with reading impairments. Dyslexia (Chichester, England) 16: 45–65.
98. Beaujean AA, Firmin MW, Knoop AJ, Michonski JD, Berry TP, et al. (2006) Validation of the Frey and Detterman (2004) IQ prediction equations using the Reynolds Intellectual Assessment Scales. Personality and Individual Differences 41: 353–357.
99. Frey MC, Detterman DK (2004) Scholastic Assessment or g? The relationship between the Scholastic Assessment Test and general cognitive ability. Psychological Science 15: 373–378.
100. Shany M, Lachman D, Shalem Z, Bahat A, Zeiger T (2005) "Aleph – Taph" – An Assessment System for Reading and Writing Disabilities. Tel Aviv: Yesod Publishing.
101. Breznitz Z, Nevo B, Shatil E (2004) ELUL: learning disabilities diagnostic test in Hebrew and Arabic languages for grades 1 to 10. Haifa: Haifa press.

9

Position of Neocortical Neurons Transfected at Different Gestational Ages with shRNA Targeted against Candidate Dyslexia Susceptibility Genes

William T. Adler[*], Maryann P. Platt[*], Alison J. Mehlhorn[*], Joshua L. Haight, Timothy A. Currier, Mikel A. Etchegaray, Albert M. Galaburda, Glenn D. Rosen*

Department of Neurology, Beth Israel Deaconess Medical Center, Boston, Massachusetts, United States of America

Abstract

Developmental dyslexia is a language learning disorder that affects approximately 4–10% of the population. A number of candidate dyslexia susceptibility genes have been identified, including *DCDC2* and *KIAA0319* on Chromosome (Chr) 6p22.2 and *DYX1C1* on Chr 15q21. Embryonic knockdown of the function of homologs of these genes in rat neocortical projection cell progenitors by *in utero* electroporation of plasmids encoding small hairpin RNA (shRNA) revealed that all three genes disrupted neuronal migration to the neocortex. Specifically, this disruption would result in heterotopia formation (*Dyx1c1* and *Kiaa0319*) and/or overmigration past their expected laminar location (*Dyx1c1* and *Dcdc2*). In these experiments, neurons normally destined for the upper neocortical laminæ were transfected on embryonic day (E) 15.5, and we designed experiments to test whether these migration phenotypes were the result of targeting a specific type of projection neuron. We transfected litters with *Dcdc2* shRNA, *Dyx1c1* shRNA, *Kiaa0319* shRNA, or fluorescent protein (as a control) at each of three gestational ages (E14.5, E15.5, or E16.5). Pups were allowed to come to term, and their brains were examined at 3 weeks of age for the position of transfected cells. We found that age of transfection did not affect the percentage of unmigrated neurons—transfection with *Kiaa0319* shRNA resulted in heterotopia formation at all three ages. Overmigration of neurons transfected with *Dcdc2* shRNA, while present following transfections at the later ages, did not occur following E14.5 transfections. These results are considered in light of the known functions of each of these candidate dyslexia susceptibility genes.

Editor: Ferdinando Di Cunto, University of Turin, Italy

Funding: The research was supported by NIH grant P01 HD057853. The funders had no role in study design, data collection and analysis, decision to publish, or preparation of the manuscript.

Competing Interests: The authors have declared that no competing interests exist.

* E-mail: grosen@bidmc.harvard.edu

[*] These authors contributed equally to this work.

Introduction

Developmental dyslexia, a language learning disorder, affects approximately 4–10% of the global population and has a strong genetic component. In the past decade, a number of candidate dyslexia susceptibility genes (CDSGs) have been identified, three of which have garnered significant support in diverse populations, including *DCDC2* and *KIAA0319* on Chromosome (Chr) 6p22.2 [1–16] and *DYX1C1* on Chr 15q21 [17–22]. Delineating the specific functions of these genes has been a target of intense investigation in recent years. For example, these three CDSGs have been shown to be involved in neocortical neuronal migration [2,23–32]. This role in neuronal migration is particularly intriguing given the association of neuronal migration disorders such as molecular layer ectopias and periventricular nodular heterotopias with developmental dyslexia in humans [33–37].

Previous work demonstrated that disruption of CDSG homolog function at embryonic day (E) 15.5 potentially yields two phenotypes in the postnatal rat. Specifically, *in utero* electroporation of plasmids encoding shRNA targeted against *Dyx1c1* at E15.5 resulted in one cohort of neurons that remained in the white matter (heterotopia) and another that migrated past their expected laminar location (overmigration) [25,26]. In contrast, only heterotopias were seen following identical transfection with plasmids encoding *Kiaa0319* shRNA [30], whereas knockdown of *Dcdc2* by the same method resulted in the overmigration phenotype only [24]. In these experiments, neurons normally destined for the upper neocortical laminæ were transfected, which raises a number of questions: Are the migration phenotypes the result of targeting a specific type of projection neuron? What would be the effect of targeting neurons destined for laminæ both below (layers 5–6) and above (layer 2)? In this experiment, we transfected litters with *Dcdc2* shRNA, *Dyx1c1* shRNA, *Kiaa0319* shRNA, or fluorescent protein (as a control) at one of three gestational ages (E14.5, E15.5, or E16.5). Pups were allowed to come to term, and their brains were examined at 3 weeks of age for the position of transfected cells. We found that age of transfection did not affect the percentage of unmigrated neurons, but did influence the overmigration phenotype.

Experimental Procedures

In utero electroporation

All procedures were approved by the Institutional Animal Care and Use Committee at Beth Israel Deaconess Medical Center. Time-mated pregnant Wistar rats (Charles River, Wilmington, MA, USA) were assigned to one of three experimental shRNA conditions: *Dcdc2* shRNA, *Dyx1C1* shRNA, or *Kiaa0319* shRNA. Each mother was also assigned to one of three transfection age conditions: E14.5, E15.5, or E16.5. Within each litter, about twice as many pups received an experimental treatment (shRNA + mRFP) as received a control treatment (eGFP). *In utero* electroporations were performed as previously described [26].

Plasmids. For the experimental shRNA condition, plasmids encoding shRNA (pU6DyxHPB, pU6shRNA-Kiaa0319, or pU6shRNA-Dcdc2A) and plasmids encoding mRFP (pCAGGS-mRFP) were co-transfected. Previous research indicates that co-transfection is highly efficient [26]. Littermates in the control condition were transfected with a plasmid encoding eGFP (pCAGGS-eGFP). The concentrations of eGFP and mRFP plasmids were 0.75 µg/ µL, and the shRNA construct concentrations used were 1.5 µg/ µL.

Histology

At postnatal day (P) 21, transfected rats were deeply anesthetized (Ketamine/Xylazine 10:1, 100 mg/mL), sacrificed, and fixed by transcardial perfusion with 0.9% saline followed by 4% paraformaldehyde. Brains were extracted, post-fixed for 24 h, and cryoprotected, first in 10% and then in 30% sucrose phosphate buffer. The tissue was frozen and sectioned at 40 µm on a sliding microtome. Sections were stored in series of every tenth section and preserved in 0.4% sodium azide/phosphate buffer. One series was then mounted and visualized under fluorescence for the presence of eGFP or mRFP. After screening, that series was stained for Nissl bodies using Thionin.

Immunohistochemistry. Immunoperoxidase activity was detected using 3,3-diaminobenzidine (DAB,Vector Labs) according to ABC protocols. One series adjacent to the Nissl-stained sections was used for the immunohistochemical detection of eGFP (AB3080, Millipore Corp., Billerica, MA, USA, 1:1800) or mRFP (18-732-292379, Genway Biotech, San Diego, CA, USA, 1:5000). Primary antibodies were labeled with biotinylated secondary antibodies (Vector Labs, Burlingame, CA, all 1:200). Immunohistochemically processed tissue was mounted, counterstained with Methyl Green/Alcian Blue, and coverslipped with Permount mounting medium (Fisher Scientific, Waltham, MA, USA). Selected tissue from transfection ages E14.5 and E16.5 was reacted for immunofluorescence of laminar markers CUX1 and FOXP2 (SC-13024, 1:1000; SC-21069, 1:50, respectively, Santa Cruz Biotechnology, Santa Cruz, CA, USA). It should be noted that although CTIP2 reliably labels neurons in layer 5 in the mouse, it is, in our hands, expressed most strongly in layer 6, and inconsistently in layers 2 and 5 (Figure S1). Primary antibodies were detected with fluorescent secondary antibodies AlexaFluor 488 or AlexaFluor 594 (Invitrogen, Carlsbad, CA, USA, all 1:200). Tissue processed for immunofluorescence were mounted, coverslipped with VECTASHIELD HardSet Mounting Medium (Vector Labs, Burlingame, CA, USA), and imaged.

Analysis

Assessment of pathology. All brains were analyzed with the experimenter blind to subject condition. Nissl-stained sections were surveyed for the presence of neocortical malformations.

Quantitative analysis of neuronal position. For each brain, four sections were chosen from the eGFP/mRFP immunostained series. The positions of immunohistochemically stained neurons were charted using Neurolucida (MBF Biosciences, Williston, VT, USA). The charted sections were then analyzed in a custom MATLAB (Mathworks, Natick, MA, USA) program that determined the location of each marked neuron as a percentage of cortical depth, with 0% corresponding to the white matter/neocortex boundary and 100% representing the pial surface [30]. The region analyzed was limited to the area of cortex that was transfected, mainly the primary somatosensory (S1) cortex. We determined the average percentage of neurons that did not migrate into the neocortex (heterotopic neurons), as well as the mean distance traveled into the neocortex for each group. Results were analyzed by ANOVA with Fisher LSD post-hoc tests.

Image processing

Fluorescent images were obtained on a Zeiss LSM 5000 confocal microscope (Carl Zeiss, Inc., Thornwood, NY). Photomicrographs were adjusted for exposure and sharpened (unsharp mask filter) with Adobe Photoshop (Adobe Inc., San Jose, CA). Brightfield images were obtained on a Nikon E800 (Nikon Corporation, Melville, NY). All figures were composited in Adobe Illustrator (Adobe Inc.).

Results

Qualitative analysis

The position of transfected neurons varied considerably based on the day of transfection, and to a lesser extent on the construct being transfected. Labeled neurons from rats embryonically transfected with *Kiaa0319*, *Dcdc2*, or *Dyx1c1* shRNA at E14.5 were found predominantly in layers 4–6 of the cortex (Fig 1A,B). The disposition of transfected neurons migrating to the cerebral cortex did not appear to differ from the controls (n = 10). White matter heterotopias were seen in 7/8 of the brains transfected with *Kiaa0319* shRNA. In contrast, none of the 5 rats embryonically transfected with *Dcdc2* shRNA and 1/7 rats transfected with *Dyx1c1* shRNA had heterotopias. There were no heterotopias in the control condition.

We examined brains from each of the E14.5 transfection conditions for the presence of CUX1 (layers 2–4) and FOXP2 (layer 6) immunopositive neurons in the somatosensory cortex (Fig 2). Of the relatively few transfected neurons that migrated to layer 4, most were co-labeled with CUX1 (Fig 2A,E,I), indicating that these neurons are expressing markers appropriate for their lamina. We found substantial numbers of CUX1+ neurons in the white matter heterotopias, only a fraction of which were transfected with shRNA (Fig 2B,J). The large number of untransfected CUX1+ neurons in these heterotopias supports the notion that there are non-cell autonomous effects of *in utero* electroporation of shRNA as we have described previously for E15.5 transfected neurons [25,30]. FOXP2+ neurons were found, as expected, in layer 6 of the neocortex in all transfection conditions. A few of these neurons were transfected (Fig 2C,G,K). In contrast to CUX1+ neurons, there was no evidence of FOXP2+ neurons in the white matter heterotopia (Fig 2D,H,L). Taken together, these results suggest that white matter heterotopias that occur following E14.5 transfection with shRNAs targeted against CDSGs are composed of late generated neurons destined for the upper laminæ.

In utero electroporation of plasmids containing shRNA targeted against *Kiaa0319*, *Dcdc2*, or *Dyx1c1* at E15.5 mostly replicated previous reports [23–26,30]. Specifically, embryonically transfect-

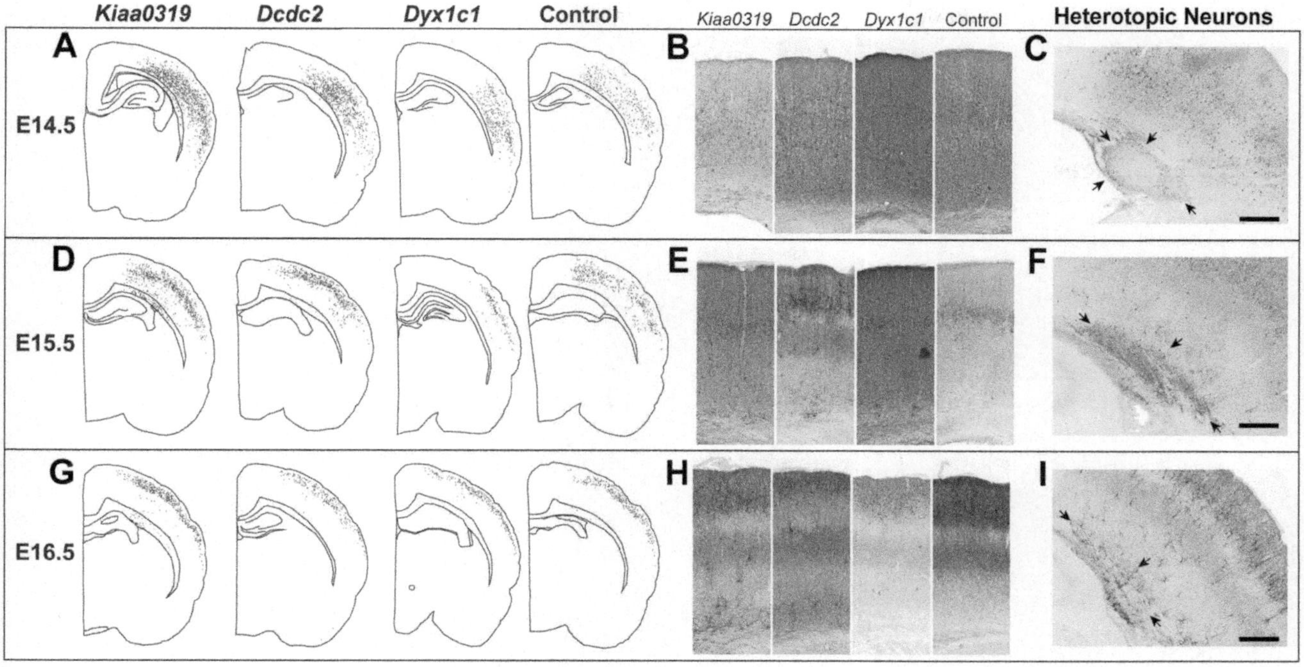

Figure 1. Hemispheric tracings (A,D,G), neocortical photomicrographs (B,E,H), and photomicrographs of white matter heterotopias (C,F,I) of rats embryonically transfected with either *Kiaa0319* shRNA, *Dcdc2* shRNA, *Dyx1c1* shRNA, or fluorescent protein (Control) at either E14.5 (A,B,C), E15.5 (D,E,F), or E16.5 (G,H,I). Bar for C,F,I = 500 μm.

ed neurons (both shRNA and control (n = 14)) that migrated into the neocortex were found predominantly in layers 2–4 (Fig 1C,D) in all conditions. White matter heterotopias were found in 6/10 of brains transfected with *Kiaa0319* shRNA, but in none of those embryonically transfected with *Dcdc2* shRNA (n = 5). Although rats *in utero* electroporated with shRNA targeted against *Dyx1c1* had scattered collections of unmigrated neurons at the border of the white matter and neocortex, only 1/5 rats had frank subcortical heterotopias, which is less than the expected incidence from previous studies [23,25,26]. The dispositions of CUX1+ and FOXP2+ neurons were identical to those previously published. Specifically, there were large numbers of transfected neurons co-labeled with CUX1 in layers 2–4 of the neocortex, whereas there were no transfected neurons co-labeled with FOXP2. In those rats with white matter heterotopias, there were large numbers of CUX1+ neurons, only a subset of which were transfected, which is consistent with there being non-cell autonomous effects of embryonic knockdown of *Kiaa0319* or *Dyx1c1* [25,26,30]. There were no FOXP2+ neurons in the heterotopia, again suggesting that heterotopic neurons are generated in the later stages of gestation.

Late transfections (E16.5) resulted in labeled neurons (both shRNA and control (n = 10)) being found almost exclusively in the upper portion of neocortical layer 2–3 (Fig 1E,F). White matter heterotopias were seen in 7/8 of the brains embryonically transfected with *Kiaa0319* shRNA, compared with 2/10 following *in utero* electroporation of *Dcdc2* and 2/6 *Dyx1c1* shRNA.

Of the E16.5 transfected neurons that migrated to layer 2–3, many (but not all) were co-labeled with CUX1, which was true for all transfection conditions. (Fig 3A,D,G). There were CUX1+ neurons in the white matter heterotopias, and some of these were embryonically transfected with shRNA (Fig 3B,E,H). FOXP2+ neurons were found, as expected, in layer 6 of the neocortex in all transfection conditions, and none of these were transfected. There were no FOXP2+ neurons in the white matter heterotopia (Fig 3C,F,I). Taken together, these results suggest that white matter heterotopias that occur following E16.5 transfection with shRNAs targeted against CDSGs, for both transfected and non-cell autonomous effects, are composed of late generated neurons destined for the upper laminæ.

Quantitative analysis

We used a customized MATLAB program to quantify the position of each transfected neuron in 4 sections taken from each case. The position of each neuron is given as a percentage of cortical depth, with 0% being the border with the white matter and 100% being the pial surface. In the E14.5 transfection group, the plot reflects the qualitative assessment, with the majority of transfected neurons in each condition found in layers 4–6 of the neocortex (Fig 4A). We computed the percentage of total transfected neurons that were unmigrated, and ran an ANOVA with Condition (4 levels) as the independent variable (Fig 4B). We found a significant main effect of Condition ($F_{2,26} = 6.6$, $P < .01$) on the average number of unmigrated neurons, and post-hoc analysis revealed that there were more unmigrated neurons in the *Kiaa0319* group as compared to the control (Fisher LSD $t = 4.3$, $P < .001$). We next computed the average distance of the neurons that migrated into the neocortex (Fig 4C). Transfected neurons were found predominantly in layers 4–6, and a one-way ANOVA revealed no significant difference in position among the four groups ($F < 1$, NS).

Neurons transfected at E15.5 were distributed predominantly in the upper laminae in a manner similar to that seen in previous reports (Fig 4D), and analyses are therefore one-tailed. There was a significant difference in the percentage of unmigrated neurons ($F_{3,30} = 7.2$, $P < .001$), with there being a significantly greater percentage of unmigrated neurons in the *Kiaa0319* group as compared to controls (Fisher LSD $t = 6.1$, $P < .001$; Fig 4E). There

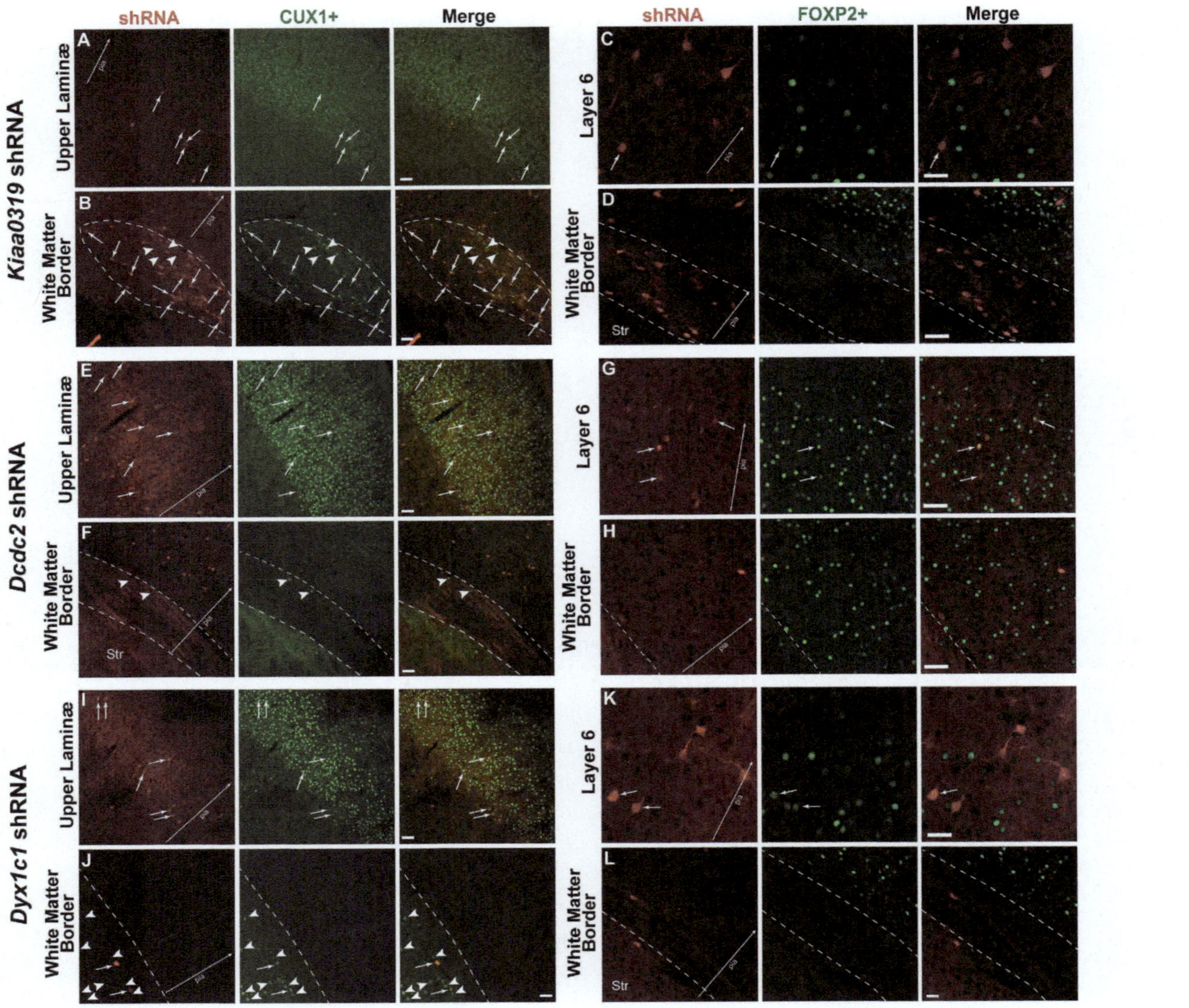

Figure 2. Confocal microscopy of laminar markers CUX1 and FOXP2 following transfection of candidate dyslexia susceptibility genes at E14.5. Small arrows indicate transfected cells co-labeled with CUX1 or FOXP2. Arrowheads indicate CUX1+ neurons that are not transfected. Large arrow for orientation with pial surface. Bar = 200 µm in all panels. **A.** Photomicrograph of upper lamina neurons from a rat transfected with *Kiaa0319* shRNA. **B.** Photomicrograph of white matter heterotopia (dotted line) from a rat transfected with *Kiaa0319* shRNA. **C.** Photomicrograph of layer 6 neurons from a rat transfected with *Kiaa0319* shRNA. **D.** Photomicrograph of white matter heterotopia (dotted line) from a rat transfected with *Kiaa0319* shRNA. **E.** Photomicrograph of upper lamina neurons from a rat transfected with *Dcdc2* shRNA. **F.** Photomicrograph of white matter border (dotted line outlines corpus callosum) from a rat transfected with *Dcdc2* shRNA. Str = Striatum. **G.** Photomicrograph of layer 6 neurons from a rat transfected with *Dcdc2* shRNA. **H.** Photomicrograph of white matter border (dotted line) from a rat transfected with *Dcdc2* shRNA. **I.** Photomicrograph of upper lamina neurons from a rat transfected with *Dyx1c1* shRNA. **J.** Photomicrograph of white matter heterotopia (dotted line is white matter border) from a rat transfected with *Dyx1c1* shRNA. **K.** Photomicrograph of layer 6 neurons from a rat transfected with *Dyx1c1* shRNA. **L.** Photomicrograph of white matter border (dotted line) from a rat transfected with *Dyx1c1* shRNA. Str = Striatum

was also a significant difference in the average location of neurons that migrated to the neocortex ($F_{3,30} = 4.9$, $P < .01$). In this case, both the *Dcdc2* and *Dyx1c1* groups migrated past the controls (Fisher LSD $t = 4.3$, $P < .01$, $t = 1.6$, $P < .06$, respectively; Fig 4F).

The migration plot for the E16.5 transfection groups reveals that nearly all neurons that migrated into the cortex were found in layer 2–3 (Fig 4G). There was a significant effect of experimental group in the percentage of unmigrated neurons ($F_{3,29} = 3.1$, $P < .05$), with both *Kiaa0319* and *Dyx1c1* having significantly higher percentage of unmigrated neurons than controls (Fisher LSD $t = 2.2$, $P < .05$, $t = 2.4$, $P < .05$, respectively; Fig 4H). Fig 4I confirms that the average position of migrated neurons in the neocortex is in layer 2–3 for all groups. There was a significant effect of group ($F_{3,29} = 5.2$, $P < .01$), with *Dcdc2* showing significant overmigration (Fisher LSD $t = 2.5$, $P < .05$).

Discussion

Previous research demonstrated that embryonic knockdown of candidate dyslexia susceptibility gene (CDSG) homologs at E15.5 results in disruption of neuronal migration, including white matter heterotopias and/or migration of transfected neurons past their expected laminar location in the neocortex. Here we report the

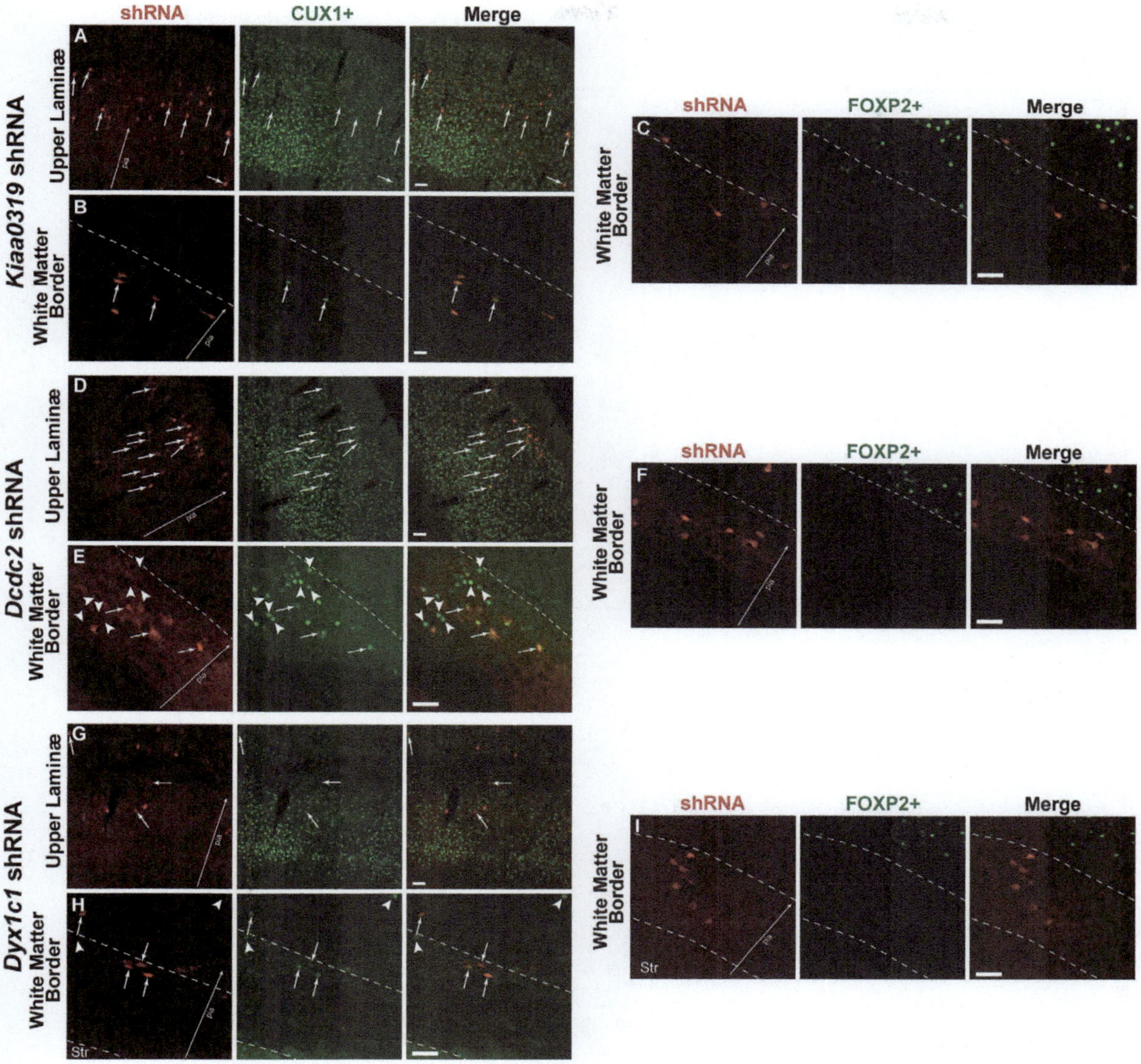

Figure 3. Confocal microscopy of laminar markers CUX1 and FOXP2 following transfection of candidate dyslexia susceptibility genes at E16.5. Small arrows indicate transfected cells co-labeled with CUX1 or FOXP2. Arrowheads indicate CUX1+ neurons that are not transfected. Large arrow for orientation with pial surface. Bar = 200 μm in all panels. **A.** Photomicrograph of upper lamina neurons from a rat transfected with *Kiaa0319* shRNA. **B.** Photomicrograph of white matter border (dotted line) from a rat transfected with *Kiaa0319* shRNA. **C.** Photomicrograph of white matter border (dotted line) from a rat transfected with *Kiaa0319* shRNA. **D.** Photomicrograph of upper lamina neurons from a rat transfected with *Dcdc2* shRNA. **E.** Photomicrograph of white matter border (dotted line) from a rat transfected with *Dcdc2* shRNA. **F.** Photomicrograph of white matter border (dotted line) from a rat transfected with *Dcdc2* shRNA. **G.** Photomicrograph of upper lamina neurons from a rat transfected with *Dyx1c1* shRNA. **H.** Photomicrograph of white matter heterotopia (dotted line) from a rat transfected with *Dyx1c1* shRNA. Str = Striatum. **I.** Photomicrograph of white matter heterotopia (dotted line) from a rat transfected with *Dyx1c1* shRNA. Str = Striatum

effects of *in utero* electroporation of plasmids encoding shRNA targeted against the CDSG homologs *Kiaa0319*, *Dcdc2*, and *Dyx1c1* at each of three embryonic ages (E14.5, E15.5, and E16.5) on the eventual disposition of transfected neurons in the neocortex. We successfully replicated the results of the previous reports using E15.5 transfection: *Kiaa0319* knockdown typically resulted in a group of unmigrated neurons in the white matter, and the neurons that did migrate into the neocortex were positioned identically to control transfected neurons [30]. Neurons embryonically transfected with *Dcdc2* shRNA, on the other hand, migrated past their expected laminar location, while few were unmigrated [24]. Transfection with *Dyx1c1* shRNA resulted in one case of white matter heterotopia, and moderate numbers of small groups or isolated unmigrated neurons that did not coalesce into a heterotopia. In addition, *Dyx1c1* shRNA transfected neurons migrated past their expected location [23,25,26]. In all cases, the majority of transfected neurons were CUX1 positive and FOXP2 negative, indicating they were mostly supragranular neurons. In cases where there were white matter heterotopias (*Kiaa0319* and *Dyx1c1* shRNA), there were no FOXP2+ neurons, and only a subset of the CUX1+ neurons in the heterotopia were transfected, with the rest showing non-cell autonomous migration defects.

Transfection with fluorescent protein alone at E14.5 generally labeled neurons in all layers of the neocortex, with the heaviest concentration in layers 5 and 6. *In utero* electroporation with shRNA targeted against *Kiaa0319* resulted in heterotopic collec-

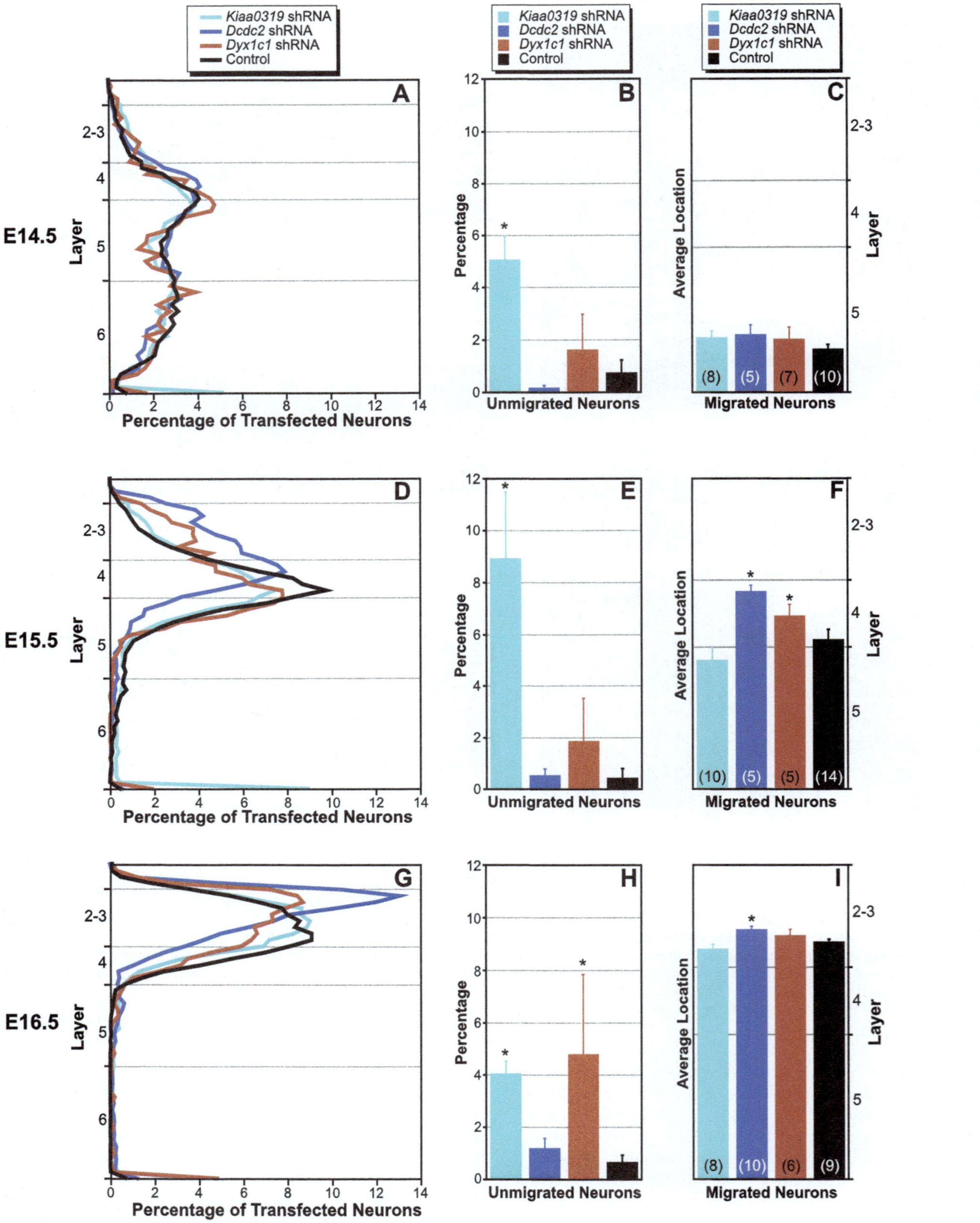

Figure 4. Quantitative analysis of transfected neuron position. A. Line chart showing mean laminar position of neurons transfected at E14.5. **B**. Histogram illustrating the mean percentage (+SEM) of transfected neurons that are unmigrated following E14.5 transfection. *Differs from control, P<.05. **C**. Histogram of mean (+SEM) average position of transfected neurons that migrated into the neocortex following E14.5 transfection. Horizontal lines indicate laminar boundaries. **D**. Line chart showing mean laminar position of neurons transfected at E15.5. **E**. Histogram illustrating the mean percentage (+SEM) of transfected neurons that are unmigrated following E15.5 transfection. *Differs from control, P<.05. **F**. Histogram of

mean (+SEM) average position of transfected neurons that migrated into the neocortex following E15.5 transfection. Horizontal lines indicate laminar boundaries. *Differs from control, P<.05. **G.** Line chart showing mean laminar position of neurons transfected at E16.5. **H.** Histogram illustrating the mean percentage (+SEM) of transfected neurons that are unmigrated following E16.5 transfection. *Differs from control, P<.05. **I.** Histogram of mean (+SEM) average position of transfected neurons that migrated into the neocortex following E16.5 transfection. Horizontal lines indicate laminar boundaries.*Differs from control, P<.05.

tions of neurons in the white matter. As with identical transfections that took place at E15.5, a subset of neurons in the heterotopias were transfected and were CUX1+, another subset were untransfected and CUX1+, and a further cohort were transfected and CUX1- [30]. In contrast, there were no large collections of unmigrated neurons following embryonic transfections with *Dcdc2* shRNA. Embryonic knockdown of *Dyx1c1* function at E14.5 resulted in white matter heterotopias in one rat, although there were clusters of transfected neurons at the white matter border in other animals. There was no evidence of an overmigration phenotype for any of the CDSGs following this early transfection—shRNA transfected neurons migrated to positions indistinguishable from those transfected with only fluorescent protein. In all CDSG conditions, subsets of neurons were co-labeled with CUX1 or FOXP2, again supporting the notion that transfection at this age labels neurons from the complete range of cortical laminæ.

Late (E16.5) transfections with fluorescent proteins labeled neurons exclusively in the upper cortical laminæ, with virtually no transfected neurons in layers 5 or 6. White matter heterotopias were seen in both the *Kiaa0319* and *Dyx1c1* conditions, and small heterotopias in 20% of the rats in the *Dcdc2* condition. There was a significant overmigration phenotype for the *Dcdc2* condition only, although there was some suggestion of supralaminar placement of *Dyx1c1* shRNA transfected neurons (Fig 4G) at this age. As with the E14.5 and E15.5 group, there were CUX1+ neurons in the heterotopias—only a subset of which were transfected—which again suggests non-cell autonomous effects of embryonic shRNA transfection on neuronal migration. There was no co-labeling of FOXP2+ and transfected neurons in any condition.

Taken together, these results suggest that disruption of neuronal migration following embryonic transfection with CDSG shRNA is partially dependent on the targeted neuronal population. In the case of white matter heterotopias, there appears to be little or no difference in incidence when age of transfection is taken into account. In the *Kiaa0319* shRNA transfected group, white matter heterotopias were seen at all transfection ages, with relatively high incidence regardless of age (~60–90%). In contrast, there were only 2 (out of 20) cases of white matter heterotopias in all the *Dcdc2* shRNA conditions, and there was never any statistical difference in the percentage of unmigrated neurons between the controls and this group for any of the three transfection ages. Although the incidence of white matter heterotopias following *Dyx1c1* transfection was relatively low when compared to previous results [23,25–28], the cases that did occur were rather large at all transfection ages and morphologically similar to previously reported findings.

In contrast, the overmigration phenotype is dependent on the age of transfection. Previous research had demonstrated that neurons embryonically transfected at E15.5 with either *Dcdc2* shRNA or *Dyx1c1* shRNA tended to migrate past their expected laminar targets [24,26], whereas those transfected with *Kiaa0319* shRNA did not [30],results that were replicated in the current study. We did not, however, find evidence of an overmigration effect for any of the CDSG groups following transfection at E14.5. Interestingly, we did see an overmigration effect following E16.5 transfection, despite the fact that the position of control transfected neurons would seemingly leave little space for overmigration.

The process of neuronal migration in the developing neocortex is a complicated series of interactions, involving many different genes and precise timing of events. Progenitor cells located in the VZ give rise to the projection cells of the neocortex as well as providing the scaffolding (radial glial fibers) by which these newly generated neurons migrate into the cortical plate. These neurons must orient properly, attach to the radial glial fibers, and then migrate into the cortical plate in an inside-out manner, and take their proper laminar position before beginning to differentiate. Disruptions of any of the genes modulating this process, however, can result in a variety of neuronal migration disorders [38].

The different functions of these CDSGs on neuronal migration may provide insight as to their roles in the different phenotypes observed. KIAA0319 encodes an integral membrane protein with a large extracellular domain, a single transmembrane domain, and a small intracellular C-terminus. There are several splice variants of this gene, one of which is secreted [11,31]. Because of its 5 polycystic kidney domains, it has been suggested that this gene plays a role in cell adhesion, and is therefore consistent with its being involved in neural cell adhesion [39]. DCDC2 is one of an eleven-member group of proteins distinguished by the presence of doublecortin domains [40–42]. The doublecortin domain is critical for binding to and stabilizing microtubules [42], and two members of this family (DCX and DCLK) have been shown to interactively affect axon outgrowth and neocortical neuronal migration [43,44]. Overexpression of the N- terminal p23 domain of DYX1C1 protein can interact with Hsp70, Hsp90 and CHIP, all of which point toward its role in degradation of unfolded proteins [45,46]. Recently, DYX1C1 has been shown to regulate estrogen receptors, which may have an impact on estrogen signaling during development [22,47,48]. Interestingly, all three CDSGs have recently been associated with cilia function [49].

KIAA0319 is a transmembrane protein that is purported to be a novel neural cell adhesion molecule. In comparison, DCDC2 is not an adhesion molecule, but is cytoplasmic and modulates microtubule function during development in a manner similar to other genes of the doublecortin family associated with neuronal migration disorders [38]. We have found that transfection with *Kiaa0319* shRNA at all three embryonic ages results in white matter heterotopias, whereas *Dcdc2* shRNA transfection rarely does. Of those *Kiaa0319* shRNA-transfected neurons that do migrate into the cerebral cortex, they do so in a manner indistinguishable from neurons transfected with fluorescent protein alone, whereas neurons that had *Dcdc2* function knocked down at E15.5 and 16.5 were positioned beyond their expected laminar location. It is therefore tempting to speculate that disruption of the purported adhesion molecule Kiaa0319 interferes with the initial attachment of some of the newly generated neurons to radial glia. In this case, those neurons would remain in the white matter, whereas the subpopulation that did attach migrated successfully into the neocortex and achieved their expected laminar position.

In contrast, almost all *Dcdc2*-transfected neurons migrated into the neocortex, and those neurons transfected at E15.5 and E16.5 tended to position themselves beyond their expected laminar position. The mechanisms that underlie this overmigration phenotype are not yet known, but any explanation must take into account a lack of this phenotype in E14.5 transfected neurons.

One possible explanation is that the earlier transfected neurons that are destined for layers 5–6, which comprise over 60% of the cortical depth, would be more difficult to demonstrate to be out of position, since they are normally located in a broad swath of cortex. Later migrating neurons (layers 2–4), which end up more restricted in upper laminæ, would be more easily identified as being in an abnormal position. This is consistent with our findings.

Overmigration could be the result of cell-autonomous or non-cell autonomous effects of the transfection. We have previously demonstrated (and have replicated here) that there are non-cell autonomous effects of *in utero* electroporation of CDSG shRNA with respect to neurons in the heterotopia and we have previously discussed possible mechanisms in detail [23,24,26,30]. One bit of evidence indicating non-cell autonomous effects is the presence of non-transfected GABAergic neurons in the heterotopia [25]. We did not find, however, any evidence of misplacement of GABAergic neurons in the cerebral cortex following embryonic transfection [25], suggesting that, at least in the case of these non-transfected neurons, there is no demonstrable evidence of non-cell autonomous effects on neuronal migration once they migrate into the cortex.

One potential mechanism of overmigration is that transfection delays the departure of transfected neurons from the ventricular zone, causing them to migrate with a cohort of later-generated neurons. Although the current study does not directly address this issue, the evidence is consistent with this hypothesis. Specifically, previous research demonstrated that there were large numbers of unmigrated *Dcdc2* shRNA-transfected neurons when examined 4 days post-transfection, with only a handful of neurons having migrated into the cortical plate [2,9,23]. This is in contrast with the controls, where most transfected neurons have migrated into the cortical plate by this time. Three weeks later, by contrast, there are relatively few unmigrated *Dcdc2* shRNA transfected neurons, but there are substantial numbers in the neocortex, and they have migrated past their expected laminar location. We therefore speculate that the embryonic disruption of Dcdc2 interferes with the normal activity of the migrating neurons, delaying their initial migration from the ventricular zone, causing them to migrate with later generated neurons and therefore taking positions beyond their expected location. Ongoing experiments documenting the developmental time course of neuronal migration following embryonic disruption of CDSGs will directly address these hypotheses.

Supporting Information

Figure S1 Laminar markers FOXP2 (A) and CTIP2 (B) in the somatosensory cortex. FOXP2+ and CTIP2+ neurons are found predominantly in layer 6, although CTIP2 inconsistently labels layer 5 and layer 2 neurons as well. Bar = 500 μm.

Author Contributions

Conceived and designed the experiments: GDR AMG. Performed the experiments: WTA MPP AJM JLH TAC MAE. Analyzed the data: WTA MPP AJM GDR. Wrote the paper: WTA MPP AJM JLH TAC MAE AMG GDR.

References

1. Cope N, Harold D, Hill G, Moskvina V, Stevenson J, et al. (2005) Strong evidence that KIAA0319 on chromosome 6p is a susceptibility gene for developmental dyslexia. American Journal of Human Genetics 76: 581–591.
2. Meng H, Smith SD, Hager K, Held M, Liu J, et al. (2005) DCDC2 is associated with reading disability and modulates neuronal development in the brain. Proc Natl Acad Sci U S A 102: 17053–17058.
3. Harold D, Paracchini S, Scerri T, Dennis M, Cope N, et al. (2006) Further evidence that the KIAA0319 gene confers susceptibility to developmental dyslexia. Mol Psychiatry11: 1085–1091, 1061.
4. Schumacher J, Anthoni H, Dahdouh F, Konig IR, Hillmer AM, et al. (2006) Strong Genetic Evidence of DCDC2 as a Susceptibility Gene for Dyslexia. Am J Hum Genet 78: 52–62.
5. Wilcke A, Weissfuss J, Kirsten H, Wolfram G, Boltze J, et al. (2009) The role of gene DCDC2 in German dyslexics. Annals of Dyslexia 59: 1–11.
6. Lind PA, Luciano M, Wright MJ, Montgomery GW, Martin NG, et al. (2010) Dyslexia and DCDC2: normal variation in reading and spelling is associated with DCDC2 polymorphisms in an Australian population sample. Eur J Hum Genet.
7. Massinen S, Hokkanen M-E, Matsson H, Tammimies K, Tapia-Páez I, et al. (2011) Increased Expression of the Dyslexia Candidate Gene DCDC2 Affects Length and Signaling of Primary Cilia in Neurons. PLoS ONE 6: e20580.
8. Francks C, Paracchini S, Smith SD, Richardson AJ, Scerri TS, et al. (2004) A 77-kilobase region of chromosome 6p22.2 is associated with dyslexia in families from the United Kingdom and from the United States. Am J Hum Genet 75: 1046–1058.
9. Paracchini S, Thomas A, Castro S, Lai C, Paramasivam M, et al. (2006) The chromosome 6p22 haplotype associated with dyslexia reduces the expression of KIAA0319, a novel gene involved in neuronal migration. Hum Mol Genet 15: 1659–1666.
10. Luciano M, Lind PA, Duffy DL, Castles A, Wright MJ, et al. (2007) A haplotype spanning KIAA0319 and TTRAP is associated with normal variation in reading and spelling ability. Biol Psychiatry 62: 811–817.
11. Velayos-Baeza A, Toma C, da Roza S, Paracchini S, Monaco AP (2007) Alternative splicing in the dyslexia-associated gene KIAA0319. Mamm Genome 18: 627–634.
12. Ludwig KU, Roeske D, Schumacher J, Schulte-Korne G, Konig IR, et al. (2008) Investigation of interaction between DCDC2 and KIAA0319 in a large German dyslexia sample. J Neural Transm 115: 1587–1589.
13. Paracchini S, Steer CD, Buckingham L-L, Morris AP, Ring S, et al. (2008) Association of the KIAA0319 Dyslexia Susceptibility Gene With Reading Skills in the General Population. Am J Psychiatry 165: 1576–1584.
14. Kirsten H, Wilcke A, Ligges C, Boltze J, Ahnert P (2012) Association study of a functional genetic variant in KIAA0319 in German dyslexics. Psychiatr Genet 22: 216–217.
15. Marino C, Meng H, Mascheretti S, Rusconi M, Cope N, et al. (2012) DCDC2 genetic variants and susceptibility to developmental dyslexia. Psychiatr Genet 22: 25–30.
16. Zuo PX, Wu HR, Li ZC, Cao XD, Pang LJ, et al. (2012) Association of polymorphisms in the DCDC2 gene with developmental dyslexia in the Han Chinese. Chin Med J (Engl) 125: 622–625.
17. Taipale M, Kaminen N, Nopola-Hemmi J, Haltia T, Myllyluoma B, et al. (2003) A candidate gene for developmental dyslexia encodes a nuclear tetratricopeptide repeat domain protein dynamically regulated in brain. Proc Natl Acad Sci U S A 100: 11553–11558.
18. Chapman NH, Igo RP, Thomson JB, Matsushita M, Brkanac Z, et al. (2004) Linkage analyses of four regions previously implicated in dyslexia: confirmation of a locus on chromosome 15q. Am J Med Genet B Neuropsychiatr Genet 131: 67–75.
19. Bates TC, Lind PA, Luciano M, Montgomery GW, Martin NG, et al. (2009) Dyslexia and DYX1C1: deficits in reading and spelling associated with a missense mutation. Mol Psychiatry.
20. Dahdouh F, Anthoni H, Tapia-Paez I, Peyrard-Janvid M, Schulte-Korne G, et al. (2009) Further evidence for DYX1C1 as a susceptibility factor for dyslexia. Psychiatr Genet.
21. Zhang Y, Li J, Tardif T, Burmeister M, Villafuerte SM, et al. (2012) Association of the DYX1C1 Dyslexia Susceptibility Gene with Orthography in the Chinese Population. PLoS ONE 7: e42969.
22. Tammimies K, Tapia-Paez I, Ruegg J, Rosin G, Kere J, et al. (2012) The rs3743205 SNP is important for the regulation of the dyslexia candidate gene DYX1C1 by estrogen receptor beta and DNA methylation. Mol Endocrinol 26: 619–629.
23. Wang Y, Paramasivam M, Thomas A, Bai J, Kaminen N, et al. (2006) Dyx1c1 functions in neuronal migration in developing neocortex. Neuroscience 143: 515–522.
24. Burbridge T, Wang Y, Volz A, Peschansky V, Lisann L, et al. (2008) Postnatal analysis of the effect of embryonic knockdown and overexpression of candidate dyslexia susceptibility gene DCDC2. Neuroscience 152: 723–733.
25. Currier TA, Etchegaray MA, Haight JL, Galaburda AM, Rosen GD (2011) The effects of embryonic knockdown of the candidate dyslexia susceptibility gene homologue DYX1C1 on the distribution of GABAergic neurons in the cerebral cortex. Neuroscience 172: 535–546.

26. Rosen GD, Bai J, Wang Y, Fiondella CG, Threlkeld SW, et al. (2007) Disruption of neuronal migration by targeted RNAi knockdown of Dyx1c1 results in neocortical and hippocampal malformations. Cerebral Cortex 17: 2562–2572.
27. Threlkeld SW, McClure MM, Bai J, Wang Y, LoTurco JJ, et al. (2007) Developmental disruptions and behavioral impairments in rats following in utero RNAi of Dyx1c1. Brain Research Bulletin 71: 508–514.
28. Szalkowski CE, Hinman JR, Threlkeld SW, Wang Y, LePack A, et al. (2011) Persistent spatial working memory deficits in rats following *in utero* RNAi of *Dyx1c1*. Genes Brain Behav 10: 244–252.
29. Tammimies K, Vitezic M, Matsson H, Le Guyader S, Burglin TR, et al. (2012) Molecular Networks of DYX1C1 Gene Show Connection to Neuronal Migration Genes and Cytoskeletal Proteins. Biol Psychiatry.
30. Peschansky VJ, Burbridge TJ, Volz AJ, Fiondella C, Wissner-Gross Z, et al. (2010) The effect of variation in expression of the candidate dyslexia susceptibility gene homolog *Kiaa0319* on neuronal migration and dendritic morphology in the rat. Cerebral Cortex 20: 884–897.
31. Velayos-Baeza A, Toma C, Paracchini S, Monaco AP (2008) The dyslexia-associated gene KIAA0319 encodes highly N- and O-glycosylated plasma membrane and secreted isoforms. Hum Mol Genet 17: 859–871.
32. Levecque C, Velayos-Baeza A, Holloway ZG, Monaco AP (2009) The dyslexia-associated protein KIAA0319 interacts with adaptor protein 2 and follows the classical clathrin-mediated endocytosis pathway. Am J Physiol Cell Physiol 297: C160–168.
33. Galaburda AM, Kemper TL (1978) Auditory cytoarchitectonic abnormalities in a case of familial developmental dyslexia. Trans Amer Neurol Assoc 103: 1–3.
34. Galaburda AM, Sherman GF, Rosen GD, Aboitiz F, Geschwind N (1985) Developmental dyslexia: Four consecutive cases with cortical anomalies. Ann Neurol 18: 222–233.
35. Humphreys P, Kaufmann WE, Galaburda AM (1990) Developmental dyslexia in women: Neuropathological findings in three cases. Ann Neurol 28: 727–738.
36. Chang BS, Katzir T, Liu T, Corriveau K, Barzillai M, et al. (2007) A structural basis for reading fluency: White matter defects in a genetic brain malformation. Neurology 69: 2146–2154.
37. Raschle NM, Chang M, Gaab N (2011) Structural brain alterations associated with dyslexia predate reading onset. Neuroimage 57: 742–749.
38. Liu JS (2011) Molecular genetics of neuronal migration disorders. Curr Neurol Neurosci Rep 11: 171–178.
39. Gabel LA, Gibson CJ, Gruen JR, LoTurco JJ (2010) Progress towards a cellular neurobiology of reading disability. Neurobiol Dis 38: 173–180.
40. Coquelle FM, Levy T, Bergmann S, Wolf SG, Bar-El D, et al. (2006) Common and Divergent Roles for Members of the Mouse DCX Superfamily. Cell Cycle 5.
41. Reiner O, Coquelle FM, Peter B, Levy T, Kaplan A, et al. (2006) The evolving doublecortin (DCX) superfamily. BMC Genomics 7: 188.
42. Gleeson JG, Minnerath SR, Fox JW, Allen KM, Luo RF, et al. (1999) Characterization of mutations in the gene doublecortin in patients with double cortex syndrome [see comments]. Ann Neurol 45: 146–153.
43. Deuel TA, Liu JS, Corbo JC, Yoo SY, Rorke-Adams LB, et al. (2006) Genetic interactions between doublecortin and doublecortin-like kinase in neuronal migration and axon outgrowth. Neuron 49: 41–53.
44. Koizumi H, Tanaka T, Gleeson JG (2006) Doublecortin-like kinase functions with doublecortin to mediate fiber tract decussation and neuronal migration. Neuron 49: 55–66.
45. Hatakeyama S, Matsumoto M, Yada M, Nakayama KI (2004) Interaction of U-box-type ubiquitin-protein ligases (E3s) with molecular chaperones. Genes Cells 9: 533–548.
46. Behrends C, Sowa ME, Gygi SP, Harper JW (2010) Network organization of the human autophagy system. Nature 466: 68–76.
47. Massinen S, Tammimies K, Tapia-Paez I, Matsson H, Hokkanen ME, et al. (2009) Functional interaction of DYX1C1 with estrogen receptors suggests involvement of hormonal pathways in dyslexia. Hum Mol Genet 18: 2802–2812.
48. Anthoni H, Sucheston LE, Lewis BA, Tapia-Paez I, Fan X, et al. (2012) The aromatase gene CYP19A1: several genetic and functional lines of evidence supporting a role in reading, speech and language. Behavior Genetics 42: 509–527.
49. Ivliev AE, t Hoen PA, van Roon-Mom WM, Peters DJ, Sergeeva MG (2012) Exploring the transcriptome of ciliated cells using in silico dissection of human tissues. PLoS ONE 7: e35618.

10

Differences in Brain Function and Changes with Intervention in Children with Poor Spelling and Reading Abilities

Daniela Gebauer[1,2], Andreas Fink[2]*, Reinhard Kargl[3], Gernot Reishofer[4], Karl Koschutnig[2], Christian Purgstaller[3], Franz Fazekas[1], Christian Enzinger[1,4]

1 Department of Neurology, Medical University of Graz, Graz, Austria, **2** Department of Psychology, Karl-Franzens-University Graz, Graz, Austria, **3** Institute for Reading and Spelling, Graz, Austria, **4** Department of Radiology, Medical University of Graz, Graz, Austria

Abstract

Previous fMRI studies in English-speaking samples suggested that specific interventions may alter brain function in language-relevant networks in children with reading and spelling difficulties, but this research strongly focused on reading impaired individuals. Only few studies so far investigated characteristics of brain activation associated with poor spelling ability and whether a specific spelling intervention may also be associated with distinct changes in brain activity patterns. We here investigated such effects of a morpheme-based spelling intervention on brain function in 20 children with comparatively poor spelling and reading abilities using repeated fMRI. Relative to 10 matched controls, children with comparatively poor spelling and reading abilities showed increased activation in frontal medial and right hemispheric regions and decreased activation in left occipito-temporal regions prior to the intervention, during processing of a lexical decision task. After five weeks of intervention, spelling and reading comprehension significantly improved in the training group, along with increased activation in the left temporal, parahippocampal and hippocampal regions. Conversely, the waiting group showed increases in right posterior regions. Our findings could indicate an increased left temporal activation associated with the recollection of the new learnt morpheme-based strategy related to successful training.

Editor: Michelle Hampson, Yale University, United States of America

Funding: The research presented in this paper was supported by grants from the Styrian government (Nr. A27214001062 - http://www.verwaltung.steiermark.at) and the Jubilee Fund of the Austrian National Bank (Nr. A26E16020013 - http://www.onb.ac.at/). The funders had no role in study design, data collection and analysis, decision to publish, or preparation of the manuscript.

Competing Interests: The authors have declared that no competing interests exist.

* E-mail: andreas.fink@uni-graz.at

Introduction

According to the ICD 10 definition [1], spelling and reading impairment (dyslexia; F 81.0) is diagnosed if reading and spelling skills are located two standard deviations below the level that might be expected based on general intelligence, age and education. The main feature of isolated spelling disorder (F 81.1) is a specific and significant impairment in the development of spelling skills in the absence of a history of specific reading disorder, which is not accounted for by age, intelligence or inadequate education. However, it has to be noted that difficulties in spelling and reading occur in various degrees of severity. Although cut points are placed to help define groups, they have been criticized for being arbitrary and lack biological validity [2]. Reading difficulties, including dyslexia, occur as the lower part of a continuum for reading ability that includes nonimpaired as well as disabled readers [2,3]. In this study we thus conceptualize spelling and reading ability as a continuum ranging from lower to higher abilities, rather than relying on categorical definitions such as "dyslexic" or "spelling impaired" children. In defining our experimental groups, we chose children exhibiting a comparatively poor performance level on this ability continuum. Discoveries about poor spelling and reading abilities may offer insights into mechanisms of normal reading acquisition and dyslexia [3].

Recent studies using functional magnetic resonance imaging (fMRI) provided important insights into potential brain mechanisms underlying reading and spelling skills and reading and spelling impairment (i.e., dyslexia; for a recent fMRI study on developmental dyslexia in the German-speaking area see e.g. [4]). Frequently, *decreased* brain activation in parieto-temporal and occipito-temporal regions of the *left* hemisphere, along with *increased* activation in frontal and right hemispheric language-related regions has been observed in individuals with reading and spelling impairment. The left parieto-temporal region (angular gyrus and supramarginal gyrus) is assumed to play a critical role in spelling in non-impaired individuals [5,6]. Decreased left parieto-temporal activation has been related to deficits in grapheme-phoneme-conversion in reading and spelling impairment [7]. The left occipito-temporal region (comprising the visual word form area) is crucial for reading processes in non-impaired individuals [8]. Decreased activation in this region is associated with impairments of automatic, fluent reading [7,9]. Also increased frontal and right hemispheric activation has been observed in individuals with reading and spelling impairment, interpreted to indicate inefficient compensatory mechanisms such as internal articulation [10,11].

Training studies using fMRI revealed changes in the above mentioned brain activation patterns in subjects with reading and spelling impairment and poor readers along with successful intervention [12–20], while only few studies focused on subjects with poor spelling ability [21].

Isolated spelling difficulties in German-speaking samples were found in about 3–6% of elementary school children [22,23]. Due to the transparent orthography in German, individuals with reading and spelling impairment manage to read slow but accurate in the course of their development, whereas spelling mistakes rather persist into adulthood [24].

Here, we used a morpheme-based spelling intervention (*Morpheus*) [25], which trains children to figure out the correct spelling of a word by separating it into specific word component parts (*morphemes*). Behavioral studies in this field provided evidence that such interventions significantly enhance reading and/or spelling ability [26–29]. Using EEG, we demonstrated a neurophysiological training effect of this intervention, by increased EEG activation in left hemispheric regions that are involved in the complex neural network subserving reading and spelling [29].

Using fMRI in a different sample, we sought to corroborate and extend these findings by more detailed functional neuroanatomical insights. We specifically tested (a) if and how brain activation patterns at baseline in children with comparatively poor spelling and reading abilities differed from controls. We hypothesized that children with poor spelling and reading abilities would show different brain activation prior to the applied spelling intervention as compared to controls. Secondly (b), we investigated whether spelling skills and brain activation can be modulated by a specific spelling intervention, comparing two groups of poor spellers (divided into a training group and into a waiting group).

Materials and Methods

Ethics Statement

The study was approved by the ethics committee of the Medical University of Graz, Austria. All children and their parents had given written informed consent.

Psychometric Tests

In an extensive pre-experimental screening, standardized tests for the assessment of reading and spelling abilities were administered in 107 children, and we explored relevant socio-demographic data such as age, sex and native language.

To assess spelling skills, we used a standardized spelling test (Hamburger-Schreibprobe, HSP) by May et al. [30]. In the HSP, words and sentences are dictated by the experimenter and have to be written next to the corresponding pictures that illustrate the respective words or sentences. This test takes about 15 minutes. Within this study, versions for $4^{th}/5^{th}$ graders and 5th to 9th graders were applied. The HSP provides measures for the number of correctly spelled words and the number of grapheme-related mistakes. The latter measure was used in this study as it provides a more precise measure of spelling ability.

Additionally, we administered the "Salzburger-Lese-Sreening" (SLS) [31,32] that measures reading speed and basic reading ability (automaticity). The SLS 1–4 was used for children up to the 4th grade, and the SLS 5–8 was applied for older children and parallel versions exist for both. In the SLS, children have to decide whether the content of a presented sentence is correct or not. Testing time is limited to three minutes. In addition, we also measured reading comprehension (i.e. comprehension of words, sentences and text) by means of a standardized German-speaking test (ELFE 1–6) [33]. Furthermore, non-verbal intelligence was measured by the Standard Progressive Matrices (SPM) by Raven [34].

Participants

Forty-two German-speaking children aged between nine and 15 years were recruited for this study based on the pre-experimental screening as described above (cf. 2.2). Three groups (training group, waiting group and control group), each comprising 14 children, were investigated. Children with overall motion >3 mm or sudden movement >1 mm during scanning were excluded from further analyses. Based on this definition, seven children had to be excluded due to movement artifacts. Furthermore, two children had to be excluded due to poor behavioral performance inside the scanner (Mean Accuracy <70%) and three children had to be excluded because they did not attend all behavioral tests and fMRI sessions, rendering a final sample of 30 children (15 males), whose age ranged from 10 to 15 years ($M = 11.80$; $SD = 1.58$, see Table 1). All participants were right-handed, healthy and had normal or corrected-to normal vision.

We formed and investigated three experimental groups: (1) Ten children with poor spelling abilities ($M = 21.0$ percent rank) were assigned to the "training group" (TG), (2) another ten children with poor spelling abilities ($M = 23.2$ percent rank) were assigned to the so-called "waiting group" (WG, receiving the training after the post-test) and (3) a control group (CG) of ten children (matched for age and intelligence) with good spelling abilities ($M = 75.7$ percent rank), were investigated. The effect of the intervention was examined in a pre-test/post-test design, comparing the two groups of poor spellers (TG and WG). The groups did not differ significantly ($p > .05$) with respect to age and non-verbal intelligence, but controls scored considerably higher in reading and spelling. Specific post-hoc comparisons by means of the Tukey HSD test revealed that controls showed significantly higher scores of reading and spelling ability than both groups of poor spellers ($p < .05$). Therefore we labeled the groups as "comparatively poor spellers and readers". However, it has to be noted that the TG and WG showed average reading scores according to age- and education-matched norms ($p < .01$; see Table 1 for details). The comparisons between the TG and the WG yielded no significant results (which appears to be particularly important in the light of the employed training design).

Intervention

The applied intervention is a computer-aided morpheme-based spelling training (*Morpheus*) [30], which has been approved as an evidence-based intervention for individuals with reading and spelling deficits by the federal ministry of Austria [35] and has shown to significantly improve spelling ability in children in a series of behavioral studies in our laboratory [36,37].

A morpheme is defined as the "smallest meaningful unit of language" [38]. Every word is built by different parts, which follow particular spellings (e.g. unforgetful = prefix (un), suffix (ful), root (forget)). Therefore, the spelling of the German verb "verfahren" can be derived by two rules: the prefix (ver) is always written with (v), the root (fahr) always with an "h". Children do not need to remember the spelling of every single word, but only to memorize the spelling of their component parts. Furthermore, morphosemantic information can support the development of a meaning-oriented decoding strategy, e.g. the correct spelling of the noun "Motor-rad" (motor-bike) can be derived by the meaning [30]. In addition, this strategy seems to be easy to apply as only "100 of the most frequent morphemes cover 70% of all written material" [39].

Table 1. Descriptive Statistics of Behavioral Measures (sex, age, non-verbal intelligence, reading- and spelling skills).

	TG	WG	CG	p
Behavioral Measures				
Sex	10 (7 males)	10 (5 males)	10 (3 males)	
Age (years)	11.5 (+/−0.7)	11.6 (+/−1.7)	12.3 (+/−2.1)	.49
Intelligence – Raven raw scores	36.7 (+/−7.7)	36.5 (+/−9.16)	43.4 (+/−5.4)	.09
Pre-Intervention				
Reading Skills -SLS*	91.4 (+/−14.3)	97.7 (+/−10.4)	115.3 (+/−15.1)	**.001**
Reading Comprehension	48.3 (+/−8.8)	50.9 (+/−5.9)	62.3 (+/−7.9)	**.001**
Spelling Skills -HSP	21.0 (+/−11.4)	23.2 (+/−14.0)	75.7 (+/−14.7)	**.000**
Post- Intervention				
Reading Skills -SLS	102.6 (+/−13.9)	100.0 (+/−9.1)	-	.53
Reading Comprehension	52.6 (+/−8.7)	50.5 (+/−5.4)	-	.62
Spelling Skills -HSP	42.3 (+/−23.0)	23.9 (+/−13.3)	-	**.04**

Means and Standard Deviations (in brackets).
Pre-Intervention: Reading Skills: SLS Reading Quotient: Average Scores range from 85–115 ($F_{(2,27)}=8.52$; $p<.001$; $\eta_p^2=.39$); Reading Comprehension: ELFE T-scores: ($F_{(2,27)}=9.57$; $p<.001$; $\eta_p^2=.42$); Spelling Skills: HSP Percent Rank: ($F_{(2,27)}=53.26$; $p<.001$; $\eta_p^2=.80$).
Post-Intervention: Reading Skills: SLS Reading Quotient ($F_{(1,18)}=0.25$; $p=.62$; $\eta_p^2=.01$); Reading Comprehension: ELFE T-scores ($F_{(1,18)}=0.42$; $p=.53$; $\eta_p^2=.02$); Spelling Skills: HSP Percent Range ($F_{(1,18)}=4.83$; $p<.05$; $\eta_p^2=.21$).
*Three out of the 20 comparatively poor spellers and readers showed below average reading scores (Reading Quotient: 83,75, 73).

The *Morpheus*-intervention consists of computerized tutorials, a book of exercises and morpheme-based games to facilitate the consolidation of the strategy. The intervention, which includes daily handwritten and computer homework along with instructor-guided courses (once a week, lasting approximately two hours), was realized within *five weeks*. These tutorials on the computer include twelve different playful exercises dealing with morphemes (e.g. recognizing and matching word families, morphological clozes, finding suffixes and prefixes). During the tutorials achieved scores are displayed on the computer screen. Participants can only reach the next difficulty level of the same exercise when they have solved at least 75% of the given problems correctly. The automatically saved score of every tutorial serves as basis for assessing training progress.

The training material of *Morpheus* consists of the most frequent morphemes of the German language and contains different levels of difficulty. The words used for the training were taken from an empirically-based collection of words (German basic vocabulary for 4th graders) [40]. *Morpheus* has been constructed on the basis of the following principles: simplicity, relief due to morpheme segmentation, rule-governed repetition, playfulness, avoidance of mistakes, individuality, productivity, and practicing handwriting.

Functional MRI (fMRI) experimental stimuli and tasks

Three different lexical decision conditions were presented during event-related fMRI (1: correctly spelled words, 2: misspelled words, 3: pseudowords). Similarly to the spelling judgment task of Richards et al. [21], children had to decide whether a presented word was spelled correctly (e.g. Bäume; trees) or if it was spelled incorrectly (e.g. Menner instead of Männer; men) or a pseudoword (e.g. Ostablast). Misspelled and Pseudowords were created by changing correctly spelled words (nouns, verbs, adjectives). The misspelled words are phonologically correct (sound exactly like the properly spelled word if spoke aloud), like the pseudohomophones [41,42], but morphematically incorrect, following the "known" pattern of german words (consonant-vocal-consonant-vocal-consonant; e.g. Negel instead of Nägel (nails); forher instead of vorher (previously)). Pseudowords included phonologically non-existing and morphematically incorrect words. A fixation cross was presented as a baseline. We found substantial correlations between spelling ability (assessed by the HSP) and performance during lexical decision tasks ($r=$ about .50) in prior studies [29]. Participants were familiarized with the task outside the scanner to ensure the instruction had been understood properly. Each condition comprised 75 words which were equal according to length and word type (25 nouns, 25 verbs, 25 adjectives; mean word length: 7 letters).

Answers were given via button presses using the right (dominant) hand, with the index finger for correctly spelled real words and the middle finger for misspelled and pseudowords (see Figure 1). Behavioral responses inside the scanner were assessed to obtain the percentage of correct responses and reaction time. Items and fixation were presented for three seconds. Each condition was directly followed by the other. The order of items and fixations was optimized by a genetic algorithm for hemodynamic response detection [43]. The total time of the fMRI experiment was 16 minutes and the entire MRI session took 30 minutes.

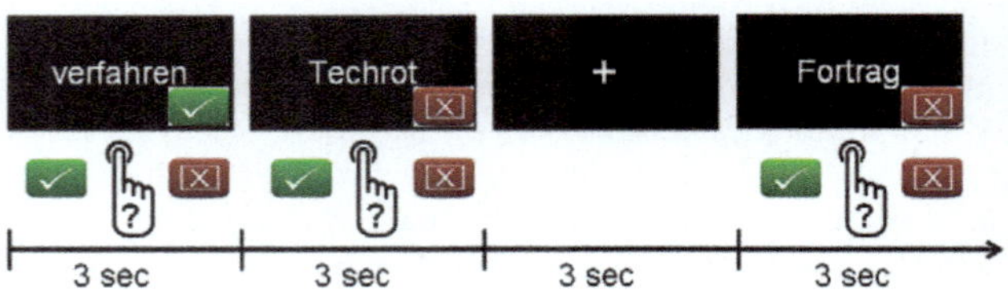

Figure 1. fMRI Paradigm. Correctly spelled words, misspelled words, pseudowords and a fixation cross were presented in a randomized order for three seconds. In each lexical decision condition, children were instructed to respond by either pressing the "correct" button with the index finger or the "misspelled/pseudoword" button with the middle finger on the response console. Responses were given with the right hand and recorded and logged for further analyses. The children did not receive feedback to their responses.

Magnetic Resonance Imaging (MRI) data acquisition and analysis

Imaging was performed on a 3.0 Tesla Trio Tim scanner (Siemens Medical Systems, Erlangen, Germany) using a 12-channel head coil. To minimize head movement, childrens' heads were stabilized with foam cushions. A high-resolution isotropic (1×1×1 mm) structural scan (TR = 1900 ms, TE = 2.2 ms) was acquired to allow precise registration of functional data to individual anatomy. Structural brain scans were reviewed by an expert and did not show morphological abnormalities. Functional images were acquired using a single-shot gradient echo EPI sequence (TR = 2190 ms, TE = 30 ms, matrix 64×64 mm, FOV = 192, Flip Angle 90°, 36 three mm thick slices). Visual stimuli were synchronized with the MR-scanner using "Presentation" (Neurobehavioral Systems, Albany, CA) and back-projected onto a translucent screen installed on the rear of the scanner bore. Participants watched the screen through a mirror attached on the top of the head coil. Answers were given via a button response box as described above.

Functional MRI data analysis was performed using FEAT (fMRI Expert Analysis Tool; Version 4.1.5., part of FMRIB's Software Library, www.fmrib.ox.ac.uk/fsl). The following preprocessing steps were applied: motion correction using MCFLIRT; non-brain removal using BET; interleaved slice time correction; spatial smoothing using a Gaussian kernel of 6 mm FWHM; and high-pass temporal filtering. Time series statistical analysis was carried out using FILM. Motion parameters were included in the model as covariates of no interest. Nonlinear registration to high-resolution and standard images (Montreal Neurological Institute (MNI) space) was carried out using FNIRT. Higher level analysis was done using FLAME (FMRIB's Local Analysis of Mixed Effects). Z statistic images were thresholded using clusters determined by $Z>2.0$ and a corrected cluster significance threshold of $p = 0.05$ (using Gaussian Random Field Theory).

Analyses for the entire group were performed by computing linear t-contrasts between selected experimental conditions for the lexical decision task for each participant, which were then entered into a random effects two-sample t-test. To examine the correlation between behavioral improvement and activation increase, as well as interaction effects between increases in the TG and WG, we ran second-level (fixed effects) analyses for each subject to calculate the differences between activation patterns (pre vs. post activation). Subsequently, group level analyses (mixed effects) were run, including the number of incorrect responses inside the scanner as variable of no interest.

Results

The main findings of this study are summarized in Figures, while the presented Tables S1 and S2 should provide additional information to the text and the Figures.

1. Baseline differences in brain activation patterns (Pre-Intervention)

To test our first hypothesis, we looked for group differences (TG, WG and CG) prior to the intervention (pre-test). Contrasts of the lexical decision tasks (1: correctly spelled words, 2: misspelled words, 3: pseudowords) versus fixation were computed. We analyzed whether the two groups with comparatively poor spelling and reading abilities (TG, WG) displayed comparable brain activation patterns before the intervention. In addition, we also investigated potential differences in brain activation between poor spellers and readers (TG, WG) and good spellers and readers (CG). The number of incorrect responses inside the scanner was included as variable of no interest. In the following section all significant differences of activation are reported:

The comparison of the two groups with comparatively poor spelling and reading abilities revealed increased activation in the left precuneus and left anterior cingulate gyrus for the TG compared to the WG during processing of misspelled words before the intervention (Figure 2; Table S1). No differences of activation between the TG and WG were found during the other conditions.

The comparison of the CG and the groups with comparatively poor spelling and reading abilities (TG and WG) revealed increased activation in left occipito-temporal regions and in the cerebellum for the CG during all three different lexical decision conditions (Figures S1, S2, S3). Beyond that, the CG exhibited increased activation in the left lateral occipital cortex, left inferior temporal gyrus, and left hippocampus relative to the TG (during processing pseudowords; Figure S2), and increased activation in the bilateral lateral occipital cortex and bilateral temporal regions compared to the WG (during processing of correctly spelled words and pseudowords; Table S1).

Furthermore, increased activation during the processing of misspelled words for the groups with comparatively poor spelling and reading abilities (TG and WG) compared to the CG was observed in the precuneus, right posterior paracingulate gyrus and in the frontal medial gyrus. Beyond that the TG exhibited increased activation in right frontal areas and right temporal regions (Table S1, Figure 3 and S3).

2. Effects of the Intervention

2.1. Behavioral Results. To investigate the behavioral effects of the intervention, we computed a 2×2 ANOVA for repeated measures on the HSP spelling scores in considering TIME (pre- and post-test) as within subjects variable and GROUP (TG and WG) as between subjects variable. We observed a significant interaction between TIME and GROUP ($F_{(1,18)} = 15.42$; $p<.001$; $\eta_p^2 = .46$), revealing increases in spelling performance only for the TG (Figure 4). With respect to reading, a 2×2 ANOVA for repeated measures on the SLS reading scores (indicative of reading speed) revealed a significant main effect of TIME ($F_{(1,18)} = 8.79$; $p<.05$; $\eta_p^2 = .33$) indicating generally higher scores in the post- than in the pre-test. No significant interaction involving experimental group emerged. For reading comprehension (ELFE), the ANOVA yielded a significant interaction between TIME and GROUP ($F_{(1,18)} = 4.52$; $p<.05$; $\eta_p^2 = .20$), revealing performance increases only for the TG (Figure 3). An overview of descriptive statistics is presented in Table 1.

2.2. Behavioral Performance during fMRI. In order to investigate task performance during fMRI (measured by response accuracy in the lexical decision tasks), a 2×2 ANOVA for repeated measures yielded a significant main effect of TIME ($F_{(1,18)} = 6.89$; $p<.05$; $\eta_p^2 = .28$), indicating generally higher scores in the post- than in the pre-test. The TIME by GROUP interaction failed to reach statistical significance, although the mean values (reported in Table 2) suggested stronger increases in accuracy for the TG than for the WG. To investigate changes in reaction time (RT in seconds) a 2×2 ANOVA for repeated measures was computed. The TIME by GROUP interaction reached statistical significance ($F_{(1,18)} = 6.4$; $p<.05$; $\eta_p^2 = .26$), indicating a stronger increase in RT for the WG (see Table 2).

2.3. Functional MRI Results. To test for changes in brain activation patterns post- compared to pre-intervention, we computed within group analyses for each group separately. Subsequently, to assess the training effects more specifically, we compared increases in activation (post>pre) for the TG, WG and CG during all lexical decision tasks. The within group comparison

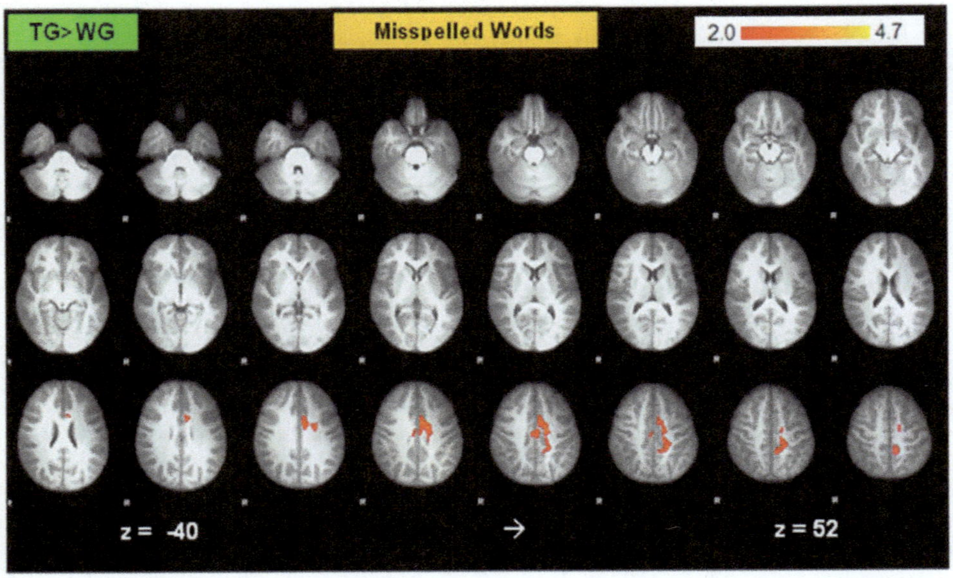

Figure 2. Baseline Comparison of the TG and WG during misspelled words. (Z>2.0; P corrected; P = 0.05). R = right.

revealed increased activation in the precuneus for *all three* groups. Beyond that, for the *TG* increased activation in the right posterior cingulate, left inferior and middle temporal gyrus and left hippocampus and parahippocampal region related intervention was found (during processing pseudowords). For the *WG*, increases in the right lateral occipital cortex and right middle temporal cortex were observed (during all three conditions; Table S2, Figure 5). In the *CG* additional increases of activation in bilateral middle temporal and occipito-temporal regions at the second scan were found (during processing misspelled and pseudowords).

To investigate the effects of the intervention with respect to potential change of brain activation patterns, we compared increases in activation (post>pre) for the TG and WG. We observed a significant interaction effect, revealing increases in activation for the TG in the bilateral parahippocampal area and in the cerebellum (extending into the brain stem) during processing misspelled words, and increased activation for the WG in the precuneus, cerebellum, left frontal pole and right lateral occipital cortex and right parieto-temporal region (Table S2, Figure 5) during processing correctly spelled and misspelled words.

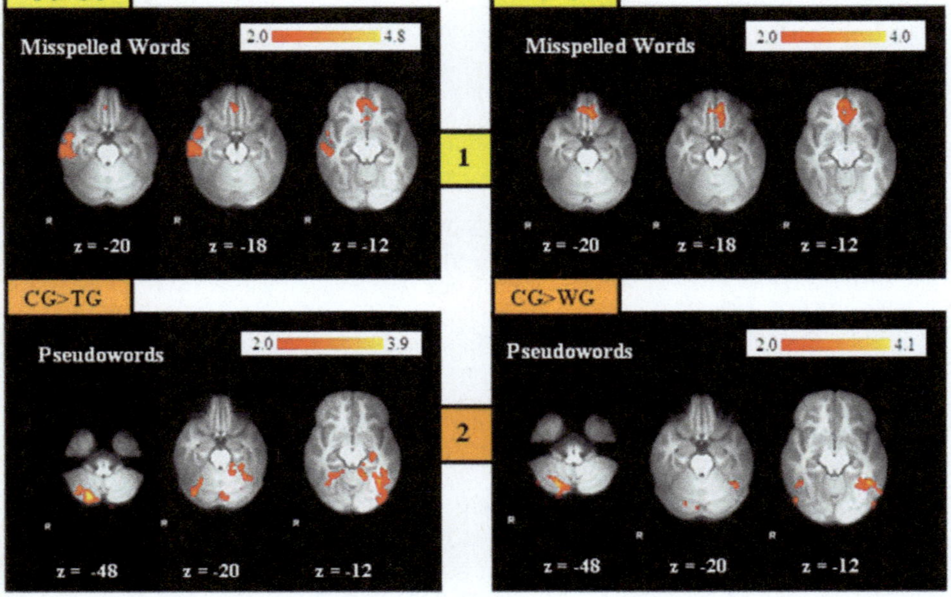

Figure 3. Baseline Comparison of Poor Spellers (Readers) vs. Controls. Pre-Intervention: 1: Activation during the condition misspelled words (relative to rest), 2: Activation during the condition pseudowords (relative to rest). Figures on the left represent contrasts between controls and the TG, and figures on the right contrasts between controls and the WG (Z>2.0; P corrected; P = 0.05). R = right. A more detailed representation of these contrasts is presented in Figure S2 and Figure S3.

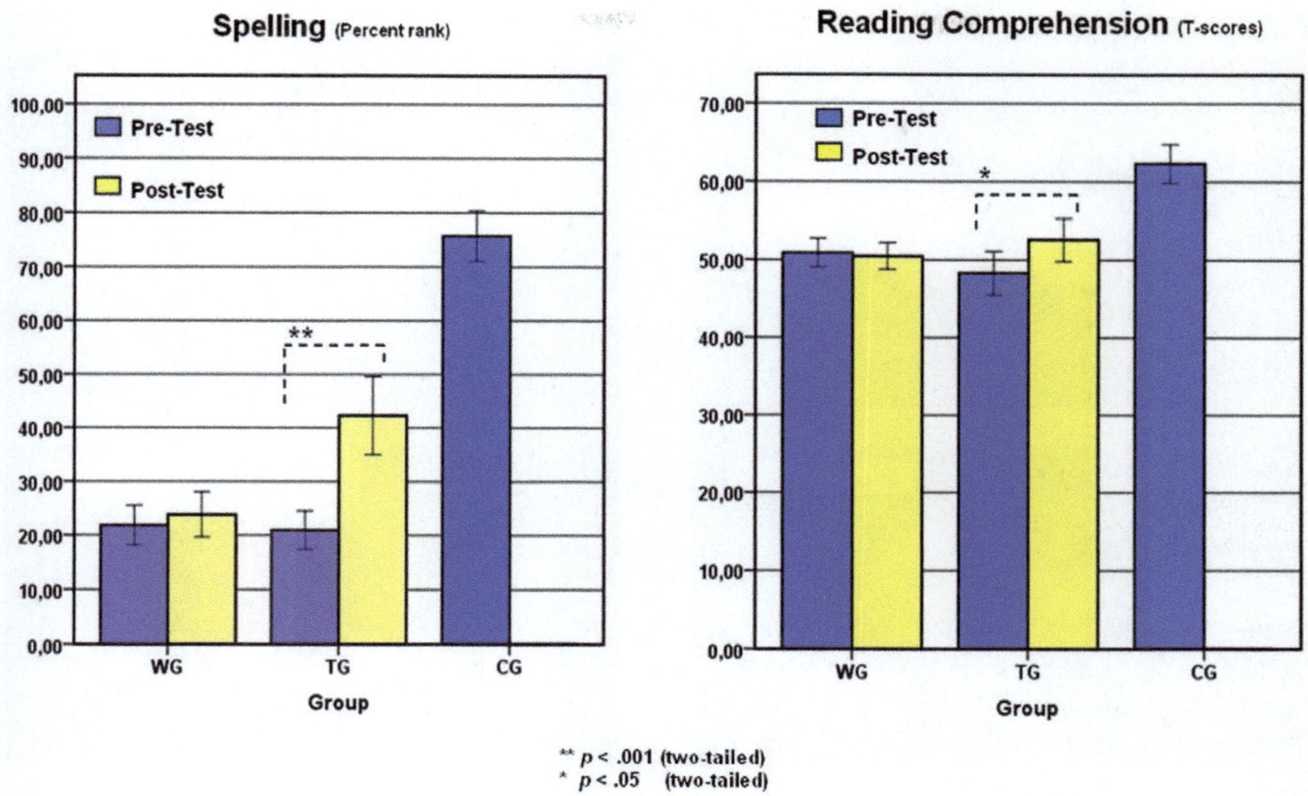

Figure 4. Behavioral Effects of the Training. Spelling (percentile rankings of the HSP) and reading comprehension (ELFE T-scores). For descriptive reasons, the pre-test scores of the CG group are presented.

To assess the relation between improvement of spelling ability and increases in brain activation patterns, we computed whole-brain correlation analyses. We found negative correlations between improvement of spelling ability and activation increase in the cerebellum and right lateral occipital cortex, right lingual gyrus and right middle temporal gyrus in the TG during all three conditions (Table 3).

Discussion

This is the first study to investigate the effects of a morpheme-based spelling intervention on patterns of brain activity in children with comparatively poor spelling reading abilities using repeated fMRI. Behavioral improvements in spelling and reading comprehension were observed in the TG. Furthermore, increased activation in left temporal, parahippocampal and hippocampal regions after five weeks of intervention were noted in the TG. We interpret these changes as related to the recollection of the new learnt morpheme-based strategy; given the hippocampus and parahippocampal gyrus have relevance for memory recollection [44,45]. In line with this notion, Krafnick et al. [46] recently reported increases in gray matter volume in the hippocampus in dyslexic children after an eight week reading intervention. The activation increases in the left inferior and middle temporal gyri could be indicative of enhanced reliance on concept retrieval, semantic processing and integration processes in the TG [47].

Conversely to *left* temporal and parahippocampal activation increases in the TG, the WG showed increases in *right* posterior regions (i.e. lateral occipital cortex, gyrus angularis, gyrus supramarginalis). Though speculative and preliminary, a possible explanation for the observed increases of activation in right posterior regions in the WG could be that they hint at (probably inefficient) compensatory cognitive mechanisms. It was found that dyslexic subjects (who represent a sample with most severe deficits in reading and spelling) showed increased activation in right posterior region [7,11], presumably reflecting a serial grapheme-phoneme decoding compensation strategy [48]. Moll and Landerl [48] report that children with poor spelling and good reading abilities (similar to our samples) named pseudohomophones as quickly as their corresponding words, and their phonological awareness skills were adequate, suggesting that good reading ability in poor spellers might be based on highly efficient grapheme-phoneme decoding procedures. Due to the asymmetry in German language (grapheme-phoneme correspondence is high,

Table 2. Performance during fMRI (correctly solved tasks as percentage and reaction time in seconds (RT).

Performance during fMRI				
Accuracy	**TG**	**WG**	**CG**	
Pre-Intervention	72.4 (+/−8.4)	70.7 (+/−10.0)	89.7 (+/−5.9)	**.000**
Post-Intervention	77.9 (+/−8.9)	73.5 (+/−12.6)	91.1 (+/−4.1)	**.001**
RT				
Pre-Intervention	1.4 (+/−0.2)	1.3 (+/−0.2)	1.3 (+/−0.2)	.282
Post-Intervention	1.6 (+/−0.3)	1.7 (+/−0.2)	1.3 (+/−0.3)	**.003**

Means and Standard Deviations (in brackets).

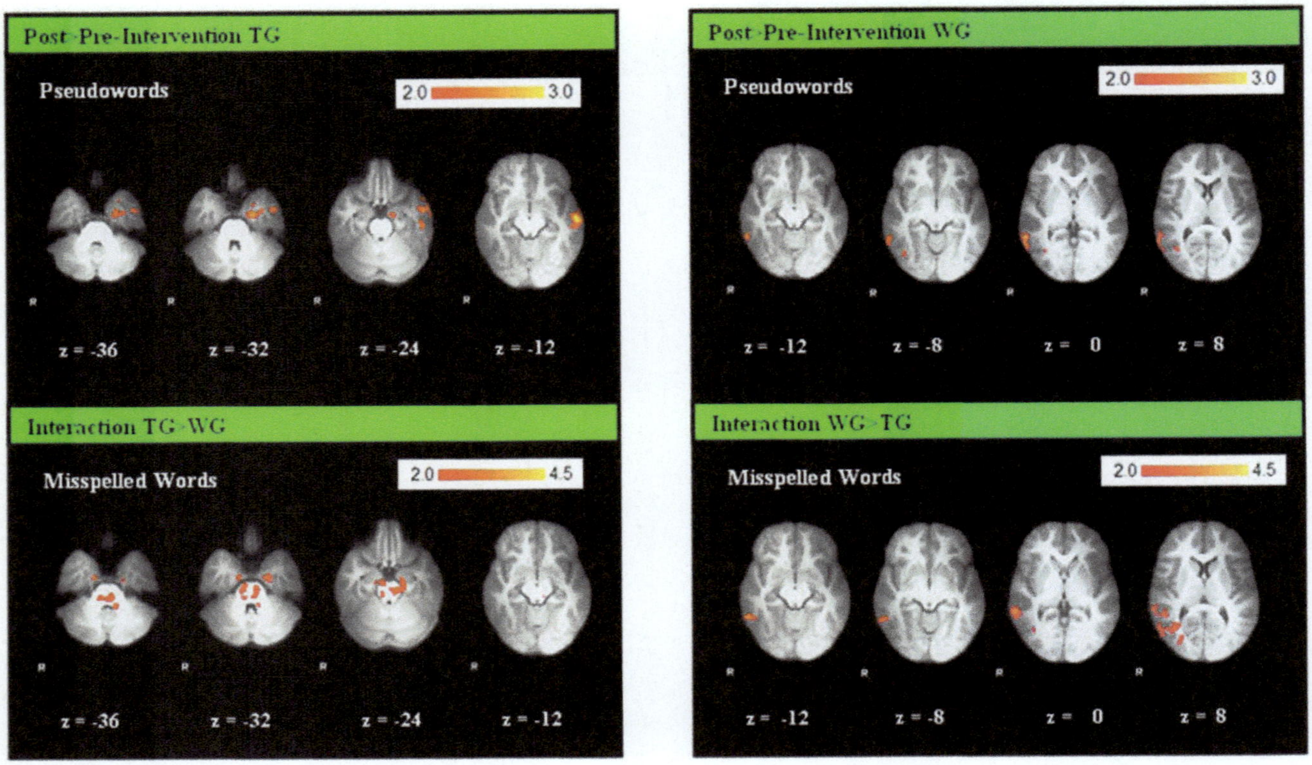

Figure 5. Changes of Activation in Poor Spellers. 1: Increases of activation after the intervention for the TG (left), compared to increases of activation without intervention for the WG (right), during the condition pseudowords. 2: Interaction Effect: Increased activation for the TG (compared to the WG) and for the WG (compared to the TG) during the condition misspelled words. ($Z>2.0$; P corrected; $P=0.05$). R = right.

but phoneme-grapheme correspondence is low) this strategy is not helpful for spelling difficulties, as different spellings for words with the same pronunciation (e.g. Wal/whale – Wahl/election) exist.

This interpretation is also strengthened by the observed negative correlations between behavioral improvement and activation increase in the cerebellum and right occipital and temporal regions in the TG. It seems that increased activation in the right posterior hemisphere correlates with less improvement of spelling ability due to intervention, which would further support the notion that reliance on the right posterior regions is probably related to inefficient compensation of poor spelling abilities.

The interpretation of these changes has to be done carefully, as the two groups of comparatively poor spellers and readers showed differences in activation patterns prior to the intervention in the precuneus and anterior cingulate. The precuneus is known to be part of the default-mode network [49]. Decreased activation in this region is related to attentive task engagement [49], reflecting rather general processing. Similarly, the anterior cingulate cortex

Table 3. Correlation: Increase of activation × less behavioral improvement in the TG.

CORRELATION: Increase of activation × less behavioral improvement in the TG

	k	Z	x	y	z
Correctly Spelled Words					
R middle temporal gyrus	6805	3.4	58	−54	−10
R lateral occipital cortex	2467	3.27	32	−72	42
Misspelled Words					
R lateral occipital cortex	1808	3.08	30	−76	44
L cerebellum	1318	2.98	−40	−64	−28
Pseudowords					
L precentral gyrus	2782	3.31	−50	−10	40
R lingual gyrus	1665	2.83	14	−84	−10
R cerebellum	1381	3.03	22	−68	−22

Coordinates (in MNI standard space) and Activation Significance (Z statistics) of Local Maxima of Clusters, $Z>2.0$, P corrected $P=0.05$.

is known as an important component of a neural network responsible for attention [50]. We therefore assume that the observed differences (TG vs. WG) at baseline are rather associated with differences in attentive task engagement than with differences in reading and spelling processes.

Remarkably, both groups of comparatively poor spellers and readers responded more slowly in the MRI session after the intervention, probably indicating that the TG and WG spent more time actually processing stimuli than the CG. However, on a purely descriptive level, there was a weak tendency towards a stronger improvement of accuracy of responses inside the scanner only for the TG (5.5%) as compared to the WG (2.8%) and CG (1.4%).

Prior to the intervention, both groups of comparatively poor spellers and readers showed increased activation in the precuneus and frontal medial cortex and relatively decreased activation of left occipito-temporal and cerebellar regions during a lexical decision task (relative to controls). Increased activation in the frontal medial region and paracingulate gyrus might be explained by a more effortful and attentionally guided reading strategy [15,51] used by the TG and WG. Increased activation of the precuneus in children with spelling and reading impairments compared to non-impaired controls has also been found by others [7,9–11,17]. In non-impaired individuals the precuneus has been associated with attention, semantic processing and most notably with the default-mode network [47,49,52]. This region is active during conscious rest and deactivated during attentive task engagement. The general increase of activation in the precuneus found in all groups at the second scan thus suggests a general decrease in attention or excitement [47,49,52].

We also observed decreased activation of left occipito-temporal and cerebellar regions in comparatively poor spellers and readers relative to controls prior to the intervention. The left occipito-temporal region has been related to automatic and fluent reading [7,9] and decreased activation has been found in multiple studies investigating dyslexia or reading impaired individuals. Several structural and functional imaging studies suggest cerebellar disruptions in individuals with dyslexia [53,54,55]. These have been related to semantic and phonological processing [56], skill automatization and learning [57–59] and linguistic performance [60,61].

Some limitations of this study also have to be considered, when interpreting our results. First, the interpretation of the interaction effect (comparing within group changes of TG *and* WG) has to be done carefully, as these two groups showed differences in activation patterns prior to the intervention. However, the comparison of activation patterns post- vs. pre-intervention for each group separately revealed increased activation in parahippocampal regions for the TG, which was also observed by the interaction analyses. Second, a sample size of ten children per group might be regarded as rather small. While this may certainly compromise statistical power, it needs to be recognized that the employed study design (requiring children to participate in the training and to take part in several behavioral and fMRI testing sessions) imposed great efforts both on participants and the resources involved, together making studies of this kind difficult and rare. Third, a follow-up assessment including fMRI several months after the intervention would have been desirable to assess potential long-term effects of training outcome. Furthermore, the application of a more elaborated research design, such as the inclusion of a control activity (e.g. reading intervention), to investigate specific intervention effects would substantially improve these kinds of studies. In addition, future studies should investigate the impact of specific cognitive strategies applied by poor spellers and good spellers during a lexical decision task. It might possibly be the case that in our study comparatively poor spellers and readers relied on visual familiarity with real words, while good spellers actually attempted to detect misspelled real words.

Nonetheless, our study provides insights into the functional correlates of poor spelling ability and preliminary evidence for training-induced changes in brain function. We hope this work encourages future investigations into this area that also seek to overcome some of these shortcomings.

Supporting Information

Figure S1 Detailed overview of all activation differences during processing of correctly spelled words. (Z>2.0; P corrected; P = 0.05). R = right.

Figure S2 Detailed overview of all activation differences during processing of pseudowords. (Z>2.0; P corrected; P = 0.05). R = right.

Figure S3 Detailed overview of all activation differences during processing of misspelled words. (Z>2.0; P corrected; P = 0.05). R = right.

Table S1 fMRI Results Pre-Intervention. Coordinates (in MNI standard space) and Activation Significance (Z statistics) of Local Maxima of Clusters, Z>2.0, P corrected P = 0.05. Comparison between the two spelling impaired groups (TG and WG), training group and controls (TG and CG) and waiting group and controls (WG and CG).

Table S2 Changes of Activation related to Intervention (Within Group Comparison). Post-Intervention vs. Pre-Intervention for the training group (TG) and waiting group (WG). Interaction effects of increases of activation (post-pre for TG vs WG). Coordinates (in MNI standard space) and Activation Significance (Z statistics) of Local Maxima of Clusters, Z>2.0, P corrected P = 0.05.

Acknowledgments

The authors wish to express their gratitude to Nadja Kozel, Bernd Schneeberger, Johanna Vogl and Stefanie Rohrer who greatly contributed to this project and to Franz Ebner, MD, for continued infrastructural support.

Author Contributions

Conceived and designed the experiments: DG AF GR KK CE. Performed the experiments: DG. Analyzed the data: DG. Contributed reagents/materials/analysis tools: DG RK CP FF CE. Wrote the paper: DG AF CE. Helped design the fMRI-paradigm: GR KK. Supported analyses of the experiment: GR KK.

References

1. Dilling H, Mombour W, Schmidt MH (2005) Internationale Klassifikation psychischer Störungen. ICD-10 V (F). Klinisch-diagnostische Leitlinien (5th ed.). Bern: Hans Huber.
2. Shaywitz SE, Morris R, Shaywitz B (2008) The education of dyslexic children from childhood to young adulthood. Annual review of psychology 59: 451–75.

3. Gabrieli JD (2009) Dyslexia: A New Synergy Between Education and Cognitive Neuroscience. Science 325: 280–283.
4. Steinbrink C, Groth K, Lachmann T, Riecker A (2012) Neural correlates of temporal auditory processing in developmental dyslexia during German vowel length discrimination. Brain & Language 121: 1–11.
5. Booth J, Burman D, Meyer J, Gitelman D, Parrish T, et al. (2002) Functional Anatomy of Intra- and Cross-Modal Lexical Tasks. NeuroImage 16: 7–22.
6. Booth J, Burman D, Meyer J, Gitelman D, Parrish T, et al. (2004) Development of Brain Mechanisms for Processing Orthographic and Phonologic Representations. Journal of Cognitive Neuroscience 16: 1234–1249.
7. Shaywitz SE, Mody M, Shaywitz B (2006) Neural Mechanisms in Dyslexia. Curr Dir Psychol Sci 15: 278–281.
8. Dehaene S, Cohen L (2011) The unique role of the visual word form area in reading. Trends in Cognitive Sciences 15: 254–262.
9. Kronbichler M, Hutzler F, Staffen W, Mair A, Ladurner G, et al. (2006) Evidence for a dysfunction of left posterior reading areas in German dyslexic readers. Neuropsychologia 44: 1822–32.
10. Richlan F, Kronbichler M, Wimmer H (2009) Functional Abnormalities in the Dyslexic Brain: A Quantitative Meta-Analysis of Neuroimaging Studies. Hum. Brain Mapp 30: 3299–3308.
11. Maisog JM, Einbinder ER, Flowers DL, Turkeltaub PE, Eden GF (2008) A Meta-analysis of Functional Neuroimaging Studies of Dyslexia. Ann N Y Acad Sci 1145: 237–259.
12. Aylward EH, Richards TL, Berninger VW, Nagy WE, Fiel KM, et al. (2003) Instructional treatment associated with changes in brain activiation in children with dyslexia. Neurology 61: 212–219.
13. Eden G, Jones KM, Cappell K, Gareau L, Wood FB, et al. (2004) Neural changes following remediation in adult developmental dyslexia. Neuron 44: 411–422.
14. Gaab N, Gabrieli J, Deutsch G, Tallal P, Temple E (2007) Neural correlates of rapid auditory processing are disrupted in children with developmental dyslexia and ameliorated with training: An fMRI study. Restor Neurol Neurosci 25: 295–310.
15. Meyler A, Keller T, Cherkassky VL, Gabrieli J, Just MA (2008) Modifying the brain activation of poor readers during sentence comprehension with extended remedial instruction: A longitudinal study of neuroplasticity. Neuropsychologia 46: 2580–2592.
16. Richards TL, Aylward EH, Berninger VW, Field KM, Grimme AC, et al. (2006) Individual fMRI activiation in orthographic mapping and morpheme mapping after orthographic or morphological spelling treatment in child dyslexics. J Neurolinguistics 19: 56–86.
17. Shaywitz B, Shaywitz S, Blachman B, Pugh K, Fulbright R, et al. (2004) Development of Left Occipitotemporal Systems for Skilled Reading in Children After a Phonologically-Based Intervention. Biol Psychiatry 55: 926–233.
18. Simos P, Fletcher J, Berman M, Breier J, Foorman B, et al. (2002) Dyslexia-specific brain activation profile becomes normal following successful remedial training. Neurology 58: 1203–1213.
19. Simos P, Fletcher J, Denton C, Sarkari S, Billingsley-Marshall R, et al. (2006) Magnetic Source Imaging Studies of Dyslexia Interventions. Dev Neuropsychol 30: 591–611.
20. Temple E, Deutsch G, Poldrack R, Miller S, Tallal P, et al. (2003) Neural deficits in children with dyslexia ameliorated by behavioral remediation: Evidence from functional MRI. PNAS USA 100: 2860–2865.
21. Richards T, Berninger V, Fayol M (2009) fMRI activation differences between 11-year-old good and poor spellers' access in working memory to temporary and long-term orthographic representations. J Neurolinguistics 22: 327–353.
22. Moll K, Landerl K (2009) Double dissociation between reading and spelling difficulties. Scientific Studies of Reading 13: 359–382.
23. Wimmer H, Mayringer H (2002) Dysfluent Reading in the Absence of Spelling Difficulties: A Specific Disability in Regular Orthographies. Journal of Educational Psychology 94: 272–277.
24. Landerl K, Klicpera C (2009) *Lese- und Rechtschreibstörung*. In F. Petermann, ed. Fallbuch der Klinischen Kinderpsychologie (3rd ed.). Göttingen: Hogrefe. pp 193–207.
25. Kargl R, Purgstaller C (2010) Morphem unterstütztes Segmentierungstraining MORPHEUS. Hogrefe, Göttingen.
26. Arnbak E, Elbro C (2000) The effect of morphological awareness training on the reading and spelling skills of young dyslexics. Scand J of Ed Res 44: 229–251.
27. Lyster SAH (2002) The effects of morphological versus phonological awareness training in kindergarten on reading development. Reading and Writing: An Interdisciplinary Journal 15: 261–294.
28. Nunes T, Bryant B, Olsson J (2003) Learning morphological and phonological spelling rules: An intervention study. Sci. Studies of Reading 7: 289–307.
29. Weiss S, Grabner RH, Kargl R, Purgstaller C, Fink A (2010) Behavioral and neurophysiological effects of morphological awareness training on spelling and reading. Reading and Writing: An Interdisciplinary Journal 23: 645–671.
30. May P, Vieluf U, Malitzky V (2000) Hamburger Schreibprobe. Diagnose orthographischer Kompetenz. Verlag für pädagogische Medien, Hamburg.
31. Mayringer H, Wimmer H (2003) Salzburger Lese-Screening für die Klassenstufen 1–4. Hans Huber, Bern.
32. Mayringer H, Wimmer H (2005) Salzburger Lese-Screening für die Klassenstufen 5–8. Hans Huber, Bern.
33. Lenhard W, Schneider W (2006) ELFE 1–6. Ein Leseverständnistest für Erst- bis Sechstklässler. Hogrefe, Göttingen.
34. Raven JC Guide to the Standard Progressive Matrices: Sets A, B, C, D and E. HK Lewis, London.
35. Website of the federal ministry of Austria. Available: http://www.schulpsychologie.at/lernen-leistung/lese-rechtschreibschwaeche/. Accessed 2011 Aug 6.
36. Kargl R, Purgstaller C, Weiss S, Fink A (2008) Effektivitätsüberprüfung eines morphemorientierten Grundwortschatz-Segementierungstrainings (MORPHEUS) bei Kindern und Jugendlichen. Heilpädagogische Forschung 31: 147–156.
37. Kargl R, Purgstaller C, Mrazek C, Ertl K, Fink A (2011) Förderung der Lese- und Rechtschreibkompetenz auf Basis des morphematischen Prinzips. Zeitschrift für Heilpädagogik 2: 61–68.
38. Bhatt C (1991) Einführung in die Morphologie. Gabel, Hürth-Efferen.
39. Scheerer-Neumann G (1979) Intervention bei Lese-Rechtschreibschwäche. Überblick über Theorien, Methoden und Ergebnisse. Kamp, Bochum.
40. Augst G (1989) Schriftwortschatz: Untersuchungen und Wortlisten zum orthographischen Lexikon bei Schülern und Erwachsenen. Peter Lang, Frankfurt am Main.
41. Kronbichler M, Bergmann J, Hutzler F, Staffen W, Mair A, et al. (2007) Taxi vs. Taksi: On Orthographic Word Recognition in the Left Ventral Occipitotemporal Cortex. J Cogn Neurosci 19: 1584–1594.
42. Van der Mark S, Bucher K, Maurer U, Schulz E, Brem S, et al. (2009) Children with dyslexia lack multiple specializations along the visual word-form (VWF) system. NeuroImage 47: 1940–1949.
43. Wager TD, Nichols TE (2003) Optimization of Experimental Design in fMRI: A General Framework Using a Genetic Algorithm. NeuroImage 18: 293–309.
44. Diana RA, Yonelinas AP, Ranganath C (2007) Imaging recollection and familiarity in the medial temporal lobe: a three-component model. Trends in Cog Sci 11: 379–386.
45. Gimbel SI, Brewer JB (2011) Reaction time, memory strength, and fMRI activity during memory retrieval: Hippocampus and default network are differentially responsive during recollection and familiarity judgments. Cog Neurosci 2: 19–23.
46. Krafnick AJ, Flowers DL, Napoliello EM, Eden GF (2011) Gray matter volume changes following reading intervention in dyslexic children. NeuroImage 57: 733–741.
47. Binder JR, Desai RH, Graves WW, Conant LL (2009) Where is the semantic system? A critical review and Meta-Analysis of 120 functional neuroimaging studies. Cereb. Cortex 19: 2767–2796.
48. Moll K, Landerl K (2009) Double dissociation between reading and spelling difficulties. Scientific Studies of Reading 13: 359–382.
49. Cavanna A, Trimble MR (2006) The precuneus: a review of its functional anatomy and behavioural correlates. Brain 129: 564–583.
50. Davis K, Hutchison W, Lozano A, Tasker R, Dostrovsky J (2000) Human Anterior Cingulate Cortex Neurons Modulated by Attention-Demanding Tasks. J Neurophysiol 83: 3575–3577.
51. Fornito A, Yücel M, Wood S, Stuart GW, Buchanan JA, et al. (2004) Individual Differences in Anterior Cingulate/Paracingulate Morphology are related to Executive Functions in Healthy Males. Cereb Cortex 14: 424–431.
52. Graves WW, Binder JR, Desai RH, Conant LL, Seidenberg MS (2010) Neural correlates of implicit and explicit combinatorial semantic processing. NeuroImage 53: 638–646.
53. Brown WE, Eliez S, Menon V, Rumsey JM, White CD, et al. (2001) Preliminary evidence of widespread morphological variations of the brain in dyslexia. Neurology 56: 780–783.
54. Brunswick N, McCrory E, Price CJ, Frith CD, Frith U (1999) Explicit and implicit processing of words and pseudowords by adult developmental dyslexics. A search for Wernicke's Wortschatz? Brain 122: 1901–1917.
55. Eckert MA, Leonard CM, Richards TL, Aylward EH, Thomson J (2003) Anatomical correlates of dyslexia: frontal and cerebellar findings. Brain 126: 482–494.
56. Fulbright RK, Jenner AR, Mencl WE, Pugh KR, Shaywitz SE, et al. (1999) The cerebellum's role in reading: a functional MR imaging study. AJNR 20: 1925–1930.
57. Nicolson RI, Fawcett AJ, Berry EL, Jenkins IH, Dean P, et al. (1999) Association of abnormal cerebellar activation with motor learning difficulties in dyslexic adults. Lancet 353: 1662–1667.
58. Nicolson RI, Fawcett AJ, Dean P (2001) Developmental dyslexia: the cerebellar deficit hypothesis. Trends Neurosci 24: 508–511.
59. Poldrack RA, Gabrieli JD (2001) Characterizing the neural mechanisms of skill learning and repetition priming. Brain 124: 67–82.
60. Riva D, Giorgi C (2000) The cerebellum contributes to higher functions during development: evidence from a series of children surgically treated for posterior fossa tumours. Brain 123: 1051–61.
61. Scott RB, Stoodley CJ, Anslow P, Paul C, Stein JF, et al. (2001) Lateralized cognitive deficits in children following cerebellar lesions. Dev Med Child Neurol 43: 685–691.

Speech Sound Processing Deficits and Training-Induced Neural Plasticity in Rats with Dyslexia Gene Knockdown

Tracy M. Centanni[1]*, Fuyi Chen[2], Anne M. Booker[2], Crystal T. Engineer[1], Andrew M. Sloan[1], Robert L. Rennaker[1], Joseph J. LoTurco[2], Michael P. Kilgard[1]

1 School of Behavioral and Brain Sciences, University of Texas at Dallas, Richardson, Texas, United States of America, **2** Physiology and Neurobiology, University of Connecticut, Storrs, Connecticut, United States of America

Abstract

In utero RNAi of the dyslexia-associated gene *Kiaa0319* in rats (KIA-) degrades cortical responses to speech sounds and increases trial-by-trial variability in onset latency. We tested the hypothesis that KIA- rats would be impaired at speech sound discrimination. KIA- rats needed twice as much training in quiet conditions to perform at control levels and remained impaired at several speech tasks. Focused training using truncated speech sounds was able to normalize speech discrimination in quiet and background noise conditions. Training also normalized trial-by-trial neural variability and temporal phase locking. Cortical activity from speech trained KIA- rats was sufficient to accurately discriminate between similar consonant sounds. These results provide the first direct evidence that assumed reduced expression of the dyslexia-associated gene *KIAA0319* can cause phoneme processing impairments similar to those seen in dyslexia and that intensive behavioral therapy can eliminate these impairments.

Editor: David S. Vicario, Rutgers University, United States of America

Funding: This work was supported by the National Institute for Deafness and Communication Disorders at the National Institutes of Health (R01DC010433 to MPK) and the National Institute of Child Health and Human Development at the National Institutes of Health (HD055655 to JJL). The funders had no role in study design, data collection and analysis, decision to publish, or preparation of the manuscript.

Competing Interests: The authors have declared that no competing interests exist.

* E-mail: tmcentanni@gmail.com

Introduction

Dyslexia is the most common developmental language disorder and affects approximately 7% of the population [1,2]. Individuals with this disorder have normal nonverbal intelligence, but score more than a standard deviation below their peers on reading tests [1,3,4]. Children and adults with dyslexia typically have deficits in phoneme perception and manipulation [5–8]. Even before learning to read, neural activation during phonological processing is impaired in young children at risk for dyslexia [9], which suggests that the neural abnormalities responsible for dyslexia are present from birth and do not reflect experience-dependent processes [10].

Dyslexia is highly heritable and at least four candidate-dyslexia genes have been identified (*KIAA0319, DYX1C1, DCDC2 and ROBO1*) [11–14]. *KIAA0319* is the most consistently associated gene and the link between *KIAA0319* and dyslexia has been replicated in many independent studies [12,15–20]. The observation that variants in *KIAA0319* impair speech evoked cortical activity [21] and cause poor speech perception and reading ability [19,22] is consistent with the earlier hypothesis that phonological processing is a core deficit in dyslexia [23–30]. We have previously shown that *in utero* RNA interference (RNAi) of the rat homolog of this gene (*Kiaa0319*) is sufficient to impair neural processing of speech sounds by elevating trial-by-trial variability in the timing of neural responses [31]. *Kiaa0319* RNAi also duplicates corpus callosum abnormalities in dyslexia [23,32,33] without changing body weight or the volume of the cortex and hippocampus [34]. Based on the similarities between this gene's apparent function in rats and humans, we hypothesized that rats with reduced expression of *Kiaa0319* would exhibit impaired learning when trained to discriminate speech sounds.

Extensive auditory therapy has been used to treat millions of children with dyslexia. Many programs use acoustically modified speech stimuli to improve phoneme awareness [35–38]. Such training can cause changes in neural responses at multiple stages of the auditory pathway [37,39]. These studies support the hypothesis that auditory training can induce therapeutic neural plasticity in dyslexia (but see [40–42]). The genotype of the participants in the intervention studies is unknown and it is not clear whether auditory training would be more or less effective in dyslexics with variants in particular dyslexia-associated genes.

In this study, we used an animal model of speech sound processing to evaluate the role of *Kiaa0319* in speech sound discrimination and training-induced plasticity. We trained control rats and rats with *in utero* RNAi of *Kiaa0319* (KIA- rats) on a variety of speech sound discrimination tasks designed to evaluate known deficits in human dyslexics, including problems with speech in noise, rapid speech sounds, and isolated phonemes. We recorded action potentials and local field potentials in primary (A1) and posterior auditory fields (PAF) after training and compared responses with untrained KIA- and control rats.

Materials and Methods

Ethics Statement

All transfection protocols were designed to minimize any animal suffering and were approved by the University of Connecticut Institutional Animal Care and Use Committee (Protocol # A12-027). All behavioral, surgical, and physiological procedures were designed to minimize any animal suffering and were approved by the University of Texas at Dallas Institutional Animal Care and Use Committee (Protocol # 99-06). Data presented in this study are available upon request.

Animals

Subjects were Wistar rats, both male and female, that were young adults at the time of study. All rats used were subjected as embryos to *in utero* electroporation targeting lateral regions of neocortex that included the auditory cortex by methods described previously [16,20,31,43–45]. In brief, pregnant Wistar rats were anesthetized on day 15 of pregnancy and the embryos were transfected with either an shRNA against *Kiaa0319* which can decrease the Kiaa0319 protein expression in cell culture (Figure S1) and can cause migration delay in neocortex in embryos. Note that this same shRNA vector and transfection procedure have been previously demonstrated to be effective at targeting and knocking down Kiaa0319 protein translation in rats [46]. Control transfection animals received a scrambled sequence control of *Kiaa0319* shRNA, also previously used, that contained 6 bases in the sequence scrambled to render the shRNA inactive in terms of reducing *Kiaa0319* expression [31]. *Kiaa0319* shRNA and scrambled shRNA constructs were injected at a concentration of 1.0 µg/µL. pB-GFP was co-transfected with the effective shRNA construct, and pB-mRFP was co-transfected with the scrambled *Kiaa0319* shRNA control construct to identify the experimental condition in post experimental histological analysis.

Analysis of Transfection Efficacy

The experimental status of the subject remained blind to experimenters throughout the behavior and electrophysiological portions of the study. Following data collection, each subject was perfused transcardially with 250 mL of 0.1 M PB solution with 0.02% heparin, followed by 500 mL of 4% formalin solution in 0.1 M PB. Sections were taken at 80 µm intervals and analyzed under a confocal microscope (Zeiss) to identify the experimental status of each subject (green florescent protein marked experimental subjects and red florescent protein marked control littermates). The number of fluorescent cells was counted in a 1 mm^2 area of layer 2/3 of primary auditory cortex bilaterally. These layers were used as this is where the highest concentration of transfected neurons were located. This number was then divided by the estimated number of cells in matching primary auditory cortex regions of this size to calculate a percentage of affected cells. The estimated number of neurons was calculated by manually counting the total number of all cells in areas of layer 2/3 auditory cortex that matched the regions used in the transfected-neuron analysis and then estimating neuron density over the 1 mm^2 area.

Behavioral Training

We trained 26 rats to discriminate a target speech sound (/dad/) in 4 different contexts. Of these rats, 16 received RNAi of *Kiaa0319* (KIA-) and 10 received scrambled RNAi and served as controls. The behavior tasks we tested are described in detail elsewhere [47–50]. Briefly, rats were trained to respond to a target sound /dad/ using either a lever press or withdrawal from an infra-red nose poke. Once rats understood the mechanism of response (either a lever press or a withdrawal from the nose poke), rats were trained to wait for the presentation of a target sound prior to making a response. Once rats reached a d' of $>= 1.5$ for 10 sessions, they were moved on to a minimum of 20 sessions of each of four discrimination tasks [51].

The isolated speech task consisted of a go-no go paradigm in which rats were trained to press a lever in response to the target sound and to reject each of seven distractors: /dad/ versus /bad/, /gad/, /sad/, /tad/, /dud/, /deed/, /dood/ [47]. Rats were rewarded with a food pellet if they pressed within 3 second (s) of the target and punished with a 6 s time out if they false alarmed. The speech in noise task used the same stimuli with the addition of four levels (0, 48, 60, 72 dB SPL) of continuous speech-shaped noise [52]. In this task, trials were presented in blocks of gradually increasing or decreasing noise to allow rats to adjust to the noise. The truncated speech task was identical to the go-no go discrimination task except that only the first 40 ms of each speech sound was presented [49]. The rapid speech task presented a random sequence of distractor sounds (/bad/, /gad/, /sad/, /tad/), with the target sound (/dad/) inserted randomly between 2–7 s from the start of the trial. Sounds were only delivered while the rat's nose was inside an infra-red nose poke [50]. Rats were rewarded with a food pellet if they removed their nose within 500 ms of the target and punished with a 6 s time out if they false alarmed. Percent correct is reported as the average hits-false alarms for each task.

Acute neural recordings

Following the approximately 4 months of training needed to complete all 4 tasks; rats were anesthetized with dilute pentobarbital and mapped. The techniques used for acute recordings are described in detail elsewhere [31,52–55]. In brief, animals were anesthetized with pentobarbital (50 mg kg^{-1}) and multi-unit recordings were acquired at cortical layer 4/5 (~600–800 µm) using four Parylene-coated tungsten microelectrodes (1–2 MΩ). We used previously recorded multiunit responses from 11 experimentally naïve rats to evaluate the effect of training on neural responses; data from 5 untrained KIA- rats and 6 naïve controls was previously published in Centanni et al. 2013a. Each experimental group (untrained, group 1 trained and group 2 trained) underwent neural recordings once for the purposes of this study. Untrained rats were recorded from as described previously [31], while group 1 and group 2 rats were recorded from following their 4 months of behavioral training.

At each site, we presented a tuning curve consisting of 90 frequencies (1–47 kHz) at 16 intensities (0–75 dB SPL) to determine the characteristic frequency (CF) of each site, trains of six broadband noise bursts (presented 4, 7, 10 and 12.5 Hz) to evaluate following ability of A1 neurons, and the speech stimuli used in our behavior tasks [31,47,49,52,55]. Speech sounds were recorded in a double-walled, soundproof booth and were spoken by a female, native English speaker. The spectral envelope was shifted up in frequency by a factor of two using the STRAIGHT vocoder [56] to better accommodate the rat hearing range (Figure S3).

Analysis of neural recordings

Though behavior did not differ between groups, we analyzed tuning curves for each group to see if the training order caused differences in the neural responses. To define A1 and PAF sites, multi-unit recording sites were manually analyzed to select the CF of each site, as well as to obtain bandwidth, latency, peak firing and end of peak response information. A1 sites were defined as having a short onset latency (~15 ms), narrow bandwidths, and tonotopic organization so that CF increased in a posterior to anterior direction. PAF sites were defined based on their long onset latency (>30 ms), broad bandwidths, and poorly defined tonotopic organization. This method of characterizing auditory fields has been previously validated [55,57–62]. Sites that were not from A1 or PAF were not analyzed further.

We trained half of the rats using one task order (group 1 rats: isolated speech, speech in noise, rapid speech, truncated speech) and the other half using a second task order (group 2 rats: truncated speech, isolated speech, speech in noise, rapid speech). This change in order was to determine if KIA- rats would benefit from specific truncated speech training, as is often used in humans with dyslexia. Control A1 and PAF sites were less variable and more accurate at the consonant classifier task following the second task order compared to control A1 and PAF sites after the first task order (unpaired t-tests for variability and classifier performance; $p<0.01$), while there was no difference in KIA- sites across training task orders. Since there were only minor differences across groups in the neural responses following training, neural activity from both groups was combined for analysis.

In response to broad band click trains, normalized spike rate (number of spikes evoked by bursts 2–6, normalized by the number of spikes to the first burst) and vector strength (VS) were calculated. VS quantifies the degree of synchronization between action potentials and repeated sounds. Mean VS is calculated with the formula:

$$VS=\frac{1}{n}\sqrt{x^2+y^2};x=\sum_{i=1}^{n}\cos\theta_i;y=\sum_{i=1}^{n}\sin\theta_i\,\theta_i=2\pi\frac{ti}{T}$$

where n = total number of action potentials, t_i is the time of occurrence of the i'th action potential, and T is the inter-stimulus interval. Perfect synchronization would result in a value of one, whereas no synchronization would result in a value of zero.

We have previously shown that neural responses in KIA- rats are poor predictors of stimulus identity, while responses in control animals are good predictors of stimulus identity. To test whether training can improve KIA- neural responses, single trial response patterns to each of the isolated speech sounds were compared using a well-documented nearest neighbor classifier [31,47,48,52,63–65]. We used Euclidean distance to compare single trial activity to the average activity (PSTH) evoked by 19 repeats each of two different stimuli. For consonants, activity was binned using 1 ms temporal precision over a 40 ms window to encompass the spike timing precision present in the initial consonant [46,48,52,54], while vowel activity was binned across a single 400 ms window so that only spike count information was preserved [47,52]. The classifier then compared the response of each single trial with the average activity template (PSTH) of each of the speech stimuli presented. The current trial being considered was not included in the PSTH to avoid artifact. The classifier attempted to identify the stimulus that evoked the current single trial activity pattern by selecting the template that was most similar to the single trial in units of Euclidean distance. ED was calculated using the formula:

$$\text{Euclidean Distance}=\sqrt{\sum\nolimits_{i=1}\#sites\sum\nolimits_{j=1}\#bins(X_{ij}-Y_{ij})^2}$$

where n_{sites} is each recording site and n_{bins} is each of 40 one-millisecond bins being compared between activity evoked by speech sound X versus speech sound Y. For vowel sounds, the classifier counted the number of action potentials over 400 ms from a single trial and compared the value to the average response to each of the sounds [47,52,64]. We used two tailed t-tests for all pairwise comparisons of the accuracy of both classifiers and for comparison of basic neural firing properties across experimental groups. One-tailed t-tests were used to evaluate behavioral ability, as our previous data suggested that KIA- animals would have impairment on speech discrimination tasks [31]. 1-way ANOVA was used to compare vector strength across groups. Bonferroni correction was used to correct for multiple comparisons.

Results

In utero RNAi of *Kiaa0319* impairs speech sound discrimination

KIA- rats (N = 16) learned to detect a target speech sound as quickly as controls (N = 10). Both groups took approximately 8 days to reach the criterion of 10 training sessions with a d' above 1.5 (Controls: 8.4±0.3 days vs. KIA-: 9.6±0.6 days; $p = 0.17$; Figure S2A). Since ADHD and dyslexia have high comorbidity in humans, we evaluated response latency across groups to ensure that RNAi of *Kiaa0319* did not also cause hyperactivity. Significantly shorter response time has been linked to the presence of ADHD in both humans [66] and in rat models [67,68]. Though on the first day of training, KIA- animals responded significantly faster, the groups were not significantly different on any other training day (Figure S2B). These results suggest that the assumed *in utero* knockdown of *Kiaa0319* does not cause significant hyperactivity, impulsivity, motor problems, or difficulty hearing speech sounds.

Five KIA- rats and five control rats next learned a speech discrimination task in which they were required to press the lever to the target sound /dad/ and withhold pressing to the distractor sounds (/bad/, /gad/, /sad/, /tad/, /dud/, /deed/, /dood/; Figure S3). On the first day, controls and KIA- rats hit to all sounds and performed at chance (56.3±2.3% correct by controls vs. 51.1±1.1% correct by KIA- compared to 50% chance; $p = 0.11$ and $p = 0.34$ respectively; Figure 1A). On each of the next 4 days of testing, KIA- rats were significantly worse than controls at performing this task (last day performance was 64.7±4.0% vs. 78.9±3.3% correct by control rats; $p<0.01$; Figure 1A). KIA- rats false alarmed to distractor sounds almost twice as often as control rats (61.3±9.3% false alarms by KIA- rats vs. 32.7±8.2% false alarms by control rats; $p = 0.04$, Figure 1B&C).

Rats with *in utero* RNAi of *Kiaa0319* remain impaired in adverse listening conditions

Dyslexia training programs often focus on intensive practice on phonological processing tasks [35–38]. We hypothesized that KIA- rats would improve on the discrimination task with additional training. After 5 additional days, all KIA- rats reached 80% correct on the full speech task (81.4±2.3% correct on the last day of training). KIA- rats took fifty percent longer to reach this criteria compared to controls (9.6±0.6 days of training vs. 6.2±0.6 days for control rats, $p<0.01$; Figure 2A). To test whether differences in RNAi transfection rate were responsible for differences in performance across rats, we compared the percent of transfected neurons with the last day performance on the full speech discrimination test. In rats with *in utero* RNAi of *Kiaa0319*, the percent of affected neurons was strongly negatively correlated with speech discrimination performance. Rats with a greater percentage of affected neurons were more impaired at the task than rats with fewer affected neurons ($R = -0.66$, $p<0.01$; Figure 3A). The percentage of transfected neurons in control rats

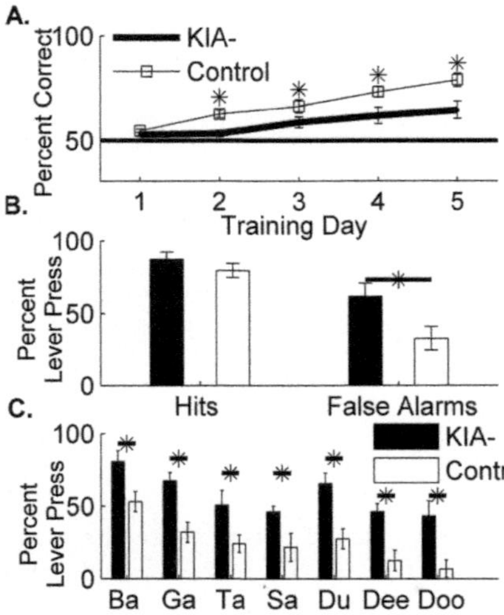

Figure 1. Rats with *in utero* RNAi of *Kiaa0319* are impaired at speech discrimination tasks. A. Performance of KIA- and control rats on the first 5 days of full length speech training. KIA- rats were significantly worse than control rats on the full speech discrimination task on 4 of the days (* = $p<0.01$). **B.** On day 5 of testing, KIA- rats hit to the target sound dad at the same rate as control rats (unpaired t-test; $p=0.33$), but false alarmed to the distractor sounds significantly more than control rats (* = $p=0.04$). **C.** Break down of lever press rates on day 5 of testing to each of the distractor sounds. KIA- rats responded to every sound significantly more than control rats (unpaired t-tests, * = $p<0.01$).

was not correlated with behavioral performance ($R= 0.88$, $p=0.12$; Figure 3B). The lack of correlation in our control rats suggests that the surgery itself did not cause the behavioral impairment, and that the deficit seen in KIA- rats was due to RNAi of the candidate-dyslexia gene *Kiaa0319*. Our results suggest that the degree of *in utero* transfection of this gene is related to each rats' aptitude for learning the full speech sound task. These results support our hypothesis that reduced expression of *KIAA0319* causes impaired phoneme discrimination.

People with dyslexia can often identify speech sounds accurately in quiet, but have a significant impairment on the same task in background noise [4,69–71]. We hypothesized that KIA- rats would also have difficulty with speech discrimination in background noise. After two weeks of discrimination training in quiet (2 sessions/day, 5 days/week), rats were subsequently trained for two weeks on a speech in noise task. The same target and distractors from the full length task were used (presented at 60 dB SPL) and were presented in continuous speech-shaped background noise at one of four intensities (0, 48, 60, or 72 dB SPL) [52].

Control rats were able to improve over the course of 10 training days (last day performance and paired t-test of last day performance vs. first day; 0 dB 91.2±1.5% $p<0.01$; 48 dB 86.9±2.3% $p<0.01$; 60 dB 72.2±2.3% $p<0.01$; 72 dB 51.9±1.5% $p=0.38$; Figure 2B&E). The inability to improve on the loudest intensity noise mimics previous chance level performance at this noise level using control rats [52]. KIA- rats were also able to significantly improve by the last day of training (last day performance and paired t-tests vs. first day performance; 0 dB 83.5±3.0% $p<0.01$; 48 dB 78.9±2.8% $p<0.01$; 60 dB 62.0±2.1% $p=0.11$; 72 dB 51.2±1.2% $p=0.96$), but remained significantly worse than control rats in both quiet and noise ($p<0.01$; Figure 2B&E). Rats with the knockdown had significantly different performance overall (2-Way ANOVA; $F(1,116) = 14.6$, $p=0.0008$), which did not change significantly over time ($F(2,116) = 1.09$, $p=0.35$). There was no significant interaction between experimental status and time ($F(8,116) = 0.80$), which is not surprising since both controls and KIA- rats were able to significantly improve over the course of training. This result suggests that although KIA- rats are able to improve with training, they remain significantly worse than control rats at speech discrimination in a variety of contexts.

As shown previously, the auditory cortex of KIA- rats is significantly worse at following repetitive stimuli compared to controls [31]. We next trained rats on a speech discrimination task made difficult by high repetition rate [72]. A target speech sound (/dad/) was inserted into a random string of distractor speech sounds, and rats were trained to respond when the target sound was presented. Since this task used an infrared nose poke instead of a lever, training time was extended to allow the rats to learn the new response mechanism (see Materials and Methods). At each training stage (marked by symbols in Figure 2C&F), rats were introduced to faster presentation rates (2, 4, 5, 6.67, 10 and 20 syllables per second; sps). KIA- and control rats performed the task equally well during these stages (Figure 2C). During the last 10 days of training, rats were trained on all 6 presentation rates within a single session (in random blocks of 20 trials per presentation rate). Control and KIA- rats were not different in their accuracy on any of the presentation rates (Figure 2F). These results suggest that either KIA- rats do not have a behavioral consequence of their temporal processing deficit or that the neural deficit has been reversed by extensive training.

KIA- rats are impaired at speech discrimination using only onset cues

Based on physiological recordings in A1 of KIA- rats, we hypothesized that rats may compensate for consonant identification deficits by using cues that occur outside the first 40 ms, such as duration or pitch [47,55]. We truncated the speech sounds so that each contained only the initial 40 ms [49] and tested KIA- and control rat discrimination of these sounds for two weeks. On the first day of testing, control rats were significantly better than KIA- rats (89.7±0.6% correct by controls vs. 72.4±0.6% correct by KIA- rats; $p<0.01$; Figure 2D). This result suggests that KIA- rats had been performing the speech discrimination task using cues not present in the onset of the sound. KIA- rats remained significantly impaired (day 1–9, $p<0.01$; day 10, $p=0.08$; Figure 2D), which suggests that KIA- rats have a persistent impairment at discriminating speech sound onsets. In spite of this persistent impairment compared to controls, KIA- rats were able to significantly improve over the course of the 10 days of training (paired t-test, $p<0.01$).

KIA- rats can learn phoneme discrimination with extensive training

Auditory training in humans with dyslexia using truncated speech sounds generalizes to other speech tasks [37,73]. We hypothesized that training KIA- rats on the truncated speech sounds from the beginning might improve performance on the other tasks since KIA- rats were able to improve on the truncated speech task over time. We trained a second group of 8 KIA- and 5 control rats on the truncated speech task for 28 days, which was the length of time needed for control rats to reach asymptotic performance [49]. This group of rats had no experimental training prior to beginning this set of tasks. All rats were first trained on shaping and detection as described above and then trained on discrimination using the truncated speech sounds. Both control

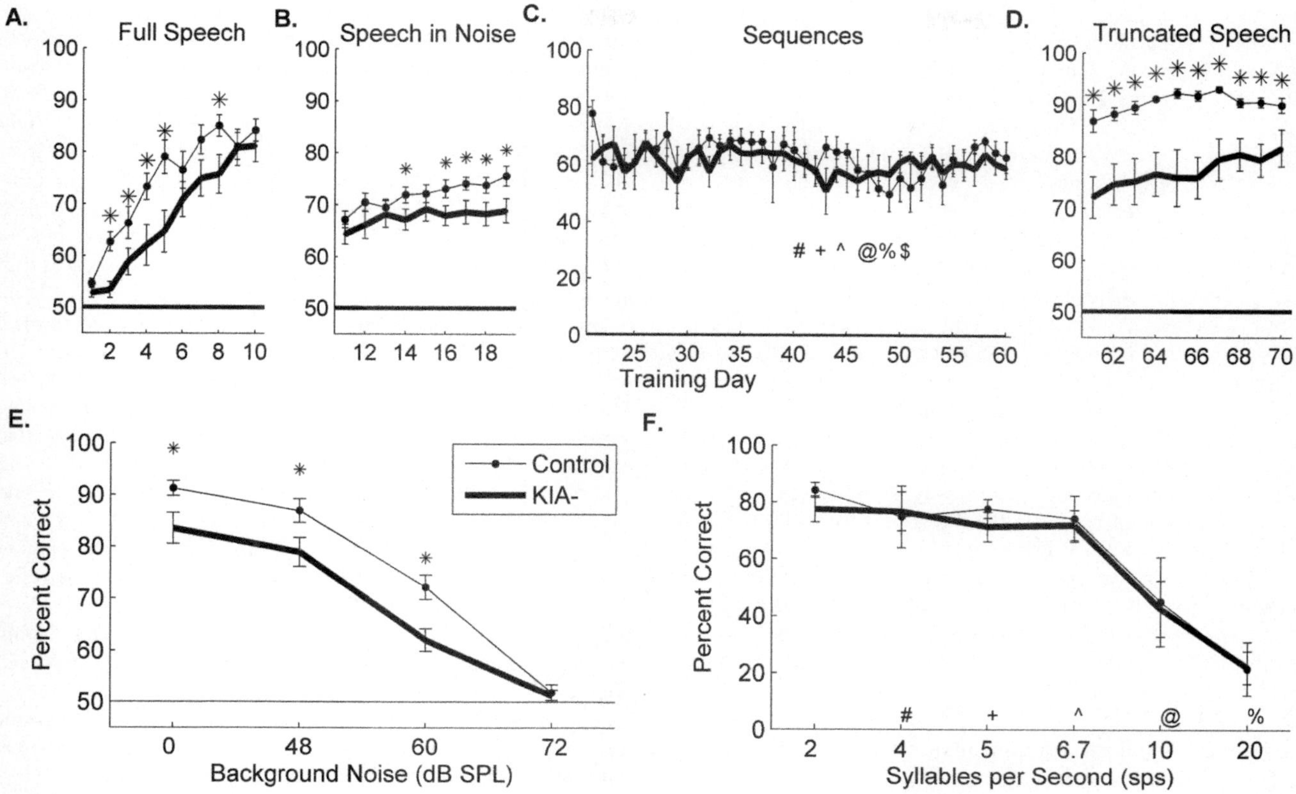

Figure 2. Extensive speech discrimination training can improve on clear speech tasks. Horizontal lines in each panel represent chance performance for that task. **A.** Timeline of performance on the full length speech task. After an additional week of training, 8 KIA- rats were able to perform the full speech task at the same level as 5 control rats (unpaired t-test, $p = 0.24$). **B.** Timeline of performance on speech in noise task. KIA- rats remained significantly below control levels at the end of training ($* = p < 0.05$). **C.** Timeline of performance on sequence task. There were no significant differences between control and KIA- rats during this 40 day training period. Symbols correspond to the first day of training at each new stage (see panel F for symbol key). **D.** Timeline of performance on truncated speech task. KIA- rats were significantly impaired at this task compared to controls until the final day of training ($* = p < 0.01$). **E.** Last day performance of rats on the speech in noise task. ($* = p < 0.01$). **F.** Last day performance of rats on the sequence task. There were no significant differences between control and KIA- rats at any presentation rate tested (2 sps, $p = 0.45$; 4 sps, $p = 0.68$; 5 sps, $p = 0.27$; 6.67 sps, $p = 0.65$; 10 sps, $p = 0.99$; 20 sps, $p = 0.74$).

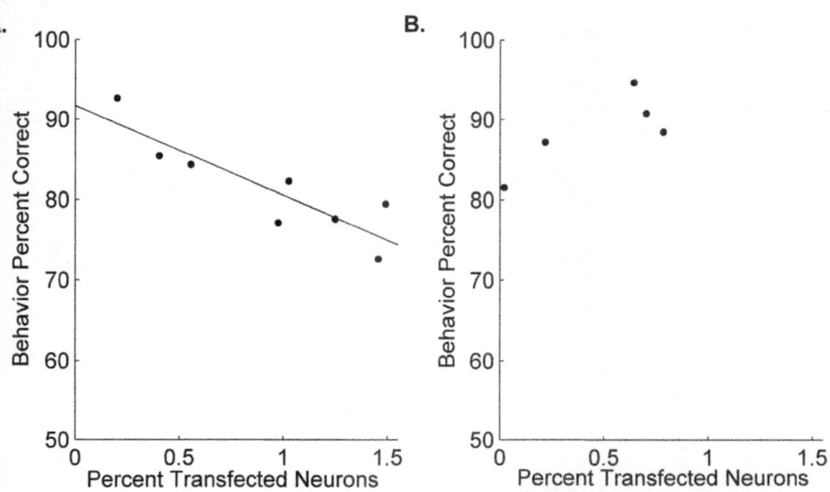

Figure 3. Percentage of transfected neurons predicts behavioral aptitude in KIA- rats. Correlation line denotes significance. **A.** The percentage of layer 2/3 pyramidal neurons affected by the transfection was calculated in A1 bilaterally. In KIA- rats, a higher percentage of transfected neurons was strongly correlated with impaired behavioral performance on the last day of full speech training ($R = -0.66$, $p < 0.01$). **B.** The percentage of transfected neurons in control animals was not correlated with performance ($R = 0.88$, $p = 0.12$).

and KIA- rats needed 7 days of training to perform above chance levels on this difficult task. KIA- rats required 33% longer to reach 80% correct, but survival curves were not statistically significant (16.3±2.1 vs. 12±1.2 days of training, survival analysis; log rank test, $X^2(1, N=13)=2.155$, $p=0.14$; Figure 4A). KIA- rats were significantly worse than controls on several training days, but performed as well as controls at the end of 28 days of training on the truncated speech task (90.8±1.9% vs. 94.5±1.6% correct, KIA- vs. controls respectively; $p=0.14$). These results suggest that KIA- rats are able to learn to discriminate truncated speech sounds when the task is introduced early in training.

We then tested these rats on the other tasks to determine whether training on isolated phonemes would generalize to full length speech sounds. KIA- rats were able to perform the full speech task as well as control rats (average percent correct in KIA- rats was 87.7±3.1% vs. 93.9±2.2% in controls, $p=0.37$; Figure 4B). KIA- rats performed as well as controls on the speech in noise task, although they were slightly worse during the blocks without background noise (0 dB $p<0.01$; 48 dB $p=0.97$; 60 dB $p=0.71$; 72 dB $p=0.53$; Figure 4C&E). KIA- rats that received truncated speech training were not significantly different from controls during the speech sequence task (Figure 4D&F). These results suggest that truncated speech sound training benefits rats with *Kiaa0319* knockdown, especially in adverse learning conditions such as speech in noise.

Extensive behavioral training restores neural firing patterns in KIA- auditory cortex

Since extensive behavioral training in normal rats and in human dyslexics can improve neural responses to speech and non-speech stimuli [37,60,74–76], we hypothesized that extensive speech training would improve neural responses in KIA- rats by reducing variability. We chose to evaluate the effect of training on neural responses in primary auditory cortex (A1) and posterior auditory field (PAF), because these fields have different response properties and training-induced plasticity may have affected these areas in unique ways [55,58,61,75]. We compared the neural data from rats acquired after 4 months of behavioral training to the neural recordings in untrained rats previously described [31]. After training, A1 neurons in KIA- rats responded to tones 7 ms faster than in untrained KIA- rats ($p<0.01$; Figure S4A). After training, PAF neurons in KIA- rats responded to tones 15 ms faster than in untrained KIA- rats ($p<0.01$; Figure S4A). Training also reduced control responses by 5 ms in A1 and 10 ms in PAF ($p<0.01$ and $p=0.11$, A1 and PAF respectively; Figure S4A).

Speech training cut the trial-by-trial variability to speech-evoked responses in half by KIA- rats in A1 (87.3±10.51 ms^2 in untrained vs. 55.3±3.5 ms^2 after training; $p<0.01$; Figures 5A and 6F) and PAF (103.2±3.9 ms^2 in untrained vs. 44.5±3.2 ms^2 after training; $p<0.01$; Figures 5A and 6H). Training also decreased trial-by-trial variability in control A1 (40.6±2.7 ms^2 in untrained vs. 31.8±3.3 ms^2 after training; $p=0.04$; Figures 5A and 6E) and control PAF (70.2±4.1 ms^2 in untrained vs. 27.9±4.4 ms^2 after training; $p<0.01$; Figures 5A and 6G). After training, the number of speech-evoked spikes in the onset response (the first 40 ms after stimulus presentation) significantly increased in control A1 and KIA- A1 and PAF sites ($p<0.04$; Figure 5B). Control PAF did not fire more spikes as a result of behavioral training ($p=0.07$; Figure 5B).

We hypothesized that the improved reliability in trial-by-trial neural firing and increased response strength to sounds to would improve neural speech discrimination ability. Using a nearest-neighbor classifier, we compared performance using trained versus untrained neural recordings (see Materials and Methods). Training did not improve classifier performance using control A1 sites (consonant tasks: $p=0.94$; vowel tasks: $p=0.33$; Figures 5C&D and S5E&G). Training improved classifier performance on consonant tasks using PAF sites in control rats ($p<0.01$;

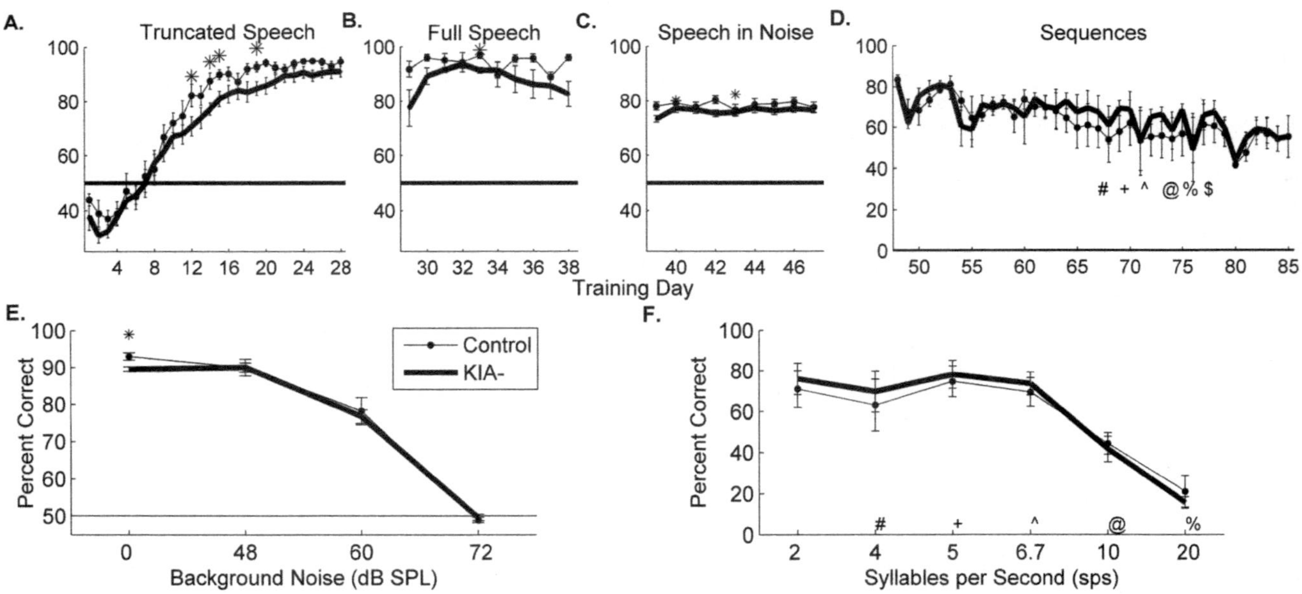

Figure 4. Extensive truncated speech training improves full speech and speech in noise performance in KIA- rats. Horizontal lines in each panel represent chance performance for that task. **A**. Timeline of group 2 rats' performance on truncated speech task. KIA- rats needed slightly longer to reach 80% correct compared to controls (unpaired 1-tailed t-test, $p=0.07$). At the end of training, there was no significant difference in performance across groups (unpaired 1-tailed t-test, $p=0.11$). **B**. Timeline of performance on full length speech task. **C**. Timeline of performance on the speech in noise task. **D**. Timeline of performance on the sequence task. Performance on this task falls slightly over time due to the addition of increased repetition rates. **E**. Last day of speech in noise performance by control and KIA- rats. **F**. Last day of sequence performance.

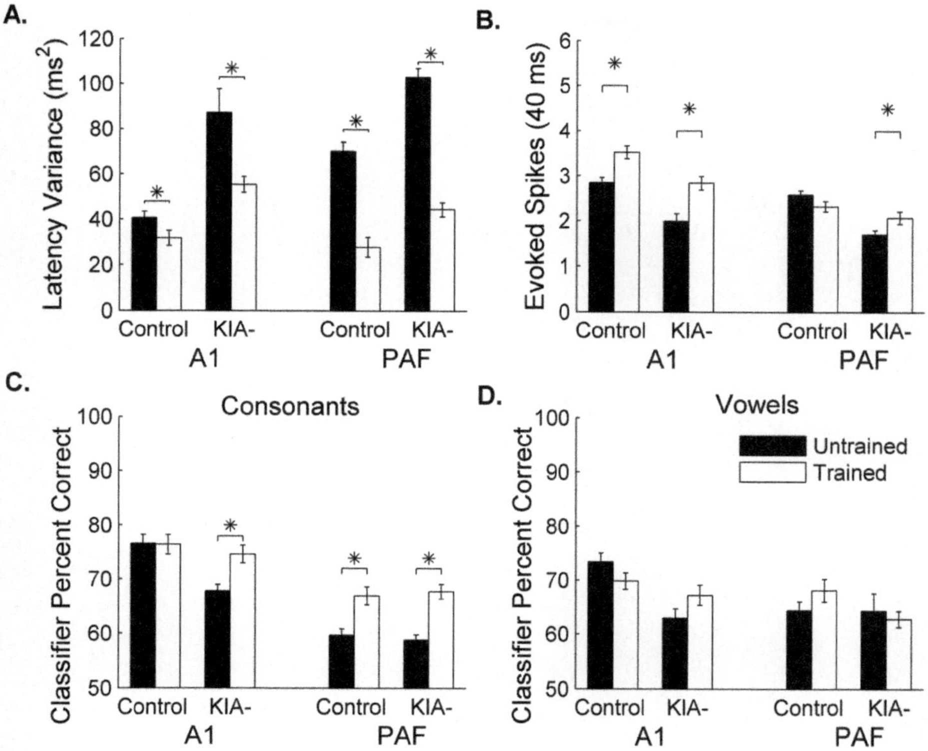

Figure 5. Extensive behavioral training improves reliability of neural firing and neural discrimination performance. A. Training significantly decreased the variability in onset latency in KIA- A1 (* = $p<0.01$) and KIA- PAF (* = $p<0.01$). Training also decreased variability in control A1 (* = $p=0.04$) and control PAF (* = $p<0.01$). **B**. Training significantly increased the number of evoked spikes (* = $p<0.04$). **C**. Consonant classifier performance before and after training. (* = $p<0.01$). **D**. Vowel classifier performance before and after training.

Figures 5C and 6G) but did not improve vowel discrimination ($p=0.97$; Figures 5D and S5G).

Training significantly improved classifier performance using A1 sites in KIA- rats on the consonant tasks ($p<0.01$; Figures 5C and 6F), but was less effective at improving vowel discrimination ($p=0.09$; Figures 5D and S5F). Neural discrimination using A1 activity from trained KIA- rats was not significantly different from that achieved using trained control A1 sites (consonants $p=0.46$; vowels $p=0.13$). Training improved KIA- PAF sites' performance on neural consonant discrimination ($p<0.01$; Figures 5C and 6H) but not neural discrimination of vowels ($p=0.52$; Figures 5D and S5H). These results suggest that extensive auditory training improves the ability of A1 and PAF in KIA- rats to accurately encode consonant speech sounds (which require temporal precision). We also noticed additional reduction in variability and additional improvement in the consonant classifier using control sites from the second group of rats as compared to the first, but did not notice any additional improvement in the second group of KIA- rats compared to KIA- rats in the first group (Figure S6). This result may suggest that there is a ceiling to the amount of training-induced neural plasticity in a brain with assumed *in utero* knockdown of *Kiaa0319* as compared to a control brain.

Extensive behavioral training improves phase-locking in KIA- rats

Auditory cortex in untrained KIA- rats had significantly lower vector strength (VS) than control rats (Figure 7A) [31]. After auditory training, VS in KIA- A1 was no longer significantly different from control rats at any speed we tested (1-way ANOVA, $F(1,6)=0.18$, $p=0.68$; Figure 7A&C). There were no significant differences in VS in PAF across control and KIA- groups (4 Hz $p=0.67$, 7 Hz $p=0.24$, 10 Hz $p=0.06$, 12.5 Hz $p=0.39$). Training did significantly improve VS in KIA- PAF (0.32 ± 0.1 in untrained KIA- PAF vs. 0.51 ± 0.1 in trained KIA- PAF; 1-way ANOVA, $F(1,6)=16.1$, $p<0.01$; Figure 7C&D), but did not affect VS in control PAF (0.45 ± 0.1 in untrained control PAF vs. 0.55 ± 0.1 in trained PAF; 1-way ANOVA, $F(1,6)=4.52$, $p=0.08$; Figure 7C&D). These results suggest that extensive speech training can improve neural firing to non-speech stimuli, which is consistent with recordings from dyslexic children before and after training [35–37,39,77,77].

Training-induced plasticity improves local field potentials as well as action potential patterns

Since earlier studies of plasticity after dyslexia therapy used EEG or fMRI, we hypothesized that the neural plasticity we observed in the action potential patterns of multi-unit recordings of rats would also be visible in the local field potentials (LFPs). After speech discrimination training, LFPs in control A1 responded faster to the onset of the speech sound /dad/ ($p<0.01$; Figure 8A). Trained KIA- A1 LFPs also responded faster compared to untrained recordings ($p<0.01$; Figure 8B). N1 amplitude was significantly increased as a result of training in control A1 (-72.4 ± 2.0 mV in untrained control A1 vs. $-82.8.3\pm20.3$ mV after training; $p<0.01$; Figure 8A) and in KIA- A1 (-41.3 ± 1.5 mV in untrained KIA- A1 vs. -69.1 ± 10.1 mV after training; $p<0.01$; Figure 8B). Latency of the N1 in control PAF was not significantly affected by training ($p=0.07$; Figure 8C). The LFP in KIA- PAF had a longer latency following training

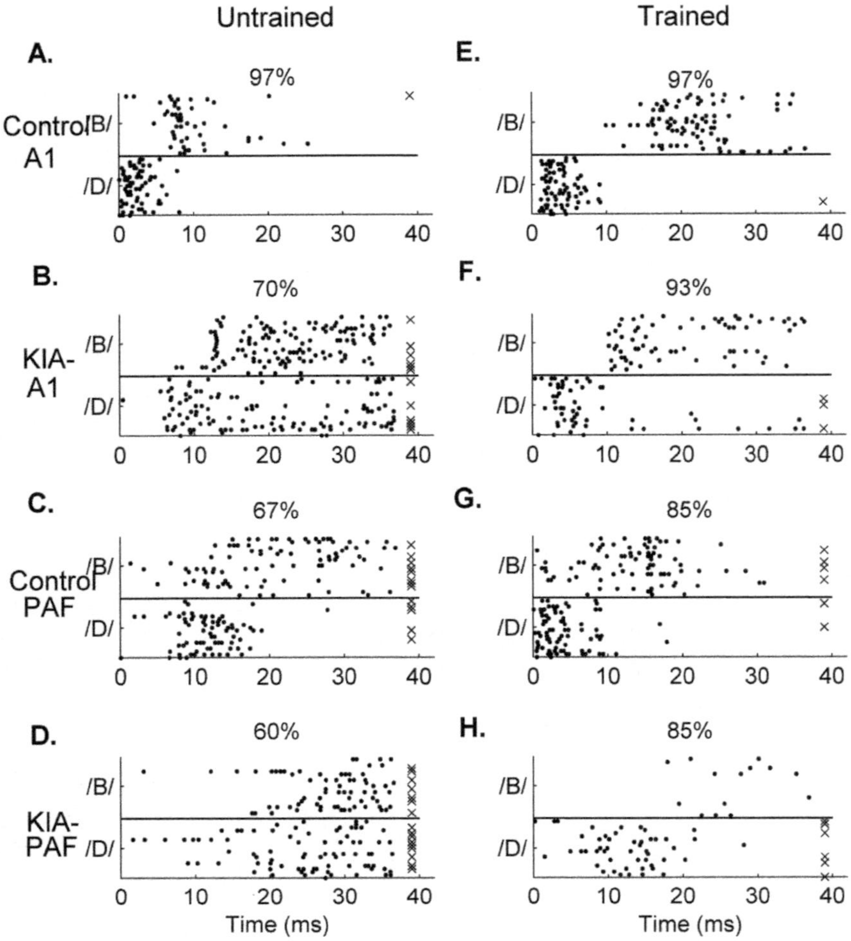

Figure 6. Training improves firing reliability in response to consonant speech sounds. Single site examples of neural responses to the consonant sounds /d/ and /b/ in every field before and after training. Classifier performance for each site is plotted on top of each panel, and trials which the classifier guessed incorrectly are marked by an 'x'. **A–D**. Representative examples of single site responses to the consonants /b/ and /d/ in A1 and PAF of untrained control or KIA- rats. **E–F**. Representative examples of single site responses to the consonants /b/ and /d/ in A1 and PAF of control or KIA- rats after training was complete.

(20.8±14.5 ms in untrained KIA- PAF vs. 42.0±0.9 ms after training; $p<0.01$; Figure 8D). After training, there was a significant increase in N1 amplitude in KIA- PAF (−18.9±3.5 mV in untrained KIA- PAF vs. −73.8±5.1 mV after training; $p<0.01$; Figure 8D). N1 amplitude in control PAF was also significantly increased by training (−42.1±5.2 mV in untrained control PAF vs. −94.6±10.4 mV after training; $p<0.01$; Figure 8C). Our observation that training induced plasticity improved neural discrimination performance of KIA- A1 and PAF sites suggests a possible neural basis for the success of current therapeutic options for humans with dyslexia.

Discussion

Summary of results

The behavioral data we collected confirmed our hypothesis that assumed *in utero* RNAi of the candidate-dyslexia gene *Kiaa0319* in rats would cause impaired speech sound discrimination in quiet and in noise. KIA- rats were significantly impaired at discriminating a target speech sound from distractor speech sounds in a variety of contexts and required twice the training time to perform at control levels. Training with truncated speech sounds led to improved performance on tasks using full length sounds in quiet and noisy conditions. KIA- rats who trained on truncated speech discrimination were more accurate on the other speech tasks compared to KIA- rats who had not trained on truncated speech. The neurophysiology data we collected demonstrates that behavioral training improved neural discrimination of consonants and reduced the neural variability in KIA- rats. Improved neural processing generalized to sounds that were not trained. These results provide a potential neural justification for the widespread use of intensive auditory training for dyslexia.

Biological basis of dyslexia

People with dyslexia have impairments in phoneme identification and manipulation that are correlated with abnormal neural responses. Dyslexics have reduced cortical and thalamic responses to non-speech sounds and speech sounds in passive and active listening conditions [21,78–80]. Auditory responses in the brainstem have similar amplitude in children with dyslexia as in normally developing children, but the trial-by-trial variability is significantly elevated [81]. Although the high heritability of dyslexia has been known for decades [14,77,82,83], the specific genes responsible have become clear only recently [11,12,22,84,85]. A growing body of evidence from human and

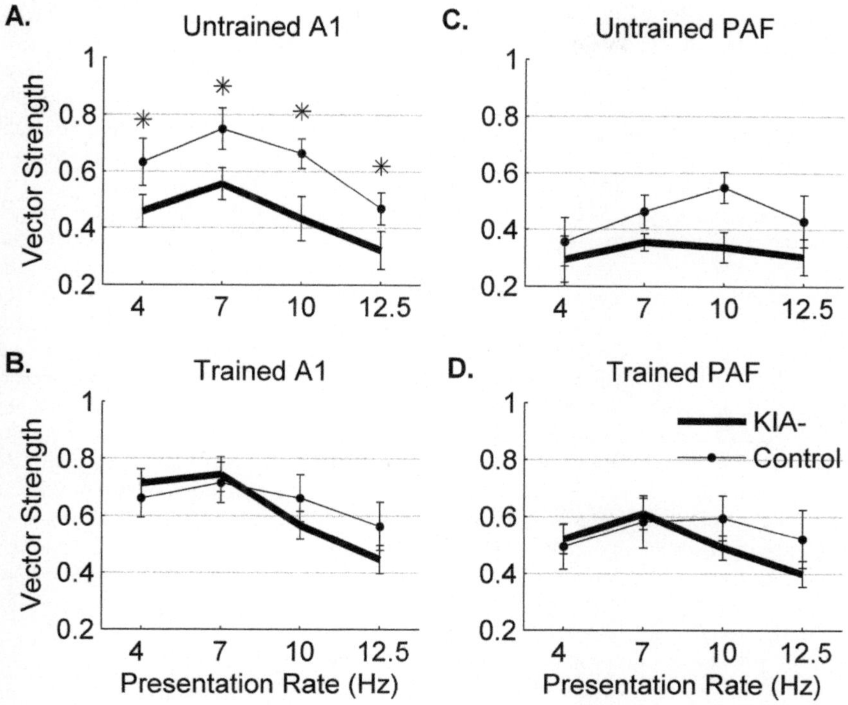

Figure 7. Training improves the ability of KIA- A1 and PAF sites to fire reliably to repetitive stimuli. **A**. Untrained KIA- A1 sites are significantly worse at following repetitive stimuli as measured by vector strength (* = $p<0.01$). **B**. Vector strength in control and KIA- A1 following auditory training. **C**. Vector strength in untrained control and KIA- PAF sites. **D**. Vector strength in control and KIA- PAF following auditory training.

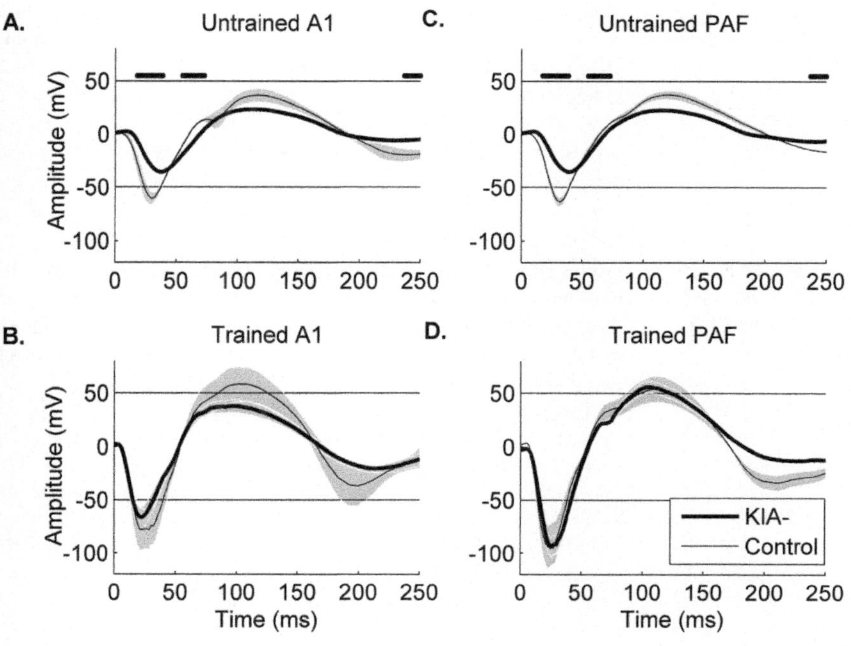

Figure 8. Extensive behavioral training shortens latency and increases amplitude of N1 component of LFP response. Responses are plotted with gray markers at −50 and 50 mV to help visualize differences across plots. Significant differences are marked by a black line. **A**. LFP response to the sound /dad/ in untrained control and KIA- A1. **B**. Extensive training improves onset latency and amplitude of the LFP response in KIA- A1. **C**. LFP response to the sound /dad/ in untrained control and KIA- PAF sites. As was seen in A1 recordings, latency and amplitude of KIA- PAF responses were significantly different from control recordings. **D**. Following training, there were not significant differences in the LFP response to the sound /dad/ between control PAF and KIA- PAF.

animal studies will establish which of these genes are responsible for the well documented impaired auditory processing impairments in dyslexia.

Variants in *KIAA0319* have been associated with dyslexia in at least nine independent studies [11,11,12,18,19,22,86,87,87–90]. None of the known human mutations in *KIAA0319* eliminate the gene, but they do reduce expression of the protein [22,90,91].The best characterized mutation causes reduced expression due to transcriptional suppression by OCT-1 [92]. Future studies should include testing of rats with full knockout of *Kiaa0319* to test the consequences of complete protein elimination, However, the rat model we describe here mimics the functional knockdown seen in human cells by suppressing Kiaa0319 protein expression in the developing brain using RNAi and is likely a more accurate model of the functional consequence of *KIAA0319* variants in humans [91].

Cortical neurons affected by *in utero* RNAi of *Kiaa0319* have significantly increased membrane resistance and are therefore hyperexcitable compared to neurons transfected with control or rescue sequences [31]. This increased excitability appears to be responsible for the increased trial-by-trial variability seen in the neural responses of KIA- rats. Variability can negatively impact the brain's ability to reliably locate a stimulus onset and determine the identity of sounds [93,94]. The increased variability in KIA- auditory cortex significantly impaired the ability of a classifier to use neural activity to identify various speech sounds [31]. These data suggested that decreased neural precision may be responsible for the impaired phonological awareness deficits in dyslexia. In the current study, we confirm that impaired neural encoding of speech sounds caused by *Kiaa0319* RNAi leads to impaired behavioral discrimination of speech sound stimuli. In addition to the 1–2% of neurons that were affected by the transfection, other studies have shown the Kiaa0319 targeting shRNA also alters non-transfected cells in cortex [16,46,95,96]. For example, non-transfected GABAergic neurons have been seen in heterotopias along with transfected cells [46,95], which suggests that more neurons in primary auditory cortex were likely affected in our study than could be visualized. The observed correlation between transfection rate and behavior suggests that the extent of the changes in non-tranfected cells is likely proportional to the number of transfected cells.

Efficacy of RNAi in the current study

In the current study, we used RNA interference, which is a common technique for knocking down protein expression in the brain [16,20,31,43,45,95,97]. Though this technique has been used and proven to be effective in countless studies with immunohistochemistry [98–100], the techniques for demonstrating effective knockdown of the Kiaa0319 protein are not yet fully developed. The success of the Kiaa0319 specific shRNA used in the RNAi procedure has been shown in culture (Figure S1). Although at least one western blot for Kiaa0319 protein has been published [46], the current antibodies available for marking this protein are not as precise as many other antibodies on the market and therefore this western does not definitively prove the efficacy of the technique used in the current study. Therefore, it is likely (but not certain) that the RNAi procedure used in this study is successful at reducing the expression of Kiaa0319 protein. Definitive confirmation of this conjecture will depend on the development of an effective antibody for Kiaa0319 protein.

A neural mechanism for training-induced plasticity

Many interventions for dyslexia focus on auditory processing to improve the mapping from phonemes to graphemes [35–38,101]. These interventions for dyslexic children can reduce the variability in speech-evoked neural responses across repeats of each stimulus [35–38,77]. The increase in firing amplitude seen after training could be due to a decrease in variability of onset latency, even if the response strength remains unchanged. Earlier studies hypothesized that the neural changes caused by training are due to a decrease in trial-by-trial variability [102].

Training could improve variability and thus improve speech sound processing through synaptic plasticity mechanisms that alter excitation and/or inhibition. Suppression of candidate-dyslexia genes affects the development of GABAergic neurons in the developing brain [97]. Normally, GABA regulates the balance between excitation and inhibition. In the dyslexic brain, improperly functioning GABA cells may contribute to the high excitability and variability of cortical neurons reported in our previous study [103]. Extensive auditory training, like the kind used in the current study, may cause LTP of GABAergic projections to cells affected by RNAi [104], which would reduce spontaneous firing and improve efficiency of downstream neurons [105,106]. We hypothesize that extensive behavioral training using complex auditory stimuli, such as speech, will reduce membrane resistance in cortical neurons and additional studies are needed to test this hypothesis.

Effect of Training on Neural Responses

There is a considerable amount of debate in the literature regarding the effect of behavioral training on neural responses to auditory stimuli. In the current study, we show that KIA- auditory cortex firing properties do change as a result of behavioral training, while control responses remain stable. Several recent studies have looked at the neural responses to auditory stimuli at various points throughout training. These studies used terminal acute recording techniques and therefore required a separate experimental group for each time point. Nevertheless, these studies clearly document the process of neural responses as they become better predictors of stimulus identity during the course of training [101,102]. Chronic recordings of non-primate animals learning motor tasks show a progression of neural plasticity throughout training [103,104]. Training studies using auditory stimuli would benefit from the use of chronic electrode implants to document the progress of neural plasticity in individual animals.

Other candidate-dyslexia genes

It is possible that candidate-dyslexia genes could interfere with reading without affecting phoneme processing by interfering with cognitive processes such as working memory or visual attention. It is interesting to note that all four of the best characterized candidate-dyslexia genes (KIAA0319, *ROBO1, DYX1C1,* and *DCDC2*) interfere with auditory processing [12,15,19,107]. Although the sequences of these genes are not related, each of these genes is required for normal neural migration [108–110]. The methods used in the current study could be used to evaluate the effect of other candidate-dyslexia genes on speech processing in rats. If future studies confirm that other genes can cause similar speech processing impairments to those described here, it will suggest that there is a common pathway to dyslexia through a variety of possible genetic mutations.

It is perhaps surprising that we can study dyslexia related genes in rats, since speech sounds have no ecological meaning to rats and rats cannot read. However, rats able to discriminate speech sounds in degraded conditions with thresholds that are indistinguishable from human participants [47,48,52,53,55]. The most likely explanation is that many of the basic auditory processing mechanisms used by mammals contribute to human speech processing. Our results suggest that assumed reduced expression of *KIAA0319* can cause dyslexia by increasing trial-by-trial variability in auditory cortex, which could impair phoneme processing and make reading more difficult because the mapping from phonemes to graphemes is compromised [81,102,111]. In addition, it is likely that trial-by-trial variability exists throughout the auditory system, and possibly even in other sensory systems. The observation that the auditory processing impairments in dyslexia are not limited to speech sounds confirms that the neural basis of dyslexia extends well beyond language-specific brain regions and is thus suitable for study in animal models [112–114]. Our observation that extensive training can significantly reduce trial-by-trial neural firing variability in our animal model suggests a possible means by which behavioral interventions could successfully treat dyslexia. Animal studies could be used to better understand how different forms of sensory and behavioral interventions impact phoneme processing. Given the substantial genetic and experiential heterogeneity among individuals with dyslexia, a simplified experimental model of the disorder is likely to prove valuable for comparing the neural and behavioral impacts of various interventions.

Supporting Information

Figure S1 In cell western assay confirming effectiveness of Kiaa0319 shRNA against rat Kiaa0319. Columns 1–4 and rows A–C show culture wells containing transfected and processed Hek293 cells in triplicate (A–C, rows) transfected with four different conditions and detected with antibodies against an mRFP epitope tag. Column 1 wells were not transfected and this is the background staining level. Column 2 cultures were transfected with pCAG-Kiaa0319-mRFP and a mutant control shRNA that does not match Kiaa0319 coding sequence. The bright red in column 2 indicates intense expression above background of Kiaa0319-mRFP. Column 3 is the same pCAG-Kiaa0319-mRFP construct transfected in 2 with the addition of the shRNA used to knockdown Kiaa0319 in this study. Column 4 is a similar co transfection with another shRNA vector based on the mir-30 system that contains the same shRNA targeting sequence as the shRNA shown in column 3 experiments.

Figure S2 *Rats with in utero* RNAi *of Kiaa0319 are able to learn a simple lever pressing task.* All rats (16 KIA- rats and 10 control rats) were first trained to press a lever, which triggered the presentation of the target sound (/dad/) and a sugar pellet reward. KIA- rats learned this task in the same amount of time as control rats (to criterion of 2 sessions of 100 presses; 113.4±14.2 minutes for KIA- rats vs. 141.5±27.2 minutes for controls; unpaired t-test, $p = 0.30$). After learning to press the lever, rats were transitioned to detection in which they were required to press the lever only when the target sound /dad/ was presented. Rats with *in utero* RNAi of *Kiaa0319* were not impaired in their ability to switch from free pressing to waiting for the target sound. Both groups were able to reach the performance criterion (10 sessions with a $d' \geq 1.5$) in approximately 5 days (Controls: 8.4±0.3 days vs. KIA-: 9.6±0.6 days; $p = 0.17$; Figure S1A). KIA- rats were not slower to respond to speech sounds compared to controls (Figure S2B). Responses by KIA- rats were faster on the first day of training, but were not different on any other training day. KIA- rats did not false alarm to silent catch trials more than control rats at any point during detection training (Figure S2C). Early in training KIA- rats missed more target sounds than controls, but were not significantly different from controls throughout the remainder of detection training (days 2 and 3 of detection training, one tailed t-test, $p < 0.01$; Figure S2C).These observations indicate that i*n utero* RNAi of *Kiaa0319* does not significantly impair gross motor, sensory or cognitive abilities, which is consistent with earlier reports that KIA- rats can hear and have normal working memory. **A.** Both KIA- and control rats were able to learn a simple speech detection task within 7 days of training (14 sessions). **B.** KIA- rats responded as quickly as control rats except on the first day of training, when they were significantly faster ($p < 0.01$). **C.** KIA- rats (thick black line) responded to the target sound (squares) less often than control rats (thin black line) during the second and third days of training (* = $p < 0.01$). The false alarm rate was not significantly different between the two groups (triangles).

Figure S3 Figure For all behavioral training, we used a set of consonant-vowel-consonant (CVC) speech sounds that have been used in many previous studies. All speech sounds were recorded in our lab by a female, native English speaker and were shifted up by an octave to better accommodate the rat hearing range (Kawahara 1997). For the truncated speech task, we used only the first 40 ms of the speech sounds, shown in the bottom panel. This figure was reprinted with permission from Porter et al., 2011.

Figure S4 *Training affects basic neural firing properties to tonal stimuli in KIA- and Control rats.* We trained rats for 4 months on a variety of speech discrimination tasks (Figures 2&4, Main Text) and evaluated the effect of such training on neural firing properties. Training reduced onset latency in both KIA- A1 (25.8±0.6 ms in untrained vs. 17.7±0.7 ms after training; $p < 0.01$) and PAF (45.6±7.1 ms in untrained vs. 29.5±2.2 ms after training, $p = 0.01$; Figure S4A). KIA- A1 neurons fired fewer evoked spikes after training (2.9±0.1 spikes in untrained vs. 2.4±0.1 spikes after training, $p < 0.01$; Figure S4D). This reduction in action potentials may be related to the decrease in neural variability we observed (Figure 5, Main Text). Training induced shorter latencies (22.3±0.7 ms in untrained vs. 17.2±0.6 spikes after training, $p < 0.01$; Figure S4A), narrower bandwidths (2.3±0.1 octaves in untrained vs. 1.9±0.1 octaves after training, $p < 0.01$; Figure S4B), and had a greater number of driven action potentials to tones (2.8±0.1 spikes in untrained vs. 3.2±0.1 spikes after training, $p < 0.01$; Figure S4D) in control rats (with scrambled shRNA). Thresholds were not affected by training in any group (Figure S4C). Following training, auditory cortex in KIA- and control rats were no longer significantly different in onset latency (A1 and PAF), bandwidth (A1 and PAF), and threshold (PAF). **A.** Training significantly shortened the onset latency in Control and KIA- A1 and KIA- PAF. No significant differences were seen in control PAF sites. **B.** Extensive behavioral training shortened bandwidths in Control A1 (2.3±0.1 octaves in untrained vs. 1.9±0.1 octaves after training, $p < 0.01$), but had no effect on bandwidths in the other fields. **C.** Extensive behavioral training had no effect on auditory thresholds in any group or field (control A1; $p = 0.72$, KIA- A1; $p = 0.06$, control PAF; $p = 0.90$, KIA- PAF; $p = 0.53$). **D.** Extensive behavioral training increased the number of tone-evoked action potentials fired in control A1 (2.8±0.1 spikes in untrained vs. 3.2±0.1 spikes after training, $p < 0.01$), but reduced the number of tone-evoked spikes fired in KIA- A1 (2.9±0.1 spikes in untrained vs. 2.4±0.1 spikes after training, $p < 0.01$).

Figure S5 *Extensive behavioral training improves neural encoding of vowel sounds in control and KIA- auditory cortex.* After training, trial-by-trial variability in onset latency across sites in KIA- A1 and PAF as well as control PAF were significantly reduced (Figure 5, Main Text). Responses to consonant speech sounds were significantly more precise following training and were better able to encode the differences between consonant sounds (Figure 6, Main Text). We saw a similar effect in the encoding of vowel sounds following training. Vowel sounds are encoded using spike count over a single 400 ms analysis window. As reported previously, untrained control and KIA- A1 responded to vowel sounds with a high degree of variability, and these two sites performed worse at the vowel task than at the consonant task (Figure S5 A&B; data originally collected for and reported in). Untrained PAF in control animals was slightly worse at the vowel task than A1 in each group. Average performance by untrained control PAF sites was 64.4±2.4% correct vs. 73.4±0.6% correct in untrained control A1 ($p<0.01$; Figure S5C). Performance in untrained KIA- PAF sites was not significantly worse than untrained KIA- A1 sites (64.3±1.4% correct in PAF vs. 62.9±0.1% correct in A1; $p=0.71$; Figure S5D). Following training, we noticed a slight (but not significant) improvement in the neural encoding of vowels. Trial-by-trial variability was reduced in every field (Figure S5 E–H and Figure 5, Main Text), which slightly improved the ability of each site to encode differences in vowel sounds. This result suggests that the specific training tasks we used benefitted consonant processing more effectively than vowel processing. **A.** A representative site from untrained control A1. The number of spikes encoded in response to each vowel sound was used to predict which sound evoked each single trial response. Data originally collected for and reported in Centanni et al. 2013. **B.** A representative site from untrained KIA- A1. The variability in neural firing was significantly higher in KIA- sites, which significantly impaired the ability of these sites to perform the vowel discrimination task. Data originally collected for and reported in Centanni et al., 2013. **C.** A representative site from untrained control PAF. **D.** A representative site from untrained KIA- PAF. **E.** A representative site from trained control A1. Though training did not have a significant impact on the classifier performance, the reduced variability in this field following training did provide some improvement on neural processing of vowels in this field. **F.** A representative site from trained KIA- A1. The improved variability in KIA- neurons after training did improve classifier performance on the vowel tasks, though this improvement was not significant. **G.** A representative site from trained control PAF. There was significant reduction in trial-by-trial variability in this field after training, and there was slight (but not significant) improvement in this fields' vowel classifier performance. **H.** A representative site from trained KIA- PAF. There was significant reduction in trial-by-trial variability in this field after training, and there was slight (but not significant) improvement in this fields' vowel classifier performance.

Figure S6 *An additional 4 weeks of behavior training causes additional plasticity in control rats.* The 4 weeks of additional training (as shown in Figure 4, Main Text) was also able to further reduce the trial-by-trial onset latency variability in control rats, but not KIA- rats as compared to group 1. In control A1, neural recordings from group 2 rats had lower trial-by-trial variability compared to group 1 (34.6±3.3 ms^2 in group 1 vs. 20.3±3.2 ms^2 in group 2; unpaired t-test, $p=0.01$; Figure S6A and Figure 6, Main Text). Control PAF in group 2 was also less variable trial-by-trial as a result of the additional training (59.4±4.3 ms^2 in group 1 vs. 29.5±2.6 ms^2 in group 2; unpaired t-test, $p<0.01$; Figure S6A). Trial-by-trial variability in KIA- rats did not decrease with additional training (A1: 27.3±4.6 ms2 in group 1 vs. 29.4±4.5 ms2 in group 2; $p=0.72$, PAF: 44.5±3.6 ms2 in group 1 vs. 44.5±3.9 ms2 in group 2, $p=0.99$; Figure S6A). We observed an increase in neural discrimination (as measured by the nearest-neighbor classifier) ability selectively in control PAF. Neural activity from group 2 control PAF sites were better able to discriminate between pairs of consonants than group 1 control PAF (65.3±2.1% correct by group 1 vs. 77.2±5.5% correct by group 2; unpaired t-test, $p<0.01$; Figure S6B). Control and KIA- A1 and KIA- PAF sites did not improve on the neural consonant discrimination task as a result of additional training (unpaired t-tests; $p=0.29$, $p=0.16$, and $p=0.88$, respectively; Figure S6B). Similarly, no group experienced an increase in neural vowel discrimination performance as a benefit of additional training (Control A1, $p=0.05$; Control PAF, $p=0.36$; KIA- A1, $p=0.42$; KIA- PAF, $p=0.70$; Figure S6C). The result that additional training did not provide additional neural plasticity in KIA- rats suggests that there may be a limit in how beneficial behavioral therapy can be in mediating the impairment caused by variants in *Kiaa0319*. **A.** The additional training received by group 2 caused a significant reduction in trial-by-trial variability in control A1 ($p=0.01$) and control PAF ($p<0.01$). No significant changes were seen in either field in KIA- rats ($p=0.72$ and $p=0.99$ in A1 and PAF respectively). **B.** Additional training improved the ability of control PAF sites to perform the consonant neural discrimination task ($p<0.01$), but this training did not improve classifier performance in control A1 ($p=0.29$), KIA- A1 ($p=0.16$), or KIA- PAF ($p=0.88$). **C.** Additional training did not improve the ability of neural activity in any group or field to perform the neural discrimination task using vowel stimuli. Control A1; $p=0.05$, KIA- A1; $p=0.42$, control PAF; $p=0.36$, KIA- PAF, $p=0.70$.

Acknowledgments

The authors would like to thank K. Im, N Moreno, K Rahebi, E Hancik, M Borland, E Buell, M Fink, and R Carraway for help with microelectrode recordings, as well as N Khodaparast, L Baxter, K Trull, and N Wasko for help with histology. We would also like to thank A. Galaburda and C. Szalkowski for their comments and suggestions on earlier versions of this manuscript.

Author Contributions

Conceived and designed the experiments: TMC MPK. Performed the experiments: TMC FC AMB CTE. Analyzed the data: TMC FC MPK. Contributed reagents/materials/analysis tools: AMS RLR. Wrote the paper: TMC JJL MPK.

References

1. Shaywitz SE, Escobar MD, Shaywitz BA, Fletcher JM, Makuch R (1992) Evidence that dyslexia may represent the lower tail of a normal distribution of reading ability. N Engl J Med 326: 145–150.
2. Shaywitz SE, Shaywitz BA, Pugh KR, Fulbright RK, Constable RT, et al. (1998) Functional disruption in the organization of the brain for reading in dyslexia. Proceedings of the National Academy of Sciences 95: 2636.
3. Tallal P (1980) Auditory temporal perception, phonics, and reading disabilities in children. Brain Lang 9: 182–198.
4. Ziegler JC, Goswami U (2005) Reading acquisition, developmental dyslexia, and skilled reading across languages: A psycholinguistic grain size theory. Psychol Bull 131: 3.
5. Boscariol M, Guimarães CA, Hage SRV, Cendes F, Guerreiro MM (2010) Temporal auditory processing: Correlation with developmental dyslexia and cortical malformation. Pró-Fono Revista de Atualização Científica 22: 537–542.
6. Tallal P, Piercy M (1974) Developmental aphasia: Rate of auditory processing and selective impairment of consonant perception. Neuropsychologia 12: 83–93.

7. Vandermosten M, Boets B, Luts H, Poelmans H, Golestani N, et al. (2010) Adults with dyslexia are impaired in categorizing speech and nonspeech sounds on the basis of temporal cues. Proceedings of the National Academy of Sciences 107: 10389.
8. Peterson RL, Pennington BF (2012) Developmental dyslexia. The Lancet.
9. Kovelman I, Norton ES, Christodoulou JA, Gaab N, Lieberman DA, et al. (2012) Brain basis of phonological awareness for spoken language in children and its disruption in dyslexia. Cerebral Cortex 22: 754–764.
10. Raschle NM, Zuk J, Gaab N (2012) Functional characteristics of developmental dyslexia in left-hemispheric posterior brain regions predate reading onset. Proceedings of the National Academy of Sciences 109: 2156–2161.
11. Zou L, Chen W, Shao S, Sun Z, Zhong R, et al. (2012) Genetic variant in KIAA0319, but not in DYX1C1, is associated with risk of dyslexia: An integrated meta-analysis. American Journal of Medical Genetics Part B: Neuropsychiatric Genetics 159: 970–976.
12. Galaburda AM, LoTurco J, Ramus F, Fitch RH, Rosen GD (2006) From genes to behavior in developmental dyslexia. Nat Neurosci 9: 1213–1217.
13. Fisher SE, DeFries JC (2002) Developmental dyslexia: Genetic dissection of a complex cognitive trait. Nature Reviews Neuroscience 3: 767–780.
14. Pennington BF, Gilger JW, Pauls D, Smith SA, Smith SD, et al. (1991) Evidence for major gene transmission of developmental dyslexia. JAMA: the journal of the American Medical Association 266: 1527–1534.
15. Bates TC, Luciano M, Medland SE, Montgomery GW, Wright MJ, et al. (2011) Genetic variance in a component of the language acquisition device: ROBO1 polymorphisms associated with phonological buffer deficits. Behav Genet 41: 50–57.
16. Burbridge TJ, Wang Y, Volz AJ, Peschansky VJ, Lisann L, et al. (2008) Postnatal analysis of the effect of embryonic knockdown and overexpression of candidate dyslexia susceptibility gene homolog Dcdc2 in the rat. Neuroscience 152: 723–733.
17. Galaburda AM, Sherman GF, Rosen GD, Aboitiz F, Geschwind N (1985) Developmental dyslexia: Four consecutive patients with cortical anomalies. Ann Neurol 18: 222–233.
18. Harold D, Paracchini S, Scerri T, Dennis M, Cope N, et al. (2006) Further evidence that the KIAA0319 gene confers susceptibility to developmental dyslexia. Mol Psychiatry 11: 1085–1091.
19. Scerri TS, Morris AP, Buckingham LL, Newbury DF, Miller LL, et al. (2011) DCDC2, KIAA0319 and CMIP are associated with reading-related traits. Biol Psychiatry 70,237–245.
20. Threlkeld SW, McClure MM, Bai J, Wang Y, LoTurco JJ, et al. (2007) Developmental disruptions and behavioral impairments in rats following *in utero* RNAi of Dyx1c1. Brain Res Bull 71: 508–514.
21. Pinel P, Fauchereau F, Moreno A, Barbot A, Lathrop M, et al. (2012) Genetic variants of FOXP2 and KIAA0319/TTRAP/THEM2 locus are associated with altered brain activation in distinct language-related regions. The Journal of Neuroscience 32: 817–825.
22. Paracchini S, Steer C, Buckingham L, Morris A, Ring S, et al. (2008) Association of the KIAA0319 dyslexia susceptibility gene with reading skills in the general population. Am J Psychiatry 165: 1576–1584.
23. Tallal P, Sainburg RL, Jernigan T (1991) The neuropathology of developmental dysphasia: Behavioral, morphological, and physiological evidence for a pervasive temporal processing disorder. In: Anonymous Reading Disabilities. Springer. pp. 175–189.
24. Farmer ME, Klein RM (1995) The evidence for a temporal processing deficit linked to dyslexia: A review. Psychon Bull Rev 2: 460–493.
25. Van Ingelghem M, Van Wieringen A, Wouters J, Vandenbussche E, Onghena P, et al. (2001) Psychophysical evidence for a general temporal processing deficit in children with dyslexia. Neuroreport 12: 3603–3607.
26. Hari R, Kiesilä P (1996) Deficit of temporal auditory processing in dyslexic adults. Neurosci Lett 205: 138–140.
27. Rey V, De Martino S, Espesser R, Habib M (2002) Temporal processing and phonological impairment in dyslexia: Effect of phoneme lengthening on order judgment of two consonants. Brain Lang 80: 576–591.
28. Bryant P, Bradley L, Maclean M, Crossland J (1989) Nursery rhymes, phonological skills and reading. J Child Lang 16: 407–428.
29. Goswami U, Bryant P (1990) Phonological skills and learning to read. Wiley Online Library.
30. Ramus F (2003) Developmental dyslexia: Specific phonological deficit or general sensorimotor dysfunction? Curr Opin Neurobiol 13: 212–218.
31. Centanni T, Booker A, Sloan A, Chen F, Maher B, et al. (2013) Knockdown of the dyslexia-associated gene Kiaa0319 impairs temporal responses to speech stimuli in rat primary auditory cortex. Cerebral Cortex doi: 10.1093/cercor/bht028
32. Paul LK (2011) Developmental malformation of the corpus callosum: A review of typical callosal development and examples of developmental disorders with callosal involvement. Journal of neurodevelopmental disorders 3: 3–27.
33. Fine JG, Semrud-Clikeman M, Keith TZ, Stapleton LM, Hynd GW (2007) Reading and the corpus callosum: An MRI family study of volume and area. Neuropsychology 21: 235.
34. Szalkowski CE, Fiondella CF, Truong DT, Rosen GD, LoTurco JJ, et al. (2012) The effects of *Kiaa0319* knockdown on cortical and subcortical anatomy in male rats. International Journal of Developmental Neuroscience 30,293–302.
35. Russo NM, Nicol TG, Zecker SG, Hayes EA, Kraus N (2005) Auditory training improves neural timing in the human brainstem. Behav Brain Res 156: 95–103.
36. Temple E, Deutsch GK, Poldrack RA, Miller SL, Tallal P, et al. (2003) Neural deficits in children with dyslexia ameliorated by behavioral remediation: Evidence from functional MRI. Proceedings of the National Academy of Sciences 100: 2860.
37. Penolazzi B, Spironelli C, Vio C, Angrilli A (2010) Brain plasticity in developmental dyslexia after phonological treatment: A beta EEG band study. Behav Brain Res 209: 179–182.
38. Lovio R, Halttunen A, Lyytinen H, Näätänen R, Kujala T (2012) Reading skill and neural processing accuracy improvement after a 3-hour intervention in preschoolers with difficulties in reading-related skills. Brain Res 1448, 42–55.
39. Tremblay KL, Kraus N (2002) Auditory training induces asymmetrical changes in cortical neural activity. Journal of Speech, Language and Hearing Research 45: 564.
40. Eden GF, Moats L (2002) The role of neuroscience in the remediation of students with dyslexia. Nat Neurosci 5: 1080–1084.
41. Lovett MW, Ransby MJ, Hardwick N, Johns MS, Donaldson SA (1989) Can dyslexia be treated? treatment-specific and generalized treatment effects in dyslexic children's response to remediation. Brain Lang 37: 90–121.
42. Schulte-Körne G (2010) The prevention, diagnosis, and treatment of dyslexia. Deutsches Ärzteblatt International 107: 718.
43. Bai J, Ramos RL, Ackman JB, Thomas AM, Lee RV, et al. (2003) RNAi reveals doublecortin is required for radial migration in rat neocortex. Nat Neurosci 6: 1277–1283.
44. Bai J, Ramos RL, Paramasivam M, Siddiqi F, Ackman JB, et al. (2008) The role of DCX and LIS1 in migration through the lateral cortical stream of developing forebrain. Dev Neurosci 30: 144–156.
45. Szalkowski CE, Fiondella CG, Galaburda AM, Rosen GD, LoTurco JJ, et al. (2012) Neocortical disruption and behavioral impairments in rats following *in utero* RNAi of candidate dyslexia risk gene *Kiaa0319*. International Journal of Developmental Neuroscience 1,116–122.
46. Peschansky VJ, Burbridge TJ, Volz AJ, Fiondella C, Wissner-Gross Z, et al. (2010) The effect of variation in expression of the candidate dyslexia susceptibility gene homolog Kiaa0319 on neuronal migration and dendritic morphology in the rat. Cerebral Cortex 20: 884–897.
47. Engineer CT, Perez CA, Chen YTH, Carraway RS, Reed AC, et al. (2008) Cortical activity patterns predict speech discrimination ability. Nat Neurosci 11: 603–608.
48. Perez CA, Engineer CT, Jakkamsetti V, Carraway RS, Perry MS, et al. (2012) Different timescales for the neural coding of consonant and vowel sounds. Cerebral Cortex 23, 670–683.
49. Porter BA, Rosenthal TR, Ranasinghe KG, Kilgard MP (2011) Discrimination of brief speech sounds is impaired in rats with auditory cortex lesions. Behav Brain Res 219: 68–74.
50. Sloan AM, Dodd OT, Rennaker RL II (2009) Frequency discrimination in rats measured with tone-step stimuli and discrete pure tones. Hear Res 251: 60–69.
51. Green DM, Swets JA (1966) Signal detection theory and psychophysics. Wiley New York.
52. Shetake JA, Wolf JT, Cheung RJ, Engineer CT, Ram SK, et al. (2011) Cortical activity patterns predict robust speech discrimination ability in noise. Eur J Neurosci 34,1823–1838.
53. Ranasinghe KG, Vrana WA, Matney CJ, Kilgard MP (2012) Neural mechanisms supporting robust discrimination of spectrally and temporally degraded speech. JARO-Journal of the Association for Research in Otolaryngology: 1–16.
54. Engineer CT, Kilgard MP, Assmann PF, Atzori M, Thompson LT (2008) Speech sound coding and training-induced plasticity in primary auditory cortex. The University of Texas at Dallas.
55. Centanni TM, Engineer CT, Kilgard MP (2013) Cortical speech-evoked response patterns in multiple auditory fields are correlated with behavioral discrimination ability. J Neurophysiol 110, 177–189.
56. Kawahara H (1997) Speech representation and transformation using adaptive interpolation of weighted spectrum: Vocoder revisited. 2: 1303–1306 vol. 2.
57. Pandya PK, Rathbun DL, Moucha R, Engineer ND, Kilgard MP (2008) Spectral and temporal processing in rat posterior auditory cortex. Cerebral Cortex 18: 301–314.
58. Polley DB, Read HL, Storace DA, Merzenich MM (2007) Multiparametric auditory receptive field organization across five cortical fields in the albino rat. J Neurophysiol 97: 3621–3638.
59. Ma H, Qin L, Dong C, Zhong R, Sato Y (2013) Comparison of neural responses to cat meows and human vowels in the anterior and posterior auditory field of awake cats. PLOS ONE 8: e52942.
60. Jakkamsetti V, Chang KQ, Kilgard MP (2012) Reorganization in processing of spectral and temporal input in the rat posterior auditory field induced by environmental enrichment. J Neurophysiol 107: 1457–1475.
61. Puckett AC, Pandya PK, Moucha R, Dai WW, Kilgard MP (2007) Plasticity in the rat posterior auditory field following nucleus basalis stimulation. J Neurophysiol 98: 253–265.
62. Doron NN, Ledoux JE, Semple MN (2002) Redefining the tonotopic core of rat auditory cortex: Physiological evidence for a posterior field. J Comp Neurol 453: 345–360.

63. Foffani G, Moxon KA (2004) PSTH-based classification of sensory stimuli using ensembles of single neurons. J Neurosci Methods 135: 107–120.
64. Foffani G, Moxon K (2005) Studying the role of spike timing in ensembles of neurons. 206–208.
65. Ranasinghe KG, Carraway RS, Borland MS, Moreno NA, Hanacik EA, et al. (2012) Speech discrimination after early exposure to pulsed-noise or speech. Hear Res 289, 1–12.
66. Coffin JM, Baroody S, Schneider K, O'Neill J (2005) Impaired cerebellar learning in children with prenatal alcohol exposure: A comparative study of eyeblink conditioning in children with ADHD and dyslexia. Cortex 41: 389–398.
67. Blondeau C, Dellu-Hagedorn F (2007) Dimensional analysis of ADHD subtypes in rats. Biol Psychiatry 61: 1340–1350.
68. Loos M, Staal J, Schoffelmeer AN, Smit AB, Spijker S, et al. (2010) Inhibitory control and response latency differences between C57BL/6J and DBA/2J mice in a Go/No-go and 5-choice serial reaction time task and strain-specific responsivity to amphetamine. Behav Brain Res 214: 216–224.
69. Nagarajan S, Mahncke H, Salz T, Tallal P, Roberts T, et al. (1999) Cortical auditory signal processing in poor readers. Proceedings of the National Academy of Sciences 96: 6483.
70. Chandrasekaran B, Hornickel J, Skoe E, Nicol T, Kraus N (2009) Context-dependent encoding in the human auditory brainstem relates to hearing speech in noise: Implications for developmental dyslexia. Neuron 64: 311–319.
71. Ziegler JC, Pech-Georgel C, George F, Lorenzi C (2009) Speech-perception-in-noise deficits in dyslexia. Developmental science 12: 732–745.
72. Ahissar E, Nagarajan S, Ahissar M, Protopapas A, Mahncke H, et al. (2001) Speech comprehension is correlated with temporal response patterns recorded from auditory cortex. Proceedings of the National Academy of Sciences 98: 13367.
73. Elbro C, Petersen DK (2004) Long-term effects of phoneme awareness and letter sound training: An intervention study with children at risk for dyslexia. J Educ Psychol 96: 660.
74. Engineer N, Engineer C, Reed A, Pandya P, Jakkamsetti V, et al. (2012) Inverted-U function relating cortical plasticity and task difficulty. Neuroscience.
75. Takahashi H, Yokota R, Funamizu A, Kose H, Kanzaki R (2011) Learning-stage-dependent, field-specific, map plasticity in the rat auditory cortex during appetitive operant conditioning. Neuroscience 199,243–258.
76. Habib M, Rey V, Daffaure V, Camps R, Espesser R, et al. (2002) Phonological training in children with dyslexia using temporally modified speech: A three-step pilot investigation. International Journal of Language & Communication Disorders 37: 289–308.
77. Hornickel J, Zecker SG, Bradlow AR, Kraus N (2012) Assistive listening devices drive neuroplasticity in children with dyslexia. Proceedings of the National Academy of Sciences 109, 16731–16736.
78. Flowers DL, Wood FB, Naylor CE (1991) Regional cerebral blood flow correlates of language processes in reading disability. Arch Neurol 48: 637.
79. Rumsey J, Horwitz B, Donohue B, Nace K, Maisog J, et al. (1997) Phonological and orthographic components of word recognition. A PET-rCBF study. Brain 120: 739–759.
80. Temple E, Poldrack RA, Salidis J, Deutsch GK, Tallal P, et al. (2001) Disrupted neural responses to phonological and orthographic processing in dyslexic children: An fMRI study. Neuroreport 12: 299.
81. Hornickel J, Kraus N (2013) Unstable representation of sound: A biological marker of dyslexia. The Journal of Neuroscience 33: 3500–3504.
82. Shaywitz SE (1998) Dyslexia. N Engl J Med 338: 307–312.
83. Castles A, Datta H, Gayan J, Olson RK (1999) Varieties of developmental reading disorder: Genetic and environmental influences. J Exp Child Psychol 72: 73–94.
84. Lind PA, Luciano M, Wright MJ, Montgomery GW, Martin NG, et al. (2010) Dyslexia and DCDC2: Normal variation in reading and spelling is associated with DCDC2 polymorphisms in an australian population sample. European Journal of Human Genetics 18: 668–673.
85. Schumacher J, Anthoni H, Dahdouh F, König IR, Hillmer AM, et al. (2006) Strong genetic evidence of DCDC2 as a susceptibility gene for dyslexia. The American Journal of Human Genetics 78: 52–62.
86. Deffenbacher KE, Kenyon JB, Hoover DM, Olson RK, Pennington BF, et al. (2004) Refinement of the 6p21. 3 quantitative trait locus influencing dyslexia: Linkage and association analyses. Hum Genet 115: 128–138.
87. Cope N, Harold D, Hill G, Moskvina V, Stevenson J, et al. (2005) Strong evidence that *KIAA0319* on chromosome 6p is a susceptibility gene for developmental dyslexia. The American Journal of Human Genetics 76: 581–591.
88. Couto JM, Livne-Bar I, Huang K, Xu Z, Cate-Carter T, et al. (2010) Association of reading disabilities with regions marked by acetylated H3 histones in KIAA0319. American Journal of Medical Genetics Part B: Neuropsychiatric Genetics 153: 447–462.
89. Czamara D, Bruder J, Becker J, Bartling J, Hoffmann P, et al. (2011) Association of a rare variant with mismatch negativity in a region between KIAA0319 and DCDC2 in dyslexia. Behav Genet 41: 110–119.
90. Francks C, Paracchini S, Smith SD, Richardson AJ, Scerri TS, et al. (2004) A 77-kilobase region of chromosome 6p22. 2 is associated with dyslexia in families from the united kingdom and from the united states. The American Journal of Human Genetics 75: 1046–1058.
91. Paracchini S, Thomas A, Castro S, Lai C, Paramasivam M, et al. (2006) The chromosome 6p22 haplotype associated with dyslexia reduces the expression of KIAA0319, a novel gene involved in neuronal migration. Hum Mol Genet 15: 1659–1666.
92. Dennis MY, Paracchini S, Scerri TS, Prokunina-Olsson L, Knight JC, et al. (2009) A common variant associated with dyslexia reduces expression of the KIAA0319 gene. PLoS genetics 5: e1000436.
93. Brasselet R, Panzeri S, Logothetis NK, Kayser C (2012) Neurons with stereotyped and rapid responses provide a reference frame for relative temporal coding in primate auditory cortex. The Journal of Neuroscience 32: 2998–3008.
94. Abbott L, Dayan P (1999) The effect of correlated variability on the accuracy of a population code. Neural Comput 11: 91–101.
95. Adler WT, Platt MP, Mehlhorn AJ, Haight JL, Currier TA, et al. (2013) Position of neocortical neurons transfected at different gestational ages with shRNA targeted against candidate dyslexia susceptibility genes. PloS one 8: e65179.
96. Dong Y, Friedrich M (2005) Nymphal RNAi: Systemic RNAi mediated gene knockdown in juvenile grasshopper. BMC Biotechnol 5: 25.
97. Currier TA, Etchegaray MA, Haight JL, Galaburda AM, Rosen GD. (2011) The effects of embryonic knockdown of the candidate dyslexia susceptibility gene homologue *Dyx1c1* on the distribution of GABAergic neurons in the cerebral cortex. Neuroscience 172: 535–546.
98. Fasano CA, Dimos JT, Ivanova NB, Lowry N, Lemischka IR, et al. (2007) shRNA knockdown of *bmi-1* reveals a critical role for p21-rb pathway in NSC self-renewal during development. Cell stem cell 1: 87–99.
99. Xia H, Mao Q, Paulson HL, Davidson BL (2002) siRNA-mediated gene silencing in vitro and in vivo. Nat Biotechnol 20: 1006–1010.
100. Hommel JD, Sears RM, Georgescu D, Simmons DL, DiLeone RJ (2003) Local gene knockdown in the brain using viral-mediated RNA interference. Nat Med 9: 1539–1544.
101. Heim S, Keil A, Choudhury N, Thomas Friedman J, Benasich AA (2013) Early gamma oscillations during rapid auditory processing in children with a language-learning impairment: Changes in neural mass activity after training. Neuropsychologia 51, 990–1001.
102. Kraus N (2012) Atypical brain oscillations: A biological basis for dyslexia? Trends Cogn Sci (Regul Ed) 16: 12–13.
103. Wang DD, Kriegstein AR (2009) Defining the role of GABA in cortical development. J Physiol (Lond) 587: 1873–1879.
104. Gaiarsa J, Caillard O, Ben-Ari Y (2002) Long-term plasticity at GABAergic and glycinergic synapses: Mechanisms and functional significance. Trends Neurosci 25: 564–570.
105. Lu YM, Mansuy IM, Kandel ER, Roder J (2000) Calcineurin-mediated LTD of GABAergic inhibition underlies the increased excitability of CA1 neurons associated with LTP. Neuron 26: 197–205.
106. Stelzer A, Slater NT, Ten Bruggencate G (1987) Activation of NMDA receptors blocks GABAergic inhibition in an in vitro model of epilepsy. 326, 698–701.
107. Marino C, Citterio A, Giorda R, Facoetti A, Menozzi G, et al. (2007) Association of short-term memory with a variant within DYX1C1 in developmental dyslexia. Genes, Brain and Behavior 6: 640–646.
108. Massinen S, Hokkanen M, Matsson H, Tammimies K, Tapia-Páez I, et al. (2011) Increased expression of the dyslexia candidate gene DCDC2 affects length and signaling of primary cilia in neurons. PLoS One 6: e20580.
109. Dijkmans TF, van Hooijdonk A, Wilhelmina L, Fitzsimons CP, Vreugdenhil E (2010) The doublecortin gene family and disorders of neuronal structure. Central Nervous System Agents in Medicinal ChemistryChemistry-Central Nervous System Agents) 10: 32–46.
110. Poon M, Chan H, Lim K, Waye MM (2011) The Dyslexia Candidate Gene KIAA0319L Encodes NGlycosylated Isoforms that Form Homeo-Dimers. Journal of Biochemistry and Molecular Biology in the Post Genomic Era: 65.
111. Snowling MJ (1980) The development of grapheme-phoneme correspondence in normal and dyslexic readers. J Exp Child Psychol 29: 294–305.
112. Nagarajan S, Mahncke H, Poeppel D, Robert T, Tallel P, et al. (1998) Neuromagnetic evidence for deficits in temporal ordering of brief tones by adult dyslexics. 96, 6483.
113. Mcanally KI, Stein JF (1996) Auditory temporal coding in dyslexia. Proceedings of the Royal Society of London.Series B: Biological Sciences 263: 961–965.
114. Schulte-Körne G, Deimel W, Bartling J, Remschmidt H (1998) Auditory processing and dyslexia: Evidence for a specific speech processing deficit. Neuroreport 9: 337–340.

12

Evidence for Deficits in the Temporal Attention Span of Poor Readers

Troy A. W. Visser*

School of Psychology, University of Western Australia, Perth, Western Australia, Australia

Abstract

Background: While poor reading is often associated with phonological deficits, many studies suggest that visual processing might also be impaired. In particular, recent research has indicated that poor readers show impaired spatial visual attention spans in partial and whole report tasks. Given the similarities between competition-based accounts for reduced visual attention span and similar explanations for impairments in sequential object processing, the present work examined whether poor readers show deficits in their "temporal attention span" – that is, their ability to rapidly and accurately process sequences of consecutive target items.

Methodology/Principal Findings: Poor and normal readers monitored a sequential stream of visual items for two (TT condition) or three (TTT condition) consecutive target digits. Target identification was examined using both unconditional and conditional measures of accuracy in order to gauge the overall likelihood of identifying a target and the likelihood of identifying a target given successful identification of previous items. Compared to normal readers, poor readers showed small but consistent deficits in identification across targets whether unconditional or conditional accuracy was used. Additionally, in the TTT condition, final-target conditional accuracy was poorer than unconditional accuracy, particularly for poor readers, suggesting a substantial cost arising from processing the previous two targets that was not present in normal readers.

Conclusions/Significance: Mirroring the differences found between poor and normal readers in spatial visual attention span, the present findings suggest two principal differences between the temporal attention spans of poor and normal readers. First, the consistent pattern of reduced performance across targets suggests increased competition amongst items within the same span for poor readers. Second, the steeper decline in final target performance amongst poor readers in the TTT condition suggests a reduction in the extent of their temporal attention span.

Editor: Suliann Ben Hamed, Centre de Neuroscience Cognitive, France

Funding: This research was funded by an Australian Research Council Discovery Grant (DP120102313). The funders had no role in study design, data collection and analysis, decision to publish, or preparation of the manuscript.

Competing Interests: The author has declared that no competing interests exist.

* E-mail: taw.visser@gmail.com

Introduction

Estimates indicate that between 5–15% of the population suffer from reading disabilities such as dyslexia [1–3]. This is a particularly alarming statistic given the increasing dominance of text-based communication such as electronic mail, instant messaging, and online social media in everyday living. The consensus opinion from decades of research is that reading problems are often underpinned by a phonological deficit [4–7]. That is, poor readers are less able to parse, process and manipulate phonemic information, leading to reduced phonemic awareness, poorer grapheme-to-phoneme conversion, and ultimately poorer text comprehension.

As well as a phonological deficit, many theorists have proposed that visual processing might be impaired in poor readers. For example, it has been argued that poor readers have a deficiency in their magnocellular system [8], a longer attentional dwell time [9,10], less-efficient attentional orienting [11–12], poorer visual search [13], and less effective inhibitory mechanisms [14,15]. Notably, however, these visual deficits are often accompanied by phonological problems [16–19]. This implies that rather than being independent problems, visual and phonological problems may spring from a common source [16,20], or at least that visual deficits may not account for unique variance in reading ability beyond known phonological problems.

One visual deficit that can be found independently from phonological problems amongst poor readers is spatial visual attention (VA) span [21–24]. Bosse et al. [21] compared children with normal reading ability and dyslexia on variations of partial- and whole-report tasks [25]. In the whole report condition, observers were asked to report all of the letters in a five-item string displayed for 200 ms. In the partial-report condition, observers were asked to report a single letter from the five-item string, indicated by a probe which appeared below the letter-to-be-reported after the offset of the string. Children with dyslexia reported fewer complete five-letter strings in the whole-report task, and fewer letters overall in both the whole- and partial-report tasks. More importantly, while some of the children with dyslexia showed both VA span and phonological deficits, a significant subset showed either phonological deficits alone or VA span deficits alone. This indicated that VA span and phonology make separate contributions to reading impairment, in at least some participants.

To explain the unique contribution of VA span to reading, Bosse et al. [21] suggested that each item in a multi-element visual array competes for access to visual short-term memory [26]. The competitive strength of items is, in turn, determined by the speed with which the item can be processed and the attentional weighting it receives. Given that single-letter reading speed was not significantly different across normal and impaired readers, Bosse et al. [21] concluded that children with dyslexia allocated attention to letter strings less efficiently than normal readers. This conjecture is supported by more recent evidence for reduced information uptake in adults and children with dyslexia [27,28], and abnormal spatial allocations of attention to letter strings amongst children with dyslexia [23].

The notion that items in multi-element spatial arrays compete for access to VSTM is very similar to some theoretical accounts of item processing during rapid serial visual presentation (RSVP) tasks in which two targets are presented in rapid succession at a single spatial location [29–31]. In this so-called attentional blink (AB), identification of the second target (T2) depends on its temporal distance (lag) from the first target (T1), with poorer T2 accuracy at shorter lags and a gradual increase in performance as lag increases. Competition accounts for the AB emphasize competition amongst T1, T2, and the RSVP items directly following them, and suggest that the AB arises because attentional resources are preferentially allocated to T1 and the item directly following it, to the detriment of T2 [29].

The notion that resource competition might underlie item identification in both spatial and temporal arrays and the existence of abnormal VA span in poor readers begs the question of whether poor readers might also allocate attention differently to sequential items presented in a rapid temporal sequence (henceforth, temporal attention span) compared to their normal reading peers. Put differently, one may ask whether poor readers have a more general problem in allocating attention to sequential stimuli in both the spatial and temporal domains. To investigate this issue, a number of studies have examined the AB in impaired readers. In general, results have shown a larger AB in readers with dyslexia [32–36] and less-skilled readers [38] (but see [37]). However, as noted by McLean and colleagues, T2 impairments in these studies have often been equivalent across inter-target intervals [39] (but see [33,34,38]). This implies that T2 deficits amongst poor readers were not the result of resource competition between T1 and T2, but rather due to a general difficulty processing T2 that occurred independently from T1 processing. On the face of it, then, it would seem that the evidence is inconclusive about whether poor readers show parallel spatial and temporal attention span difficulties.

Before making this conclusion, however, it is important to note that there are significant problems with interpreting results from AB studies as a measure of temporal attention span. Whereas spatial span tasks call for observers to process all items on the display, the AB involves selection of two target items, separated from each other by a number of non-target distractors. Thus, the AB requires not just encoding of potential targets as in spatial span tasks, but also selection of relevant information and inhibition of irrelevant inputs. This point is particularly critical when interpreting existing AB experiments because many researchers have shown that the nature of distractors significantly modulates T2 performance [40–44]. The upshot of this is that AB performance likely reflects selection performance just as much, if not more, than inter-item competition, and thus may make a relatively insensitive index of temporal attention span.

In light of this argument, and the lack of clear evidence from existing AB studies on the nature of temporal attention span in poor readers, the present work focuses instead on a modified AB task where targets appeared in direct succession, rather than on measuring T2 performance across a breadth of lags, separated by distractors, as has been done in previous work. The resulting paradigm thus more closely resembled the demands of partial and whole report tasks used to assess spatial VA span. Of course, many AB studies have included some trials with directly consecutive targets. This work has shown T2 performance is largely unimpaired when it follows T1 directly [45,46], and that this so-called "lag-1 sparing" can extend out to as many as five consecutive targets ("extended sparing") [40,47]. Importantly, like spatial VA span, theoretical accounts of sparing suggest T1 initiates an attentional episode that can encompass multiple additional target items as long as they continue to match a target template [40,42,46,48–49]. Moreover, there is good evidence for inter-item competition amongst items entering this attentional episode. For example, T2 sparing is often accompanied by significant decrements in T1 accuracy (e.g., [49–53]), while experimental manipulations designed to enhance T1 processing often diminish later sparing [54–55].

The methodology here closely followed that of Di Lollo et al. [40]. Observers were presented with a series of trials in which two (TT condition) or three (TTT condition) targets appeared in succession. These conditions were designed to elicit lag-1 sparing and extended sparing respectively. In addition, trials with two consecutive targets separated by a single distractor (TDT condition) were also included in order to verify that the presentation conditions used here produced similar results to previous AB studies. The key question was whether the performance of poor readers in the TT and TTT conditions would differ from that of normal readers, implying differences in their temporal span of attention analogous to those found for VA span [21].

Methods

Participants

Eighty-five university students (61.2% women; 38.8% men) participated in the study. Ages ranged from 16 to 63 years ($M = 23.24$, $Mdn = 21.00$, $SD = 9.20$; women: $M = 22.92$, $Mdn = 21.00$, $SD = 9.32$; men: $M = 23.73$, $Mdn = 21.00$, $SD = 9.13$). Participants received course credit in exchange for participation in a one hour session. All participants reported normal or corrected-to-normal (i.e., eye glasses or contact lenses) vision and English as their first language.

Ethics Statement

All experimental procedures were conducted in accordance with the principles expressed in the Declaration of Helsinki, and were approved by the University of Queensland Ethics Committee. Written informed consent was obtained from each participant (and their parents/guardian where applicable) prior to participation.

Apparatus and Stimuli

Reading efficiency. The phonemic decoding efficiency subtest from the Test of Word Reading Efficiency (TOWRE) was used [56]. This test measured observers' ability to rapidly name as many non-words as possible (top score of 63) without errors in 45 seconds. Non-words were divided into three equal lists printed vertically on a white form. Participants were instructed to read down each list, pronouncing items based on their common sounds, and skipping any items they could not pronounce. Participants were asked to stop reading after 45 seconds and a line was drawn after the last non-word read.

Nonverbal intelligence. Nonverbal intelligence was assessed using the nonverbal subtest of the Kaufman Brief Intelligence Test [57]. This subtest was composed of 46 matrices involving meaningful and abstract visual stimuli. Participants were required use fluid thinking and problem solving abilities to identify relationships and complete visual patterns in either 2×2 or 3×3 matrices. Each matrix had one missing item and participants were instructed to choose one of six possible items to complete it. A score out of 46 was recorded.

Rapid Automatised Naming (RAN). Processing speed was assessed using the rapid letter naming subtest from the Comprehensive Test of Phonological Processing [58]. Participants were asked to read aloud, as quickly as possible, 72 items composed of six black randomly arranged letters (*a*, *c*, *k*, *n*, *s*, and *t*) divided into 4 rows and 9 columns on two white pages. Participants were instructed to read across the top row of the first page from left to right before going onto the second row and so on. Once each letter on the first page was named, the same procedure was completed with the second page. The cumulative time taken to name both pages was recorded, along with the number of errors.

Temporal attention span task. All stimuli were presented on an Acer AC915 monitor running at a refresh rate of 100 Hz, and connected to a Windows-based computer, using Presentation software (Version 12.4, Neurobehavioral Systems). Targets were the digits 1–9. Distractor items were all letters (except I, O, Q, Z due to their similarity to digits). All items were presented in a light gray (RGB: 170, 170, 170) Arial font (Sz 28; approximately 1°×1° of visual angle) on a black background.

A schematic outline of the events on each trial can be seen in Figure 1. Each trial began with a central fixation cross. Participants were then instructed to focus their gaze at fixation, and press the space bar to begin the trial. Following a 300 ms blank screen, a rapid-serial visual presentation (RSVP) stream was presented at fixation. Each item in the stream was presented for 30 ms and followed by a blank screen for 70 ms. After 5 to 8 distractors, T1 was presented, and then followed by: a) T2 (TT condition); b) one distractor and T2 (TDT condition); or, c) T2 and then a third target (T3). Distractors were chosen randomly with replacement, with the proviso that identical distractors could not appear consecutively. The final item in the RSVP was always a distractor that acted as a mask for the last target. After a 200 ms pause, during which the display was blank, participants were prompted to identify the target digits by typing them into the keyboard in any order. Following these responses, the fixation reappeared, indicating the next trial was ready to begin. Each participant completed 25 trials in the TT, TDT, and TTT conditions, yielding a total of 75 trials.

Procedure

Participants completed the battery of written, verbal and computerized tasks during a one-hour experimental session. All tasks were completed in a quiet dimly-lit room, with participants seated comfortably at a desk or computer workstation. To control for the effects of presentation order, the computerized and non-computerized tasks were counterbalanced separately, with approximately half of participants receiving the non-computerized tasks first, while the other half received the computerized task first.

Results

Mean target accuracy was calculated without consideration of response order, as is customary in studies of the AB [59] and extended sparing [40]. In addition, both unconditional and conditional accuracy scores were calculated for each target. Unconditional accuracy scores convey the absolute ability of observers to identify each target without consideration of whether they were also able to accurately identify preceding targets. Conditional accuracy, on the other hand, estimates the ability of observers to identify targets, given correct identification of preceding items, and thus provides a way of assessing how processing one target in an attentional episode impacts the ability for additional targets to be processed within that same episode.

To create reading efficiency groups, norms from the TOWRE were used to classify participants as poor or normal readers based on their standard scores. Normal readers were classified as those whose standard scores were greater than 90 (n = 74); poor readers were classified as those whose standard scores fell below the cut-off point (<90) for average reading skill (n = 11). It is worth noting that the proportion of poor readers (12.9%) mirrors the prevalence of reading disabilities in the population. This is in keeping with the fact that the research did not target individuals with reading disabilities, but rather recruited a large sample from the broader undergraduate population in order to capture normal and poor readers.

Mean age, IQ, and RAN scores for both reading groups can be seen in Table 1. Independent-samples t-tests showed no significant differences between age (p>.77) or IQ scores (>.42). However, the difference between mean RAN scores approached significance (p = .07). In addition, there was a significant correlation between TOWRE standard scores and RAN scores (r = −.42, p<.001). For these reasons, we included RAN scores as a covariate in all of the ANOVAs reported below.

TDT Condition

Mean target accuracy scores were analyzed in a 2 (Conditionality: conditional vs. unconditional accuracy) × 2 (Target: T1 vs. T2) × 2 (Reading Group: normal vs. poor) mixed-design ANOVA. Here, and in subsequent analyses, multivariate statistics are reported for within-subjects effects due to unequal sample sizes and violations of sphericity assumptions. The results revealed significant effects of Target, $\underline{F}(1, 82) = 17.12$, $\underline{p}<.001$, $\eta_p^2 = .173$, and Reading Group, $\underline{F}(1, 82) = 4.96$, $\underline{p}<.03$, $\eta_p^2 = .057$. No other main effects or interactions were significant (all $\underline{p}$'s >.19, η_p^2's < .01). Examination of Figure 2 (Panel A) suggests that the main effect of Target reflected generally poorer performance on T2 than T1, consistent with the AB deficit typically obtained when T1 and T2 are separated by one non-target item [40]. These results are broadly in keeping with previous studies that have examined the link between the AB and reading [39], and validate the general paradigm used here. In addition, the main effect of Reading Group indicates that poor readers had lower overall target accuracy. The possible implications of this finding will be discussed in greater detail after reporting the results from the remaining conditions.

TT Condition

Mean accuracy scores were analyzed in a 2 (Conditionality) × 2 (Target) × 2 (Reading Group) mixed-design ANOVA. This analysis revealed a significant main effect of Reading Group, $\underline{F}(1,82) = 5.14$, $\underline{p}<.03$, $\eta_p^2 = .06$, but no other significant main effects or interactions (all $\underline{p}$'s >.17, η_p^2's <.03). In sharp contrast to the TDT condition, examination of the results in Figure 2 (Panel

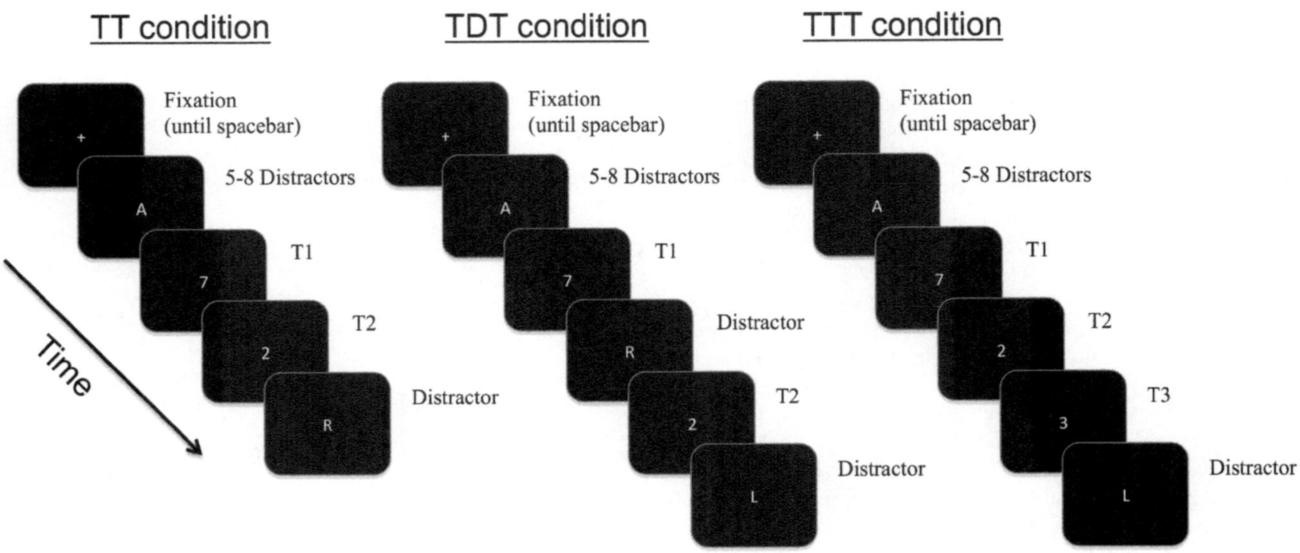

Figure 1. Schematic diagram of TT, TDT, and TTT conditions (not to scale).

B) suggests that sparing was evident across all participants with similar levels of accuracy on T1 and T2. However, the main effect of Target indicates that poor readers again demonstrated significantly impaired target identification across both items.

TTT Condition

Mean accuracy scores were analyzed in a 2 (Conditionality) × 3 (Target: T1, T2, T3) × 2 (Reading Group) mixed-design ANOVA. This analysis revealed significant main effects of Target, $F(2, 81) = 8.25$, $p < .01$, $\eta_p^2 = .17$, and Reading Group, $F(1, 82) = 12.87$, $p < .001$, $\eta_p^2 = .14$, as well as a Conditionality × Reading Group interaction, $F(1, 82) = 8.18$, $p < .01$, $\eta_p^2 = .09$, and a Conditionality × Target × Reading Group interaction, $F(2, 81) = 5.39$, $p < .01$, $\eta_p^2 = .12$. All other main effects and interactions were non-significant (all p's >.17, η_p^2's <.03). Examination of Figure 2 (Panel C) suggests that, as in the other conditions, poor readers showed worse performance across all targets, particularly for T1 and T3. This is further evidence for increased competition amongst items in the same attentional episode. Moreover, as suggested by the three-way interaction, poor readers showed greater deficits in T3 performance than normal readers when accuracy scores were calculated conditionally compared to when they were calculated unconditionally (i.e., when T3 accuracy was calculated only on trials where prior targets had been successfully encoded versus trials when accuracy was calculated without regard for whether previous targets had been encoded).

To verify this impression, the three-way interaction was followed with a pair of 3 (Target) × 2 (Reading Group) mixed-design ANOVAs conducted separately for unconditional and conditional accuracy scores. For unconditional scores, this analysis revealed significant main effects of Target, $F(2, 81) = 7.69$, $p < .01$, $\eta_p^2 = .16$, and Reading Group, $F(1, 82) = 12.02$, $p < .01$, $\eta_p^2 = .13$, but no interaction, $F(2, 81) = 2.02$, $p > .14$, $\eta_p^2 = .05$. In contrast, for conditional scores, there were main effects of Target, $F(2, 81) = 8.05$, $p < .01$, $\eta_p^2 = .17$, Reading Group, $F(1, 82) = 13.03$, $p < .01$, $\eta_p^2 = .14$, and a Target ×The follow-up analyses confirm the graphical impression that poor readers showed significantly reduced T3 performance on trials where they accurately encoded T1 and T2 within the same attentional episode, and that this deficit is greater than that found in normal readers. The contrast with results in the TT condition, where no additional deficit was seen for conditional accuracy relative to unconditional accuracy scores, implies that the ability for items to enter the same attentional episode is reduced in poor readers. That is, successful entry of one item into an attentional episode does not impair encoding a further item (TT condition), while the entry of two items into an attentional episode does impair encoding of a further item (TTT condition).

Discussion

Reading problems are a significant disability that has persisted at relatively high levels for the last thirty years. Moreover, with the dramatic increase in the importance of text-based media in the past decade, this is a problem that is likely to have even greater consequences in the future. While, a large body of research has shown a connection between phonological processing and reading impairment, more recent experiments have also shown significant deficits in spatial VA span amongst impaired readers [21–23] that

Table 1. Mean Age, IQ, and RAN scores (in seconds) as a function of reading group (poor vs. normal).

Reading Group	Age	IQ	RAN
Poor	24.00 (2.99)	106.36 (5.23)	27.12 (2.05)
Normal	23.12 (1.06)	110.16 (1.65)	24.33 (0.50)

Numbers in parentheses indicate standard error.

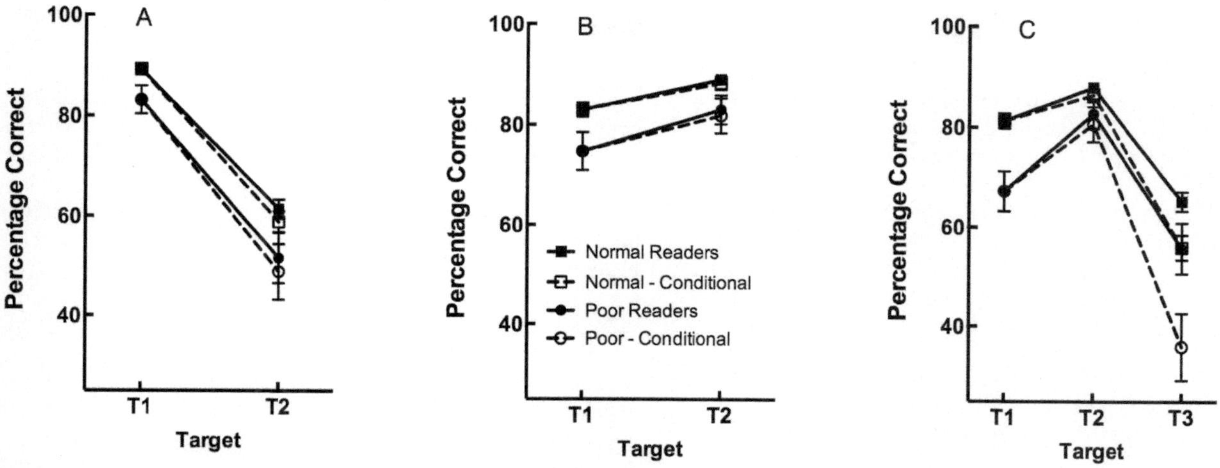

Figure 2. Mean target accuracy in TDT (Panel A), TT (Panel B), and TTT (Panel C) conditions. Dashed lines and open symbols represent conditional target accuracy, while solid symbols and lines represent unconditional target accuracy. Error bars represent one standard error of the mean.

predict reading performance over and above the presence of phonological deficits.

The present work examined whether deficits similar to those seen in spatial VA span could be found in the temporal attention span of poor readers. A number of studies have examined a similar issue in the past using the AB paradigm. However, the results have been distinctly mixed [39], and it is unclear whether the AB taps into a temporal analog of the spatial VA span, because targets are often interspersed with distractors, requiring additional processes of selection and/or inhibition not required in spatial VA tasks, and because processing occurs across significantly longer time spans than in tasks used to estimate VA span [27].

To address these shortcomings, the present work employed a modified AB paradigm in which observers viewed two (TT condition) or three (TTT condition) consecutive targets, as well as control trials in which two targets were separated by a single distractor (TDT condition) as in the conventional AB. Of chief interest was whether poor readers would show reduced target accuracy across consecutive targets, indicating a difference in their temporal span of attention. Consistent with this possibility, two key results emerged. First, across all conditions, poor readers showed an overall reduction in target accuracy compared to their normal-reading peers. Second, when presented with three consecutive targets, poor readers showed distinctly poorer T3 performance when accuracy was calculated conditional on accurate identification of preceding targets compared to when accuracy was calculated without consideration of accuracy on preceding targets (unconditional accuracy). This implies that poor reader's ability to process successive inputs within the same attentional episode is significantly curtailed beyond two items, indicating a temporal span deficit analogous to the VA span deficit shown in previous studies [21–25].

What are the origins of this temporal span deficit? Theoretical accounts suggest that VA span is determined by inter-item competition for entry into VSTM and that impaired readers differentially distribute attention amongst items compared to normal readers [26] as a result of reductions in processing speed and abnormal allocation of attention across items [23,27,28]. Theoretical accounts from the AB literature also suggest that inter-item competition plays a key role in determining consecutive target performance [29]. This conjecture has been bolstered by numerous studies showing changes in performance on one target are mirrored by concomitant variations in performance on other targets when items are presented in direct sequence [49–55]. Taken together, then, it seems reasonable to hypothesize that reductions in temporal span were the result of increased inter-item competition in poor readers.

One possible source of increased competition would arise if poorer readers were less efficient at filtering out the distractors that preceded target sequences in the TT and TTT conditions. This would result in additional distractor items competing for VSTM access, thereby reducing target accuracy. While this is plausible, several previous studies have failed to show reduced T1 performance in the AB deficit amongst poor readers [10,38] even when target-distractor similarity was quite high, implying that their target selection was unimpaired. In addition, this account would seem to predict a larger T2 accuracy difference between poor and normal readers in the TDT condition relative to the TT condition, given the additional distractor interposed between T1 and T2. However, comparison of performance across these conditions shows no interaction between condition and reading ability, $F(1,\ 83) = .21$, $p > .64$, $\eta_p^2 < .01$. Lastly, it is difficult to explain how inadvertent processing of distractors presented prior to T1 would yield a significant difference between reading groups on T3 in the TTT condition, but not on T2.

A second possible explanation for increased competition amongst poor readers is that they have slower processing speed, rendering them less able to adequately process the rapid visual inputs presented on each trial. While there is evidence for the role of processing speed in VA span, at least two points would seem to countermand this as a possible explanation here. First, previous work has suggested that processing speed is unrelated to the magnitude of the AB per se, but rather to the ability of observers to filter out distractors [60]. As noted above, given that there is little evidence that poor readers are less able to filter out distractors, either in the present study or in previous experiments, this would imply that differences in processing speed cannot account for the present differences in temporal attention span. More importantly, analyses were conducted using RAN performance as a covariate, thus obviating processing speed as the source of statistical differences between reading groups.

Another option to consider is that competition is less important in determining temporal attention span. Rather, reduced target accuracy reflects impairments in working memory capacity. Such reductions have been repeatedly demonstrated amongst poor readers [61–64]. Moreover, a reduced ability to store information would provide a plausible reason for the failure to report T3 in the TTT condition. One way to test this explanation is by comparing the TT and TTT conditions. If inter-target competition was responsible for reduced T3 accuracy amongst poor readers then other targets in the TTT condition should also show performance changes. On the other hand, if the decrease in T3 performance were simply due to the addition of another target, thereby exceeding working memory capacity, then we might expect only T3 accuracy to suffer. Consistent with the former option, T1 performance was significantly lower amongst poor readers in the TTT condition compared to the TT condition, $t(10) = 2.44$, $p < .04$. It is also notable that T2 accuracy amongst poor readers was not significantly different in the TTT condition compared to the TT condition, $t(10) = 0.45$, $p > .66$. This rules out the option that the addition of a third target led to a global decline in working memory capacity that affected encoding of all targets amongst poor readers.

Having considered explanations for the present results, it is also important to compare these findings to outcomes of previous studies. One similar study is that of Lassus-Sangosse, N'guyen-Morel & Valdois who presented multiple consecutive target items in a single spatial location [65]. Unlike the current findings, however, they obtained no differences between normal readers and those with dyslexia. Critically, Lassus-Sangosse et al. [65] used a much longer inter-target interval of 200 ms between items. This may be particularly important because studies of the temporal parameters of lag-1 sparing suggest that this longer interval is outside the temporal span of a single attentional episode [31].

Additionally, several previous studies that have examined the relationship between AB and reading have contained lag-1 trials with consecutive targets as in the TT condition used here [34,38]. To my knowledge, only Laasonen et al. [34] compared lag-1 sparing across reading groups, and they found no differences. However, given that there was also no evidence for sparing across any of the reading groups in this study, this result is difficult to interpret in the present context. In general, it would seem that additional work would be important to further examine the processing of consecutive targets across different experimental contexts.

Although the present findings are intriguing, it is also critical to consider potential limitations of the current study. One set of limitations stem from the characteristics of the participants which included eleven poor readers drawn from a pool of undergraduate psychology students who were predominately young adult, relatively affluent, female and had somewhat higher IQs than those in the population. This opens up the possibility that the results here would not extend to larger samples with more diverse characteristics and academic backgrounds. That said, while such generalizability must be demonstrated in future work, there are some suggestions that this is likely to occur. First, despite the small sample size, the differences seen between poor and normal readers were highly statistically significant and obtained reliably across experimental conditions. Second, the sample size of poor readers is consistent with studies using similar paradigms [10,32,38,66,67] and studies examining spatial VA span [22,23,27,33]. Finally, previous work has shown considerable overlap between RSVP task performance in poor readers drawn from university, community and child samples [10,38,39], suggesting broad similarities exist between participants with diverse backgrounds, ages, and cognitive abilities.

Another potential limitation of the study is that it did not assess whether poor readers met criteria for a diagnosis of dyslexia nor whether they had other co-morbid clinical conditions, such as attention-deficit-hyperactivity disorder or depression that might have contributed to task performance. As a result, the present experiment cannot speak to whether temporal attention span would also be impaired in a group of readers with dyslexia compared to their normal-reading peers, nor whether temporal attention span is related directly to reading or indirectly via a comorbid condition. Clearly, these are both important questions to be answered in future research if we are to fully characterize the relationship between temporal attention span and reading disability. However, the unique evidence presented here for a link between reductions in temporal attention span and reading proficiency still has important implications for understanding poor reading. In addition, as noted above, past studies suggest broad similarities in RSVP task performance across poor readers and readers with dyslexia. This bolsters the likelihood that temporal attention span deficits will also be implicated other instances of reading impairment.

In sum, while it is widely accepted that reading impairments often have a phonological basis, there is persistent and growing evidence that visual processes may also play a role in many instances. In particular, recent evidence has suggested that poor readers often have impaired spatial VA spans, even when no phonological impairment is present. This work provides the first evidence that poor readers may have analogous impairments in temporal attention span. In particular, the results here suggest a reduced capacity for simultaneous item processing within attentional episodes arising from increased inter-item competition. It remains for future work to confirm, clarify and expand upon these initial indications, and examine how temporal attention span impairments may impact upon reading performance in more severely impaired readers.

Author Contributions

Conceived and designed the experiments: TV. Performed the experiments: TV. Analyzed the data: TV. Contributed reagents/materials/analysis tools: TV. Wrote the paper: TV.

References

1. Shaywitz SE, Shaywitz BA, Fletcher JM, Escobar MD (1990) Prevalence of reading disability in boys and girls. JAMA 264: 998–1002.
2. Shaywitz SE (1998) Dyslexia. N Engl J Med 338: 307–312.
3. Fluss J, Ziegler J, Ecalle J, Magnan A, Warszawski J, et al. (2008) Prevalence of reading disabilities in early elementary school: Impact of socioeconomic environment on reading development in three different educational areas. Arch Pediatr 15: 1058–1067.
4. Frith U (1997) Brain, mind and behavior in dyslexia. In: Hulme C, Snowling M, editors. Dyslexia: Biology, cognition and intervention. London: Whurr. 1–19.
5. Vellutino FR, Fletcher JM, Snowling MJ, Scanlon DM (2004) Specific reading disability (dyslexia): What have we learned in the past four decades? J Child Psychol Psychiatr 45: 2–40.
6. Ramus F, Rosen S, Dakin SC, Day BL, Castellote JM, et al. (2003) Theories of developmental dyslexia: insights from a multiple case study of dyslexic adults. Brain 126: 841–865.
7. Snowling MJ (2001) From language to reading and dyslexia. Dyslexia 7: 37–46.
8. Stein J, Walsh V (1997) To see but not to read; the magnocellular theory of dyslexia. Trends Neurosci 20: 147–152.
9. Hari R, Renvall H (2001) Impaired processing of rapid stimulus sequences in dyslexia. Trends Cogn Sci 5: 525–532.
10. Visser TAW, Boden C, Giaschi DE (2004) Children with dyslexia: Evidence for visual attention deficits in perception of rapid sequences of objects. Vision Res 44: 2521–2535.
11. Brannan JR, Williams MC (1987) Allocation of visual attention in good and poor readers. Percept Psychophys 41: 23–28.

12. Facoetti A, Turatto M, Lorusso ML, Mascetti GG (2001) Orienting of visual attention in dyslexia: Evidence for asymmetric hemispheric control of attention. Exp Brain Res 138: 46–53.
13. Marendaz C, Valdois S, Walch JP (1996) Developmental dyslexia and visuospatial attention. Annee Psychol 96: 193–224.
14. Rayner K, Murphy LA, Henderson JM, Pollatsek A (1989) Selective attentional dyslexia. Cogn Neuropsychol 6: 357–378.
15. Facoetti A, Lorusso ML, Paganoni P, Cattaneo C, Galli R, et al. (2003) Auditory and visual automatic attention deficits in developmental dyslexia. Cogn Brain Res 16: 185–191.
16. Slaghuis WL, Lovegrove WJ, Davidson JA (1993) Visual and language processing deficits are concurrent in dyslexia. Cortex 29: 601–615.
17. Borsting E, Ridder WH, Dudeck K, Kelley C, Matsui L, et al. (1996) The presence of a magnocellular defect depends on the type of dyslexia. Vision Res 36: 1047–1053.
18. Slaghuis WL, Ryan JF (2006) Directional motion contrast sensitivity in developmental dyslexia. Vision Res 46: 3291–3303.
19. Cestnick L (2001) Cross-modality temporal processing deficits in developmental phonological dyslexics. Brain Cogn 46: 319–325.
20. McAnally KI, Castles A, Stuart GW (2000) Visual and auditory processing impairments in subtypes of developmental dyslexia: A discussion. J Dev Phys Disabil 12: 145–156.
21. Bosse ML, Tainturier MJ, Valdois S (2007) Developmental dyslexia: The visual attention span deficit hypothesis. Cogn 104: 198–230.
22. Hawelka S, Wimmer H (2005) Impaired visual processing of multi-element arrays is associated with increased number of eye movements in dyslexic reading. Vision Res 45: 855–863.
23. Valdois S, Bosse ML, Ans B, Carbonnel S, Zorman M, et al. (2003) Phonological and visual processing deficits can dissociate in developmental dyslexia: Evidence from two case studies. Read Writ 16: 541–572.
24. Lobier M, Dubois M, Valdois S (2013) The role of visual processing speed in reading speed development. PloS One, 8(4), e58097.
25. Averbach E, Coriell AS (1961) Short-term memory in vision. Bell System Technical Journal 40: 309–328.
26. Bundesen C (1990) A theory of visual attention. Psychol Rev 97: 523–547.
27. Dubois M, Kyllingsbæk S, Prado C, Musca SC, Peiffer E, et al. (2010) Fractionating the multi-character processing deficit in developmental dyslexia: Evidence from two case studies. Cortex 46: 717–738.
28. Stenneken P, Egetemeir J, Schulte-Körne G, Müller HJ, Schneider WX, et al. (2011) Slow perceptual processing at the core of developmental dyslexia: A parameter-based assessment of visual attention. Neuropsychologia 49: 3454–3465.
29. Shapiro KL, Raymond JE, Arnell KM (1994) Attention to visual pattern information produces the attentional blink in RSVP. J Exp Psychol Hum Percept Perform 20: 357–371.
30. Raymond JE, Shapiro KL, Arnell KM (1995) Similarity determines the attentional blink. J Exp Psychol Hum Percept Perform 21: 653–662.
31. Potter MC, Staub A, O'Connor DH (2002) The time course of competition for attention: attention is initially labile. J Exp Psychol Hum Percept Perform 28: 1149–1162.
32. Hari R, Valta M, Uutela K (1999) Prolonged attentional dwell time in dyslexic adults. Neurosci Lett 271: 202–204.
33. Lallier M, Donnadieu S, Berger C, Valdois S (2010) A case study of developmental phonological dyslexia: Is the attentional deficit in the perception of rapid stimuli sequences amodal? Cortex 46: 231–241.
34. Laasonen M, Salomaa J, Cousineau D, Leppämäki S, Tani P, et al. (2012) Project DyAdd: visual attention in adult dyslexia and ADHD. Brain Cogn 80: 311–327.
35. Lum JA, Conti-Ramsden G, Lindell AK (2007) The attentional blink reveals sluggish attentional shifting in adolescents with specific language impairment. Brain Cogn 63: 287–295.
36. Buchholz J, Aimola Davies A (2007) Attentional blink deficits observed in dyslexia depend on task demands. Vision Res 47: 1292–1302.
37. Lacroix GL, Constantinescu I, Cousineau D, de Almeida RG, Segalowitz N, et al. (2005) Attentional blink differences between adolescent dyslexic and normal readers. Brain Cogn 57: 115–119.
38. La Rocque CL, Visser TAW (2009) Sequential object recognition deficits in normal readers. Vision Res 49: 96–101.
39. McLean GM, Castles A, Coltheart V, Stuart GW (2010). No evidence for a prolonged attentional blink in developmental dyslexia. Cortex 46: 1317–1329.
40. Di Lollo V, Kawahara JI, Ghorashi SS, Enns JT (2005) The attentional blink: Resource depletion or temporary loss of control? Psychol Res 69: 191–200.
41. Olivers CN, Meeter M (2008) Feature priming in visual search does not depend on the dimensional context. Vis Cogn 16: 785–803.
42. Chun MM, Potter MC (1995) A two-stage model for multiple target detection in rapid serial visual presentation. J Exp Psychol Hum Percept Perform 2: 109–127.
43. Visser TAW, Bischof WF, Di Lollo V (2004) Rapid serial visual distraction: Task-irrelevant items can produce an attentional blink. Percept Psychophys 66: 1418–1432.
44. Tang MF, Badcock DR, Visser TAW (2013) Training and the attentional blink: Limits overcome or expectations raised? Psychon Bull Rev: in press.
45. Potter MC, Chun MM, Banks BS, Muckenhoupt M (1998) Two attentional deficits in serial target search: the visual attentional blink and an amodal task-switch deficit. J Exp Psychol Learn Mem Cogn 24: 979–992.
46. Visser TAW, Bischof WF, Di Lollo V (1999) Attentional switching in spatial and nonspatial domains: Evidence from the attentional blink. Psychol Bull 125: 458.
47. Olivers CN, van der Stigchel S, Hulleman J (2007) Spreading the sparing: Against a limited-capacity account of the attentional blink. Psychol Res 71: 126–139.
48. Sperling G, Weichselgartner E (1995) Episodic theory of the dynamics of spatial attention. Psychol Rev 102: 503–532.
49. Visser TAW, Ohan JL (2011) Is all sparing created equal? Comparing lag-1 sparing and extended sparing in temporal object perception. J Exp Psychol Hum Percept Perform 37: 1527–1541.
50. Ferlazzo F, Lucido S, Di Nocera F, Fagioli S, Sdoia S (2007) Switching between goals mediates the attentional blink effect. Exp Psychol 54: 89–98.
51. Dell'Acqua R, Jolicoeur P, Pascali A, Pluchino P (2007) Short-term consolidation of individual identities leads to Lag-1 sparing. J Exp Psychol Hum Percept Perform 33: 593–609.
52. Olivers CN, Nieuwenhuis S (2006) The beneficial effects of additional task load, positive affect, and instruction on the attentional blink. J Exp Psychol Hum Percept Perform 32: 364–379.
53. Visser TAW, Davis C, Ohan JL (2009) When similarity leads to sparing: Probing mechanisms underlying the attentional blink. Psychol Res 73: 327–335.
54. Dux PE, Asplund CL, Marois R (2008) An attentional blink for sequentially presented targets: evidence in favor of resource depletion accounts. Psychon Bull Rev 15: 809–813.
55. Dux PE, Asplund CL, Marois R (2009). Both exogenous and endogenous target salience manipulations support resource depletion accounts of the attentional blink: A reply to Olivers, Spalek, Kawahara & Di Lollo (2009). Psychon Bull Rev 16: 219–224.
56. Torgesen JK, Wagner R, Rashotte C (1999) TOWRE–2 Test of Word Reading Efficiency. Austin, TX: Pro-Ed.
57. Kaufman AS, Kaufman NL (2004) Kaufman Brief Intelligence Test. 2nd. Circle Pines, MN: AGS Publishing.
58. Wagner RK, Torgesen JK, Rashotte CA (1999) Comprehensive test of phonological processing. CTOPP: Pro-Ed.
59. Raymond JE, Shapiro KL, Arnell KM (1992) Temporary suppression of visual processing in an RSVP task: An attentional blink? J Exp Psychol Hum Percept Perform 18: 849–860.
60. Visser TAW, Ohan JL (2012) How does information processing speed relate to the attentional blink? PloS One 7: e33265.
61. de Jong PF (1998) Working memory deficits of reading disabled children. J Exp Child Psychol 70: 75–96.
62. Swanson HL, Zheng X, Jerman O (2009) Working memory, short-term memory, and reading disabilities a selective meta-analysis of the literature. J Learn Disabil 42: 260–287.
63. Bacon AM, Parmentier FB, Barr P (2013) Visuospatial memory in dyslexia: Evidence for strategic deficits. Memory 21: 189–209.
64. Wang S, Gathercole SE (2013) Working memory deficits in children with reading difficulties: Memory span and dual task coordination. J Exp Child Psycho 115: 188–197.
65. Lassus-Sangosse D, N'guyen-Morel M-A, Valdois S (2008) Sequential or simultaneous visual processing deficit in developmental dyslexia? Vision Res 48: 979–988.
66. Lallier M, Donnadieu S, Berger C, Valdois S (2010) A case study of developmental phonological dyslexia: Is the attentional deficit in the perception of rapid stimuli sequences amodal? Cortex 46: 231–241.
67. Buchholz J, Aimola Davies A (2007) Attentional blink deficits observed in dyslexia depend on task demands. Vision Res 47: 1292–1302.

Association of the *DYX1C1* Dyslexia Susceptibility Gene with Orthography in the Chinese Population

Yuping Zhang[1]◑, Jun Li[1]◑, Twila Tardif[2], Margit Burmeister[3,4,5], Sandra M. Villafuerte[3,4], Catherine McBride-Chang[6], Hong Li[7], Bingjie Shi[1], Weilan Liang[8], Zhixiang Zhang[8], Hua Shu[1]*

1 State Key Laboratory of Cognitive Neuroscience and Learning, Beijing Normal University, Beijing, China, **2** Department of Psychology, University of Michigan, Ann Arbor, Michigan, United States of America, **3** Molecular and Behavioral Neuroscience Institute, University of Michigan, Ann Arbor, Michigan, United States of America, **4** Department of Psychiatry, University of Michigan, Ann Arbor, Michigan, United States of America, **5** Department of Human Genetics, University of Michigan, Ann Arbor, Michigan, United States of America, **6** Department of Psychology, The Chinese University of Hong Kong, Hong Kong, China, **7** Department of Psychology, Beijing Normal University, Beijing, China, **8** Peking University First Hospital, Beijing, China

Abstract

Several independent studies have supported the association of *DYX1C1* with dyslexia, but its role in general reading development remains unclear. Here, we investigated the contribution of this gene to reading, with a focus on orthographic skills, in a sample of 284 unrelated Chinese children aged 5 to 11 years who were participating in the Chinese Longitudinal Study of Reading Development. We tested this association using a quantitative approach for Chinese character reading, Chinese character dictation, orthographic judgment, and visual skills. Significant or marginally significant associations were observed at the marker rs11629841 with children's orthographic judgments at ages 7 and 8 years (all P values$<$0.020). Significant associations with Chinese character dictation (all P values$<$0.013) were also observed for this single-nucleotide polymorphism (SNP) at ages 9, 10, and 11 years. Further analyses revealed that the association with orthographic skills was specific to the processing of specific components of characters (P values$<$0.046). No association was found at either SNP of rs3743205 or rs57809907. Our findings suggest that *DYX1C1* influences reading development in the general Chinese population and supports a universal effect of this gene.

Editor: Trevor Bruce Penney, National University of Singapore, Singapore

Funding: This research was supported by a grant from the Natural Science Foundation of China (30870758), by the Fundamental Research Funds for the Central University, and by BCS-0350272 from the U.S. Natural Sciences Foundation. Funding was also provided by the Research Grants Council of the Hong Kong Special Administrative Region (project reference #448907). The funders had no role in study design, data collection and analysis, decision to publish, or preparation of the manuscript.

Competing Interests: The authors have declared that no competing interests exist.

* E-mail: shuh@bnu.edu.cn

◑ These authors contributed equally to this work.

Introduction

Dyslexia (reading disability), which affects 5–10% of school-aged children across populations, is a specific impairment in learning to read that is independent of educational opportunities and general cognitive abilities [1,2,3]. Dyslexia is generally identified by gross difficulties in reading and spelling [4,5,6] and has moderate-to-high heritability, ranging from 43–73% for reading to 55–75% for spelling [7,8,9]. Although the etiology for dyslexia is not clear, behavioral studies have suggested that there are several cognitive factors underlying dyslexia, such as orthographic skills [4,10,11,12]. Indeed, the heritability of orthographic skills, or the ability to recognize specific letter patterns (orthography) of whole words, has been reported to range from 20–67% [7,8,12]. Recent molecular genetic studies have revealed several susceptibility candidates for dyslexia, including variants in the *DYX1C1* gene, which is one of the most robustly reproduced findings [4,5]. However, only a few studies have reported a significant association between *DYX1C1* and orthographic skills [13,14].

DYX1C1 (dyslexia susceptibility 1 candidate 1) was first identified as a candidate gene for dyslexia susceptibility in a Finnish family transmitting a chromosome translocation [t(2; 15)(q11; q21)] that segregated with dyslexia [15]. Subsequently, multiple studies have supported the association between *DYX1C1* and dyslexia, although not all [13,14,16–26]. The most widely replicated SNPs are rs3743205 (-3G/A) and rs57809907 (1249G/T) [13,14,15,17,20,21]. The rs3743205 SNP has been found to be associated with several phenotypes, including spelling, with the "G" allele specified as the risk allele, and the common haplotype rs3743205/rs57809907 (G/G) associated with dyslexia [17]. The SNP rs57809907 and the haplotype rs3743205/rs57809907 (G/G) have also been reported to be associated with a measure of orthographic coding choice (OC-choice), with the "G" allele rs57809907, in particular, with poor OC-choice performance in individuals from 264 nuclear families with dyslexia [14]. Nonetheless, conflicting results have also been found for both rs3743205 and rs57809907, with the opposite allelic association with dyslexia [15,21]. Moreover, recent studies have also supported the role of *DYX1C1* in normal reading variations, albeit with different SNPs (e.g., rs17819126). In these studies [16,18], as in the present study, children with dyslexia were neither specifically selected for, nor were they screened out, and thus they are assumed to represent the low tail of the normal distribution of reading ability in the population. Although *DYX1C1* has been reproducibly reported to be significantly associated with dyslexia, there are few studies of its association with orthography [13,14], a phenotype that varies between languages. In alphabetic languages (e.g., English), words consist of letter strings, which directly represent sounds, and orthographic coding can be measured by tasks such as OC-choice, which taps the ability to recognize orthographic representations of whole words and retrieve appropriate phonological representations from a mental lexicon [14]. In contrast, Chinese writing is striking in its visual complexity and its more abstract relation between the visual representation of a word and its pronunciation. All characters are square shapes comprised of different components; a component usually involves a fixed internal structure and a legal position within a character [10,27,28]. Knowledge of orthography is developed gradually over the primary school years and beyond [28,29,30]. Indeed, with reading experience, the internal structures of Chinese characters are fairly predictable [30]. Thus, orthography skills in Chinese are based on two primary aspects [28,31,32]: the ability to master the rules in combining different components into characters [27] and awareness of internal structure and positions of components. However, to our knowledge, only one recent study has investigated the genetic association between *DYX1C1* variants and dyslexia in the Chinese population [13]. Specifically, Lim et al. [13] genotyped eight SNPs for 393 individuals from 131 Chinese families with dyslexia and reported a significant association of rs3743205, but not rs57809907, to several phenotypes of reading, including orthographic skills.

Here we report data examining the association of polymorphisms in *DYX1C1* with reading, spelling, and orthographic skills in a general population of Chinese children. Since the present data is part of a large longitudinal study, we were able to test this association in relation to children's reading development over time. We were especially interested in the association between *DYX1C1* and orthographic skills, including awareness of internal structures and positions of components, as children go through the stages of becoming fluent readers. In contrast to reading, spelling requires the retrieval of sound to print correspondences and, therefore, encompasses a higher level of orthographic involvement [33,34]. To rule out the possibility that basic visual skills play a major role in the *DYX1C1*-orthography relationship, we also examined the association between *DYX1C1* and visual skills. Thus, in our study, four quantitative traits were measured at critical ages (between 5 and 11 years of age) during reading development: a) Chinese character reading, b) Chinese character dictation (spelling), c) visual-related skills, and d) orthographic judgment. We examined three SNPs that were previously found to be associated with dyslexia in previous studies [13,14,15,17,20,21], including the two SNPs (rs3743205 and rs57809907) originally reported by Taipale et al. [15] and replicated by Wigg et al. and Scerri et al. [14,17] and another SNP (rs11629841) that was also reported by Wigg et al. [17].

Methods

Subjects

We used data from a general population cohort of 284 unrelated children who were recruited from maternal-child health care clinics to develop the Chinese Communicative Development Inventory (CCDI) in 2000 [35] and were demographically representative of the city of Beijing. All of these children were tested annually on a variety of tasks as part of a large longitudinal study and all met the following inclusion criteria: native Mandarin speakers, no known intellectual disability, and a nonverbal IQ within normal limits as assessed by the Raven's Standard Progressive Matrices [36] (i.e., a score $\geq 16^{th}$ percentile, corresponding to approximately ≥ -1 SD from the population average of the 50th percentile). Informed written consent was obtained from the parents of all children. Ethical approval for the present study was obtained from the Institutional Review Board (IRB) of Beijing Normal University Imaging Center for Brain Research, the State Key Laboratory of Cognitive Neuroscience and Learning, and from the Health Sciences and Behavioral Sciences Institutional Review Boards (IRB-HSBS) of the University of Michigan.

Phenotype measures

The selection of tasks for the present study was based on the criterion that each had been administered for at least three years (except for the visual-spatial relationship subtest) and appeared to make use of some visual or orthographic skills. These included tests of single Chinese character reading and dictation, visual-related skills, and orthographic awareness.

Chinese character reading. This test was administered when children were aged 7, 8, 9, and 10 years old. This single character reading test has been successfully used in previous studies [28,37,38] and is comparable with tests of single word reading commonly used in genetic association studies of dyslexia for English and other languages [6]. During the test, children were asked to read a list of characters of increasing difficulty at their own pace and were allowed self-corrections and guessing. The final score for this test was the total number of correctly pronounced characters. A simple version consisting of 100 single Chinese characters was used for children 7 years of age, while another more difficult version consisting of 150 single characters was used for children older than age 8.

Chinese character dictation. This test was used to measure children's spelling ability at from ages 9 to 11 years. Children were required to write down target characters that were orally presented. Characters were all familiar and presented within the context of two- to four-character words. All target characters were listed in order of increasing difficulty. The final score of this dictation test was the total number of characters correctly written down. Children were tested on 32 items at ages 9 and 10 and on 40 items at age 11. A similar task has been successfully used in a previous study examining children's spelling ability [39].

Visual-related skills. Three tests of visual-related skills were used in this study: a) the Visual-Spatial Relationships test, b) Visual Matching, and c) Cross Out. Each of these three tests has been successfully used in other studies of Chinese children [28,40].

Visual-spatial skill. The visual-spatial relationships subtest from the Gardner's [41] Test of Visual-Perceptual Skills (non-motor) Revised was used to assess visual-spatial skill. This test consisted of one practice item and 16 test items, and each trial consisted of five black-and-white line drawings. Children were asked to distinguish which of the drawings was oriented differently from the others. The final score of this test was the total number of correct responses. Due to subsequent ceiling effects with older children, this test was used only when children were 5 years old.

Processing speed. Two subtests from the Woodcock-Johnson Test of Cognitive Ability [42] were used to assess processing speed. We conceptualized both of these tasks as involving visual manipulations, since each requires visual analysis and identification. The Visual Matching test measures the ability to quickly locate and circle the 2 identical digits out of 6 in each row (e.g., 8 9 5 2 9 7) within 3 minutes. The whole test consists of 60 rows, and one practice trial was given before the formal test. The task advanced in difficulty from single-digit numbers to triple-digit numbers.

The Cross Out test measures the ability to quickly scan and compare visual information. In this task, children were asked to mark 5 out of 20 drawings in a row that were identical to the target drawing at the left end of the row in 3 minutes and the whole test was comprised of 30 rows. One practice trial was given before the formal test. For both subtests, correct responses were tallied as 1 point per row. These two tests were administered at ages 6, 7, and 8 years old.

Orthographic judgment. This test is aimed at measuring orthographic awareness and has been successfully used in a previous study examining predictors of reading in Chinese children [28]. In this test, children were asked to decide whether the visually presented items were real characters or not in a list of 70 items that included 40 test items and 30 real Chinese character fillers. Of the 40 test items, 10 were black-and-white drawings with no conventional stroke pattern used (Figure S1-A, Supporting Information) and 10 were ill-formed structure non-characters with real radicals in illegal positions (Figure S1-B, Supporting Information). Another 10 compound non-characters were ill-formed components with pseudo components or subcomponents from the Chinese writing system (Figure S1-C, Supporting Information). In addition, there were 10 well-formed structured pseudo-character items consisting of real components with components in their legal position (Figure S1-D, Supporting Information). The performance score was the number of items correctly rejected amongst the 40 test items. This test was used when the children were 6, 7, and 8 years old.

Descriptive statistics for all quantitative measures at each time point are presented in Table S1, with obvious increases with age observed in Visual Matching, Cross Out, orthographic judgment, Chinese character reading, and Chinese character dictation, with no floor or ceiling effects. Data for the Cross Out task for children at 7 years of age showed a poor distribution and was log-transformed to generate a more normal distribution. Table S2 presents the correlation coefficients between phenotypic measures and all significant correlations. The Chinese character reading and Chinese character dictation tests were strongly correlated across all test points (all correlation coefficients >0.63). Both Visual Matching and Cross out measured across children's test sessions from 6- to 8-year-old were significantly and moderately correlated with the Visual-Spatial Relationship test measured at age 5, providing support that these measures share the same visual construct. These visual-related tests and orthographic judgment tests were also found to correlate significantly with the reading measures.

Genotyping

The three SNPs (rs3743205, rs11629841, and rs57809907) that showed significant associations in previous studies [15,17] were genotyped using the MassArray system (Sequenom) with primers and probes shown in Table S3. The sample success rates for all three SNPs reached 100%. Four samples were genotyped twice and the reproducibility of the genotyping was 100%.

Statistical analyses

The PLINK program version 1.07 [43] was used to carry out the Hardy-Weinberg Equilibrium (HWE) test of all three SNPs and to examine the association between SNPs or haplotypes and the quantitative measures. In line with previous studies [15,18], additive models were considered and were evaluated against the null hypothesis of no association. As the three SNPs were low in linkage disequilibrium (LD) (Table S4, r^2 ranged from 0.002 to 0.054), only the widely reported haplotype spanning rs57809907/rs3743205 [14,15,17] was analyzed in the present study. Linkage disequilibrium of the SNPs was estimated using Haploview Version 4.2 [44]. The SPSS 13.0 program was used to perform descriptive statistics and Pearson correlations. SNP association was performed with Chinese character reading and Chinese character dictation in the first step. SNPs that showed significant association in the first step were then further explored with visual-related measures and orthographic judgment. Finally, SNPs that showed significant association with orthographic judgments were then tested for associations with each of the four orthographic conditions. In all analyses, both age and sex were specified as covariates. We corrected for the number of SNPs, which yielded a significance level of 0.0167 after Bonferroni correction. Since all quantitative phenotypes were highly correlated (see Table S2), we did not correct for multiple phenotypes tested.

Results

No deviation from HWE was found at any of these SNPs (Table S4). Allele frequencies for rs3743205 and rs57809907 were consistent with previous studies [15,17,18]. However, a minor allele frequency of 0.081 was observed for rs11629841, which is lower than that reported by Wigg et al. (MAF = 0.336) [17].

In the single-marker analyses, association signals were found between rs11629841 and Chinese character dictation at all three test points ($P = 0.012$, 0.009, and 0.013 for 9-, 10-, and 11-year-olds, respectively) and remained significant after correcting for multiple comparisons, with the minor allele "G" associated with poor performance (Table 1 and Figure 1). However, no significant association with this SNP was found for Chinese character reading (all P values>0.05). Further analyses with orthographic skills showed a significant or marginally significant association between the same SNP and orthographic judgment at ages 7 and 8 ($P = 0.0003$ and $P = 0.0198$, respectively), although only the results at age 7 remained significant after correcting for multiple comparisons, with the minor allele "G" significantly associated with poor performance (Table 2 and Figure 2-A). A similar trend was also found at age 6 ($P = 0.109$). No association was found between rs11629841 and visual-related skills for ages 5 to 8 (all P values>0. 05). Of the four conditions in the orthographic judgment test, a significant association was found for the condition of illegal position (Figure 2-B) at age 7 ($P = 0.0002$) and a similar association trend was found for the other two test points ($P = 0.082$ and $P = 0.098$ for ages 6 and 8, respectively). Significant or marginally significant associations were also found for the condition of ill-formed components (Figure 2-C) for two test points ($P = 0.0004$ and $P = 0.029$ for ages 7 and 8, respectively), and the same association trend was found at age 6 ($P = 0.096$). No association was found for the other two conditions for any of the three test points (all P values>0.05). In addition, no associations, even at the nominal level, were observed for the other two markers, rs3743205 and rs57809907 (all P values>0.10).

We also performed a haplotypic analysis for the two-marker combination, namely rs3743205/rs57809907. Similar haplotype frequencies were observed: G/C (0.938), G/T (0.041), T/C (0.013) and T/T (0.008), but neither the rare haplotype nor the common haplotype that has been previously reported [14,15,17,21] to influence dyslexia was found in association with our sample (all P values>0.10).

Discussion

We investigated the association between *DYX1C1* and reading skills in a general population of Chinese children followed from

Table 1. Association of *DYC1C1* with reading and dictation.

	Reading								Dictation					
	Age 7 CCR		Age 8 CCR		Age 9 CCR		Age 10 CCR		Age 9 CCD		Age 10 CCD		Age 11 CCD	
	B	*P*	β	*P*	β	*P*	β	*P*	β	*P*	β	*P*	β	*P*
rs3743205	−1.66	0.543	0.29	0.936	−0.52	0.887	0.95	0.736	−0.09	0.933	−0.72	0.540	−0.16	0.909
rs11629841	−4.17	0.058	−5.61	0.059	−5.64	0.053	−3.80	0.093	−2.24	0.012**	−2.47	0.009**	−2.82	0.013**
rs57809907	−1.73	0.670	−0.86	0.875	1.67	0.756	1.56	0.707	−0.62	0.707	−1.45	0.405	−1.41	0.502

Note. CCR, Chinese character reading; CCD, Chinese character dictation.
*P<0.05,
**P<0.0167.

ages 5 to 11. The study is significant in its utilization of a longitudinal design in examining this association over multiple time points in relation to general reading abilities in the Han population. Support was found for an association between rs11629841 and Chinese character dictation, but not Chinese character reading, at all three test points (ages 9, 10, and 11 years), with the "G" allele associated with poor performance. Given that spelling ability is both dependent on and a reflection of orthographic skills [33], further analyses were done with orthographic skills. We found a significant association between the same SNP and orthographic judgment at two out of three test points (ages 7 and 8 years, but not 6 years), particularly with the two conditions that involved component processing of characters that were illegally positioned or ill-formed. An association for visual-related skills was also tested, but as expected, no association signal was observed between rs11629841 and basic visual skills throughout all ages tested (5 to 8 years). Together these results suggest a possible role for this SNP in the etiology of orthographic skills and, therefore, spelling skills.

The significant associations between rs11629841 and orthographic skills and spelling support its role in reading and are consistent with a study reporting biased transmission of the "G" allele of this SNP in a sample of 148 Caucasian families with dyslexia [17]. However, in another study of 247 parent-proband trios from the UK [23], Cope et al. failed to find any association between rs11629841 and dyslexia or varied reading measures, including spelling and orthography [23]. This discrepancy between our findings and those of Cope et al. [23] may be due to many factors.

First, the nature of orthography was different in our study, when compared with the English language study of Cope et al. [23]. Based on previous behavioral, patient, and brain studies,

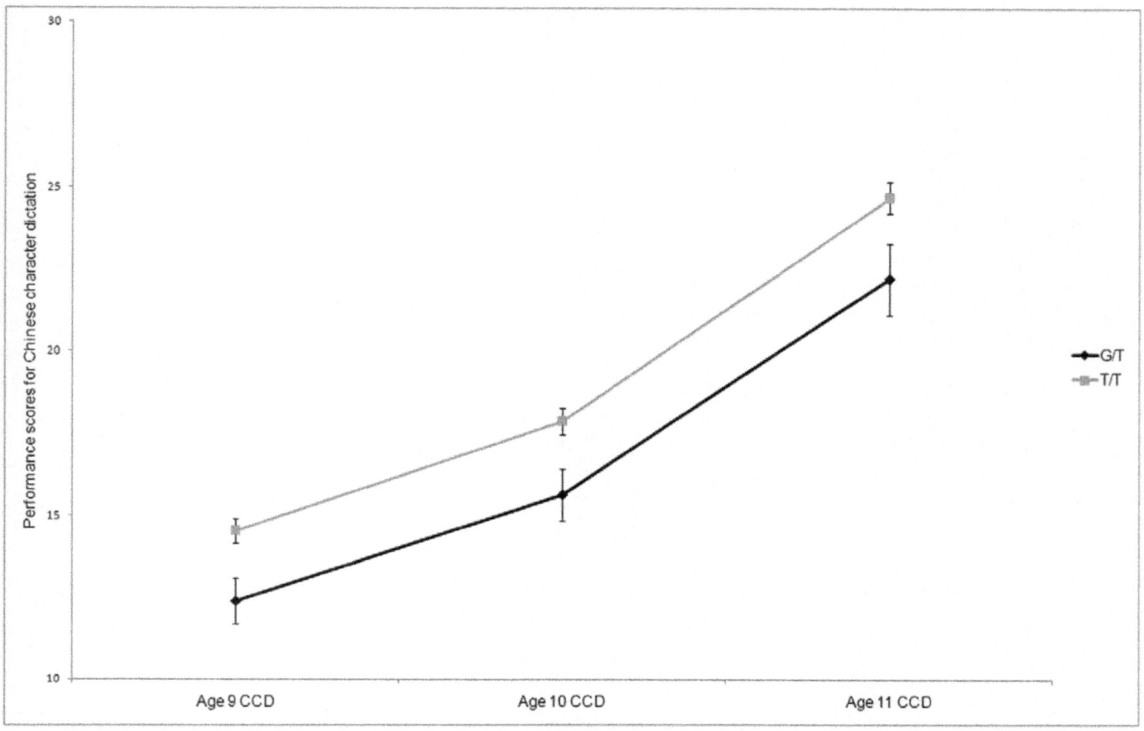

Figure 1. Performance of different genotypic groups of rs11629841 in Chinese character dictation. *N* = 0, 46, and 238 for the three genotypes of G/G, G/T, and T/T respectively. X-lab = test time (in years), Y-lab = performance scores for Chinese character dictation. CCD = Chinese character dictation.

Table 2. Association of *DYC1C1* with visual and orthographic skills.

	rs11629841							
	Age 5		**Age 6**		**Age 7**		**Age 8**	
	β	*P*	β	*P*	β	*P*	β	*P*
Visual-related skills								
VSR	−0.60	0.306	NA	NA	NA	NA	NA	NA
VM	NA	NA	−0.35	0.683	−0.69	0.391	−1.49	0.089
VC	NA	NA	−0.20	0.664	−0.29	0.541	−0.55	0.295
Orthographic judgment								
OJ	NA	NA	−1.84	0.109	−4.40	0.0003**	−1.76	0.0189*
OJ (black-and-white drawings)	NA	NA	0.025	0.844	−0.17	0.067	−0.024	0.746
OJ (illegal position)	NA	NA	−0.84	0.082	−1.97	0.0002**	−0.39	0.098
OJ (ill-formed component)	NA	NA	−0.73	0.096	−1.50	0.0004**	−0.56	0.028*
OJ (pseudo-character)	NA	NA	−0.30	0.358	−0.75	0.103	−0.78	0.092

Note. VSR, the visual spatial relationship test; VM, Visual Matching; VC, Cross Out; OJ, orthographic judgment.
NA, Not available.

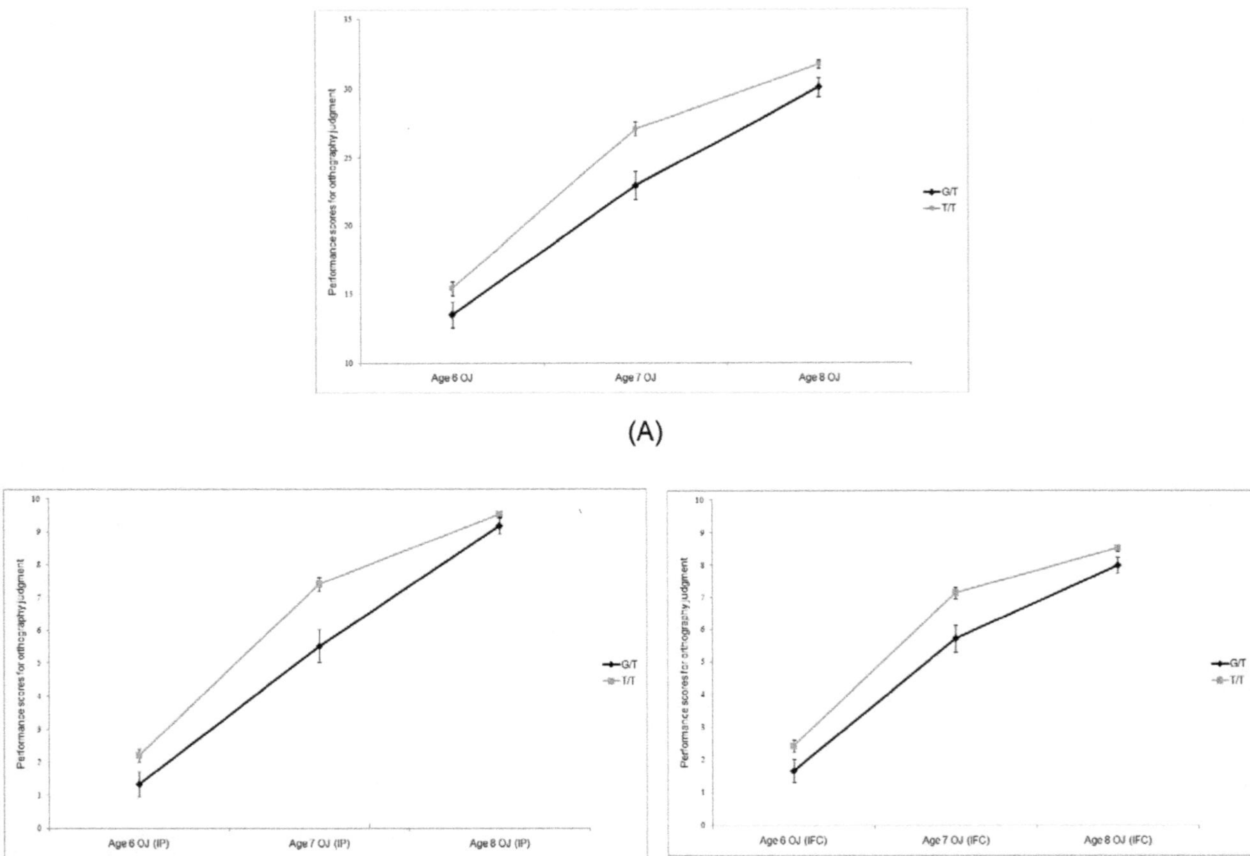

Figure 2. Performance of different genotypic groups of rs11629841 in orthographic judgment. Orthographic judgment (all four conditions combined) (A), illegal position (B), and ill-formed component (C). $N=0$, 46, and 238 for the three genotypes of G/G, G/T, and T/T respectively. X-lab = test time (in years), Y-lab = performance scores for orthographic judgment. OJ = orthographic judgment, IP = illegal position, IFC = ill-formed component.

awareness of internal structure and position of components are the basic orthographic skills necessary for the Chinese language [10,28,30,31,32,45], which are quite different from those for the English language. Moreover, different biological and neural mechanisms underlie the processing of these two languages [31,32,46]. Han et al. [31] reported a Chinese dysgraphic patient whose errors in the delayed copy task were mostly at the logographeme level, suggesting the component level of processing can be selectively impaired in the brain. Another study found significantly greater activation in the left middle fusiform gyrus (MFG), the Visual Word Form Area (VWFA) [32], during real and pseudo character processing compared to artificial characters, suggesting a crucial role of the VWFA in orthography or component processing of Chinese characters. Combined, we agree that these findings, together with our association results, imply a possible role of rs11629841 in the etiology of orthography. Nonetheless, given that the present study is the first of its kind to examine genetic association orthographic in Chinese, further research in this area that allows for functional analyses is required before a strong conclusion can be drawn.

Second, compared with the wide age range (6–17 years) in Cope et al.'s sample population, we assessed children's reading skills longitudinally with all children almost at the same ages in the present study and reported significant associations at specific ages during development.

Third, differences in the MAF between samples may also be a reason for a discrepancy in findings (8.1% in the present sample vs. about 32% in reported samples). Although the lower MAF may reduce the reliability of the present findings, this genuinely reflects the cases of different populations as shown by the MAF based on the Hapmap data, with about 35% in Caucasian, 17% in African American, but only 9% in Chinese, and 2% in Japanese.

Finally, other factors may also have contributed, such as different samples (families with dyslexia probands in Cope et al.'s study vs. general population in the present study), sex effects (with a ratio of about 2:1 for male and female in samples of dyslexia vs. about 1:1 in the general population). At this point, it is not possible to determine the precise reasons for the discrepancies. Nonetheless, the present results, together with those of Cope et al. [23] suggested several important directions for future research.

In contrast, SNP rs3743205 was not associated with any measure in this study, which is inconsistent with a recent dyslexia study of Hong Kong Chinese that reported a significant association with multiple reading skills, including orthographic skills [13]. There are several factors that may explain this discrepancy between the study with Hong Kong Chinese children and our study with Mandarin Chinese children. As stated earlier, the characteristics of the research samples (dyslexia vs. general sample; more heterogeneous Han population in our sample) may result in different findings. It is possible that this SNP (rs3743205) only influences reading skills in dyslexia since no association was found in two previous studies on general populations [16,18]. In addition, the previous study focused on children learning to read traditional Chinese characters, whereas the present study included only children reading simplified characters. Since less information is provided by fewer strokes and simpler structure, mastering simplified Chinese used in Mainland China may require slightly different visual and orthographic analyses than those required for traditional Chinese characters [47]. Finally, the clear differences in educational practices and language environment (bilingual vs. monolingual) between the two cultures may also contribute to this discrepancy. Although a number of previous studies have discussed the role of rs3743205, its association with either orthographic skills or spelling abilities has only been found in two other studies [14,17] while six other studies failed to find any association, even with dyslexia [16,18,19,22,23,24]. The lack of association with rs3743205 does not preclude our findings with rs11629841 that supporting the association between *DYX1C1* and orthographic skills. It is possible that there is a third SNP, in high LD with both rs3743205 and rs11629841, that contributes to the association between *DYX1C1* and orthography.

We also failed to find an association between rs57809907 and any of our reading measures in this study, which is consistent with the study of Hong Kong Chinese dyslexic readers [13]. Several previous studies of dyslexia also failed to find any association with this SNP [18,22,23,25,26], although some studies on Caucasian populations that use an alphabetic language reported a positive association [14,15,19,21]. As mentioned above, discrepancies between these studies may due to language differences, sex effects, and many other factors. It is also possible that this SNP is simply not associated with reading abilities in the Chinese population.

We are aware that the present study may have been potentially hampered by several limitations, for example, the small sample size, exploratory analysis of the *DYX1C1* effect in the Han population, and limited *DYX1C1* marker coverage. Although our study suggests that a longitudinal design may be advantageous in identifying additional causal alleles for reading phenotypes, further research using a larger sample of Chinese children is still needed in replicating these findings. Nonetheless, our findings are consistent with previous reports in supporting the role of the dyslexia candidate gene of *DYX1C1* in general reading variation [16,18]. In particular, they provide new evidence on the associations between rs11629841 and orthographic skills and spelling in a non-European population.

Supporting Information

Figure S1 Examples of the orthographic judgment test, black-and-white drawing (A), illegal position (B), ill-formed component (C), and pseudo characters (D).

Table S1 Descriptive statistics of phenotype measures. *The absolute scores were log-transformed for Age 7 cross out to achieve suitable skewness and kurtosis values.

Table S2 Pearson correlations between phenotype measures. VSR- the Visual-Spatial Relationship test, VM-Visual Matching, VC-Cross Out, OJ-orthographic judgment, CCR-Chinese character reading, CCD-Chinese character dictation. Correlation coefficients above 0.19 are significant at $P<0.001$, correlation coefficients above 0.15 are significant at $p<0.01$, and correlation coefficients above 0.12 are significant at $p<0.05$, $N=284$.

Table S3 Markers genotyped by MassArray system (sequenom) probes.

Table S4 Linkage disequilibrium. MAF, minor allele frequency. D′ values are shown in the upper half of the table, and r^2 values in the lower half of the table.

Acknowledgments

The authors thank all participating children and parents.

Author Contributions

Conceived and designed the experiments: YZ JL TT MB SV HS. Performed the experiments: YZ JL HL BJS WL ZZ. Analyzed the data: YZ JL MB SV BS HS. Contributed reagents/materials/analysis tools: YZ TT MB SV CM HL HS. Wrote the paper: YZ JL TT MB SV CM HL HS.

References

1. Shaywitz SE, Shaywitz BA, Fletcher JM, Escobar MD (1990) Prevalence of reading disability in boys and girls. Journal of the American Medical Association 264: 998–1002.
2. Fisher S, DeFries J (2002) Developmental dyslexia: genetic dissection of a complex cognitive trait. Nature Reviews Neuroscience 3: 767–780.
3. Stevenson HW, Stigler JW, Lucker GW, Lee S, Hsu C, et al. (1982) Reading Disabilities: The Case of Chinese, Japanese, and English. Child Development 53: 1164–1181.
4. Poelmans G, Buitelaar JK, Pauls DL, Franke B (2011) A theoretical molecular network for dyslexia: integrating available genetic findings. Molecular Psychiatry 16: 365–382.
5. Kere J (2011) Molecular genetics and molecular biology of dyslexia. Wiley Interdisciplinary Reviews: Cognitive Science 2: 441–448.
6. Shaywitz SE (1998) Current Concepts: Dyslexia. The New England Journal of Medicine 338: 307–312.
7. Gayán J, Olson RK (2001) Genetic and environmental influences on orthographic and phonological skills in children with reading disabilities. Developmental Neuropsychology 20: 483–507.
8. Chow BWY, Ho CSH, Wong SWL, Waye MMY, Bishop DVM (2011) Genetic and Environmental Influences on Chinese Language and Reading Abilities. PloS ONE 6: e16640.
9. Stevenson J, Graham P, Fredman G, McLoughli V (1987) A twin study of genetic influences on reading and spelling ability and disability. Journal of Child Psychology and Psychiatry 28: 229–247.
10. Ho CSH, Chan DWO, Lee SH, Tsang SM, Luan VH (2004) Cognitive profiling and preliminary subtyping in Chinese developmental dyslexia. Cognition 91: 43–75.
11. Hultquist AM (1997) Orthographic processing abilities of adolescents with dyslexia. Annals of dyslexia 47: 89–114.
12. Olson RK (2002) Dyslexia: nature and nurture. Dyslexia 8: 143–159.
13. Lim CKP, Ho CSH, Chou CHN, Waye MMY (2011) Association of the rs3743205 variant of DYX1C1 with dyslexia in Chinese children. Behavioral and Brain Functions 7: 16.
14. Scerri TS, Fisher SE, Francks C, MacPhie IL, Paracchini S, et al. (2004) Putative functional alleles of DYX1C1 are not associated with dyslexia susceptibility in a large sample of sibling pairs from the UK. Journal of Medical Genetics. 41: 853–857.
15. Taipale M, Kaminen N, Nopola-Hemmi J, Haltia T, Myllyluoma B, et al. (2003) A Candidate Gene for Developmental Dyslexia Encodes a Nuclear Tetratricopeptide Repeat Domain Protein Dynamically Regulated in Brain. Proceedings of the National Academy of Sciences of the United States of America 100: 11553–11558.
16. Paracchini S, Ang QW, Stanley FJ, Monaco AP, Pennell CE, et al. (2010) Analysis of dyslexia candidate genes in the Raine cohort representing the general Australian population. Genes, Brain and Behavior 10: 158–165.
17. Wigg KG, Couto JM, Feng Y, Anderson B, Cate-Carter TD, et al. (2004) Support for EKN1 as the susceptibility locus for dyslexia on 15q21. Molecular Psychiatry 9: 1111–1121.
18. Bates TC, Lind PA, Luciano M, Montgomery GW, Martin NG, et al. (2009) Dyslexia and DYX1C1: deficits in reading and spelling associated with a missense mutation. Molecular Psychiatry 15: 1190–1196.
19. Brkanac Z, Chapman NH, Matsushita MM, Chun L, Nielsen K, et al. (2007) Evaluation of candidate genes for DYX1 and DYX2 in families with dyslexia. American Journal of Medical Genetics Part B: Neuropsychiatric Genetics 144: 556–560.
20. Dahdouh F, Anthoni H, Tapia-Páez I, Peyrard-Janvid M, Schulte-Körne G, et al. (2009) Further evidence for DYX1C1 as a susceptibility factor for dyslexia. Psychiatr Genet. 19: 59–63.
21. Marino C, Citterio A, Giorda R, Facoetti A, Menozzi G, et al. (2007) Association of short-term memory with a variant within DYX1C1 in developmental dyslexia. Genes, Brain and Behavior 6: 640–646.
22. Bellini G, Bravaccio C, Calamoneri F, Cocuzza MD, Fiorillo P, et al. (2005) No evidence for association between dyslexia and DYX1C1 functional variants in a group of children and adolescents from Southern Italy. Journal of Molecular Neuroscience 27: 311–314.
23. Cope NA, Hill G, van den Bree M, Harold D, Moskvina V, et al. (2005) No support for association between dyslexia susceptibility 1 candidate 1 and developmental dyslexia. Molecular Psychiatry 10: 237–238.
24. Marino C, Giorda R, Lorusso M, Vanzin L, Salandi N, et al. (2005) A family-based association study does not support DYX1C1 on 15q21.3 as a candidate gene in developmental dyslexia. European Journal of Human Genetics 13: 491–499.
25. Meng H, Hager K, Held M, Page G, Olson RK, et al. (2005) TDT-association analysis of EKN1 and dyslexia in a Colorado twin cohort. Human Genetics 118: 87–90.
26. Saviour P, Kumar S, Kiran U, Ravuri RR, Rao VR, et al. (2008) Allelic variants of DYX1C1 are not associated with dyslexia in India. Indian Journal of Human Genetics 14: 99–102.
27. Shu H, Chen X, Anderson RC, Wu N, Xuan Y (2003) Properties of school Chinese: Implications for learning to read. Child Development 74: 27–47.
28. Li H, Shu H, McBride-Chang C, Liu H, Peng H (2012) Chinese children's character recognition: Visuo-orthographic, phonological processing and morphological skills. Journal of Research in Reading 35: 287–307.
29. Pak AKH, Cheng-Lai A, Tso IF, Shu H, Li W, et al. (2005) Visual chunking skills of Hong Kong children. Reading and Writing 18: 437–454.
30. Shu H, Anderson RC (1999) Learning to read Chinese: The development of metalinguistic awareness. In: J. Wang, A. W. Inhoff, H.-C. Chen (eds.). Reading Chinese script: A cognitive analysis. Mahwah, NJ: Lawrence Erlbaum. pp.1–18.
31. Han Z, Zhang Y, Shu H, Bi Y (2007) The orthographic buffer in writing Chinese characters: Evidence from a dysgraphic patient. Cognitive neuropsychology 24: 431–450.
32. Liu C, Zhang W, Tang Y, Mai X, Chen H, et al. (2008) The visual word form area: evidence from an fMRI study of implicit processing of Chinese characters. Neuroimage 40: 1350–1361.
33. Ouellette G, Sénéchal M (2008) Pathways to literacy: A study of invented spelling and its role in learning to read. Child Development 79: 899–913.
34. Yang J, McCandliss BD, Shu H, Zevin JD (2009) Simulating language-specific and language-general effects in a statistical learning model of Chinese reading. Journal of Memory and Language 61: 238–257.
35. Tardif T, Fletcher P, Zhang ZX, Liang WL, Zuo QH (2008) The Chinese Communicative Development Inventory (Putonghua and Cantonese versions): Manual, forms, and norms: Beijing: Peking University Medical Press.
36. Raven J, Court J, Raven J (1996) Standard Progressive Matrices. Oxford: Oxford Psychologists Press.
37. Lei L, Pan J, Liu HY, McBride-Chang C, Li H, et al. (2011) Developmental trajectories of reading development and improvement from ages 3 to 8 years in Chinese children. Journal of Child Psychology and Psychiatry 52: 212–220.
38. Lin D, McBride-Chang C, Shu H, Zhang Y, Li H, et al. (2010) Small wins big: Analytic Pinyin skills promote Chinese word reading. Psychological Science 21: 1117–1122.
39. Shu H, McBride-Chang C, Wu S, Liu H (2006) Understanding Chinese Developmental Dyslexia: Morphological Awareness as a Core Cognitive Construct. Journal of Educational Psychology 98: 122–133.
40. McBride-Chang C, Kail RV (2002) Cross-Cultural similarities in the predictors of reading acquisition. Child Development 73: 1392–1407.
41. Gardner MF (1996) Tests of Visual-Perceptual SKills (n-m) revised manual: New York: Psychological and Educational Publications.
42. Woodcock RW, Johnson MB (1989) Woodcock-Johnson Tests of Cognitive Ability: TX: DLM Teaching Resources.
43. Purcell S, Neale B, Todd-Brown K, Thomas L, Ferreira MAR, et al. (2007) PLINK: a tool set for whole-genome association and population-based linkage analyses. The American Journal of Human Genetics 81: 559–575.
44. Barrett JC, Fry B, Maller J, Daly MJ (2005) Haploview: analysis and visualization of LD and haplotype maps. Bioinformatics 21: 263–265.
45. Li H, Peng H, Shu H (2006) A study on the emergence and development of Chinese orthographic awareness in preschool and school children. Psychological Development and Education (in Chinese) 18: 35–38.
46. Tan L, Liu H, Perfetti CA, Spinks JA, Fox PT, et al. (2001) The neural system underlying Chinese logography reading. Neuroimage 13:836–846.
47. McBride-Chang C, Chow BWY, Zhong Y, Burgess S, Hayward W (2005) Chinese character acquisition and visual skills in two Chinese scripts. Reading and Writing 18: 99–128.

14

The Effect of Learning on Feedback-Related Potentials in Adolescents with Dyslexia: An EEG-ERP Study

Dror Kraus[1], Tzipi Horowitz-Kraus[2,3]*

1 Department of Pediatric Neurology, Cincinnati Children's Hospital Medical Center, Cincinnati, Ohio, United States of America, **2** Pediatric Neuroimaging Research Consortium, Cincinnati Children's Hospital Medical Center, Cincinnati, Ohio, United States of America, **3** Edmond J. Safra Brain Research Center for the Study of Learning Disabilities, Faculty of Education, University of Haifa, Haifa, Israel

Abstract

Introduction: Individuals with dyslexia exhibit associated learning deficits and impaired executive functions. The Wisconsin Card Sorting Test (WCST) is a learning-based task that relies heavily on executive functioning, in particular, attention shift and working memory. Performance during early and late phases of a series within the task represents learning and implementation of a newly learned rule. Here, we aimed to examine two event-related potentials associated with learning, feedback-related negativity (FRN)-P300 complex, in individuals with dyslexia performing the WCST.

Methods: Adolescents with dyslexia and age-matched typical readers performed the Madrid card sorting test (MCST), a computerized version of the WCST. Task performance, reading measures, and cognitive measures were collected. FRN and the P300 complex were acquired using the event-related potentials methodology and were compared in early vs late errors within a series.

Results: While performing the MCST, both groups showed a significant reduction in average reaction times and a trend toward decreased error rates. Typical readers performed consistently better than individuals with dyslexia. FRN amplitudes in early phases were significantly smaller in dyslexic readers, but were essentially equivalent to typical readers in the late phase. P300 amplitudes were initially smaller among readers with dyslexia and tended to decrease further in late phases. Differences in FRN amplitudes for early vs late phases were positively correlated with those of P300 amplitudes in the entire sample.

Conclusion: Individuals with dyslexia demonstrate a behavioral and electrophysiological change within single series of the MCST. However, learning patterns seem to differ between individuals with dyslexia and typical readers. We attribute these differences to the lower baseline performance of individuals with dyslexia. We suggest that these changes represent a fast compensatory mechanism, demonstrating the importance of learning strategies on reading among individuals with dyslexia.

Editor: Zhong-Lin Lu, The Ohio State University, Center for Cognitive and Brain Sciences, Center for Cognitive and Behavioral Brain Imaging, United States of America

Funding: This study was supported by the Edmond J Safra foundation. The funders had no role in study design, data collection and analysis, decision to publish, or preparation of the manuscript.

Competing Interests: The authors have declared that no competing interests exist.

* Email: Tzipi.Horowitz-Kraus@cchmc.org

Introduction

Dyslexia is a neurodevelopmental disorder characterized by difficulties in accurate and/or fluent word recognition and by poor spelling and decoding abilities. It is the most common specific learning impairment with an estimated prevalence of 5–6% among school-aged children in the United States. It is believed that dyslexia is mainly caused by a deficit in the phonological component of language [1].

Despite being a specific learning impairment, dyslexia has been associated with a range of deficits that extend beyond the verbal domain. These include nonverbal deficits such as sequential, visuomotor, implicit and procedural learning [2], [3], [4], as well as in executive functions such as speed of processing and performance monitoring [5], [6], [7].

The Wisconsin Card Sorting Test (WCST) is a well-validated neuropsychological task that assesses both learning and executive functioning. It was developed by Grant and Berg in 1948 [8] and was originally introduced as a measure of frontal lobe function by Milner [9]. It has been validated in children in several age groups [10], [11] and has been used clinically in children with ADHD [10], [12], Pervasive Developmental Disorder [12], temporal lobe epilepsy [13] and traumatic brain injury [14]. In the context of the WCST, learning consists of how fast a participant finds the card sorting rule and whether he is able to maintain it (see Methods below) [15]. Thereby, the main executive functions tested by the WCST are set-shifting (the ability to switch rules following a negative feedback) and working memory (the capacity to memorize previously tested rules and maintain a given rule).

Other executive functions tested include attention, inhibition, and speed of processing [16].

Individuals with dyslexia do not seem to exhibit a consistent pattern of reading errors, which interferes with their potential to learn from previously made mistakes [17], [18]. In the context of the WCST, both adults and children with dyslexia were reported to commit more errors, complete fewer categories, and have longer reaction times as compared to age-matched typical readers [16], [19], [20].

Event-related potentials (ERPs) are stereotyped electrophysiological responses to a given stimulus. ERPs are measured using electroencephalography (EEG) and provide a non-invasive, objective and easily reproducible measure of processing by linking a series of stimuli and responses. Another advantage over behavioral measures is their sensitivity, i.e. the ability to measure processing of stimuli as well as providing information regarding cognitive processes/underlying mechanism even in the absence of a behavioral change [21].

Our previous study examined ERPs during performance of the Madrid Card Sorting Test (MCST), a computerzied version of the traditional WCST, in 12-year-old adolescents with dyslexia compared to age-matched typical readers [16]. Adolescents with dyslexia demonstrated smaller target-locked potentials. This was manifested by ERPs reflecting decreased attention/perception (smaller target-locked N100) and speed of processing and working memory abilities (demonstrated by smaller target-locked P300). This difference was particularly pronounced toward the end of a series [16].

While the previous study examined responses to stimulus processing (i.e., the presentation of cards in the MCST), the current study focused on cognitive processing following feedback perception (i.e. following the response). This can be assessed electrographically by measuring the feedback-related negativity event-related potential. Feedback-related negativity is a fronto-central negative potential, which is evoked 200–300 ms after an external feedback of an erroneous response is given. It originates presumably from the Anterior Cingulate Cortex [22]. Several studies linked the FRN to the P300 component, and referred to it as the FRN-P300 complex, which reflects learning ability [23], [24], [25]. The centro-parietal P300 cue-locked component provides complementary information about the learning process. It is thought to represent attentive processes [23] and the rapid shift of attention toward unexpected stimuli [26], [27], [28].

The effect of learning on cue (performance)-locked components has been the subject of debate. While some studies showed a decrease in both FRN and P300 amplitudes following learning [24], others found only P300 amplitudes to be decreased [25]. Another study [23] demonstrated changes in FRN-P300 amplitudes occurring in the course of a task. Comparing subjects who learned a task to those performing it for the first time, FRN amplitudes in the late phase were smaller than during early phases of the task in both groups, whereas P300 amplitudes in the late phase decreased only in trained subjects.

Such differences between early and late phases in a learning task were suggested to exist also in the MCST. Barcelo & Knight (2002) found that healthy adults were found to commit fewer errors in late than in early stages of MCST series (7–8 items per series) [29]. Subjects with frontal lobe dysfunction did not demonstrate a similar decrease in errors. The researchers also suggested that higher error rates during early responses in older vs. younger participants were due to working memory overload [29].

In the current study, we sought to characterize learning within MCST series among adolescents with dyslexia by examining FRN and P300. Specifically, we sought to monitor the evolution of these markers in early vs late trials. Assuming that readers with dyslexia have an impaired ability to learn from previous mistakes [18], we hypothesized that 1) Reaction times (RT) and error rates will decrease in late phases for both groups, but to a lesser extent in individuals with dyslexia; 2) In the early phases of individual series, individuals with dyslexia will exhibit decreased FRNs and P300 components compared to typical readers; 3) When comparing early and late phases of series, differences in FRN amplitudes will be correlated with differences in P300 amplitudes. These changes will be more pronounced among individuals with dyslexia; 4) FRN-P300 complex amplitudes will be associated with speed of processing, working memory and reading scores.

Methods

2.1. Participants

All participants gave their informed written assent and their parents provided informed written consents prior to inclusion in the study. The experiment was approved by the University of Haifa Ethical Committee (number 009\09\09) based on the principles of the Helsinki declaration. Fifty-eight adolescents participated in the current study: 27 individuals with dyslexia (16 males, mean age 12.84±0.55 years old) and 31 age-matched typical readers (18 males, mean age 12.8±0.47 years old). All participants were eighth-grade students from a junior high school in the center of Israel, who volunteered for the study.

Participants with dyslexia and typical readers did not differ in their nonverbal IQs [all were within the normal range (90 and above) $t(57) = -1.934$, n.s)] as measured by the TONI-III general ability task [30] and normal attention skills as measured by two visual screening tests. In these tests the participants had to scan a page and circle specific targets (e.g., the three digits "592" or a shape of a diamond) (after [31]). Attention abilities did not differ between the two [592:t $(57) = -.553$, n.s; diamond: $t(57) = -.447$ n.s]. All were native Hebrew speakers from a middle-class background, right-handed, displayed normal or corrected-to-normal vision in both eyes, and were found on screening to have normal hearing. None of the participants had a history of neurological or emotional disorders. Participants with dyslexia had been diagnosed at least two years prior to the study and were found to meet the criteria of dyslexia as described below. The experiments were carried out at the school. All participants were compensated with a special pen.

2.2 Behavioral and Experimental Measures

Prior to the MCST, several cognitive and reading measures were assessed in all participants (see Table 1). Participants were assigned to the dyslexia group if they achieved a standard score of <-1 on standard normative one-minute words and nonwords (or pseudowords) reading tests in Hebrew (reading speed and accuracy). Additional descriptive measures included fluency in an oral reading passage [32] and reading comprehension measures. The behavioral testing lasted 1.5 hours.

2.2.1 The Madrid Card Sorting Test. Executive abilities were examined using the Madrid Card Sorting Test (MCST), a computerized version of the WCST adapted from Barcelo [38]. The MCST is a standardized tool that measures ERP components elicited during task-shifting. Stimuli were presented by Presentation® software (Neurobehavioral Systems Inc., Albany CA). MCST stimuli were all presented at a visual angle of 4° horizontally and 3.5° vertically, and remained on the screen until the participant responded. The colored geometrical figures were outlined in black against a white background and were identical in luminance.

Table 1. Behavioral measures administered to all participants.

	Description
Reading measures	A. Decoding — One-minute words/nonwords test for children [32]
	B. Oral reading task for children [32].
	D. Comprehension [33].
Cognitive measures	A. Short term memory and capacity — Digit span subtest from the WAIS-III [34].
	B. Coding WAIS-III [34].
	C. Symbol search WAIS-III [34].
	D. Naming letters, objects and Rapid Alternate Stimuli naming (RAS) [modeled after [35], [36].
	E. Trial making test [37].

MCST cards contain geometrical shapes that differ in three dimensions: color, shape and quantity. Each card can have one of 4 possible characteristics in each dimension (e.g possible colors were red, green, blue and yellow, see figure 1). The MCST stimuli consisted of 24 of the original 62 WCST cards that were to be matched with four target cards (Figure 1). In each trial, subjects had to select which of the 4 target cards matched the single stimulus card below. The trials, totaling 137, were semi-randomly arranged into 18 series, varying in length from 6 to 8 trials per series to avoid rule-switch anticipation.

The instructions to the subjects were to match the stimulus card with one of the target cards (without mentioning how to match them). They had to discover the matching rule (whether according to shape, color, or quantity of elements) by trial and error and then maintain the rule for several repetitions. The only feedback given during the test was whether each matching was right or wrong.

After a varying number of correct responses, the rule changed unpredictably, and the participant had to adjust to a new rule (e.g., from shape to color or number). There was a fixed interval of 1400 msec between the feedback onset and the onset of the next trial. The MCST design employed in this study is depicted in Figure 1 (modeled after [38]).

The MCST included feedback on the subject's performance. A "stay" indicated that the stimulus card was matched with the correct target card (and that the same matching rule was to be used in the next trial). A "shift" cue indicated that a target card was matched incorrectly; indicating that a different matching rule was to be used with the next stimulus card. The cues were delivered 1500–2000 msec after a response (200 msec duration, 10 msec rise/fall times; 65 dB SPL; 1000 Hz for "stay" cues, 500 Hz for "shift" cues).

We defined three types of errors leading to "shift" feedbacks, using Barcelo's terminology [38]:

1) The first erroneous response following a rule change was termed "shift-3D", as the subject had to handle 3 different dimensions in the working memory (discard the previously used rule and choose between two others).
2) In the trial following the shift-3D cue, the subject had a 50% chance of choosing the correct rule. An incorrect choice would result in a second consecutive shift cue termed "shift-

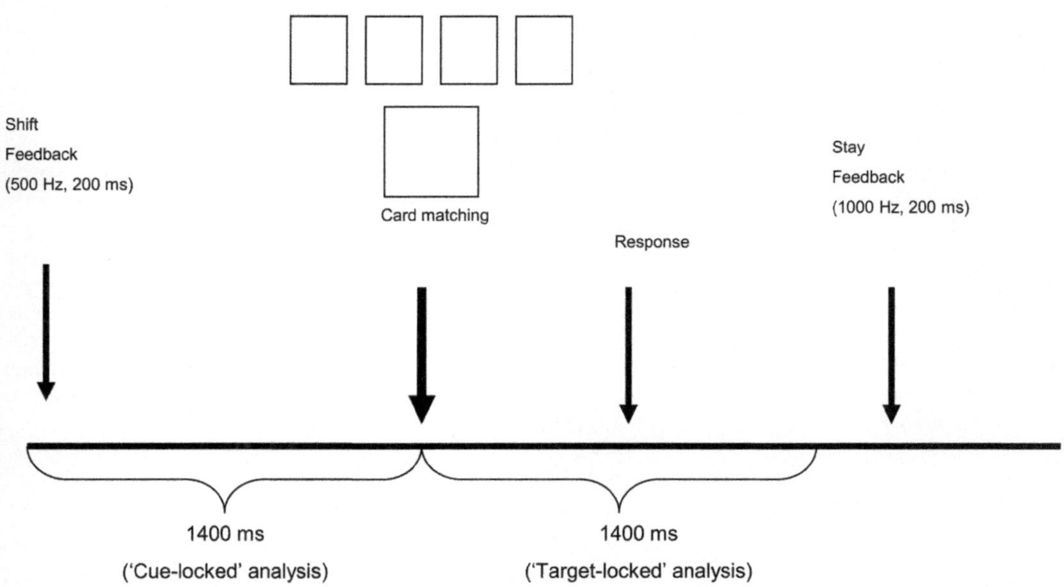

Figure 1. MCST task design and time windows for analysis (modeled after Barcelo, [38]). The data used for the current study's analysis were "cue-locked" only.

2D", as the subject now had to handle only two matching rules after rejecting the previous rule.

3) Any additional errors occurring within a series were termed random errors.

Our analysis compared shift-3D and shift-2D errors to random errors in the last 2 trials of a series.

2.2.2. Experimental measures. Mean RTs and mean accuracy were obtained from correct and error trials. Error trials were ones in which the subject failed to select the correct target response when the rule changed, or when the subject failed to follow the instruction to switch/repeat the previous trial [38].

2.2.3 Electrophysiological measures. The EEG was recorded continuously via 64 electrodes mounted on a custom-made cap (Bio-logic Ltd, Claix, France), according to the international 10/20 system [39] and sampled at a rate of 2048 Hz with an analog band pass filter of 0.1 to 70 Hz and 12-bit A/D converter, and stored for off-line analysis. Horizontal eye movements were recorded by electro-oculogram (EOG) electrodes placed on the right and left temples. Vertical eye movements were recorded by an electrode placed under the right eye. All electrode impedances were maintained at or below 5 kΩ.

The EEG was corrected for horizontal and vertical eye movements using Gratton, Coles & Donchin's algorithm (1983) [40] as implemented in the Vision Analyzer (version 1.05) program (Brain Products, Freiburg, Germany), and filtered with a 25 Hz filter. ERP epochs time-locked to "Cues" for early and late errors were averaged separately. An average reference was placed on the chin/nose and was used to reject artifacts. ERPs were epoched into 1400 msec segments with a 200 msec baseline for all conditions. Since we were interested in cognitive processes following an error commission rather than guessing a new rule, only error trials that followed correct responses were segmented and epoched. All epochs were subsequently inspected visually to ensure that they were free of residual artifacts. A grand-average was obtained separately for each condition.

The components were chosen in accordance with the global field power (GFP) measured over the scalp. The time window of each peak corresponded with the time-window observed visually in the GFP for each condition. We used semi-automatic peak detection to mark the ERPs. Since the GFP map demonstrated a fronto-central distribution both components, they were inspected in Fz, FCz and Cz.

2.2.4. Data analyses. Mean RTs and accuracy were obtained only for error trials. Error trials were those in which the participant failed to select the correct response when s/he had to repeat the rule from the previous trial. We included only error trials that followed a correct response. Early errors were considered as an average of errors in the first and second trials whereas late errors were an average of the two last trials (after Barcelo & Knight) [29]. All responses were included in the analyses.

The feedback stage was termed the "cue-locked" condition and card presentation the "target/stimulus-locked" condition (for more details see [38]). In the current study only cue-locked data was analyzed.

Prior to data analyses, we verified that there are no significant differences between number of early and late errors using *t*-tests analyses (see Table 2 for details). See Figure 2 for analyses illustration.

2.3 Research design and procedure

All behavioral and electrophysiology testing took place in a dark, quiet room at the participants' school. Participants sat at a distance of about 80 cm from a video display. They were instructed to match the choice-card (target) to one of four presented cards according to one of three rules: the color, shape, or number of objects on the key cards. They were told that when they found the correct rule they would hear a high frequency sound. However, when the rule changed or in a case of an error, they would hear a low-frequency sound. Participants used the index and middle fingers of both hands to press numbers 1 to 4 on the keyboard corresponding to the four presented cards on the screen (the "1" key represented the card on the left of the screen, "2" the second from the left, and so on). The task took about 10 minutes. Participants practiced five series that differed from those employed in the task to make sure they understood the instructions. Speed and accuracy were recorded for all task conditions. The entire task and recordings lasted approximately 45 minutes.

2.4. Statistical analyses

Mean error rates and mean reaction times were subjected to two separate two-way repeated-measures analyses of variance (RM-ANOVA) with Phase (early, late errors) as a within-subjects factor and Reading Group (readers with dyslexia, typical readers) as between-subjects factor. Independent *t*-tests were used in order to determine differences error responses between groups.

The mean amplitudes were submitted to two three-way RM-ANOVA with Phase (early, late errors) and Electrodes Site (Fz,FCz,Cz) as the within-subjects variable, and Reading Group (readers with dyslexia, typical readers) as the between-subjects variables for FRN and P300, separately.

In order to find the relations between the cognitive processing following feedback and executive abilities underlying it, Pearson correlation was performed. The relation between cognitive ability underlies cue-evaluation (measured by FRN amplitude) and attentional set shifting (measured by P300) in early and late phases was examined by correlating the differences in FRN and P300 amplitudes for early and late erroneous responses. We also wanted to examine the relations between reading ability and learning and therefore these abilities were also correlated with ERPs using the Pearson correlation.

Bonferroni correction for multiple comparisons was applied for all statistical analyses.

Results

3.1 Background measures

Significant differences were found between individuals with dyslexia and typical readers on reading and cognitive tasks: individuals with dyslexia read fewer words and made more reading errors for words/pseudowords and in oral reading text than typical readers. Individuals with dyslexia exhibited lower digit-span (backward, forward and general), symbol search, coding, and shifting. They also were slower in letters, objects, and RAS naming tasks. The groups were comparable in terms of their reading comprehension ability (see Table 3 for reading ability and Table 4 for cognitive measures).

3.2. Behavioral results

Accuracy. No differences in errors for the early and late phases between or within the groups were found. See Table 5 for the direction of these results.

Reaction time. Main effect of reading group was observed [$F(1,53) = 4.618$, $P < .05$, $\eta_p^2 = .08$], indicating longer RTs for individuals with dyslexia than for typical readers. A main effect of phase was observed [$F(1,53) = 5.791$, $P < .05$, $\eta_p^2 = .099$], with

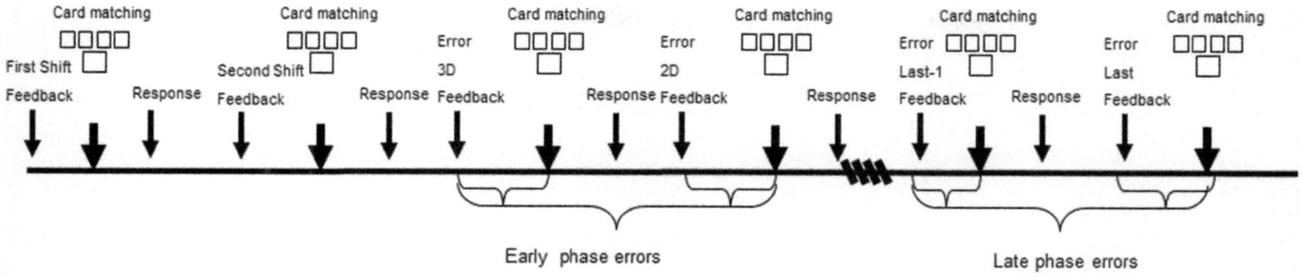

Figure 2. An illustration of the EEG data-analyses.

longer RTs for early vs. late errors. No significant phase X reading group interaction was found. Data are presented in Table 5.

3.3. Electrophysiology

3.3.1. FRN component. FRN components were defined as the most negative deflections occurring between 100 and 250 msec after the feedback. In order to explore whether differences in early and late phase conditions are reflected also in FRN components, several RM-ANOVAs were performed. A main effect of reading group was found [$F(1,56) = 4.799$, $P<.05$, $\acute{\eta}_p^2 = .079$] at the Cz electrode, indicating a slightly smaller FRN in individuals with dyslexia as compared to typical readers. A main effect of phase was also observed [$F(3,54) = 3.722$, $P<.05$, $\acute{\eta}_p^2 = .171$] in all electrodes; this resulted from a larger FRN for the late phase versus the early phase. The significant phase × reading group interaction [$F(3,54) = 3.517$, $P<.05$, $\acute{\eta}_p^2 = .163$] pointed at slightly larger differences between FRN for early versus late phases in individuals with dyslexia than in typical readers. Within-subjects RM-ANOVA analysis suggested that this main effect resulted from larger FRN for late than for early phases only in individuals with dyslexia [$F(3,24) = 9.291$, $P<.001$, $\acute{\eta}_p^2 = .537$]. See Table 6 and Figure 3 for details.

3.3.2. P300 component. P300 was defined as the most positive deflection occurring between 250 and 400 msec after a feedback. We examined whether the same effect of phase (early vs late) was observed in P300 component. Main effect for group was observed [$F(3,54) = 5.372$, $P<.05$, $\acute{\eta}_p^2 = .23$], implying smaller P300 amplitudes in individuals with dyslexia compared to typical readers (Table 6 and Figure 3). No significant main effect for within-group analyses was found.

To summarize, both groups exhibited larger FRN amplitudes for late compared to early phases. However, the difference between early and late phases was more pronounced in individuals with dyslexia. This was accompanied by a trend of shorter RTs and decreased error rates in the late phase. P300 amplitudes decreased more in individuals with dyslexia than in typical readers. The relations between the FRN and P300 were demonstrated by the positive correlation in the late phase (for Cz electrode: $r = .394$, $P<.01$, for Fz electrode: $r = .368$, $P<.01$) indicating that larger FRNs were associated with smaller P300s. Changes between early and late FRN amplitudes were correlated with changes in P300 in all participants ($r = .461$, $p<.001$).

3.4. Correlations

Correlations between P300 and reading measures are given in table 7. The correlation of P300 for the late phase with reading measures showed that greater P300 amplitudes were associated with more accurate and fluent reading. Faster speeds of processing and better memory measures were associated with higher accuracy scores and faster words/pseudowords and oral reading.

Discussion

The current study aimed to examine learning within a series among adolescents with dyslexia during the MCST.To do so, we examined performance on the MCST using FRN and P300. Learning was assessed as a function of change in ERP components and in behavioral performance between early and late phases of individual series within the task. To the best of our knowledge, this is the first study to evaluate these components within MCST series in individuals with dyslexia.

Behavioral measures

In line with our hypothesis, the main behavioral difference between both groups was in reaction times (RTs). Individuals with dyslexia exhibited longer RTs than typical readers. In the MCST, a change in rule requires the participant to shift attention to a different characteristic of the stimulus, to keep it in the working memory and to inhibit the previous response [27]. Speed of processing plays an important role in such activities: when speed of processing is slow, the working memory is more likely to be

Table 2. Number of early and late errors among dyslexic and skilled readers adolescents.

	Early errors		Late errors			
	Individuals with dyslexia (A)	Typical readers(B)	Individuals with dyslexia (C)	Typical readers(D)	*P*	Contrasts
Measure	**M(SD)**	**M(SD)**	**M(SD)**	**M(SD)**		
Number of trials	52(1.57)	48(1.56)	66(2.43)	70(1.69)	1.446, ns	A>B
					0.883, ns	D>C

ns = nonsignificant.

Table 3. A comparison of individuals with dyslexia and typical readers on reading measures (M = mean, SD = standard deviation).

Measures		Individuals with dyslexia (A) M (SD)	Typical readers (B) M (SD)	*t*	Contrasts
One-minute test for words	Speed (number)	57.4 (19.18)	76.6 (21.94)	−3.621**	B>A
	Accuracy (error percentage)	15.78 (6.71)	10.52 (5.38)	3.396**	A>B
One-minute test for nonwords	Speed (number)	26.1 (10.53)	31.32 (12)	0.458 *	B>A
	Accuracy (error percentage)	49.02 (21.33)	25.31 (14.31)	5.162***	A>B
Oral reading	Speed (seconds per word)	0.73 (0.18)	0.56 (0.13)	4.059***	A>B
	Accuracy (error percent)	7.18 (4.54)	3.87 (2.42)	3.462**	A>B
Comprehension (standard score)	Accuracy	0.08 (0.8)	0.55 (0.79)	ns	B>A

$^{*}P<.05$;
$^{**}P<.01$;
$^{***}P<.001$, ns = nonsignificant.

overloaded and the attention required is higher [41]. We therefore suggest that slower RTs achieved by readers with dyslexia represent reduced speed of processing. This has already been demonstrated in this group of readers [5].

The fact that both groups showed similar accuracy rates is of potential interest, as one would expect typical readers to perform better than their peers with dyslexia. While performing the task, individuals with dyslexia may have recruited brain regions outside the prefrontal cortex to compensate for their executive deficit [19] such as parietal regions involved in cognitive control (see the dual-network model [42]). Furthermore, the MCST relies on spatial abilities (i.e., the participant has to recognize the characteristics of a stimulus card and to categorize it), which localize to the right hemisphere [43]. Functional magnetic resonance imaging would be a suitable tool to characterize the entire network contributing to MCST performance in individuals with dyslexia.

Participants in both groups showed decreased error rates in late phases of individual series, which confirmed our hypothesis. Yet, the differences between early and late phases did not reach statistical significance in either group. Previous studies (e.g [29]) have shown a significant reduction in errors during late phases, when adults performed the test. The relative absence of effect can be attributed to the fact that executive functions assessed by the MCST localize to frontal brain regions, which complete maturation in the late 20s [44]. In the current study, participants in both groups were young adolescents, who might have not been able to perform at an adult level. This is a possible limitation of the current study.

Electrophysiological measures

Our second hypothesis was that in early phases of individual series, individuals with dyslexia would exhibit decreased FRNs and

Table 4. A comparison of individuals with dyslexia and typical readers on cognitive measures (M = mean, SD = standard deviation).

Measures		Individuals with dyslexia (A) M (SD)	Typical readers (B) M (SD)	*t*	Contrasts
Coding (standard score)	Speed	6.03 (1.93)	8.06 (2.26)	−3.72***	B>A
Symbol search (standard score)	Speed	7.82 (2.76)	10.45 (3.2)	3.405***	B>A
Digit span forward (number of items)	Accuracy	8.07 (1.84)	9.75 (1.58)	−2.507*	B>A
Digit span backward (number of items)	Accuracy	5.39 (1.96)	6.54 (1.62)	−3.844***	B>A
Digit span total (standard score)	Accuracy	6.67 (3.07)	9.21 (2.38)	−3.545**	B>A
Letter naming (seconds)	Speed	29.25 (4.4)	26.48 (3.99)	2.291**	A>B
Object naming (seconds)	Speed	37.53 (6.1)	34.15 (5.86)	2.205*	A>B
RAS naming (seconds)	Speed	30.64 (5.51)	27.39 (5.45)	2.307*	A>B
Trail making — part A (sec)	Speed	30.48 (6.7)	28.96 (9.29)	ns	A>B
Trail making — part A (number of errors)	Accuracy	0.04 (0.2)	0.06 (0.25)	ns	B>A
Trail making — part B (sec)	Speed	87.16(32.58)	65.1(17.4)	3.032**	A>B
Trail making — part B (number of errors)	Accuracy	1.04(2.44)	0.82(1.69)	ns	A>B
Trail making time ratio (A/B)	Speed	2.89(.93)	2.46(1.05)	ns	A>B

$^{*}P<.05$;
$^{**}P<.01$;
$^{***}P<.001$, ns = nonsignificant.

Table 5. A comparison of individuals with dyslexia and typical readers in terms of accuracy (error rates) and reaction times in the Madrid card-sorting test.

Measure	Early phase		Late phase		*t*	Contrast
	Individuals with dyslexia (A)	Typical readers (B)	Individuals with dyslexia (C)	Typical readers (D)		
Accuracy/% errors – mean (SD)	6.5 (4.55)	5.14 (5.71)	6.65 (5.37)	5.13 (3.71)	ns	
Reaction times in msec – mean (SD)	2327.76 (1213.64)	1985.53 (589.61)	2192.65 (922.4)	1684.72 (365.98)	2.547*	A>B
					2.514*	B>D

*$P<.05$.

P300 amplitudes compared to typical readers. The results of the current study confirm our hypothesis: individuals with dyslexia showed decreased FRNs in the early phase, which then increased to levels comparable to those of typical readers towards the end of a series. We suggest this increase might represent a distinct learning pattern that occurs preferentially in individuals with dyslexia with repetition of a task.

This pattern of "normalization" of an ERP component related to the error monitoring system has been observed in previous studies dealing with individuals with dyslexia [6], [7], [45], [46],

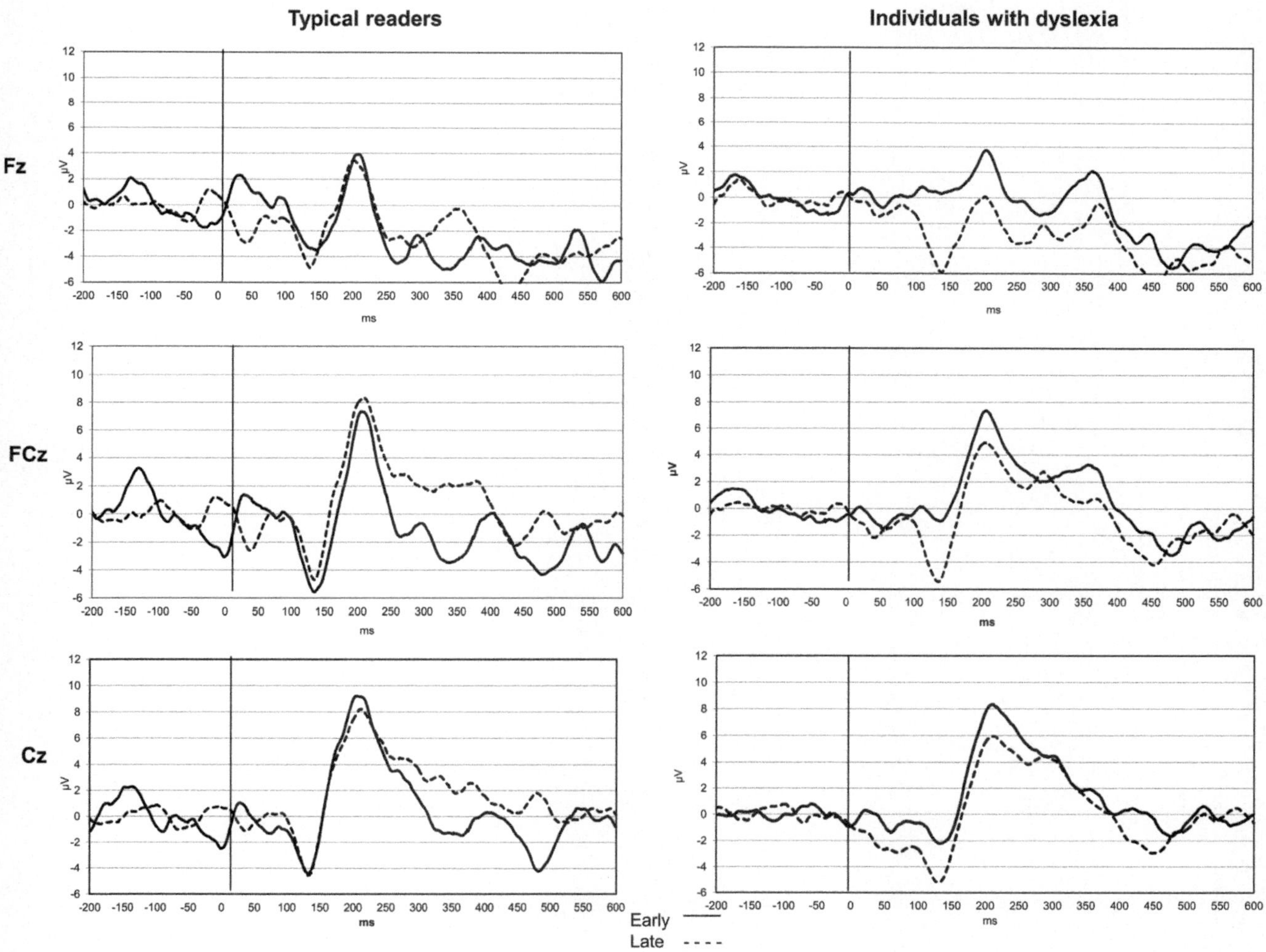

Figure 3. FRN and P300 cue-locked Event-related components. Elicitation of ERPs following cue presentation for individuals with dyslexia (right column) and typical readers (left column). Upper rows: frontal region (Fz electrode); middle rows: fronto-central regions (FCz electrode) bottom rows: central regions (Cz electrode). Smooth line: "early phase"; dashed line: "late phase." FRN was identified as the most negative peak at 100–250 msec and P300 as the most positive peak at 250–400 msec. X axis: time in msec; Y axis: amplitude in μV. Note that the negative axis is plotted down.

Table 6. Amplitudes (in µV) of FRN and P300 cue-locked components for individuals with dyslexia and typical readers for early and late errors conditions.

		Early errors		Late errors			
		Individuals with dyslexia (A)	Typical readers (B)	Individuals with dyslexia (C)	Typical readers(D)	*t*	Contrast
		M(SD)	M(SD)	M(SD)	M(SD)		
Component	Electrode						
FRN	Fz	−2.73(5.22)	−6.7(5.29)	−7.47(6.69)	−6.64(5.15)	2.859**	B>A
						ns	C>D
						−3.458**	C>D
	FCz	−4.77(6.11)	−7.91(6.78)	−7.6(4.5)	−7.87(7.06)	1.838*	B>A
						ns	D>C
						2.204*	C>A
	CZz	−2.99(4.1)	−6.08(3.72)	−6.39(3)	−6.25(4.26)	2.996**	B>A
						ns	C>D
						−3.12**	C>A
P300	Fz	4.2(4.02)	7.66(6.53)	2.37(4.8)	7.16(5.49)	−2.385*	B>A
						−3.513**	D>C
	FCz	9.5(6.77)	10.42(7.78)	6.89(5.7)	11.58(9.43)	−2.245*	D>C
						ns	B>A
						−2.203*	A>C
	Cz	10.53(5.04)	11.45(5.87)	8.35(6.42)	11.81(6.99)	−1.948*	D>C
						ns	F>E

*$P<.05$;
**$P<.01$, ns = nonsignificant.

Table 7. Correlations of ERPs and cognitive abilities with reading measures.

Cognitive ability	Measure	Reading measures	Correlation (r)
Attention set shifting	P300 amplitude in the late phase (μV)	Number of correct words read per minute	.34**
		Oral reading time (sec)	.27*
		Reading comprehension score	.26*
Speed of processing	Object naming time (sec)	Number of erroneous words per minute	.33**
		Oral reading time (sec)	.45***
	Symbol search standard (standard score)	Number of correct words read per minute	.466***
		Number of correct pseudowords read per minute	.27*
		Oral reading time (sec)	-.43***
Memory	Digit span (standard score)	Number of erroneous words per minute	-.41**
		Number of correct pseudowords per minute	.3*
		Oral reading time (sec)	-.38*

*$P<.05$;
**$P<.01$;
***$P<.001$. Data were corrected for multiple comparisons.

[47]. These studies utilized the Error-Related Negativity (ERN) as a marker for the function of this system. Following a working memory intervention, adults with dyslexia demonstrated a similar increase of ERN amplitudes to typical reader levels that was associated with improved working memory measures [7]. The possible association between these findings is intriguing in light of the commonalities between the ERN and the FRN: both are part of the learning circuit [25], [48] and increase in amplitude preferentially in response to feedback stimuli associated with unfavorable outcomes (in our case — an erroneous choice of a card) [49]. According to this hypothesis, FRN is the cue-locked variant of the response-locked ERN. The fact that the interaction between these components seems to depend on the specific task further complicates any clear conclusions at this time. Examination of ERN and FRN characteristics in the same group of individuals with dyslexia could fill this knowledge gap.

The control group of typical readers showed only minor reductions in FRN amplitudes. Previous studies have shown a general reduction in FRN throughout the performance of a task [23], [24], [25]. These apparent inconsistencies might be related to the nature of the current study task. We have assessed learning within a series of the MCST rather than throughout the entire test. It is possible that the learning effect during a repetition of a single rule was not large enough to produce an electrographic change. However, the current study focused on short-term rather than long-term learning-related changes in performance, which were expected to be more limited than the changes observed in studies examining learning in its more conventional sense. Yet, it would be interesting to examine whether a card-sorting task consisting of longer series will have a larger impact on these measures.

An analogous phenomenon was observed in P300 amplitudes during individual MCST series. During early phases, individuals with dyslexia showed smaller P300 amplitudes compared to typical readers. However, during late phases individuals with dyslexia showed a further decrease in P300 amplitudes, while amplitudes among typical readers remained essentially constant throughout a series. Larger P300 amplitudes were associated with increased reading and cognitive abilities.

In the process of learning a task, P300 amplitudes were expected to decrease [23], [24], as the amount of novelty diminishes and the attentional resources required by the task decrease [50]. As was postulated in our third hypothesis, such a decrease showed a significant correlation with the increase in FRN amplitudes in the study group, which strengthen the correspondence between FRN and P300 as a "complex". These results imply that repetition of a rule within a series had a beneficial effect on individuals with dyslexia, but not on typical readers. In contrast to FRN, the amplitude difference between early and late phases rather than the absolute values are of significance in the case of individuals with dyslexia.

We suggest that the current results may represent a rapid compensation phenomenon that leads to more efficient performance during late phases of MCST series. Even repetition of a single matching rule resulted in decreased RTs as well as in ERP changes related to learning mechanisms. While these changes were insufficient to lead to decreased error frequency, the stable accuracy rates rule out increased impulsivity as a possible explanation for the reduced RTs.

These results do not imply that individuals with dyslexia have superior capabilities to adjust performance based on errors compared to typical readers. As exemplified by the changes in FRN amplitudes, they merely show that the lower one's baseline, the higher the chance to benefit from an appropriately designed intervention. Based on our results, we hypothesize that in the case of individuals with dyslexia, the lower the baseline performance in a given task, the larger the potential for rapid improvement following a targeted intervention.

In summary, the current study supports previous findings associating dyslexia with a top-down processing impairment [16].It also highlights the role of neuroimaging in providing information about cognitive mechanisms. From a clinical point of view, our findings support the notion that repetitions and rehearsals of a task seem to benefit these adolescents almost immediately. This may encourage educators and parents to repeat instructions and learning materials for students with dyslexia.

Author Contributions

Conceived and designed the experiments: THK. Performed the experiments: THK. Analyzed the data: THK DK. Contributed reagents/materials/analysis tools: THK. Wrote the paper: THK DK.

References

1. International Dyslexia Association (2011) Definition of dyslexia. Available: http://interdys.org/DyslexiaDefinition.html Based in the initial definition of the Research Committee of the Orton Dyslexia Society, former name of the IDA, done in 1994.
2. Menghini D, Hagberg GE, Caltagirone C, Petrosini L, Vicari S (2006) Implicit learning deficits in dyslexic adults: An fMRI study. Neuroimage 33: 1218–1226. doi: http://dx.doi.org/10.1016/j.neuroimage.2006.08.024
3. Nicolson RI, Fawcett AJ, Berry EL, Jenkins IH, Dean P, et al. (1999) Association of abnormal cerebellar activation with motor learning difficulties in dyslexic adults. The LANCET 353: 1662–1667.
4. Vicari S, Finzi A, Menghini D, Marotta L, Baldi S, et al. (2005) Do children with developmental dyslexia have an implicit learning deficit? J Neurol Neurosurg Psychiatry, 76: 1392–1397. doi: 10.1136/jnnp.2004.061093
5. Breznitz Z, Misra M (2003) Speed of processing of the visual-orthographic and auditory-phonological systems in adult dyslexics: the contribution of "asynchrony" to word recognition deficits. Brain and Language 85: 486–502. doi: doi: org/10.1016/S0093-934X(03)00071-3 Accessed 2014 June 1.
6. Horowitz-Kraus T, Breznitz Z (2008) An error-detection mechanism in reading among dyslexic and regular readers—an ERP study. Clinical Neurophysiology 119: 2238–2246. doi: http://dx.doi.org/10.1016/j.clinph.2008.06.009 Accessed 2014 June 1.
7. Horowitz-Kraus T, Breznitz Z (2009) Can the error detection mechanism benefit from training the working memory? A comparison between dyslexics and controls—an ERP study. PLoS One 4(9): e7141.
8. Grant DA, Berg EA (1948) A behavioral analysis of degree of reinforcement and ease of shifting to new responses in a Weigl-type card-sorting problem. Journal of Experimental Psychology 38(4): 404–411.
9. Milner B (1963) Effects of different brain lesions on card sorting. Archives of Neurology 9: 100–110.
10. Romine CB, Lee D, Wolfe ME, Homack S, George C, et al. (2004) Wisconsin Card Sorting Test with children: a meta-analytic study of sensitivity and specificity. Archives of Clinical Neuropsychology 19(8): 1027–1041.
11. Bujoreanu IS, Willis WG (2008) Developmental and neuropsychological perspectives on the Wisconsin Card Sorting Test in children. Developmental Neuropsychology 33(5): 584–600.
12. Kado Y, Sanada S, Yanagihara M, Ogino T, Ohno S, et al. (2012) Executive function in children with pervasive developmental disorder and attention-deficit/hyperactivity disorder assessed by the Keio version of the Wisconsin card sorting test. Brain Development 34(5): 354–359.
13. Igarashi K, Oguni H, Osawa M, Awaya Y, Kato M, et al. (2002) Wisconsin card sorting test in children with temporal lobe epilepsy. Brain Development 24(3): 174–178.
14. Greve KW, Love JM, Sherwin E, Mathias CW, Ramzinski P, et al. (2002) Wisconsin Card Sorting Test in chronic severe traumatic brain injury: factor structure and performance subgroups. Brain Injury 16(1): 29–40.
15. Ritter FF, Schooler LJ (2001) The learning curve. In International Encyclopedia of the social and behavioral sciences (pp. 8602–8605). Amsterdam: Pergamon.
16. Horowitz-Kraus T (2012) Pinpointing the deficit in executive functions in teenage dyslexic readers: an ERP study using the Wisconsin Card Sorting Test, Journal of Learning Disabilities. Aug 18. [Epub ahead of print]
17. Breznitz Z (2006) Fluency in Reading: Synchronization of Processes. Mahwah, NJ: Lawrence Erlbaum and Associates.
18. Crutch SJ (2006) Qualitatively different semantic representations for abstract and concrete words: further evidence from the semantic reading errors of deep dyslexic patients. Neurocase;12(2):91–97. PubMed PMID: 16714241.
19. Helland T, Asbjornsen A (2000) Executive functions in dyslexia. Child Neuropsychology 6(1): 37–48. doi: 10.1076/0929-7049(200003)6: 1;1-B;FT037
20. Stoet G, Markey H, Lopez B (2007) Dyslexia and attentional shifting. Neuroscience Letters 427(1): 61–65. doi: http://dx.doi.org/10.1016/j.neulet.2007.09.014
21. Henson R (2005) What can functional neuroimaging tell the experimental psychologist? The quarterly journal of experimental psychology, 58A (2), 193–233.
22. Holroyd CB, Coles MG (2002) The neural basis of human error processing: reinforcement learning, dopamine, and the error-related negativity. Psychological Review 109(4): 679–709. doi: 10.1037/0033-295X.109.4.679
23. Sailer U, Fischmeister FS, Bauer H (2010) Effects of learning on feedback-related brain potentials in a decision-making task. Brain Research 1342: 85–93. doi: http://dx.doi.org/10.1016/j.brainres.2010.04.051
24. Bellebaum C, Daum I (2008) Learning-related changes in reward expectancy are reflected in the feedback-related negativity. Eur. J. Neurosci 27: 1823–1835. doi: 10.1111/j.1460-9568.2008.06138
25. Groen Y, Wijers AA, Mulder LJ, Minderaa RB, Althaus M (2007) Physiological correlates of learning by performance feedback in children: a study of EEG event-related potentials and evoked heart rate. Biological Psychology 76(3): 174–187. doi: http://dx.doi.org/10.1016/j.biopsycho.2007.07.006 Accessed 2014 June 1.
26. Courchesne E, Hillyard SA, Galambos R (1975) Stimulus novelty, task relevance and the visual evoked potential in man. Electroencephalography and Clinical Neurophysiology 39: 131–143.
27. Barcelo F, Perianez JA, Knight RT (2002) Think differently: a brain orienting response to task novelty. Neuroreport 13(15): 1887–1892.
28. Kopp B, Tabeling S, Moschner C, Wessel K (2006) Fractionating the Neural Mechanisms of Cognitive Control. Journal of Cognitive Neuroscience 18(6): 949–965.
29. Barcelo F, Knight RT (2002) Both random and perseverative errors underlie WCST deficits in prefrontal patients. Neuropsychologia 40: 349–356. doi: http://dx.doi.org/10.1016/S0028-3932(01)00110-5 Accessed 2014 June 1.
30. Brown L, Sherbenou RJ, Johnsen SK (1997) TONI-3 form a picture book test of nonverbal intelligence, third edition.
31. Rudel RG, Denckla MB, Broman M (1978) Rapid silent response to repeated target symbols by dyslexic and non-dyslexic children. [Comparative Study]. Brain and Language 6(1): 52–62. doi: http://dx.doi.org/10.1016/0093-934X(78)90043-3
32. Shany M, Lachman D, Shalem Z, Bahat A, Zeiger T (2006) "Aleph-Taph" A test for the diagnosis of reading and writing disabilities, based on national Israeli norms. Tel Aviv: Yesod Publishing.
33. Shatil E, Nevo B, Breznitz Z (2008) Elull learning disabilities diagnostic test — The reading sub-test. University of Haifa, Haifa.
34. Wechsler D (1997) Wechsler adult intelligence scale — third edition (WAIS-III). New York: The Psychological Corporation.
35. Denckla MB, Rudel RG (1976) Rapid "automatized" naming (R.A.N): dyslexia differentiated from other learning disabilities. Neuropsychologia 14(4): 471–479. doi: http://dx.doi.org/10.1016/0028-3932(76)90075-0 Accessed 2014 June 1.
36. Wolf M, Bally H, Morris R (1986) Automaticity, retrieval processes, and reading: a longitudinal study in average and impaired readers. Child Development 57(4): 988–1000. doi: http://www.jstor.org/stable/1130373
37. Reitan RM, Wolfson D (1985) The Halstead–Reitan Neuropsycholgical Test Battery: Therapy and clinical interpretation. Tucson, AZ: Neuropsychological Press.
38. Barcelo F (2003) The Madrid card sorting test (MCST): a task-switching paradigm to study executive attention with event-related potentials. [Research Support, Non-U.S. Government]. Brain research. Brain research protocols 11(1): 27–37. doi: http://dx.doi.org/10.1016/S1385-299X(03)00013-8
39. Jasper HH (1958) The ten-twenty electrode system of the International Federation of Societies for Electroencephalography: Appendix to report of the committee on methods of clinical examination in electroencephalography. EEG Clinical Neurophysiology 10: 371–375. doi: 10.1016/0013-4694(58)90053-1
40. Gratton G, Coles MG, Donchin E (1983) A new method for off-line removal of ocular artifact. Electroencephalography and Clinical Neurophysiology 55(4): 468–484. doi: http://dx.doi.org/10.1016/0013-4694(83)90135-9
41. Jacobson LA, Ryan M, Martin RB, Ewen J, Mostofsky SH, et al. (2011) Working memory influences processing speed and reading fluency in ADHD. Child Neuropsychology 17: 209–224. doi: 10.1080/09297049.2010.532204
42. Dosenbach NUF, Fair DA, Cohen AL, Schlaggar BL, Peterson SE (2008) A dual-networks architecture of top-down control. Trends in Cognitive Sciences.12: 99–105.
43. Witelson D F (1976) Sex and the single hemisphere: Specialization of the right hemisphere for spatial processing. Science 193: 425–427.
44. Segalowitz SJ, Davies PL (2004) Charting the maturation of the frontal lobe: An electrophysiological strategy. Brain and Cognition 55: 116–133. doi: http://dx.doi.org/10.1016/S0278-2626(03)00283-5 Accessed 2014 June 1.
45. Horowitz-Kraus T (2011) Does Development Affect the Error-related Negativity of Dyslexic and skilled readers in Reading? An ERP study. Developmental Neuropsychology 36: 914–932. doi: 10.1080/87565641.2011.606415
46. Horowitz-Kraus T, Breznitz Z (2011) Error Detection Mechanism at Words and Sentences: A Comparison Between Readers with Dyslexia and Skilled Readers, The international journal of developmental disabilities and education 58: 33–45.
47. Horowitz-Kraus T, Cicchino N, Breznitz Z, Holland SK (2012) "More than Words": Training Improves Reading and Executive Functions in Children with Dyslexia: an ERP and fMRI study. International Dyslexia Association Conference, Baltimore, USA.
48. van Noordt SJ, Segalowitz SJ (2012) Performance monitoring and the medial prefrontal cortex: a review of individual differences and context effects as a window on self-regulation. Front Hum Neurosci 6: 197.
49. Nieuwenhuis S, Yeung N, Holroyd CB, Schurger A, Cohen JD (2004) Sensitivity of electrophysiological activity from medial frontal cortex to utilitarian and performance feedback. Cerebral Cortex 14: 741–747. doi: 10.1093/cercor/bhh034.
50. Polich J (2007) Updating P300: an integrative theory of P3a and P3b. Clin Neurophysiol 118: 2128–2148.

15

Segregation of Lexical and Sub-Lexical Reading Processes in the Left Perisylvian Cortex

Franck-Emmanuel Roux[1,2]*, Jean-Baptiste Durand[3], Mélanie Jucla[1,4], Emilie Réhault[1], Marion Reddy[2], Jean-François Démonet[1,2]

1 UMR Unité 825, Faculté Paul Sabatier, IFR 96, Toulouse, France, **2** Pole Neurosciences, Centres Hospitalo-Universitaires, Toulouse, France, **3** Centre de Recherche Cerveau et Cognition, Toulouse, France, **4** U.R.I. Octogone-Lordat 4156, Université de Toulouse II, Toulouse, France

Abstract

A fundamental issue in cognitive neuroscience is the existence of two major, sub-lexical and lexical, reading processes and their possible segregation in the left posterior perisylvian cortex. Using cortical electrostimulation mapping, we identified the cortical areas involved on reading either orthographically irregular words (lexical, "direct" process) or pronounceable pseudowords (sublexical, "indirect" process) in 14 right-handed neurosurgical patients while video-recording behavioral effects. Intraoperative neuronavigation system and Montreal Neurological Institute (MNI) stereotactic coordinates were used to identify the localization of stimulation sites. Fifty-one reading interference areas were found that affected either words (14 areas), or pseudo-words (11 areas), or both (26 areas). Forty-one (80%) corresponded to the impairment of the phonological level of reading processes. Reading processes involved discrete, highly localized perisylvian cortical areas with individual variability. MNI coordinates throughout the group exhibited a clear segregation according to the tested reading route; specific pseudo-word reading interferences were concentrated in a restricted inferior and anterior subpart of the left supramarginal gyrus (barycentre $x = -68.1$; $y = -25.9$; $z = 30.2$; Brodmann's area 40) while specific word reading areas were located almost exclusively alongside the left superior temporal gyrus. Although half of the reading interferences found were nonspecific, the finding of specific lexical or sublexical interferences is new evidence that lexical and sublexical processes of reading could be partially supported by distinct cortical sub-regions despite their anatomical proximity. These data are in line with many brain activation studies that showed that left superior temporal and inferior parietal regions had a crucial role respectively in word and pseudoword reading and were core regions for dyslexia.

Editor: Antoni Rodriguez-Fornells, University of Barcelona, Spain

Funding: The authors have no support or funding to report.

Competing Interests: The authors have declared that no competing interests exist.

* E-mail: franck_emmanuel.roux@yahoo.fr

Introduction

In neurocognitive models, word reading has been supposed to rely on two distinct processes that allow orthographic information to be matched to homologous phonological information. 'Dual-route' models proposed that words can be read either by an "indirect", sub-lexical route, using grapheme to phoneme correspondence rules, or a "direct", lexical route, in which words are directly recognized as lexicon members and associated with verbal semantic representations [1,2,3]. For instance, the sub-lexical route would be used to process new orthographic forms such as previously unknown words (i.e. rare words, foreign words, or experimental pseudo-words). The lexical route would be used to read common words, thought to be stored in an orthographic lexicon.

The dual-route models of reading originated from cases of dissociated reading disorders observed in patients with acquired dyslexia. Indeed, some alexic patients, presenting with phonological dyslexia, were found to name irregular words flawlessly but not pseudo-words [4,5] whereas others, known as surface dyslexia patients, could process pseudo-words but not irregular words [1,6,7,8]. According to lesion anatomy studies, different neural pathways and cortical areas could be associated with these lexical and sub-lexical processes. For instance, phonological acquired dyslexia has been linked to damage to left inferior-parietal [9] or left inferofrontal regions [10].

In brain imaging experiments, it has been shown that the phonological store (crucial to the efficient correspondence between orthographic sequences to their phonological counterparts) was localized in the supramarginal gyrus [11,12] or in the left posterior superior temporal gyrus [13]. In a meta-analysis of 35 previous neuroimaging studies of reading, Jobard et al. [14] dissociated a lexicosemantic route involving the left basal temporal language area, the posterior part of the middle temporal gyrus, and the inferior frontal gyrus (pars triangularis) and a sublexical route involving left lateralized superior temporal areas, supramarginal gyrus, and the opercular part of inferior frontal gyrus. Nevertheless, controversies still exist about the anatomical substrates involved in lexical and sublexical reading routes [14,15].

Direct cortical electrostimulation for neurosurgical cases offers researchers an invaluable technique to study human brain functions as it induces on-line transient inhibitory lesion-like effects on association areas. Stimulation-induced impairment of language performance during a given task indicates that the small area beneath the electrode is involved in the function elicited by the task. It has been shown that naming [16] or reading [17] are clinically relevant tasks during brain mapping. Our group previously studied some aspects of the organization of reading processes [18,19,20,21,22] showing that various reading scripts as musical score, Arabic numbers or alphabetic scripts from different languages could be anatomically segregated within left posterior Sylvian cortex. Another team, using words versus pseudo-words tasks, Simos et al. [23,24] supported the existence of two different brain mechanisms for phonological processing in word reading; one in the posterior part of superior temporal gyrus subserving assembled phonology and a second, lexical mechanism that could be responsible for pronouncing words with rare print-to-sound correspondences depending on middle temporal gyrus. Beyond the scientific aspect, this finding could be important in practice when removing brain lesions within left posterior Sylvian region; it would imply that brain mappings should be performed using lexical and sublexical reading tasks.

In order to identify the perisylvian areas involved in reading and to spare them during surgery, cortical electrical stimulation mapping was used intraoperatively in 14 patients during the removal of brain tumours. Direct electrostimulation gave us opportunity to study the neural basis of reading processes in such crucial regions as the left perisylvian fissure and to address whether the two major, sub-lexical and lexical, reading processes are anatomically partially or entirely segregated within this region.

Materials and Methods

Patients

In this study, 14 patients (11 men - mean age: 42 year-old – Standard deviation: 18.6 - all right handed) underwent surgical resection of brain tumours or arteriovenous malformations (**Table 1**). In critical regions such as the posterior Sylvian fissure, electrostimulation was used in patients with deep seated cavernomas or metastasis to choose the best cortical approach (i.e. sparing functional areas). The surgical approach was modified according the functional data obtained by electrostimulation. Our surgical concept of tumour removal was to resect only tissue located within one centimeter of functional areas detected by electrostimulation. However, this principle approach was occasionally broken, if essentially necessary, to achieve tumour resection. All patients were French speakers and fulfilled the following criteria (1) had no language deficit pre-operatively, and (2) had a lesion located close to the left posterior Sylvian fissure. Language abilities were tested by one of us (ER, a speech therapist) in all subjects pre- and postoperatively, with standardized tests of visual naming, written and oral understanding, oral fluency, reading, dictation, repetition, written transcription, and object handling [25,26] and handedness was assessed using the Edinburgh Inventory [27]. Patients with pre-operative language disorders were excluded from this study.

All the patients and their families gave their verbal and written informed consent to study their language areas by direct brain mapping. The National consultative committee of INSERM (Institut National de la Santé et de la Recherche Médicale) gave its approval for the storage of patients' data and preservation of their anonymity. Data from these successive brain mappings were collected prospectively by the same team using the same protocol over throughout this three year-long period.

Cortical Mapping: Tasks

We used 3 language tasks to map cortical areas: picture naming, word reading, pseudoword reading. Initially, the patients were asked to perform the naming task (visual naming task using drawings of various objects), followed by the word task and the pseudoword reading task. Each stimulation site was tested systematically with these 3 tasks. For each site, 4 or 5 word or pseudoword reading items were used in order to avoid "single" errors during brain mapping. Word reading considered of paramount importance by multiple testing to be certain that the tests were reproducible.

An assistant alerted the surgeon whenever performance impairments were induced by stimulation. When a functional site was found, it was marked by a sterile ticket of.25 cm^2. Sub-cortical mapping was performed when appropriate but only with naming tasks.

To evaluate the use of each route, lexical and sublexical, we respectively used two sets of 36 stimuli: one of frequent French words and one of pronounceable pseudowords (see the full list of items in Table 2). The items were selected from a list of materials used in preoperative language tests. In order to maximize the use of the lexical route, the words selected were a) frequent words (median *freqlemlivres* = 32, Lexique 3, New, B. & Pallier, C., www.lexique.org); b) contained at least one irregular/inconsistent segment whose correct pronunciation cannot be obtained by using the most frequent segment-phoneme correspondence. Irregularities were due to different factors: irregular grapheme-phoneme mapping (se**c**ond, m**on**sieur, **oi**gnon), inconsistent rhyme orthography (n**erf**, g**ars**, n**et**) or loanwords (s**qu**are, pi**zz**a, f**oo**tb**all**). In order to maximize the use of the indirect, phonological route, without possible orthographic/semantic interaction, we selected pseudwords that could be pronounced in French but that do not have close orthographic neighbours. In order to compare results in word and pseudoword reading, we paired the stimuli for length (number of letter and syllable) and bigram frequency (see Table 3 for a statistical description of the material used).

The task for word reading was performed first, and, after completion, patients performed the pseudo-word reading task. We chose orthographically irregular French words and phonologically legal pseudowords to contrast two modes of accessing output phonology. Reading irregular words elicits access to phonological output lexicon and assembled phonological representations. Pseudoword reading requires sub-lexical orthography-to-phonology mapping and segmented phonological processing [28].

Cortical Mapping: Procedure

As described in previous studies [19], the cortex was directly stimulated using the bipolar electrode of the "Nimbus" cortical stimulator (1 mm wide electrodes separated by 6 mm: Newmedic®, Toulouse, France). The current amplitude was started at 2 mA, and progressively increased by 1 mA, using biphasic square wave pulses of 1 ms at 60 Hz. Care was taken to avoid electrical diffusion and afterdischarges by stimulating under the level of stimulation generating afterdischarges. So, intraoperative cortical stimulation was used to localize the areas of the functional cortex after determination of the afterdischarge threshold roughly one second by electrocorticography.

Accuracy of Electrostimulation Mapping

Electrostimulation is the oldest technique of brain mapping [16]. The main advantage of this technique is its high level of accuracy [29]. We used a low stimulation frequency known to activate preferentially cortical local cells [30] or afferent inputs of the stimulated area. The peak current density is localized in a small spherical region around the bipolar electrodes [31]. Indeed, the signal remains tangentially located in the immediate vicinity of the electrode which deters the cortical functions located in less than 1 cm^2 under the probes [29]. During stimulation, we often observe that the displacement of the electrode to an adjacent

Table 1. Demographics and topography of explored brain regions - 14 patients.

Patient	Gender/Age/Occupation/Handedness (Edinburgh score)	Brain Lesion Treated
1	M/54/technician/Right Handed (+90)	High grade Glioma
2	M/23/student/Right Handed (+85)	High grade Glioma
3	M/22/student/Right Handed (+65)	Low grade Glioma
4	M/73/retired/Right Handed (+80)	Cavernoma
5	F/36/nurse/Right Handed (+65)	Cavernoma
6	M/14/student/Right Handed (+90)	Low Grade Glioma
7	M/32/technician/Right Handed (+70)	Low Grade Glioma
8	M/28/technician/Right Handed (+75)	Low Grade Glioma
9	F/48/social worker/Right Handed (+70)	Metastasis
10	M/34/computer engineer/Right Handed (+90)	Low Grade Glioma
11	M/62/retired/Right Handed (+80)	High grade Glioma
12	F/33/secretary/Right Handed (+80)	High grade Glioma
13	M/55/technician/Right Handed (+90)	High grade Glioma
14	M/70/notary/Right Handed (+90)	High grade Glioma

region located 1 cm apart from the initial area results in strikingly different effects.

Extent and Localization of Stimulated Sites

Stimulation was guided by a neuronavigational system, with 3D reconstructions of the brain (Stealth Station, Sofamor Danek, Surgical navigation technologies, Broomfield, CO, USA) to localize brain gyri. Each 3D brain volume was normalized in the MNI space, and parameters were used to obtain normalized coordinates from stimulation site locations, which were intraoperatively visualized and positioned on 3D original images provided by a neuronavigation software (Medtronic, Minneapolis, MN). The sites of cortical stimulation were 1 cm apart. The cortical surface tested was divided into several squares of 1 cm^2. The extent and the number of cortical stimulation sites varied from one patient to another depending on the size of craniotomy.

Conditions of Validation

Criteria for validation of interference sites can be summarized in 3 points:

1) We think that video recording is crucial to data monitoring so that observations can be validated or discarded from the analysis. All patients of this series had their cortical mapping procedures video recorded. Video recordings were especially helpful to improve postoperative analysis of type of interference (phonemic substitution, jargon, etc…) obtained during reading tasks.
2) To be accepted as "word reading site" or "pseudo word reading site", the identified interference sites were meticulously tested at least 3 times (not consecutively). Cortical sites showing no 3 reproducible task interferences were not included in this study. In cases of ambiguity, a site could be tested more than 3 times.
3) Finally, it must be emphasized that, when we qualified a reading site as "pseudo word-specific reading" it meant that neither naming nor word reading interferences were found in this area. We could not exclude, however, that this site defined as "specific" may lead to stimulation interference for other functions not tested in this study.

Results

No general complications were noted in this series during operation. Current intensity that did not evoke afterdischarges ranged from 4.1 to 5.6 mA in this study. None of the patients had generalized seizures intra-operatively. We found reading interferences in all patients (3.6 reading interference per patient; Standard deviation: 2.3) but one (patient 14). Overall, a total of 51 reading interference sites were detected, common to both reading tasks (26 sites) or specific to one reading task (25 sites). These interference sites were detected in small cortical patches of 1, 2 or 3 cm^2. Individualized reading maps were generated in terms of number, size, type and localization of reading interference sites.

Number and Size of Reading Interference Areas

Group analysis on 14 patients showed that the mean area of cortical surface tested and calculated on operative 3D MRI reconstructions was 29 cm^2 (range, 22 to 36 cm^2 – Standard deviation, 4.24). Interferences for reading were observed for stimulation of discrete, highly localized patches of cortex. Twenty-six areas were "single" sites (i.e. sites occupying a surface of 1 cm^2 with intervening areas evoking no reading interferences). The margins of these sites were distinct, the displacement of the electrode into an adjacent cortical area located in the same gyrus producing no reading interference. Reading interferences found varied from 0 to 7 (mean: 3.3 interferences per subject). The range of the cortex involved in word and pseudo-word reading routes for each patient was 3.64 cm^2 (range, 0 cm^2 to 7 cm^2– standard deviation, 2.34). Neural structures found by electrostimulation and involved in reading occupied only 12.5% of the surface tested. **Figure 1a** details the surface of the cortical gyri studied in each patient and **Figure 1b** illustrates the variability of the number and surface of the positive reading areas found.

Type and Localization of Interference of the Cortex Areas Involved in Reading

Table 4 summarizes the type and the localization of interference found during reading mapping by direct stimulation in the 13 patients with positive results. Results of stimulations were

Table 2. List of words and pseudowords used in this study.

Words	Pseudowords
deuxième	moube
nerf	butiro
chaos	dasul
sculpture	adrile
choix	écine
second	tople
longtemps	birzouko
gars	cande
square	tribul
oignon	voral
respect	durche
franc	atrul
orgueil	dipulo
football	énoure
gentil	nacide
violemment	toupre
net	nochir
aiguille	sinope
patience	nurin
flux	afnur
banc	cipre
pizza	jamik
chronique	pudiro
hall	covulta
oeil	égibe
maximum	dripul
août	chulo
examen	filchon
six	cuifle
orchestre	saille
ville	pitode
dessous	prapou
poêle	bultir
choeur	pogide
monsieur	simade
poing	tanepi

divided in: 1) common interference areas for word and non word reading and 2) specific interference areas for either word or pseudo word reading. Over 51 reading interference sites, 26 common interference sites for word and pseudo word reading were found. Fourteen specific word interference areas and 11 specific pseudo-word interferences were detected. Interferences specific to pseudo words were detected in 6 patients (patients 1, 2, 5, 6, 8, and 13). Interferences specific to words were found in another group of 6 patients (patients 3, 5, 7, 8, 9, and 13) with partial overlap between the two groups, i.e. patients 5, 8 and 13 showed each interference sites specific to either words or pseudo-words. In cortical areas where word and pseudo-word reading interferences were observed (common areas), types of reading disorders observed during electrostimulation were similar for both tasks. The 51 positive interferences either elicited by pseudo-word and word reading tasks, 41 (80%) corresponded clearly to the impairment of the phonological level of reading processes (i.e. electrostimulation elicited jargon, neologism, substitution of syllabes, syllabation). Other interferences were reading arrest (blockade) or various phenomena such as hesitations or auto corrections.

Figure 2 summarizes the results of reading mapping by direct stimulation obtained in the patients. In group analysis, specific word or pseudo word reading areas exhibited a clear topographical segregation; pseudoword reading interferences were located in the anterior part of the supramarginal gyrus or the posterior part of postcentral gyrus (Brodmann's area 3, 40 or 43) and word reading areas in the superior temporal gyrus (Brodmann's area 22 and 42) or a more posterior part of the supramarginal gyrus. Common interferences for word and pseudo word reading were mainly observed in superior temporal gyrus and anterior part of the supramarginal gyrus. In the 3 patients (Patients 5, 8, and 13) showing interferences of each of the two reading processes, the specific sites were clearly segregated in anatomical terms; pseudo-word reading interferences were concentrated in the inferior/ anterior part of the left supramarginal gyrus, while word interference sites were more distributed, being found either in the posterior part of the supramarginal gyrus or the superior temporal gyrus (**Figure 3**).

Discussion

In this study, we found that reading processes involved discrete, highly localized left perisylvian cortical areas with individual variability. Partial segregation of the pseudo-word and word reading routes was detected, specific pseudo-word reading interferences being concentrated in a restricted inferior and anterior subpart of the left supramarginal gyrus while specific word reading areas were located almost exclusively alongside the left superior temporal gyrus. Despite their anatomical proximity, lexical and sublexical processes of reading could be supported by distinct cortical sub-regions, at least partially. Moreover, the literature on brain-damaged patients suggests that these pathways are not fully independent but instead interact [32]. It is worth to note that pseudo-word/word anatomical segregation has also been described in left occipitotemporal cortex [7,8,22,33,34,35]. This partial dissociation between pseudo-word reading and irregular

Table 3. Comparative description of words and non words lists.

Items	Number of letters *(SD)*	Number of syllables *(SD)*	Mean bigram frequency *(SD)*
Words	5,75 *(0,7)*	1,9 *(0,6)*	2211 *(779)*
Non words	6 *(1,9)*	1,6 *(0,6)*	2455 *(1218)*
p-value	*0,74*	*0,07*	*0,32*

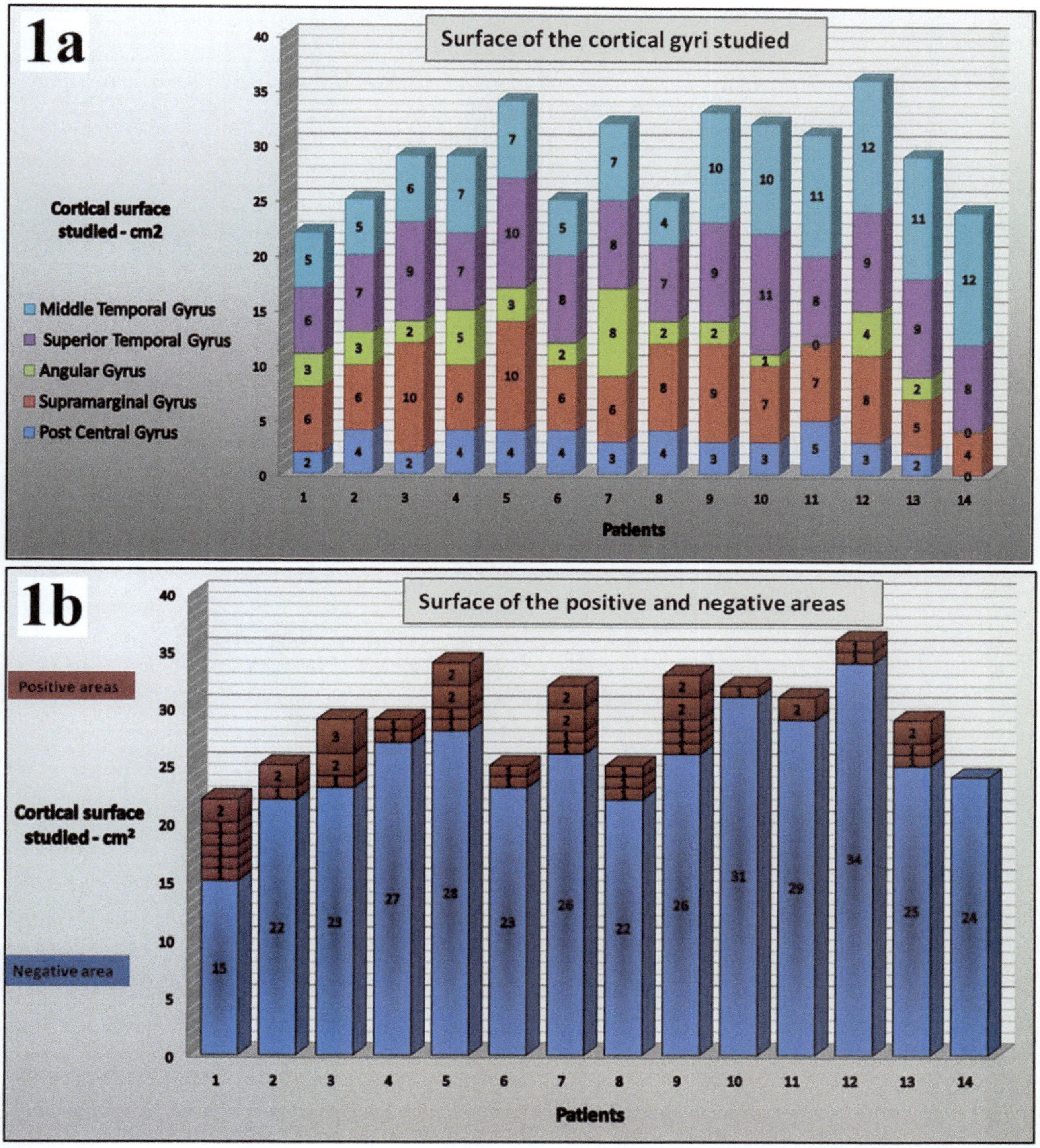

Figure 1. Number and size of reading interference areas. Figure 1a shows in each patient the surface of the cortical gyri studied with some variations according to the tumor location and size of bone flap. Figure 1b illustrates the variability of the number and surface of the positive reading areas among this group of patient. A majority of positive areas were discrete (1 cm^2) cortical areas; adjacent sites (2 cm^2) found to be both involved in reading was observed 11 times, and only in a single case did we find a positive area of 3 cm^2.

word reading suggests that the left inferior-parietal cortex could be more involved in pseudo-word reading than the left temporal cortex that is thought to relate to lexical long-term memory and therefore might be more involved in the processing of irregular words. Patients with acquired phonological dyslexia are poor at reading pseudo-words, whereas their word reading is relatively spared [5]. This could possibly result from impairment in graphemic-phonologic conversion, which is thought to depend mainly on functions of the left inferior-parietal [9] and inferior frontal regions [10].

Table 4. Intraoperative Talairach's coordinates (MNI) of sites showing interference upon stimulation in the explored group of 14 patients.

Patient	MNI coordinates of detected interference area			Word, non-word or common interference	Type of reading interference	Anatomical Area/BA
	X	Y	Z			
1	−70	−47	5	Common	Auto-corrections	Superior Temporal Gyrus/22
1	−70	−36	2	Common	Hesitation	Middle Temporal Gyrus/22
1	−70	−24	−1	Common	Letter -level errors	Superior Temporal Gyrus/22
1	−68	−8	−3	Common	Blockade	Superior Temporal Gyrus/21
1	−70	−20	12	Common	Blockade	Superior Temporal Gyrus/42
1	−68	−14	11	Non-Word	Letter -level errors	PostCentral Gyrus/43
1	−69	−14	16	Non-Word	Slowing/Syllabations	PostCentral Gyrus/43
2	−66	−40	27	Common	Letter -level errors	Supramarginal Gyrus/40
2	−65	−36	37	Non-Word	Letter -level errors	Supramarginal Gyrus/40
2	−61	−36	52	Common	Slowing/syllabation	PostCentral Gyrus/40
3	−68	−32	8	Common	Blockade	Superior Temporal Gyrus/42
3	−68	−45	9	Word	Neologism/jargon	Superior Temporal Gyrus/22
3	−68	−37	20	Word	Neologism/jargon	Superior Temporal Gyrus/22
3	−64	−48	26	Word	Letter -level errors	Supramarginal Gyrus/40
3	−65	−37	29	Common	Articulation/voice alteration	Supramarginal Gyrus/40
3	−65	−31	31	Word	Neologism/jargon	Supramarginal Gyrus/40
4	−68	−39	30	Common	Blockade	Supramarginal Gyrus/40
4	−70	−48	−10	Common	Blockade	Middle Temporal Gyrus/21
5	−65	−32	43	Non-Word	Letter -level errors	Supramarginal Gyrus/40
5	−68	−31	36	Non-Word	Letter -level errors	Supramarginal Gyrus/40
5	−68	−23	36	Non-Word	Slowing/syllabations	PostCentral Gyrus/2
5	−71	−25	6	Word	Letter -level errors	Superior Temporal Gyrus/42
5	−66	−42	40	Word	Letter -level errors	Supramarginal Gyrus/40
5	−65	−46	35	Word	Neologism/jargon	Supramarginal Gyrus/40
6	−68	−36	32	Non-Word	Letter -level errors	Supramarginal Gyrus/40
6	−70	−26	31	Non-Word	Letter -level errors	Supramarginal Gyrus/40
7	−65	−36	42	Common	Letter -level errors	Supramarginal Gyrus/40
7	−67	−29	42	Common	Letter -level errors	Supramarginal Gyrus/40
7	−69	−21	33	Common	Slowing/syllabation	PostCentral Gyrus/2
7	−70	−25	22	Common	Autocorrections	PostCentral Gyrus/40
7	−71	−36	21	Word	Neologism/jargon	Superior Temporal Gyrus/22
7	−71	−39	27	Word	Word-level	Supramarginal Gyrus/40
8	−67	−36	30	Word	Slowing/syllabation	Supramarginal Gyrus/40
8	−65	−49	17	Common	Neologism/jargon	Superior Temporal Gyrus/22
8	−68	−21	36	Non-Word	Slowing/syllabation	PostCentral Gyrus/3
9	−68	−30	24	Word	Blockade	Supramarginal Gyrus/40
9	−65	−17	26	Common	Letter -level errors	PostCentral Gyrus/43
9	−70	−12	20	Common	Letter -level errors	PostCentral Gyrus/43
9	−68	−6	19	Common	Letter -level errors	PostCentral Gyrus/43
9	−72	−20	5	Word	Neologism/jargon	Superior Temporal Gyrus/22
9	−71	−13	4	Word	Slowing/syllabation	Superior Temporal Gyrus/22
9	−62	0	−6	Common	Neologism/jargon	Superior Temporal Gyrus/22
10	−68	−18	26	Common	Letter -level errors	PostCentral Gyrus/2
11	−68	−23	36	Common	Neologism/jargon	PostCentral Gyrus/2
11	−65	−24	41	Common	Letter -level errors	PostCentral Gyrus/2
12	−69	−43	22	Common	Letter -level errors	Supramarginal Gyrus/40

Table 4. Cont.

Patient	MNI coordinates of detected interference area			Word, non-word or common interference	Type of reading interference	Anatomical Area/BA
	X	Y	Z			
12	−69	−49	12	Common	Letter -level errors	Superior Temporal Gyrus/22
13	−72	−20	9	Common	Letter -level errors	Superior Temporal Gyrus/42
13	−69	−5	1	Word	Slowing/syllabation	Superior Temporal Gyrus/22
13	−70	−26	23	Non-Word	Letter -level errors	Supramarginal Gyrus/40
13	−70	−26	31	Non-Word	Letter -level errors	Supramarginal Gyrus/40
14	No interference detected					

BA: Brodmann's areas. Each site had a cortical surface of 1 cm^2. Sites in dotted square are adjacent sites (2 or 3 cm^2).

However, the numerous neuroimaging studies [21,36,37,38] on this topic yield rather controversial conclusions in establishing the organization of lexical and sublexical processes within the posterior Sylvian region [14,15]. Main difficulties arose from the fact that words and pseudowords differ in more than one way (length, familiarity, access to semantics and phonological decoding) and because differences in activation were often relative within detected areas [14,15]. The supramarginal gyrus seems especially involved in studies dealing with pseudo-words or unfamiliar letter combinations [39]. A recent study [35], taking into account many psycholinguistic parameters that could be responsible for differential activations during word versus pseudo-word reading, put forward specific brain regions involved in direct orthography to phonology mapping (including the left

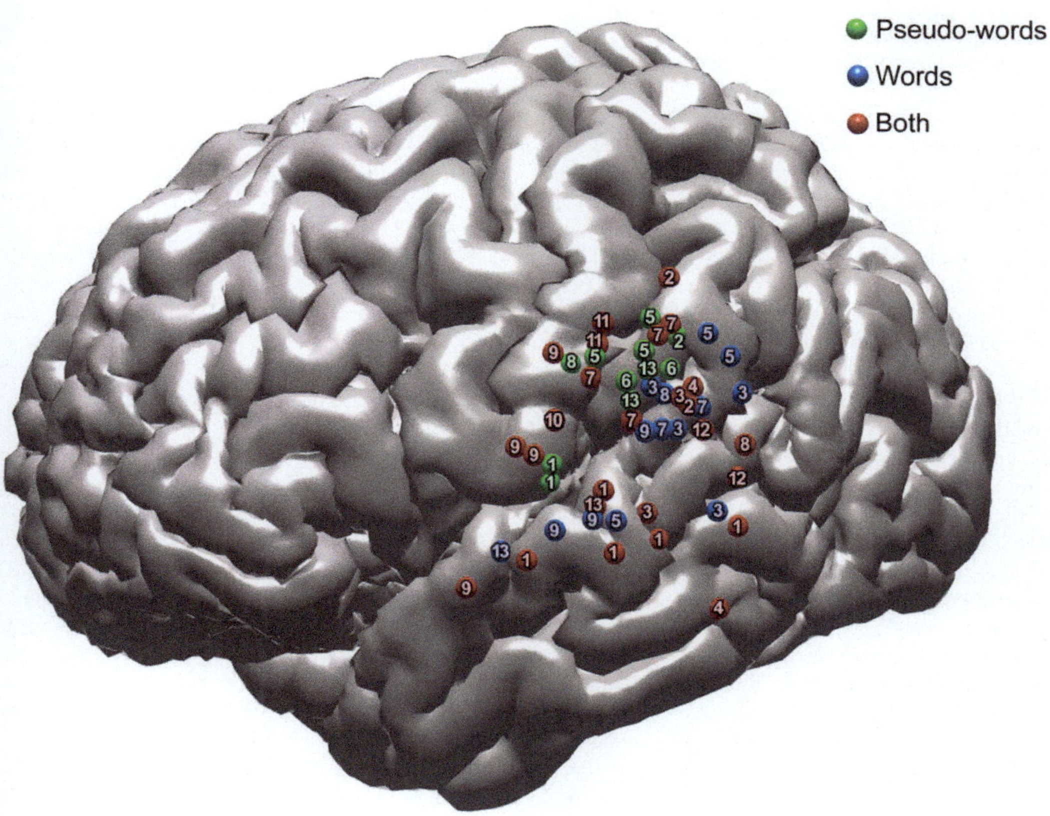

Figure 2. Localization of the word and pseudo word sites. Figure 2 shows the localization of word and pseudo word reading stimulation sites positioned in the standard normalized Montreal Neurological Institute (MNI) space (listed in Table 3 - Numbers inside the dots refer to patient number listed in this table). Overall, 26 common words and pseudo word reading interferences (red) were found in different regions of posterior Sylvian fissure. Fourteen specific word reading (blue) and 11 specific pseudo word reading were detected (green). Group analysis demonstrated that specific word or pseudo word reading areas exhibited a clear somatotopy, pseudo-word reading interferences being located in the anterior part of the supramarginal gyrus (barycentre: $x = -68.1$; $y = -25.9$; $z = 30.2$; Brodmann's area 40) and word reading areas in the temporal gyrus (barycentre: $x = -68.3$; $y = -32.4$; $z = 19.9$ Brodmann's area 42).

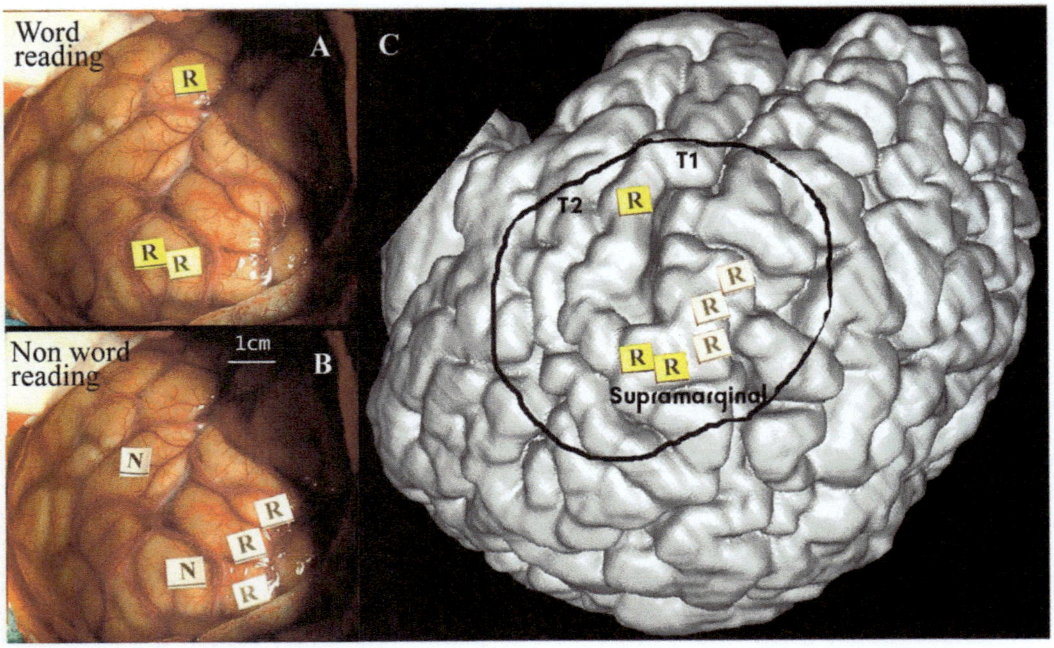

Figure 3. Example of cortical mapping in patient 5. Figure 3 shows in patient 5 the results of word (R yellow) and pseudo word reading (R white) mapping in a patient who had an arteriovenous malformation within the posterior part of the Sylvian fissure. Word reading (A) involved the posterior part of supramarginal gyrus and T1 gyrus whereas pseudo word reading (B) involved anterior part of supramarginal gyrus. To improve the understanding of the intraoperative pictures, cortical sites producing no reading interference (Negative area = N) were not systematically noted by a sterile ticket. These sites were extremely localized in small areas of the cortex. In this case, as seen in the 3D reconstruction of patient's brain (in C) strict segregation of the areas involved in word or pseudo-word reading was found.

supramarginal gyrus) or lexical/semantic processing (left middle and inferior temporal regions, bilateral angular gyri). Other authors have challenged these conclusions, pointing the fact that, overall, pseudo-words and real-words recruit the same neural areas [15,21,40,41] maybe with some differences in terms of spatiotemporal dynamic of activation between the two word classes [41]. Other claimed that the very small number of subjects of some case report studies do not allowed reaching clear conclusions [15].

Regarding the connectivity between these areas, the reading process could be mediated by the temporo-parietal section of the arcuate fasciculus from the inferior temporal lobe to inferior-parietal region [42]. The superior longitudinal fasciculus could also convey reading information from inferior-parietal region to dorsal prefrontal cortex [21]. Overall, both ventral and dorsal pathways could process frequent regular words [1]. Levy et al., investigated the use of these two pathways in an effective connectivity study during word or pseudo-word reading [22]. They showed that both routes could be involved in processing both types of stimuli and that using the appropriate route was predictive of better reading performance. The use of both ventral and dorsal pathways in word and pseudo-word reading could partly explain the composite reading maps generated within the left perisylvian cortex in our population.

In this study, we found that pseudo-word and word reading could involve discrete, highly localized (often limited to small neuronal patches less than 1 cm^2) perisylvian cortical areas with some individual variability. Composite and individual reading maps generated in this study may be linked to cytoarchitectonic studies showing high variability of cortical microstructures within the inferior parietal lobe [43]. Other hypotheses could be raised to explain this variability such as the influence of epileptic activity (although none of our patients had chronic epilepsy) as well as the individual variability in the type of brain disease treated; slow-growing tumors (5 patients in this study) in areas which could lead to a local potential re-organization of higher cortical functions.

This variability did not prevent us to observe that not only the left perisylvian cortex was crucial to the phonology-level coding of verbal stimuli but that both sublexical and lexical reading routes could be anatomically segregated within this region. Although, at the individual level, an overlap may exist in this region between pseudo-word and word processing, group analysis reveals a certain degree of topographical segregation between sub-lexical and lexical types of language processes. The grapho-phonological conversion linked to the sublexical reading process seems to involve the anterior part of the left supramarginal gyrus. This is in line with our previous works describing the involvement of the supramarginal gyrus in phonological processing of sentence reading [19] and with the existence of a spatial segregation of the phonological process for the 2 different types of script (alphabetic versus arabic number) in this gyrus [18]. This study and the current psycholinguistic models of reading also suggest that the superior temporal gyrus and the more posterior part of the supramarginal gyrus are involved in the phonological output level of the lexical reading process. Indeed, irregular word reading interferences found in this region stand at the border of the angular gyrus (BA 39) whose specific implication in the lexical route of reading, has been frequently described [13,44], although its lexical and/or semantic specificity is still controversial [14]. These data are congruent with 2 recent meta-analysis on brain activation studies on normal reading and dyslexia [45,46]. In a meta-analysis on functional imaging data of reading, Cattinelli et al. claimed that reading involves a pseudoword-related network in the left inferior parietal cortex and a word-related network in the left temporal lobe [45]. Analyzing 17 neuroimaging studies on dyslexia, Richlan et al. found that these left inferior parietal and superior temporal regions were underactivated in dyslexic readers [46]. Moreover, white matter abnormalities were also detected in developmental dyslexic in these regions [47].

Conclusion

Data from literature suggest that segregation between both reading routes could involve the left lateral superior temporal cortex with the left ventral inferior frontal gyrus for the lexicosemantic route and the postero-superior temporal and anterior inferior parietal cortices for a non-semantic phonological decoding route. As shown in this study, these pathways can overlap in the left posterior Sylvian region but also dissociate. With the previous electrostimulation studies on the same topic [23,24], these findings could be clinically relevant. The cortical and subcortical individual variability seen during surgery is an essential factor and plays a significant role in map reading and tumour resection in each patient. Nevertheless, in the frame of this study, we could not show that individual word and non word testing during surgery were essential for the functional prognosis of patients (i.e. is removing of those specific areas during a tumor resection, lead to significative and permanent language disturbances?). However, we believe that patients with tumors or arteriovenous malformations in this left posterior Sylvian region could be tested with different reading tasks in order to effectively preserve, as much as possible, these functional areas. Finally, we hypothesized that the individual pattern of the organization of reading within the posterior Sylvian fissure and the discrete spatial segregation of these cortical neuronal structures sometimes separated by less than 1 cm could explain the difficulties in reaching a consensus within the numerous brain imaging studies that have been devoted to reading.

Acknowledgments

The authors thank Denise Géblé for her help in supplying them with the references for this article. The authors are also grateful to Catherine Raux for editorial assistance.

Author Contributions

Performed the experiments: FER JBD. Analyzed the data: FER JBD ER JFD. Contributed reagents/materials/analysis tools: MR MJ. Wrote the paper: FER MJ JFD.

References

1. Coltheart M, Patterson K, Marshall JC (1980) Deep dyslexia. London, Eng.: Routledge & K. Paul.
2. Coltheart M, Rastle K, Perry C, Langdon R, Ziegler J (2001) DRC a dual route cascaded model of visual word recognition and reading aloud. Psychol Rev, 108: 204–256.
3. Morton J, Patterson KE (1980) A new attempt at an interpretation, or an attempt at a new interpretation. In: Coltheart M, Patterson KE, Marshall JC, eds. Deep Dyslexia. London: Routledge and Keagan Paul.
4. Beauvois MF, Dérouesné J (1979) Phonological alexia: three dissociations. J Neurol Neurosurg Psychiatry, 42: 1115–1124.
5. Funnell E (1983) Phonological processes in reading: new evidence from acquired dyslexia. Br J Psychol, 74: 159–180.
6. Marshall JC, Newcombe F (1973) Patterns of paralexia: A psycholinguistic approach. Journal of Psycholinguistic Research, 2: 175–199.
7. Patterson K, Hodges JR (1992) Deterioration of word meaning: implications for reading. Neuropsychologia, 30: 1025–1040.
8. Hodges JR, Patterson K (2007) Semantic dementia: a unique clinicopathological syndrome. Lancet Neurol, 6: 1004–1014.
9. Rapcsak SZ, Beeson PM, Henry ML, Leyden A, Kim E et al. (2009) Phonological dyslexia and dysgraphia: cognitive mechanisms and neural substrates. Cortex, 45: 575–579.
10. Feiz JA, Tranel D, Seager-Frerichs D, Damasio H (2006) Specific reading and phonological processing deficits are associated with damage to the left frontal operculum. Cortex, 42: 624–643.
11. Démonet JF, Chollet F, Ramsay S, Cardebat D, Nespoulous JL et al. (1992) The anatomy of phonological and semantic processing in normal subjects. Brain, 115: 1753–1768.
12. Paulesu E, Frith CD, Frackowiak RS (1993) The neural correlates of the verbal component of working memory. Nature, 362: 342–345.
13. Graves WW, Grabowski TJ, Mehta S, Gupta P (2008) The left posterior superior temporal gyrus participates specifically in accessing lexical phonology. J Cogn Neurosci, 20: 1698–1710.
14. Jobard G, Crivello F, Tzourio-Mazoyer N (2003) Evaluation of the dual route theory of reading: a metanalysis of 35 neuroimaging studies. Neuroimage, 20: 693–712.
15. Mechelli A, Gorno-Tempini ML, Price CJ (2003) Neuroimaging studies of word and pseudoword reading: consistencies, inconsistencies, and limitations. J Cogn Neurosci, 15: 260–271.
16. Penfield W, Robert L (1959) Speech and brain mechanisms. Princeton: Princeton University press.
17. Ojemann G (1989) Intraoperative investigations of the neurobiology of reading In: Von Euler, Lundberg, Llinas, eds. Brain mechanisms in cognition and language: Elsevier Science.
18. Roux FE, Lubrano V, Lauwers-Cances V, Giussani C, Demonet JF (2008) Cortical areas involved in Arabic number reading. Neurology, 70: 210–217.
19. Roux FE, Lubrano V, Lauwers-Cances V, Tremoulet M, Mascott CR et al. (2004). Intra-operative mapping of cortical areas involved in reading in mono- and bilingual patients. Brain, 2127: 1796–1810.
20. Roux FE, Lubrano V, Lotterie JA, Giussani C, Pierroux C et al. (2007) When "abegg" is read and ("A, B, E, G, G") is not: a cortical stimulation study of musical score reading. J Neurosurg, 106: 1017–1027.
21. Levy J, Pernet C, Treserras S, Boulanouar K, Berry I et al. (2008) Piecemeal recruitment of left-lateralized brain areas during reading: a spatio-functional account. Neuroimage, 43: 581–591.
22. Levy J, Pernet C, Treserras S, Boulanouar K, Aubry F et al. (2009) Testing for the dual-route cascade reading model in the brain: an fMRI effective connectivity account of an efficient reading style. PLoS One, 4:e6675.
23. Simos PG, Breier JI, Wheless JW, Maggio WW, Fletcher JM et al. (2000) Brain mechanisms for reading: the role of the superior temporal gyrus in word and pseudoword naming. Neuroreport, 11: 2443–2447.
24. Simos PG, Breier JI, Fletcher JM, Foorman BR, Castillo EM et al. (2002) Brain mechanisms for reading words and pseudowords: an integrated approach. Cereb Cortex. 12: 297–305.
25. Nespoulous JL, Joanette Y, Lecours AR (1992) Protocole Montréal-Toulouse d'examen linguistique de l'aphasie (MT86). Isbergues: L'Ortho-Edition.
26. Deloche G, Metz-Lutz M, Kremin H (1997) Test de dénomination orale de 80 images: DO 80. Paris: ECPA.
27. Oldfield RC (1971) The assessment and analysis of handedness: the Edinburgh inventory. Neuropsychologia, 9: 97–113.
28. Binder JR, Medler DA, Desai R, Conant LL, Liebenthal E (2005) Some neurophysiological constraints on models of word naming Neuroimage, 27: 677–693.
29. Haglund MM, Ojemann GA, Blasdel GG (1993) Optical imaging of bipolar cortical stimulation. J Neurosurg, 78: 785–793.
30. McIntyre CC, Richardson AG, Grill WM (2002) Modeling the excitability of mammalian nerve fibers: influence of afterpotentials on the recovery cycle. J Neurophysiol, 87: 995–1006.
31. Nathan SS, Sinha SR, Gordon B, Lesser RP, Thakor NV (1993) Determination of current density distributions generated by electrical stimulation of the human cerebral cortex. Electroencephalogr Clin Neurophysiol, 86: 183–192.
32. Hillis AE, Caramazza A (1995) Converging evidence for the interaction of semantic and sublexical phonological information in accessing lexical representations for spoken output. Cognitive Neuropsychology, 12: 187–227.
33. Nosarti C, Mechelli A, Green DW, Price CJ (2010) The impact of second language learning on semantic and nonsemantic first language reading. Cereb Cortex, 20: 315–327.
34. Woollams AM, Silani G, Okada K, Patterson K, Price CJ (2011) Word or word-like? Dissociating orthographic typicality from lexicality in the left occipito-temporal cortex. J Cogn Neurosci, 23: 992–1002.
35. Graves WW, Desai R, Humphries C, Seidenberg MS, Binder JR (2010) Neural systems for reading aloud: a multiparametric approach. Cereb Cortex, 20:1799–1815.
36. Petersen SE, Fox PT, Snyder AZ, Raichle ME (1990) Activation of extrastriate and frontal cortical areas by visual words and word-like stimuli. Science, 249: 1041–1044.
37. Horwitz B, Rumsey JM, Donohue BC (1998) Functional connectivity of the angular gyrus in normal reading and dyslexia. Proc Natl Acad Sci USA, 95: 8939–8944.
38. Xu B, Grafman J, Gaillard WD, Ishii K, Vega-bermundez F et al. (2001) Conjoint and extended neural networks for the computation of speech codes: the neural basis of selective impairment in reading words and pseudowords. Cerebral Cortex, 11: 267–277.

39. Price CJ (1998) The functional anatomy of word comprehension and production. Trends Cogn Sci, 2: 281–288.
40. Price CJ, Winterburn D, Giraud AL, Moore CJ, Noppeney U (2003) Cortical localisation of the visual and auditory word form areas: a reconsideration of the evidence. Brain Lang 86: 272–286.
41. Wilson TW, Leuthold AC, Moran JE, Pardo PJ, Lewis SM et al. (2007) Reading in a deep orthography: neuromagnetic evidence for dual-mechanisms. Exp Brain Res, 180: 247–262.
42. Mandonnet E, Nouet A, Gatignol P, Capelle L, Duffau H (2007) Does the left inferior longitudinal fasciculus play a role in language? A brain stimulation study. Brain, 130: 623–629.
43. Caspers S, Geyer S, Schleicher A, Mohlberg H, Amunts K et al. (2006) The human inferior parietal cortex: cytoarchitectonic parcellation and interindividual variability. Neuroimage, 33: 430–448.
44. Joubert S, Beauregard M, Walter N, Bourgouin P, Beaudoin G et al. (2004) Neural correlates of lexical and sublexical processes in reading. Brain Lang, 89: 9–20.
45. Cattinelli I, Borghese NA, Gallucci M, Paulesu E Reading the reading brain: A new meta-analysis of functional imaging data on reading. Journal of Neurolinguistics. In press.
46. Richlan F, Kronbichler M, Wimmer H Structural abnormalities in the dyslexic brain: A meta-analysis of voxel-based morphometry studies. Hum Brain Mapp. In press.
47. Peterson RL, Pennington BF (2012) Developmental dyslexia. Lancet. 2012, 379: 1997–2007.

16

Immaturity of the Oculomotor Saccade and Vergence Interaction in Dyslexic Children: Evidence from a Reading and Visual Search Study

Maria Pia Bucci[1]*, Naziha Nassibi[1], Christophe-Loic Gerard[2], Emmanuel Bui-Quoc[3], Magali Seassau[4]

1 Laboratoire de Psychologie et Neuropsychologie Cognitives, FRE 3292 CNRS - Université Paris Descartes, Boulogne Billancourt Cedex, France, **2** Service de Psychopathologie de l'enfant et de l'adolescent, Hôpital Robert Debré, Paris, France, **3** Service d'Ophtalmologie, Hôpital Robert Debré, Paris, France, **4** e(ye)BRAI, Ivry-sur-Seine, France

Abstract

Studies comparing binocular eye movements during reading and visual search in dyslexic children are, at our knowledge, inexistent. In the present study we examined ocular motor characteristics in dyslexic children *versus* two groups of non dyslexic children with chronological/reading age-matched. Binocular eye movements were recorded by an infrared system (mobileEBT®, e(ye)BRAIN) in twelve dyslexic children (mean age 11 years old) and a group of chronological age-matched (N = 9) and reading age-matched (N = 10) non dyslexic children. Two visual tasks were used: text reading and visual search. Independently of the task, the ocular motor behavior in dyslexic children is similar to those reported in reading age-matched non dyslexic children: many and longer fixations as well as poor quality of binocular coordination during and after the saccades. In contrast, chronological age-matched non dyslexic children showed a small number of fixations and short duration of fixations in reading task with respect to visual search task; furthermore their saccades were well yoked in both tasks. The atypical eye movement's patterns observed in dyslexic children suggest a deficiency in the visual attentional processing as well as an immaturity of the ocular motor saccade and vergence systems interaction.

Editor: John E. Mendelson, California Pacific Medicial Center Research Institute, United States of America

Funding: These authors have no support or funding to report.

Competing Interests: The authors have declared that no competing interests exist.

* E-mail: maria-pia.bucci@parisdescartes.fr

Introduction

The term "dyslexia" has its origins in 1887 when an ophthalmologist described reading difficulty; after more than a century of research it is still unclear what dyslexia exactly is [1].

Reading is a higher cognitive process depending on multiple processes: sensorial perception, eye movements, linguistic and semantic capacities. Deficits in one or more of such mechanisms could be at the origin of dyslexia. Despite intensive research on such issues the origin of dyslexia is still debated, and many theories have been proposed [2].

For instance, a large amount of data has shown that eye movements during reading are abnormal in dyslexia and this has been reported in different languages. Pavlidis [3] was the first to show a high number of regressive saccades and unstable fixation in dyslexic population; Rayner [4] reported frequent saccades of smaller amplitude as well as longer duration fixation in dyslexic children; similarly, De Luca et al. [5] observed frequent fixations with longer duration in Italian dyslexic children and Hutzler & Wimmer [6], also showed a high number of fixations and short duration in dyslexic children. Furthermore, in Chinese dyslexic children, Li et al. [7] reported abnormal eye movements in picture searching, slow and more fixations and frequent saccades of small amplitude. Recently, Trauzettel-Klosinski et al. [8] reported in German dyslexic children slower reading speed and high number of saccades and regressions; similar findings have been also reported in Greek dyslexic children by Hatzidaki et al. [9].

Taken together all these findings suggest that the abnormal eye movement performance observed in dyslexic children could be due to poor ability and strategy of visual information processing. Recently Jainta & Kapoula [10] reported in dyslexics poor binocular coordination of saccades during reading as well as in non reading task (while exploring a painting), while other studies on dyslexic children comparing reading and non reading tasks found ocular motor deficits in the reading task only and made the hypothesis of a deficiency of a higher psycholinguistic level of processing [11],[12].

The presence of a poor visual system in dyslexics has been suggested since many years [13] who first reported dysfunction at the level of the magnocellular system in dyslexics. Following this work, many studies confirmed this hypothesis showing in dyslexic children poor binocular coordination during prolonged fixations [14], visual confusion during reading [15] and poor eye alignment during fixation after the saccade [16]. Iles et al. [17] also reported an impairment in visual search performance in a group of dyslexic adults with a motion coherence deficit confirming and extending the magnocellular hypothesis of dyslexia. Despite these results, recent research did not share the hypothesis of poor visual system, and the existence of a deficiency in the magnocellular system in dyslexia is still under debate [18],[19]. Maybe as suggested by

Vidyasagar & Pammer [20] deficit in dyslexia could be localized anywhere along the dorsal stream.

Furthermore, one should also mention that apart from the visual perceptual deficiencies, visual attentional processes are involved in reading and they could be responsible for altered eye movements' performance in dyslexic population. In this line of thinking, Bosse et al. [21] reported that some dyslexic children have a reduced visual attentional window size leading to a limitation in the number of letters which can be processed in parallel. A consequence of such a disorder is that dyslexics will make shorter saccades and frequent fixations with respect to non dyslexic children not only during reading task but also during visual search [22]. A recent fMRI study of this group [23] provided evidence on the role of parietal regions, particularly the left superior parietal area, in the visual attentional span and its deficiency in dyslexics.

In the present study, we wonder to assess the quality of ocular motor coordination in reading and visual search tasks. Studies comparing binocular eye movements during reading and visual search in dyslexic children are, at our knowledge, inexistent.

Ocular motor coordination in dyslexic children will be compared with that observed in a group of non dyslexic children of similar chronological age, and also in a group of non dyslexic children of similar reading age. Indeed, according to our previous studies exploring binocular coordination in normal [24] as well as in children with vergence abnormalities [25],[26] we made the hypothesis that the poor quality of binocular coordination of saccades could be related to immaturity of normal ocular motor learning mechanism responsible of a fine control between the saccades and the vergence command. Such learning mechanisms could grow up with visual experiences during daylife leading to an improvement in binocular coordination during childhood [27]. Our driven hypothesis is that the saccade and vergence interaction in dyslexic children is immature with respect to their chronological age. To test this hypothesis we explored whether ocular motor performance of dyslexic children was more similar to those of a group of younger children (reading age matched) rather than to those of a group of chronological age matched children.

Materials and Methods

Subjects

Twelve dyslexic children participated in the study. Dyslexic children were recruited from the pediatric hospital where they were referred for a complete evaluation of their dyslexia state with an extensive examination including neurological/psychological and phonological capabilities. For each child the time of reading a text, its comprehension, and the capacity of reading word/pseudowords were evaluated by using the L2MA battery [28]. This is the standard test developed by the Centre de Psychologie appliquée de Paris, often used in France and already employed in our previous studies for selecting dyslexic population [26],[29]. Inclusion criteria were: scores of this test beyond 2 standard deviations; a normal mean intelligence quotient (IQ, evaluated with WISC-IV; between 80 and 115). The mean age of the dyslexic children was 11±0.6 years, the mean IQ was 100±7 and the mean reading age was 8.8±1 years. A carefully selected chronological age-matched group (mean age: 11±0.9 years) of 9 non-dyslexic children and reading age-matched group of 10 non-dyslexic children (age: 8.3±0.9 years) were selected. Both groups of non dyslexic children had to satisfy the following criteria: no known neurological or psychiatric abnormalities, no history of reading difficulty, no visual impairment or difficulty with near vision. Also, their reading capabilities were in normal range. Both the similitude test of the WISC IV assessing the verbal capability, and the matrix test of the WISC IV assessing the logic capability were performed. Normal range for both tests is 10±3 (Wechsler intelligence scale for children—fourth edition, 2004). The selected reading age-matched group was normal for verbal (11.78±0.8) and for logic (9.97±0.6) capabilities. The selected age-matched group was also normal (10.36±0.4 for verbal and 11.89±0.5 for logic).

Both non-dyslexic and dyslexic children underwent an ophthalmologic examination of their visual sensorial and motor function (mean values showed in Table 1). All children had normal binocular vision (mean value of 55 s of arc or better), which was evaluated with the TNO random dot test. Visual acuity was normal (≥20/20) for all children, dyslexic as well as non dyslexic. The near point of convergence was normal for all three groups of children tested (mean value of 2 cm). Heterophoria at near distance (i.e. latent deviation of one eye when the other eye is covered, using the cover-uncover test) was normal for all three groups of children tested (≤exophoria of 3.5 prism D). Moreover, an evaluation of vergence fusion capability using prisms and Maddox rod was done at near distance. The divergence and convergence amplitudes were significantly different in the dyslexic group with respect to the other two groups of non dyslexic children. ANOVA showed a significant group effect for the divergence and convergence amplitudes (respectively, $F_{(2,28)} = 4.74$, $p<0.01$ and $F_{(2,28)} = 4.47$, $p<0.02$). The LSD test showed that the dyslexic group had significantly smaller values of divergence with respect to the reading age-matched group ($p<0.005$) while they had significantly smaller values of convergence amplitudes with respect to the two groups of non dyslexic children (younger, $p<0.02$ and older, $p<0.01$).

In summary, orthoptic evaluation showed a tendency of poor divergence and convergence amplitude in dyslexic children.

The investigation adhered to the principles of the Declaration of Helsinki and was approved by our Institutional Human Experimentation Committee (CPP Ile de France I, Hôpital Hotel-Dieu). Written consent was obtained from the children's parents after an explanation of the experimental procedure.

Ocular motor paradigms

Stimuli were presented on a PC screen of 22″, its resolution was 1920×1080 and the refresh rate was 60 Hz. Note that even if it is well known that intermittent illumination could affect saccade accuracy and visual assessment [30], such refresh rate was sufficient to assure a normal saccade performance.

Table 1. Clinical characteristic of the three groups of children examined (dyslexic, D 10–12; non dyslexic children reading age matched, ND 7–9; and non dyslexic children chronological age matched, ND 10–12).

	TNO	NPC	Heterophoria	Divergence	Convergence
D 10–12	55	2	Exo 3.5	10	24
ND 7–9	48	2	Exo 2	16*	38*
ND 10–12	35	2	Exo 2	12	39*

Mean values of: binocular vision (Stereoacuity test, TNO measured in seconds of arc; near point of convergence, NPC measured in cm; Heterophoria at near distance measured in prism diopters; Exo = exophoria; Vergence fusional amplitudes (divergence and convergence) at near distance measured in prism diopters. Asterisks indicate that value is significantly different with respect to the group of dyslexic children (p≤0.01).

The reading and visual search tasks are similar to those used by Prado et al. [22] and are described below.

Reading: A text of four lines taken from a book for children. The paragraph contained 40 words and 174 characters. The text was 29° wide and 6.4° high; mean character width was 0.5° and the text was written in black "courier" font on a white background. Text was different for the two different ages of children examined. Figure 1 A and B shows the text presented to children with reading age of 7–9 years (extract from '*Jojo Lapin fait des farces*', Gnid Bulton, Hachette) and that presented to children with reading age of 10–12 years (extracted from '*Bagarres à l'école*', Marc Cantin et Eric Gasté, Castro Cadet). Children were asked to read the text silently.

Visual search: The same text presented in the reading task was used for such task but vowels were replaced by consonants (see Figure 1 C and D). Children were asked to count the number of 'r' occurring in the text.

In both tasks stimuli were presented without time limitation. The recording of each task stopped when child raised one finger.

Eye movement recordings

Eye movements were recorded with the Mobile Eyebrain Tracker (Mobile EBT®, e(ye)BRAIN, www.eye-brain.com), an eye-tracking device CE marked for medical purpose. The Mobile EBT® benefits from cameras that capture the movements of each eye independently. Recording frequency was set up to 300 Hz. The precision of this system is typically 0.5° and in controlled condition 0.25° (see www.eye-brain.com, for more details). There is no obstruction of the visual field with the recording system.

Procedure

Children were seated in a chair in a dark room, with the head stabilized by a forehead and chin support; viewing was binocular; the viewing distance was 58 cm. Calibration was done at the beginning of eye movements recordings. The best calibration could be an haploscopic arrangement. However, it should be noted that binocular vision was normal for all children tested (see stereoacuity scores in Table 1), suggesting that they were fixating targets with both eyes. A previous study from Bucci et al. [31] comparing normal and strabismic children confirmed that in the absence of strabismus either type of calibration (under monocular or binocular viewing) was valid.

During the calibration procedure, children were asked to fixate a grid of 13 points (diameter 0.5 deg) mapping the screen. Each calibration point required a fixation of 250 ms to be validated. A polynomial function with five parameters was used to fit the calibration data and to determine the visual angles. After the calibration procedure, the reading or visual search tasks were presented to the child. Duration of the each task was kept short (lasting a couple of minutes) allowing an accurate evaluation of eye movement recordings.

Data analysis

Calibration factors for each eye were determined from the eye positions during the calibration procedure. The software MeyeAnalysis (provided with the eye tracker, e(ye)BRAIN, www.eye-brain.com, France) was used to extract saccadic eye movements from the data. It determines automatically the onset and the end of each saccade by using "built-in saccade detection algorithm". All detected saccades were verified by the investigator and corrected/discarded if necessary.

For each saccade recorded in the two tasks (reading and visual search) we examined the amplitude of the conjugate [(left eye+right eye)/2], and the disconjugate components (left eye - right eye) during the saccade. The disconjugacy was measured as the change in vergence between the beginning and the end of each saccade [24], [25], [26]. We also examined the disconjugate component of the post-saccadic drift over the period between two saccades. The duration and the number of those fixations were also evaluated.

Statistical analysis was performed by the three-way ANOVAs using the three groups of children (dyslexics and non-dyslexics, chronological and reading age-matched) as inter-subject factor and the two conditions (reading text and visual search) as within subject factor. The effect of a factor is significant when the p-value is below 0.05.

Results

Eye movement pattern during reading and visual search

Figure 2 shows an example of eye movement patterns from a dyslexic child (11 years old), a non dyslexic child with similar reading age (9 years old) and a non dyslexic child with similar age (11 years old), during the reading task and the visual search task.

Reading task:

A)

Frère ours n'en écouta pas plus. Il s'enfuit chez lui en se
bouchant les oreilles. Là, furieux, il se mit à
réfléchir. Ce soir décida-t-il, j'irai me cacher sous la
fenêtre. Dans le noir, il ne pourra pas me voir.

B)

Hugo sort de chez lui par la porte de derrière. Il traverse
le jardin. Il ressort de l'autre côté, la tête entre les
feuilles. Personne à droite, personne à gauche. Il bondit
hors de sa cachette et remonte la rue.

Visual search task:

C)

Fmcrc cnrs n'cn cccnts pss plns. ll s'cnfnlt chcz lrl cn sc
bcnchsnt lcs crclllcs. Ls, fnrlcnx, ll sc mlt s
mcflrchlm. Cc sclm dcclds-t-ll, j'lrsl mc cschcr scns ls
fcnctrc. Dsns lc nclm, ll nc pcrmms prs mc vmlc.

D)

Hngc scrt dc chcz lnl psr ls pcrtc dc dcmmlcmc. ll tmsvcmsc
lc jsrdln. ll mcsscmt dc l'sntmc cctc, ls tctc cntrc lcs
fcnlllcs. Pcrscnnc s dmcltc, pcrscnnc s gsnchc. ll bcrdlt
hcrs dc ss cschcttc ct mcmcntc ls nrc.

Figure 1. Oculomotor paradigms. Reading (A and B) and visual search (C and D) task respectively used for children with reading age of 7–9 and 10–12 years, respectively.

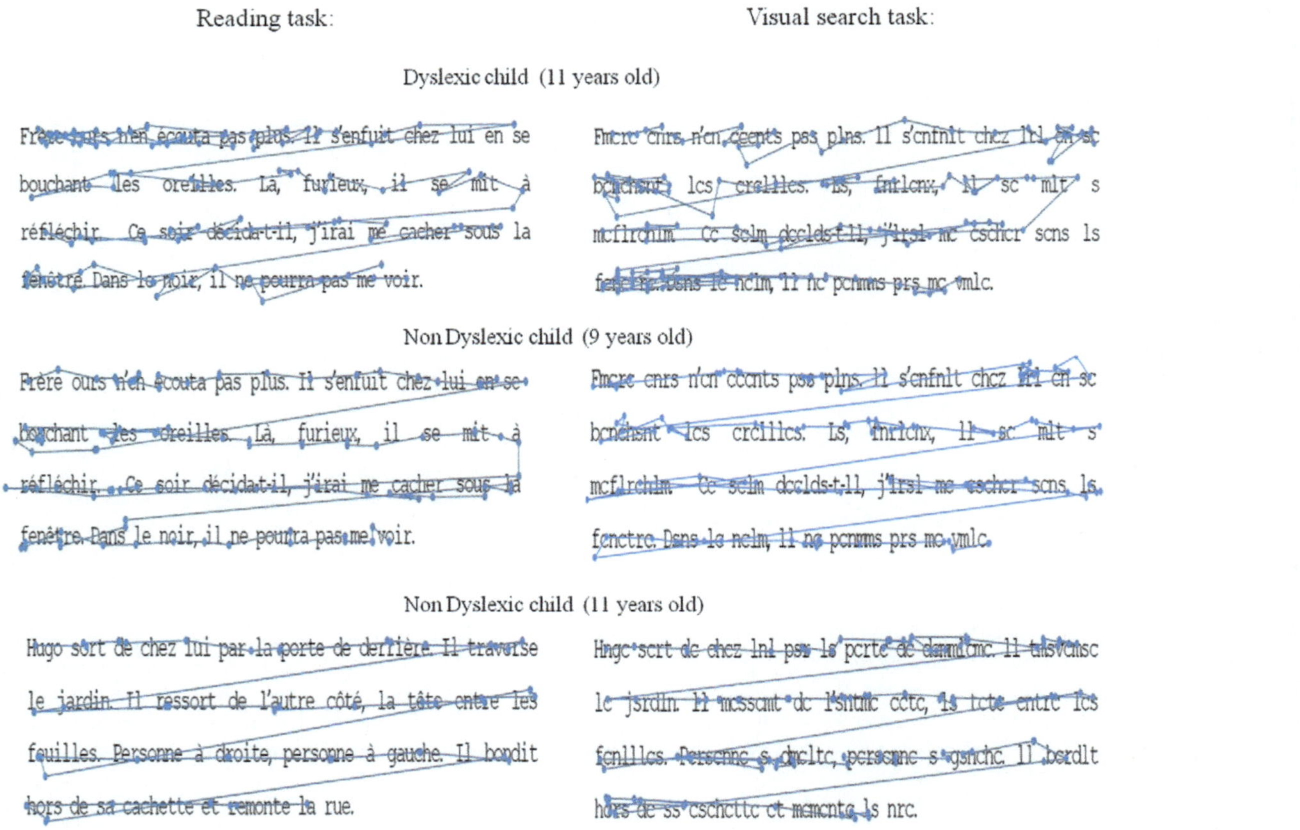

Figure 2. Eye movement pattern during reading and visual search. Number and duration of fixations from dominant right eye the in x- and y-coordinates from a dyslexic child (11 years old) from a non dyslexic child (9 years old) and from a non dyslexic child (11 years old).

The dyslexic child showed many fixations independently of the task (reading or visual search); furthermore, he also made frequent backward saccades. The non dyslexic child of 9 years old showed a pattern similar to that of the dyslexic child: many fixations in both tasks. In contrast, the non dyslexic child with similar age (11 years old) showed few fixations in the reading task, suggesting that reading capabilities are working well at that age; while in the visual search task he made many fixations.

In Table 2 the number of fixations assessed during reading and visual search is shown for the three groups of children examined. The ANOVA showed a significant group effect ($F_{(2,28)} = 16.64$, $p<0.0001$). Post hoc comparison showed that the number of fixations for the older group of non dyslexic children was significant smaller with respect to that of the dyslexic group ($p<0.001$) and of the younger group of non dyslexic children ($p<0.007$).

Table 2. Mean number of fixations (± their standard error) in the reading and visual search task for the three groups of children examined (dyslexic, D 10–12; non dyslexic children reading age matched, ND 7–9; and non dyslexic children chronological age matched, ND 10–12).

	Reading	Visual search
D 10–12	95±9	100±11
ND 7–9	80±6	83±5
ND 10–12	36±3	73±6

We found also a significant effect of the task ($F_{(2,28)} = 13.24$, $p<0.001$), meaning that the number of fixations was larger in the visual search task with respect to the reading task. Finally, a significant interaction between group and task has been also reported ($F_{(2,28)} = 4.05$, $p<0.03$): the older group of non dyslexic children made less fixations during reading than during visual search.

In order to assess more information about fixations, we also measured the average duration of fixations, which is the time period between two saccades (see Figure 3). The ANOVA showed a significant group effect ($F_{(2,28)} = 8.40$, $p<0.001$): the duration of fixation of the older group of non dyslexic children was significantly shorter with respect to the dyslexic group of children ($p<0.0003$) and to the younger group of non dyslexic children ($p<0.01$).

We found a significant interaction between group and task ($F_{(2,28)} = 6.27$, $p<0.005$); more precisely, the older group of non dyslexic children showed shorter duration of fixations in reading task with respect to the visual search task ($p<0.04$). The ANOVA did not show a significant task effect ($F_{(2,28)} = 3.00$, $p<0.94$).

Finally, the performance in the visual search task has been also measured (see Method section) by asking to the child the number of 'r' read in the text. Such performance was similar in dyslexic children and in the other two groups of non dyslexic children (younger and older) suggesting that all children accomplished this

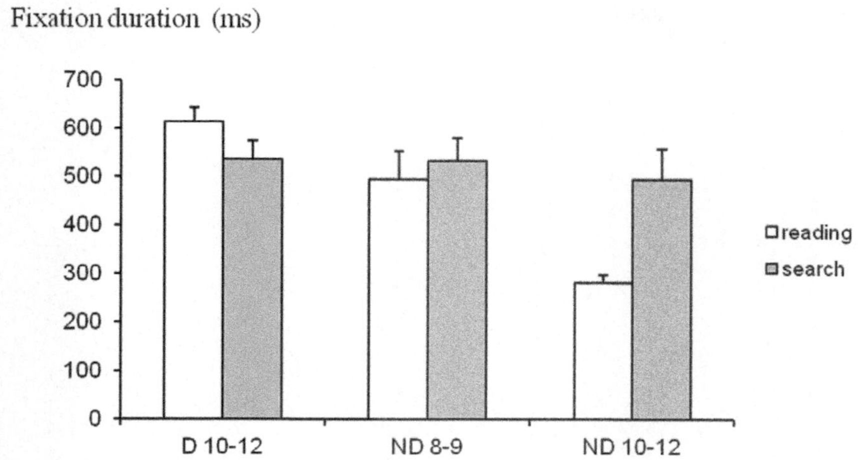

Figure 3. Fixation duration ata. Mean values of fixation duration (in ms) during reading and during visual search for the three groups of children tested. Vertical lines indicate the standard error.

task in a similar way. The mean value of their performance was 8.9±0.2, 8.7±0.4, 9.1±0.4, respectively in the three groups of children examined.

Saccade amplitude

The absolute mean amplitude of saccades during reading and visual search task for each group of children is shown in Figure 4. The ANOVA showed a significant group effect ($F_{(2,28)} = 4.78$, $p < 0.01$) and a significant interaction between groups of children and the tasks ($F_{(2,28)} = 3.53$, $p < 0.04$). Post hoc comparison showed that the amplitude of saccades of the younger group of non dyslexic children was significant smaller with respect to the dyslexic group ($p < 0.01$) and to the older group of non dyslexic children ($p < 0.008$). The amplitude of saccades during reading task for the older group of non dyslexic children was significantly larger with respect to the other groups of children in both reading and visual search tasks ($p < 0.001$). The ANOVA failed to show any significant task effect ($F_{(2,28)} = 1.41$, $p < 0.24$).

Disconjugacy during and after the saccades

Given that saccade disconjugacy depends on the saccade amplitude, the values on dysconjugacy during and after the saccades are presented as the percentage of ratio of the disconjugacy on the saccade amplitude.

In Figure 5 the disconjugacy assessed during (A) and after the saccade (B) is shown. For the disconjugacy values reported during the saccade, the ANOVA showed a significant group effect ($F_{(2,28)} = 19.71$, $p < 0.00001$). Post hoc comparison showed that the saccades disconjugacy of the older group of non dyslexic children was significant smaller with respect to the dyslexic group ($p < 0.0001$) and to the younger group of non dyslexics ($p < 0.0001$). The ANOVA did neither show a significant task effect ($F_{(2,28)} = 0.24$, $p < 0.63$) nor a significant interaction between the groups of children and task ($F_{(2,28)} = 0.38$, $p < 0.69$).

Similar statistical results were reported for the values of the disconjugacy measured after the saccade. The ANOVA showed a significant group effect ($F_{(2,28)} = 10.16$, $p < 0.004$). Post hoc comparison showed that the disconjugacy after the saccades of the older group of non dyslexic children was significant smaller with respect to the dyslexic group ($p < 0.0001$) and to the younger group of non dyslexics ($p < 0.005$). The ANOVA failed to show both a significant task effect ($F_{(2,28)} = 0.86$, $p < 0.36$) and a significant interaction between the groups of children ($F_{(2,28)} = 1.38$, $p < 0.27$).

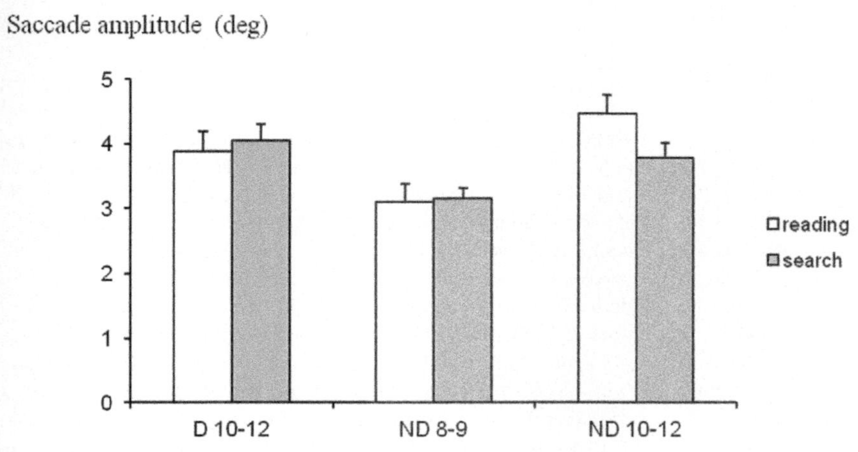

Figure 4. Amplitude of saccades. Mean values of amplitude of saccades (in deg) during reading and during visual search for the three groups of children tested. Vertical lines indicate the standard error.

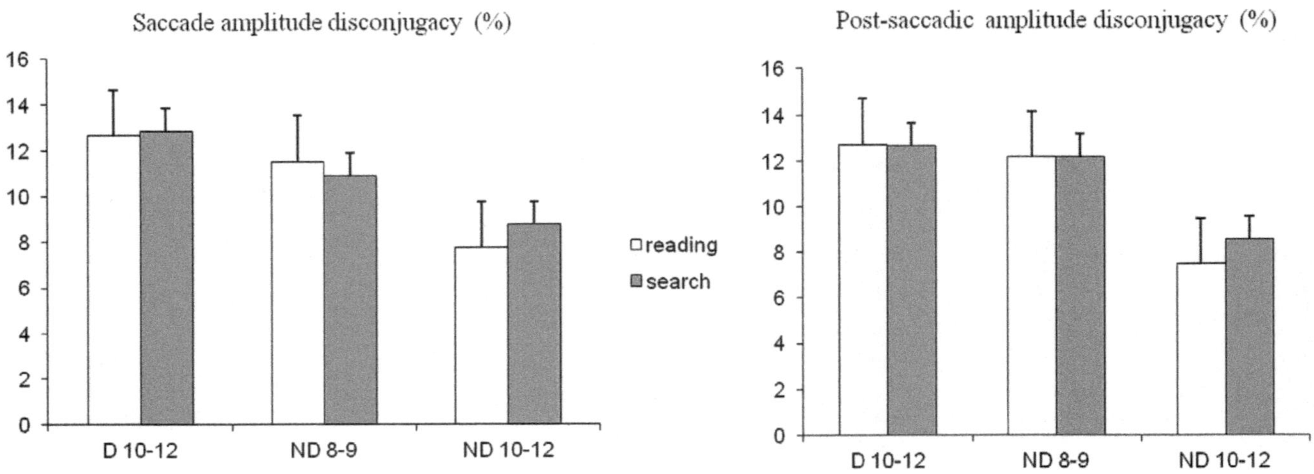

Figure 5. Disconjugacy during and after the saccades. Mean values of disconjugacy (measured as the percentage of ratio of the disconjugacy on the saccade amplitude) during (A) and after (B) the saccades during reading and during visual search for the three groups of children tested. Vertical lines indicate the standard error.

Finally, we have to note that we did not found out any correlation between subjective measures of vergence clinically assessed and ocular motor measures. However a previous work of Bucci et al. [25] showed that binocular coordination of saccades at reading distance in children with limited range of fusional vergence was poor and it was improved significantly after orthoptic training. Such finding suggests a relationship between saccade performance and subjective vergence capabilities (see also [32]) that, however, need to be explored further.

Discussion

At our knowledge, it is the first time that the ocular motor behavior of dyslexic children is compared to that of reading age-matched and chronological age-matched non dyslexic children. This study shows that ocular motor characteristics of dyslexic children are impaired with respect to those reported in non dyslexic children with comparable chronological age. This finding is in agreement with many previous studies on dyslexic children. In contrast, here we reported that fixation's pattern and disconjugacy assessed during and after the saccades in dyslexic children is similar to those observed in reading age-matched non dyslexic children. Finally, another finding of this study is that for dyslexic children and for reading age-matched non dyslexic children the ocular motor behavior is similar in the two tasks, reading a text and visual search. Each of these findings is discussed.

Pattern of fixations

Many fixations and longer duration, during reading and visual search, could be due to an immaturity of visual attentional strategies, leading to reduced visual attentional span, which corresponds to the number of elements that can be processed in parallel according to Bosse et al. [21]. Such a limitation leads to a higher number of fixations and longer fixation duration that, at least for the reading task, suggest that the child will read the text analytically. In normal children, fixation duration, during reading, decreases with age and reaches the adult level at 11 years of age [33]. On the other hand, the brain activity (frontal and parietal cortex) in children during saccade task is low relative to adults and it increases until the adolescence [34]. Furthermore, cortical structures (e.g. left temporal and parietal cortex) involved in linguistic processes are also developing with age [35], [36]. Based on all these findings, the pattern of fixation reported here in dyslexic children, as well as in reading age-matched non dyslexic children, could be related to general cortical development that is not yet completed. This hypothesis is corroborated by the pattern of fixations found in the group of chronological age-matched non dyslexic children, whose reading capabilities are well developed, and the number and the duration of fixations decreased drastically in reading task with respect to the two other groups of children.

Disconjugacy during and after the saccades

The poor quality of binocular coordination in dyslexic children, during and after the saccades, suggests an immaturity of ocular motor learning mechanisms, at central/cortical level responsible of saccade yoking. Fioravanti et al. [37] were the first to show that saccades to LEDs in young children (<9 years old) are poorly coordinated while for older children (>11 years old), disconjugacy was smaller and similar to that observed in adults. Subsequently, Bucci & Kapoula [24] reported that in a simplified reading task (single word reading) the binocular coordination during and after the saccades in a group of 7 years old children was also significantly worse compared to that of adults. These authors suggested that the interaction between the saccade and vergence ocular motor system responsible for the execution of yoked saccades is still immature in 7 years old children. It has also been mentioned that in dyslexic children the clinically assessed limited vergence capabilities (see Table 1) could be responsible for such a deficient interaction between saccadic and vergence movements and thus lead to disconjugate saccades as those reported in the group of younger (reading age-matched) non dyslexic children. We could make the hypothesis that, as reported in children with vergence deficiencies [25] that vergence training could help dyslexic children improve the quality of their saccade coordination. This hypothesis, however, needs further exploration.

Finally with respect to magnocellular theory cited in Introduction this study does not show convincing evidences in favor of this theory; indeed our data are more in line with the hypothesis of an immaturity of learning mechanisms responsible of the fine binocular coordination of saccades. Such mechanisms could involve the magnocellular network and also the cerebellum according to the study of Nicolson et al. [38]. However, according to Iles et al. [17], deficits in the magnocellular network involving the parietal cortex could be related to poor visuo-attentional capabilities already reported in dyslexic children. Further studies by combining neuroimaging techniques and visuo-attentional tasks will be necessary to test the different hypothesis on the origin of dyslexia.

Task effect

For dyslexic children and for reading age-matched non dyslexic children, the two tasks produced similar effects in terms of fixation as well as in terms of binocular coordination. This finding is in line with the study of Prado et al. [22] according to which a reduced visual attentional span could have a similar impact on reading and on visual search, because of the similar visual attentional demand in the two tasks. Most likely, at least for these two groups of children, for who the reading capabilities are not well structured yet, reading and visual search had similar demands in visuo-perceptual, attention and spatial processing.

In contrast, for the group of chronological age-matched non dyslexic children, the results found for the two tasks differ in the number and the duration of the fixations. Indeed, the pattern of fixation is different in the two tasks because they correspond to different cognitive demands in the case of well-reading children. For instance, in visual search task, child is required to identify and count a single target, and has to see all the letters. In contrast, in reading task, because the linguistic processing is well developed, the child can skip letters. Consequently, for these children, reading is an easier task than the visual search.

Finally, it should be pointed out that the two tasks did not show any difference regarding the binocular coordination of saccades. This is in line with previous works from Bucci [24], [26] showing that the quality of binocular coordination during and after the saccades does not depend on the stimulus used (single word reading or fixation of LEDs), and also with the study of Jainta & Kapoula [10] comparing binocular saccade coordination during reading and free exploration of painting. The present study brings new evidence on the fact that reading a text does not interfere with the quality of binocular coordination and contrasts earlier [39] and recent [12] reports suggesting that reading itself induces impairment in the binocular saccade control and fixation instability.

We should also mention that the type of the word and its font may have an influence in the vergence error recording in a reading task as shown by the study of Jainta et al. [40]. Indeed, these authors reported larger vergence error while adult subjects were fixating words with high auto-correlation (see also Wilkins et al. [41]). As suggested by these authors [40] maybe words with low auto-correlation could be easily read by dyslexic population having poor vergence control. This issue, however, need to be tested.

Conclusion and future directions

Deficits in ocular motor behavior reported in dyslexic children seem to be due to the immaturity of their mechanism, responsible for the precise controlled interaction between the saccade and the vergence systems. Although no correlations could be found between oculomotor measures and clinical assessments, poor fusional vergence capabilities in dyslexic children may add to poor binocular coordination; this issue has to be investigated in further studies. Also, even if in the present study we did not measured the spatio-attentional capabilities of children we agree with the studies of Valdois's group [21], [22], [23] suggesting that a reduced visual attention span could be at the origin of the pattern of fixation found out in dyslexic children.

We believe that orthoptic vergence training, together with specific visual attentional training and reading tasks, could be useful tools in dyslexic children to improve visual attentional span, vergence capabilities as well as saccade yoking.

Acknowledgments

The authors thank the medical doctors and nurses of "Service de Psychopathologie de l'enfant et de l'adolescent", Robert Debré Hospital (Paris, France); the directors and the teachers of the Collège Saint André (Saint Maur des Fossés) and of the elementary school Saint François (Paris) for allowing oculomotor tests in non dyslexic children; Camille de Solages for revising the English version of the manuscript; and the parents and children for their kind participation.

Author Contributions

Conceived and designed the experiments: MPB MS. Performed the experiments: MBP NN MS. Analyzed the data: MPB MS. Contributed reagents/materials/analysis tools: Selected dyslexic children: CLG. Did visual examination for children: EBQ. Wrote the paper: MPB NN EBQ CLG MS.

References

1. Angelakis E (2012) What is dyslexia? Insights from electrophysiology. Clinical Neurophysiology 121: 1792–1793.
2. Habib M (2000) The neurological basis of developmental dyslexia. An overview and working hypothesis. Brain 123: 2373–2399.
3. Pavlidis GT (1981) Do eye movements hold the key to dyslexia? Neuropsychologia 19(1): 57–64.
4. Rayner K (1985) Do faulty eye movements cause dyslexia? Developmental Neuropsychology 1: 3–15.
5. De Luca M, Di Pace E, Judica A, Spinelli D, Zoccolotti P (1999) Eye movement patterns in linguistic and non-linguistic tasks in developmental surface dyslexia. Neuropsychologia 37(12): 1407–1420.
6. Hutzler F, Wimmer H (2004) Eye movements of dyslexic children when reading in a regular orthography. Brain and Language 89(1): 235–242.
7. Li XH, Jing J, Zou XB, Huang X, Jin Y, et al. (2009) Picture perception in Chinese dyslexic children: an eye-movement study. Chin Med J (Engl) 122(3): 267–271.
8. Trauzettel-Klosinski S, Koitzsch AM, Dürrwächter U, Sokolov AN, Reinhard J, et al. (2010) Eye movements in German-speaking children with and without dyslexia when reading aloud. Acta Ophthalmol 88(6): 681–691.
9. Hatzidaki A, Gianneli M, Petrakis E, Makaronas N, Aslanides IM (2011) Reading and visual processing in Greek dyslexic children: an eye-movement study. Dyslexia 17(1): 85–104.
10. Jainta S, Kapoula Z (2011) Dyslexic children are confronted with unstable binocular fixation while reading. PLoS One 6(4): e18694.
11. Hutzler F, Kronbichler M, Jacobs AM, Wimmer H (2006) Perhaps correlational but not causal: No effect of dyslexic readers' magnocellular system on their eye movements during reading. Neuropsychologia 44(4): 637–648.
12. Kirkby JA, Blythe HI, Drieghe D, Liversedge SP (2011) Reading Text Increases Binocular Disparity in Dyslexic Children. PLoS ONE 6(11): e27105.
13. Galaburda AM, Sherman GF, Rosen GD, Aboitiz F, Geschwind N (1985) Developmental dyslexia: four consecutive patients with cortical anomalies. Ann Neurol 18(2): 222–233.
14. Stein JF, Fowler MS (1993) Unstable binocular control in dyslexic children. Journal of Research in Reading 16: 30–45.
15. Stein J, Walsh V (1997) To see but not to read; the magnocellular theory of dyslexia. Trends Neurosci 20(4): 147–152.
16. Eden GF, Stein JF, Wood HM, Wood FB (1994) Differences in eye movements and reading problems in dyslexic and non-dyslexic children. Vision Res 34(10): 1345–1358.
17. Iles J, Walsh V, Richardson A (2000) Visual search performance in dyslexia. Dyslexia 6(3): 163–77.
18. Skottun BC (2010) Rats, dyslexia, and the magnocellular system. Cortex 46(6): 799.
19. Dhar M, Been PH, Minderaa RB, Althaus M (2010) Of rats and men: A reply to Skottun. Cortex 46(6): 800–801.
20. Vidyasagar TR, Pammer K (2010) Dyslexia: a deficit in visuo-spatial attention, not in phonological processing. Trends Cogn Sci 14(2): 57–63.
21. Bosse ML, Tainturier MJ, Valdois S (2007) Developmental dyslexia: the visual attention span deficit hypothesis. Cognition 104(2): 198–230.
22. Prado C, Dubois M, Valdois S (2007) the eye movements of dyslexic children during reading and visual search: Impact of the visual attention span. Vision Res(47): 2521–2530.

23. Peyrin C, Démonet JF, N'guyen-Morel MA, Le Bas JF, Valdois S (2010) Superior parietal lobule dysfunction in a homogeneous group of dyslexic children with a visual attention span disorder. Brain Lang 118(3): 128–38.
24. Bucci MP, Kapoula Z (2006) Binocular coordination of saccades in 7 years old children in single word reading and target fixation. Vision Res 46(4): 457–466.
25. Bucci MP, Kapoula Z, Bremond-Gignac D, Wiener-Vacher S (2006) Binocular coordination of saccades in children with vertigo: dependency on the vergence state. Vision Res 46: 3594–3602.
26. Bucci MP, Kapoula Z, Brémond-Gignac D (2008) Poor binocular coordination of saccades in dyslexic children. Graefe's Archive for Clinical and Experimental Ophthalmology 246(3): 417–428.
27. Yang Q, Kapoula Z (2003) Binocular coordination of saccades at far and at near in children and in adults. J Vis 3(8): 554–561.
28. Chevrie-Muller C, Simon AM, Fournier S (1997) Batterie Langage oral écrit. Mémoire. Attention (L2MA) Paris, Editions du Centre de Psychologie appliquée.
29. Bucci MP, Vernet M, Gerard C, Kapoula Z (2009) Normal speed and accuracy of saccades, vergence and combined saccades vergence movements in dyslexic children. Journal of Ophthalmology ID 325214.
30. Kennedy A, Brysbaert M, Murray WS (1998) The Effects of Intermittent Illumination on a Visual Inspection Task. The Quarterly Journal of Experimental Psychology 51A(1): 135–151.
31. Bucci MP, Kapoula Z, Yang Q, Roussat B, Bremond-Gignac D (2002) Binocular coordination of saccades in strabismic children before and after surgery. Investigative Ophthalmology, Visual Science 43(4): 1040–1047.
32. Bucci MP, Kapoula Z, Bui-Quoc E, Bouet A, Wiener-Vacher S (2011) Saccades and vergence performance in a population of children with vertigo and clinically assessed abnormal vergence capabilities. PLoS One 6(8): e23125.
33. Levy-Schoen A, O'Regan J (1979) The control of eye movements in reading. In Processing of visible language HBPA. Kolers, ME. Wrolstand, eds. Plenum Press: NY & London.
34. Luna B, Velanova K, Geier CF (2008) Development of eye-movement control. Brain and Cognition 68: 293–308.
35. Simos PG, Breier JI, Fletcher JM, Foorman BR, Mouzaki A, et al. (2001) Age-related changes in regional brain activation during phonological decoding and printed word recognition. Dev Neuropsychol 19(2): 191–210.
36. Turkeltaub PE, Gareau L, Flowers DL, Zeffiro TA, Eden GF (2003) Development of neural mechanisms for reading. Nat Neurosci 6(7): 658–663.
37. Fioravanti F, Inchingolo P, Pensiero S, Spanio M (1995) Saccadic eye movement conjugation in children. Vision Research 35: 3217–3229.
38. Nicolson RI, Fawcett AJ, Berry EL, Jenkins IH, Dean P, et al. (1999) Association of abnormal cerebellar activation with motor learning difficulties in dyslexic adults. Lancet 353: 1662–1667.
39. Heller D, Radach R (1999) Eye movements in reading. In E. Becker, ed. Current oculomotor research. New York: Plenum Press.
40. Jainta S, Jaschinski W, Wilkins AJ (2010) Periodic letter strokes within a word affect fixation disparity during reading. J of Vision 10(13): 2, 1–11.
41. Wilkins AJ, Smith J, Willison CK, Beare T, Boyd A, et al. (2007) Stripes within words affect reading. Perception 36(12): 1788–1803.

17

Strategy Choice Mediates the Link between Auditory Processing and Spelling

Tru E. Kwong*, Kyle J. Brachman

Department of Psychology, Mount Royal University, Calgary, Alberta, Canada

Abstract

Relations among linguistic auditory processing, nonlinguistic auditory processing, spelling ability, and spelling strategy choice were examined. Sixty-three undergraduate students completed measures of auditory processing (one involving distinguishing similar tones, one involving distinguishing similar phonemes, and one involving selecting appropriate spellings for individual phonemes). Participants also completed a modified version of a standardized spelling test, and a secondary spelling test with retrospective strategy reports. Once testing was completed, participants were divided into phonological versus nonphonological spellers on the basis of the number of words they spelled using phonological strategies only. Results indicated a) moderate to strong positive correlations among the different auditory processing tasks in terms of reaction time, but not accuracy levels, and b) weak to moderate positive correlations between measures of linguistic auditory processing (phoneme distinction and phoneme spelling choice in the presence of foils) and spelling ability for phonological spellers, but not for nonphonological spellers. These results suggest a possible explanation for past contradictory research on auditory processing and spelling, which has been divided in terms of whether or not disabled spellers seemed to have poorer auditory processing than did typically developing spellers, and suggest implications for teaching spelling to children with good versus poor auditory processing abilities.

Editor: Sygal Amitay, MRC Institute of Hearing Research, United Kingdom

Funding: The authors have no support or funding to report.

Competing Interests: The authors have declared that no competing interests exist.

* Email: tkwong@mtroyal.ca

Introduction

Does what people hear affect how they spell? Certainly in an extreme case, such as when one mistakes one word for another (e.g., thinking one has heard the word *train* when the speaker has actually said *chain*), accurate spelling is unlikely. What, however, of less extreme cases? For instance, what should one expect from a person who does not distinguish between two different phonemes (speech sounds) as accurately as does another person? Will this inability to make a phonemic distinction affect an individual's ability to spell words containing those phonemes? Will it affect the individual's ability to spell in general?

Moreover, if linguistic auditory processing *does* affect spelling ability, the question remains as to why. Are such problems specific to language, or does this difficulty have roots in more basic level sounds? If one person is better at discriminating among auditory frequencies than is another, does this discriminative ability provide information about these individuals' respective spelling abilities? The ability to distinguish between two tones may seem quite removed from the ability to perceive and spell phonemes. However, could this basic auditory ability (or disability) be representative of some lower level of processing? In the case where basic auditory processing is compromised, this issue may be considered a possible underlying cause for linguistic auditory processing difficulties and may result in spelling difficulties. The goals of the current research were threefold: to determine whether or not there is a basic link between nonlinguistic and linguistic auditory processing, to look for links between these types of processing and spelling ability, and to determine whether or not spelling strategy choice mediates those links.

Much of the research in this area has been conducted with children learning to spell and with children and adults experiencing reading difficulties. The present study extends these lines of research to examine the role of auditory processing in spelling for nondisabled adults.

Linguistic Auditory Processing

The literature concerning the effects of linguistic auditory processing on spelling is largely clear and consistent, at least with regard to learning to spell in English. Researchers [54] compared speakers of different English dialects and found that differing pronunciations of certain words led to differing spellings among beginning spellers. Research [51] has found that the effect of pronunciation on spelling may persist into adulthood. She compared a group of college students who spoke African American vernacular English (AAVE) to a group of Caucasian students, and found that differences in pronunciation of the final/ d/(often pronounced more as/t/in AAVE) influenced spelling in these adult participants.

The effects of pronunciation on spelling in other contexts have also been examined. For instance, researchers have studied children's spellings of syllabic consonants; that is, cases in which the rime of a syllable is similar or identical to the letter-name of the final consonant [40], [52]. In these studies, it was found that beginning spellers often omitted the preceding vowel in cases like this (e.g., spelling *car* without the *a*), presumably because the presence of the vowel is not clear to them in the pronunciation of the words.

Such research shows that there are conditions that can be present in dialect or in a word's structure that can cause letters to be inserted or omitted in spelling and pronunciation. How common is it, though, for two phonemes to be confused? In cases where the pronunciation of two phonemes differs only in one characteristic, such as voicing (whether or not the vocal cords vibrate during articulation), young children often have difficulty distinguishing between the two [53]. Is it reasonable to assume, then, that these confusions affect their spelling? Other researchers [55] found that children who had difficulty discriminating between confusable phonemes had lower spelling accuracy, not only when attempting to spell words that contained those phonemes, but also for other words.

It has been found that phonological awareness, measured in preschool children, predicted reading and spelling in Grade 1 in Both English and Dutch children [19]. A study with English-speaking Grade 1 children, showed a relationship between phonemic segmentation ability and spelling [16]. It has also been found that early phonological awareness (tested in preschoolers) correlated with spelling skills at school age [33].

When considering research focused on reading, much of it focusing on reading disabilities, we see perhaps an even clearer influence of auditory processing than when looking at spelling. For instance, it has been repeatedly demonstrated different ERP responses to presentation of phonemes for infants who are at familial risk for dyslexia and those who are not [21], [22], [30–32], [39]. This indicates differences in the brain's processing of phonemes before an individual even begins learning to read and write.

A longitudinal study of children with familial risk for dyslexia yielded evidence of a relationship between linguistic auditory processing and literacy skills. The 5-year-olds included in the initial study were more likely to show deficits in speech-in-noise perception if they were from families with risk of dyslexia [6]. The children's phonological awareness was later tested in terms of their ability to parse out the different sounds in words [8]. Their performance on these tasks not only correlated with their literacy skills at that point in time, but predicted literacy skills in Grade 1. In another follow-up with the same participants, the researchers found that impaired phonological awareness in Kindergarten predicted the diagnosis of dyslexia by Grade 3 [7].

Researchers working with English-speaking adults have found deficits on almost all measures of speech perception among reading disabled participants [57]. In one study, children with reading disabilities performed more poorly on phoneme discrimination tasks than did those with no disabilities [10]. In another, children who were poor (but not necessarily diagnosed as disabled) readers, showed deficits in phoneme discrimination as well [15]. It has also been shown that children who are poor readers have more difficulty in phoneme discrimination than do good readers [37]. In fact, one study indicated that reading problems could be predicted with 92% accuracy using a combination of several measures of phonological awareness [20].

Taken together, the presented research suggests a general agreement that baseline linguistic auditory processing is lower in individuals diagnosed with disabilities in reading or spelling. In the case of nonlinguistic auditory processing, however, there is considerably less agreement.

Nonlinguistic Auditory Processing

There is considerably less agreement concerning the effects of nonlinguistic auditory processing on spelling than there is concerning linguistic auditory processing. Researchers' lack of agreement concerning the effects of nonlinguistic auditory processing on spelling ability is not due to a lack of research in the field. Over 30 years ago, Tallal and her colleagues were investigating possible links between nonlinguistic auditory processing and reading and writing skills

Studies finding an effect. Tallal found that primary school children with reading disabilities performed as well as normal readers when the tones were presented relatively slowly, but not when tones were presented rapidly [48]. Working with colleagues, she found that performance on auditory tasks could be used to classify primary school children as having or not having language impairments with near-perfect accuracy [50]. Children who had language impairments almost always performed significantly more poorly on the task than did those who did not.

Since then, researchers have found differences between individuals with and without reading or language impairment in terms of ability to detect frequency changes in a sound [7–8], ERP (event-related potential) responses to tones differing in rise times [25], performance on tasks involving rise time and temporal order of sounds [41], frequency discrimination [24], [27], [36].

In a study with university students, adults with good auditory temporal processing ability (as determined by tasks such as gap detection and determining the order in which two tones have been presented) were better readers and spellers than those with poor auditory temporal processing [3].

Both of the auditory impairments (i.e., discrimination and sequencing) that Tallal and her colleagues reported in children who had reading disabilities and language impairments have been replicated. One group of researchers found that adults with dyslexia were less able to discriminate between tones of differing frequencies; they required larger differences between two tones, on average, in order to detect a difference [34], [46]. Others found that adults with dyslexia had more trouble with pitch discrimination tasks when the interstimulus interval (ISI) was brief [17]. Another group found that 7- to 13-year-old children who had language impairments were less accurate in their recollection of tone sequences than were unimpaired controls [5]. Several other research groups have found similar impairments when, as in [17], the ISI is brief, e.g., [9], [11]. However, a closer look at Stein and McAnally's [34], [46] results reveals that there were some mixed results in terms of which tasks elicited differential performance. Specifically, they did not find significant differences between readers with dyslexia and normal readers in the ability to detect very brief gaps between presentations of a tone, contrary to another of their predictions. Also, as discussed below, other researchers have reported evidence that contradicts their findings.

Studies finding no effect. Attempts have been made to replicate McAnally and Stein's [34] findings [28]. These researchers found that, once outliers were removed, most significant differences between participants with and without dyslexia disappeared; with the exception of a subgroup of participants with dyslexia, all of the differences disappeared. They concluded that any phonological deficit that may exist in dyslexia could not be reasonably connected to a low-level auditory deficit based on current evidence [28]. Some other researchers [10], [37] found no evidence of impaired frequency discrimination or temporal order judgment of non-speech sounds in reading disabled children compared to controls.

Some researchers have found no difference between the gap-detection threshold for groups with spelling disabilities and for control groups [44]. Others have found that children with dyslexia performed significantly worse than did the control group children on speech segmentation, but not on the non-speech tasks [38].

Some of the contradictory results reported regarding the effects of nonlinguistic auditory processing on reading and spelling may be due to different measures of nonlinguistic auditory processing. Nonlinguistic auditory processing has been operationalized in terms of frequency discrimination, temporal order judgment, gap detection, and rise time discrimination, to name just a few. However, there has not been complete agreement of results even when similar measures have been used. Some researchers [28], for instance, were unable to completely replicate McAnally and Stein's [34] results. Their discovery of a subgroup of individuals with dyslexia for which there was a significant correlation, though, does suggest that the conflicting results could be explained, at least partially, by differences in participant groups. Specifically, participants who have less accurate nonlinguistic auditory processing may be compensating for this impairment to different degrees. Another possibility is that different ISI lengths contributed to different results, and that temporal issues (determining order of presentation, or length of gap between tones), rather than simple discrimination (whether or not two tones are of the same frequency) are responsible for some of the results.

Spelling Strategy as a Possible Mediating Variable

One possible reason why, some researchers find a correlation between auditory processing and spelling ability while others do not may be that some individuals with less accurate auditory processing are compensating for processing deficits. One form of compensation is strategy choice. This idea is supported by findings obtained when researchers had children with and without dyslexia (matched for reading level) read information from a computer screen at different speeds and in both a quiet condition and a condition in which auditory masking (that is, white noise presented via headphones) was used [12]. Both auditory masking and reading acceleration can function to shift the reader's focus away from linguistic auditory processing and towards other strategies. These conditions combined served to enhance the reading performance of children with dyslexia only. It seems plausible that these children may have had less accurate nonlinguistic and/ or linguistic auditory processing and thus may have performed better when using strategies other than phonology. For individuals with more accurate auditory processing, phonology may be a more viable choice, so shifting attention away from phonological strategies would thus not be helpful. Given the connection between reading and spelling, it also seems plausible that this phenomenon may generalize to spelling ability. Also, McAnally and Stein [35] found their hypothesized differences between individuals with and without dyslexia in terms of amplitude modulation following response (AMFR; that is, a change in the potential recorded at the scalp following response to a tone stimulus) in only one of three frequency ranges when the two groups of participants were matched for hearing sensitivity. Thus, it is reasonable to ask if something other than auditory acuity is also influencing the difference in their reading and spelling abilities. The possibility exists that it stems from differences in the strategies the participants were using to perform these tasks. Specifically, we might expect to find differences based on whether or not individuals are relying heavily on phonological, or "sounding out" strategies.

The extent to which individuals who choose adaptively among spelling strategies (e.g., avoiding phonological strategies if auditory processing is less accurate) versus those who do not are included in a sample may have considerable implications for the results of that study. Research on strategy choice, e.g., [45] suggests that people are more likely to employ strategies that have been successful in the past, so we may expect that many individuals with less-accurate auditory processing will use strategies that are not based on phonology. However, that is not likely the case for all. If more of the participants in a study who have less-accurate auditory processing are also less-adaptive spellers, any link between auditory processing and spelling is likely to be clear. People who fail to "sound out" words accurately, but continue to try, are likely to show deficits in spelling. If more of the participants in a study who have less-accurate auditory processing are adaptive spellers, they presumably do not "sound out" many words. Thus, they are less likely to show a deficit in spelling, as they have found ways to compensate for this potential source of spelling difficulty. In this case, even if there is a link, or potential link, between auditory processing and spelling accuracy, it would not be evident by testing these participants.

Research Needs

While there is a plethora of literature on the subject of auditory processing and its connection to reading and spelling accuracy, there are several conspicuous holes in the research. Particularly unclear is the relationship between linguistic and nonlinguistic processing. That is, it is unclear whether or not individuals with less accurate nonlinguistic auditory processing are also likely to have less accurate linguistic auditory processing.

Also, nonlinguistic auditory processing, as it relates to literacy skills, has been studied almost exclusively in individuals who have reading and/or language impairments, e.g., [17], [23] [46], [49]. In an exception, one group of researchers found that children with better nonlinguistic auditory processing (as demonstrated in a frequency discrimination task) did show better literacy skills [47]. However, even this study may have been measuring a distinction between participants with and without impairments; the effect related specifically to readers in the lower quartile of their participant group, and they did not exclude participants on the basis of learning disabilities. The literature on linguistic auditory processing has been expanded to include individual differences within typically-developing populations. It has been shown that linguistic auditory processing skills affect spelling even within normal readers and spellers [55]. Light may be shed on the area of nonlinguistic auditory processing if such differences are investigated.

In addition, other variables may mediate the effect of auditory processing on spelling. It is possible that there is a mediating variable, such as spelling strategy use, influencing the link between auditory processing and spelling ability. As described above, an argument can be made for the viability of strategy choice as a means through which a person may circumvent auditory processing difficulties. It is also possible that there are other mediating variables that have not been explored.

We are left with indications that the different types of auditory processing are quite possibly linked to one another, clear indications of links between linguistic auditory processing and spelling, and less clear indications of links between nonlinguistic auditory processing and spelling. There is reason to believe spelling strategy may mediate these links, but little to no direct assessment of this likelihood. There has also been very little research exploring whether or not auditory processing influences individual differences in spelling for typically-developing individuals. Thus, the specific questions addressed in the present study are: a) whether or not the different types of auditory processing even correlate with one another, b) which (if any) of the types of auditory processing correlate with spelling ability in a group of individuals without reading disabilities, and c) whether or not strategy choice mediates any relationship between auditory processing and spelling ability.

Rationale for Measures

Both auditory processing tasks were chosen largely for their simplicity. Although some very important work is being done to determine the exact nature and origin of any auditory processing deficits, at least among individuals with dyslexia, e.g., [1–2], [56], the purpose for the present study is best served by using the simplest measures possible. Our interest in nonlinguistic auditory processing here was in tone discrimination, rather than temporal ability. That is to say that we are interested in this initial exploration in participants' ability to distinguish tones of different frequencies, rather than in their ability to detect small gaps between tones or the temporal order of tones. In many studies of nonlinguistic auditory processing, ISI has not been reported. When it has, e.g., [17], the studies have involved brief ISIs for study of temporal processing. This does not necessarily allow temporal processing effects (e.g., is there a gap between the tones?) to be teased apart from discrimination (are the tones the same or different?). For this reason, our measure (described below) involves two-tone stimuli with a relatively long (0.5sec) ISI. A significant correlation between nonlinguistic auditory processing and spelling ability should clearly indicate an effect that is specific to frequency perception. A lack of correlation may suggest that past findings have been based on temporal processing, rather than problems with frequency perception.

Our test of nonlinguistic auditory processing was based on the tone discrimination task used by McAnally and Stein [34], but unlike that study, we presented all tones to all participants, regardless of performance. McAnally and Stein used the method of limits, starting with larger frequency differences, decreasing the difference when participants answered correctly. However, in an initial pilot trial of this task, we noticed that participants sometimes erred on a judgment for a larger frequency difference, only to perform much better on subsequent trials with smaller differences. Rather than indicating a participant's just noticeable difference, our method indicates a total number of correct response, allowing participants the opportunity to give correct answers on more difficult pairs even if they have given incorrect answers on simpler pairs.

One measure of linguistic auditory processing was phoneme perception, conducted in much the same way as was done by Varnhagen et al. [55]. Participants' scores were based on their percentage of correctly identified phonemes, to mirror the process used for nonlinguistic auditory processing. A second linguistic auditory processing task was a mirror of the "same/different" paradigm used in the nonlinguistic task. Because the phonemes were recorded for natural sound, rather than computer-generated, this task carries the disadvantage of the possibility of factors *other than* linguistic auditory processing (e.g., differences in white noise or tone of voice from one recording to the next) affecting performance. However, this task is arguably easier to compare to the "same/different" frequency discrimination task than is the letter-choice task.

We obtained strategy reports, while participants completed the spelling subtest of the *Wide Range Achievement Test 3 (WRAT 3)* [58], to determine participants' preferred strategies. Past research, e.g., [29], [42], [43] supports the use of self-reports of strategy use. We expected that participants' preferences for phonological or nonphonological strategies would affect the degree to which their nonlinguistic and linguistic auditory processing skills influenced their spelling ability. Assignment to a preferred-strategy category was based on a median split. Previous research [29] demonstrated that most individuals have some clear preference in terms of spelling strategy.

We measured participants' spelling ability using words taken from the vocabulary tests that are included in the *Test of Written Language – 4th Edition (TOWL 4)* [26]. Because the tasks were being completed by a university student population, it was necessary to make the task challenging; many of the vocabulary words from the TOWL 4 were more difficult than were those from the standardized spelling test, and were thus compiled into a test. As participants were all adults with comparable levels of education, unstandardized scores should still yield usable results.

Method

Ethics Statement

Ethics approval was obtained from Mount Royal University's Human Research Ethics Board, application number 2011–38. Written consent was obtained from all participants.

Participants

Participants were 63 undergraduate students (50 female, 13 male) enrolled in introductory psychology courses in an undergraduate university in Alberta, Canada. Participants received course credit for participation. Criteria for participation included requirements that participants have English as their first language and not be diagnosed with any type of disability affecting literacy. An additional five female participants were excluded from analysis because they did not meet the criteria for the study or because they spoke accented English that could have potentially influenced their phoneme perception. Ages were not collected, as none of the tests used were standardized.

Materials

Nonlinguistic auditory processing. Tones for the nonlinguistic auditory processing task were presented via headphones on computer. There were three groups of tones: one in the range of 1000 Hz, one in the range of 1500 Hz, and one in the range of 2000 Hz. For each pair of tones, one tone was exactly 1000, 1500, or 2000 Hz. For two presentations within the set, the tones would match (two ones at 1000 Hz, for example). Within each range, there were two presentations in which the tones differed by 2 Hz, two in which the tones differed by 4 Hz, with the difference increasing by 2 Hz intervals up to a maximum of 20 Hz. At each difference level, one of these tones was lower than the baseline and one was higher (e.g., one set pairing 1000 Hz with 1002 Hz, and one set pairing 1000 Hz with 998 Hz). This resulted in a total of 66 tone pairs presented to each participant (Appendix S1 lists all tone pairs); the task was scored in terms of total number of pairs correctly identified as same or different, and also in terms of median reaction time (RT) for items. The order in which the tone pairs were presented was randomized for each participant. Three practice pairs (either identical or very different) were presented as well, to ensure all participants understood instructions.

Linguistic auditory processing. Phonemes were presented via headphones on computer. For the phoneme discrimination task, participants heard pairs of phonemes. The phonemes were sometimes identical, sometimes similar, and sometimes dissimilar. For similar phonemes, or confusable phonemes, the phonemes always differed in a single feature of articulation. For most of these pairs, one phoneme was voiced and one was unvoiced. There were several pairs for which the difference was between fricative and lateral fricative or between dental and labiodental. For each pair, participants were required to indicate whether they were hearing two different phonemes ('different') or the same phoneme twice ('same'). Each participant heard a total of 43 pairs of phonemes (see Appendix S2 for a complete list of phonemes pairs); 41 of these pairs were heard twice, while 2 pairs that were part of multiple confusable phoneme sets (b/b, which was part of the b-d and b-p pairs; and f/f, which was part of the f-v and f-θ pairs) were heard four times, for a total of 92 trials. The task was scored in terms of total number of pairs correctly identified as either same or different, and also in terms of median RT for responses.

For the phoneme spelling task, participants heard single phonemes. For each, they were asked to choose among three potential spellings: one correct, one spelling for a similar phoneme, and one spelling for a dissimilar phoneme. The confusable phoneme pairs were the same as for the "same/different" task. There were 20 sets of phonemes and spellings (see Appendix S3 for a complete list of phonemes and response options); each was presented twice, for a total of 40 trials. The task was scored in terms of total number of correct responses, and also in terms of median RT for responses.

Practice items, presented to ensure that all participants understood instructions, consisted of pairs of words or sounds that either matched or were dissimilar.

Strategy choice. Words selected from the WRAT 3 [58] were used to obtain strategy reports. Fifteen words, selected to represent words whose spellings probably were and probably were not in participants' long-term memories (i.e., words that are quite common or very uncommon), were read aloud by one of the researchers. Strategy reports were ultimately scored as being phonological (based entirely or mostly on "sounding out" the word) or nonphonological (based mostly on strategies that do not involve "sounding out" the word, such as using orthographic conventions).

Spelling ability. Thirty-three words and sample sentences taken from the vocabulary tests of the *TOWL-4* [26] were read aloud to participants for the test of spelling ability. Only raw scores were used for this test.

Procedure

Participants completed all tasks in individual sessions that took approximately 35 minutes. No feedback was provided on any task except for the practice trials that were presented at the beginning of each auditory processing task. Participants began with the nonlinguistic auditory processing task. They wore headphones to ensure standardized noise and volume conditions. Tones pairs were randomized throughout. Participants were to determine, for each pair, whether or not the tones matched; they responded to each tone pair by clicking either "same" or "different" on the computer screen.

Following completion of the nonlinguistic auditory processing task, participants began the phoneme discrimination task. Again, they wore headphones to ensure standardized presentation. Phoneme pairs were presented in random order. Participants again responded to each pair by clicking either "same" or "different" on the computer screen.

Third, participants completed the phoneme spelling task. Phonemes were presented in random order. For each phoneme, participants saw three spelling choices, also presented in random order. Participants used the mouse to select the spelling that they thought represents the presented phoneme.

The fourth task was the strategy choice task. One of the researchers read participants a word, a sentence containing the word, and the word again. Participants wrote the word using pencil and paper. After spelling each word, participants were asked to describe their strategies (e.g., "How did you decide how that word should be spelled?"). Non-leading probing was used for participants who did not give full explanations of spelling (e.g., "Is there anything else?", "That explains how you spelled the beginning of the word. Can you tell me how you figured out how to spell the end?").

The spelling ability tasks were presented last. For each word, the experimenter read a word, a sentence containing the word, and then the word again. Participants were given time to complete each spelling before moving on to the next word.

Statistical Analyses

Data were analyzed in two ways: using correlations and a regression analysis. Pearson's correlations were conducted to investigate relationships among the three measures of auditory processing, and to investigate the relationship between each measure of auditory processing and spelling ability for each strategy grouping. A regression was used to investigate the potential influence of each auditory processing measure and of strategy choice on spelling ability.

Results

Strategy Scoring

Strategy reports, collected orally and retrospectively for each individual word, were assigned to one of several categories (see Table 1). Although responses were categorized by specific strategy or combination of strategies, the only categorization that is meaningful for our purposes is whether or not participants used *phonology*, sounding out a word. Strategy reports for any given word were designated as follows: "phonology", "half phonology" (if a participant sounded out part of a word, but spelled part using another strategy), or "not phonology". Inter-rater reliability was checked by having 10% of the strategy reports scored independently by both raters. Raters agreed fully on 96% of the reports, partially agreed (e.g., agreeing on one strategy a participant described for a particular word, but disagreeing on another) on 2.8% of the others. Agreement was 100% for the extent to which any given word was spelled phonologically. For the purposes of further testing, a median split was used to divide participants into phonological (6 or more of 15 words spelled using phonology only) versus nonphonological (5 or fewer) spellers.

Descriptive Statistics

Scores on auditory processing measures are given in terms of number of correct responses. For nonlinguistic auditory processing, the maximum possible score was 66. For the phoneme discrimination task, the maximum possible score was 92. For the phoneme spelling task, the maximum possible score was 40. Reaction times were also recorded, and are presented as average time (in seconds) per item. There were four cases in which one of the tasks failed to record results (one nonlinguistic auditory processing, one phoneme discrimination, and two phoneme spelling); the participants in these cases were dropped from analyses including these tasks, but still included in the remainder of analyses. Spelling scores are also given in terms of total number correct, with a maximum possible score of 33. Table 1 shows the means and standard deviations for accuracy on the auditory processing tasks and the spelling ability task. Table 2 shows means and standard deviations for reaction times on the auditory processing tasks. Nonphonological spellers performed significantly better on the spelling test than did phonological spellers ($t(61) = 2.33$, $p = .023$), and slightly but significantly better on the phoneme spelling task ($t(39) = 2.20$, $p = .034$), but the two groups were otherwise comparable. Both groups showed ceiling effects for

Table 1. Means and Standard Deviations for Accuracy in Auditory Processing and Spelling Tasks.

	Phonological Spellers		Nonphonological Spellers		Combined	
	M	*SD*	*M*	*SD*	*M*	*SD*
Nonlinguistic	29.00	13.02	29.06	11.02	29.03	11.96
Phon. Discrimination	86.53	7.44	86.34	11.29	86.44	9.55
Phoneme Spelling	39.4	0.93	39.81	0.40	39.61	0.74
Spelling Ability	24.77	4.57	27.09	3.23	25.95	4.09

both linguistic auditory processing tasks (phoneme discrimination and phoneme spelling). These tasks are thus analyzed in terms of Reaction Time (RT) rather than accuracy.

Linguistic Versus Nonlinguistic Auditory Processing

None of the auditory processing tasks correlated with one another when analyzed in terms of accuracy. When analyzed in terms of (RT), all were moderately to strongly correlated. Nonlinguistic auditory processing was significantly correlated with both the phoneme discrimination measure ($r(59) = .60, p< .001$) and the phoneme spelling measure ($r(58) = .45, p< .001$). The two linguistic auditory processing measures correlated significantly with one another, $r(59) = .52$, $p< .001$. In short, all of the measures of auditory processing correlated with one another in terms of speed of processing, but not in terms of accuracy of responses (see Figures 1–3 for scatterplots of reaction times). No corrections were used for multiple tests.

Linguistic Auditory Processing and Spelling

Correlational analyses were conducted both for the group as a whole, and for phonological and nonphonological spellers separately. We did not find any significant correlations when assessing accuracy of responses, but found more interesting results when considering RT. Looking at the group as a whole, RT for the phoneme discrimination task did not correlate significantly with spelling ability, $r(60) = .098$, $p = .447$. RT for the phoneme spelling task did not correlate significantly with spelling, $r(59) = -.187$, $p = .149$.

When we divided the participants by spelling strategy, a slightly different picture emerged. RTs for the phoneme discrimination task did not correlate significantly with spelling ability for nonphonological spellers ($r(30) = -.06$, $p = .728$) or for phonological spellers ($r(28) = .184$, $p = .330$). RTs for the phoneme spelling task did not correlate significantly with spelling ability for nonphonological spellers, $r(29) = .009$, $p = .960$ (see Figure 4). However, the correlation between the phoneme spelling task spelling ability for phonological spellers was significant, $r(28) = -.353$, $p = .028$ (1-tailed) (See Figure 4). So, among phonological spellers only, there was a slight tendency for those who were quicker in the phoneme spelling task to be better spellers. No corrections were used for multiple tests.

A regression analysis was conducted to shed more light on these correlations. As predicted, the nonphonological spellers did not demonstrate a relationship between auditory processing and spelling ($F(6,23) = .378$, $p = .885$). Phonological spellers showed several notable trends in our analysis. The RT for both the phoneme discrimination and for the phoneme spelling approached significance ($b = .586$, $t(30) = 1.720$, $p = .100$ and $b = -.446$, $t(30) = -1.987$, $p = .060$, respectively). Thirty-seven percent of the variability in spelling ability was accounted for by the auditory processing factors combined ($R^2 = .372$).

Nonlinguistic Auditory Processing and Spelling

For the group as a whole, accuracy on the nonlinguistic auditory processing task did not significantly correlate with spelling, $r(60) = .165$, $p = .200$.

Accuracy on the nonlinguistic auditory processing task did not correlate significantly with spelling for nonphonological spellers, $r(29) = -.179$, $p = .335$ (See Figure 5). Accuracy on the nonlinguistic auditory processing task did, however, correlate significantly with spelling for phonological spellers, $r(29) = .385$, $p = .032$ (See Figure 5). Among phonological spellers only, there was a tendency for those who performed better on the nonlinguistic auditory processing task to be better spellers. No corrections were used for multiple tests.

Discussion

The present study combines areas of research linking linguistic auditory processing to spelling, e.g., [33], conflicting research investigating links between nonlinguistic auditory processing to spelling (e.g., [34] v. [28]), and studies suggesting that strategy choice may impact these links, e.g., [12]. The current effort represents the first study in which both auditory processing and strategy choice are considered, and performance on both is compared. This unique approach adds to the literature and serves

Table 2. Means and Standard Deviations for Reaction Time (in seconds) in Auditory Processing Tasks.

	Phonological Spellers		Nonphonological Spellers		Combined	
	M	*SD*	*M*	*SD*	*M*	*SD*
Nonlinguistic	4.43	0.66	4.75	1.09	4.58	0.91
Phon. Discrimination	4.71	0.66	4.79	0.58	4.75	0.62
Phoneme Spelling	3.10	0.39	3.08	0.42	3.09	0.40

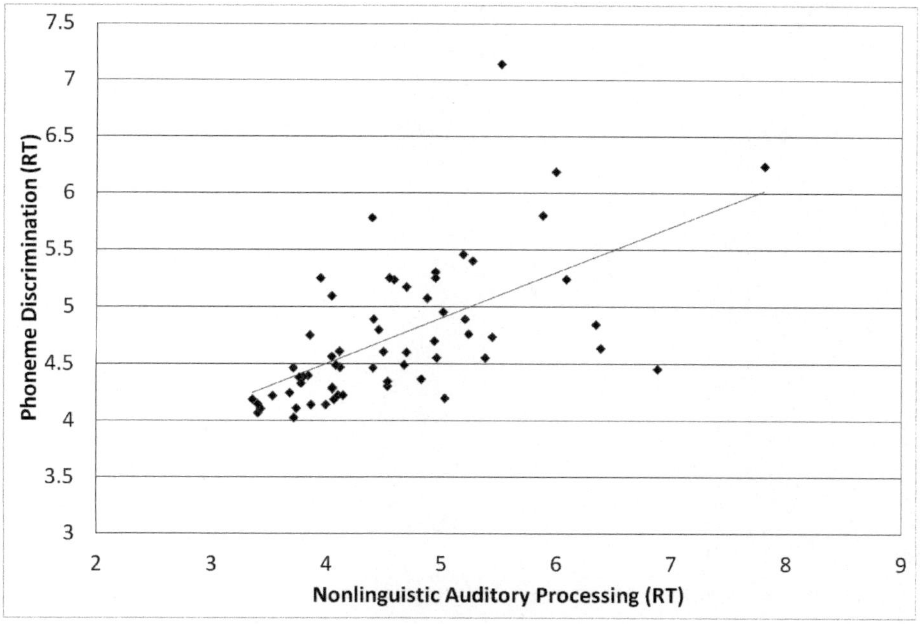

Figure 1. Correlations between RTs on nonlinguistic auditory processing and phoneme discrimination, $r(59) = .60$, $p < .001$.

as a foundation for research in these areas in the future. Based on the analyses, in sum, the answers to our research questions are: a) the different types of auditory processing appear to be somewhat related to one another, b) both linguistic and nonlinguistic processing appear related to spelling, and c) the relationship between auditory processing and spelling appears to hold for individuals who rely heavily on phonological strategies but not for those who do not.

Linguistic Versus Nonlinguistic Auditory Processing

Although the results from this study do not provide definitive proof that nonlinguistic auditory processing underlies linguistic auditory process, the results of this study do indicate a possible relationship between linguistic and nonlinguistic auditory processing. This finding provides potential support for the idea of lower-level auditory skills being at the root of the phonological processing problems often reported in those with low literacy skills. It may not be possible to tease linguistic and nonlinguistic auditory processing apart to a sufficient extent to determine that one is the cause of the other. However, at the very least, this result suggests that linguistic and nonlinguistic auditory processing are connected, and that both are important for spelling. These findings could have implications for screening for future spelling ability and also for identifying different developmental ability and disabilities. That is, if there is a sufficiently strong overlap between linguistic and nonlinguistic

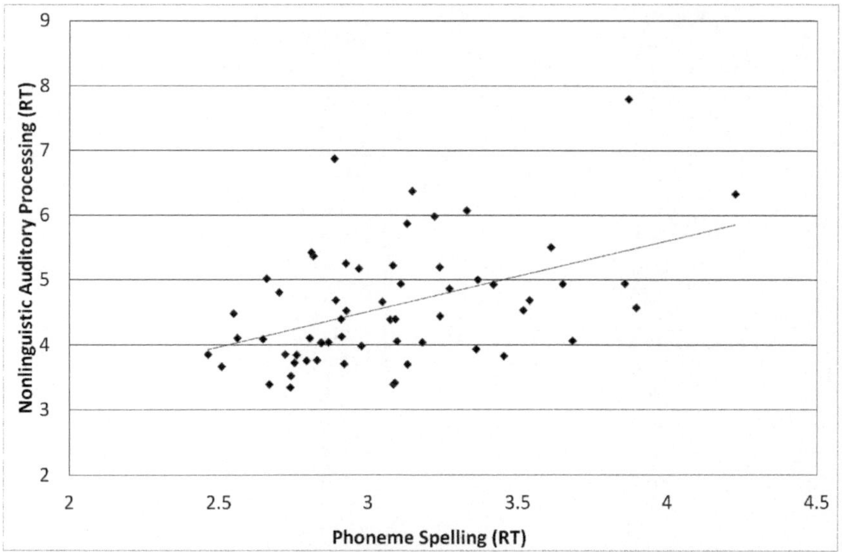

Figure 2. Correlation between RTs on nonlinguistic auditory processing and phoneme spelling, $r(58) = .45$, $p < .001$.

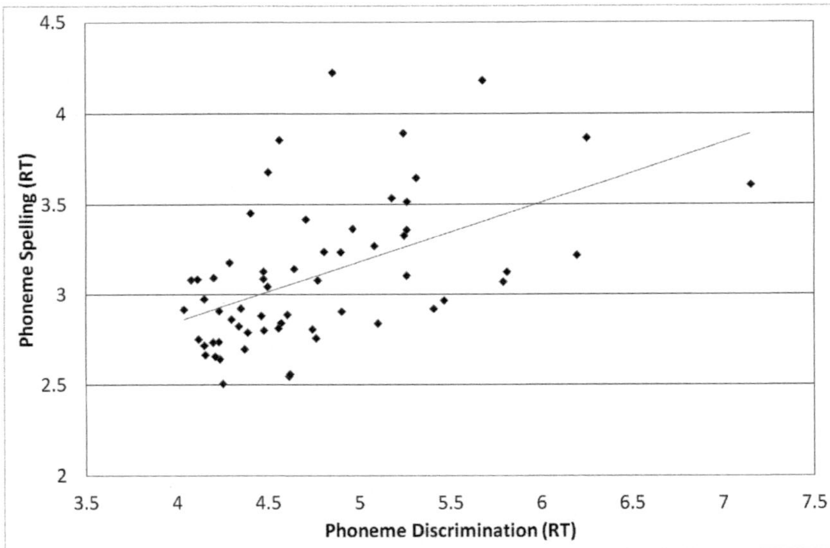

Figure 3. Correlation between phoneme discrimination and phoneme spelling, $r(59) = .52$, $p < .001$.

auditory processing, it may not be necessary to test both when screening.

We found correlations for RTs only, rather than for accuracy scores; this result could have at least two potential explanations. One possibility is that there may have been ceiling and floor effects (scores were, in general, quite high on the linguistic tasks and fairly low on the nonlinguistic tasks), thus making RT the only indicator with enough variability to show results. Another possibility is that individual differences in participants' general speed of processing may have contributed significantly to this result. Thus, this particular result should be regarded with caution.

Linguistic Auditory Processing and Spelling

Analyses yielded a moderate correlation between linguistic auditory processing and spelling for phonological spellers. On the phoneme spelling task, this correlation was for RT only. While the lack of a significant correlation for accuracy on the phoneme spelling task may have been due to the ceiling effects seen on this test, the significant correlation with RT on this same task is still informative. This finding suggests that rapid linguistic auditory processing is important for efficient use of phonological strategies, even for adults who are experienced spellers. It is therefore possible that more challenging linguistic auditory processing tasks would produce different results. In accordance with the correlational findings, our regression model also indicated that a marked proportion of the variance in spelling ability among phonological spellers was accounted for by auditory processing.

While significant in terms of the correlations, and approaching significance in terms of the regression analysis, note that the relationship between linguistic auditory processing and spelling is not as strong as those reported in past studies, for instance [7–8]. Of note, these studies focused on differences between participants with and without reading disabilities, and although further research would be necessary to draw any definitive conclusions, a probable explanation is that auditory processing plays a smaller role in influencing individual differences within a nondisabled population than it does in the differences between groups that do or do not have reading disabilities.

Nonlinguistic Auditory Processing and Spelling

A significant correlation between frequency discrimination and spelling ability for phonological spellers was identified. This

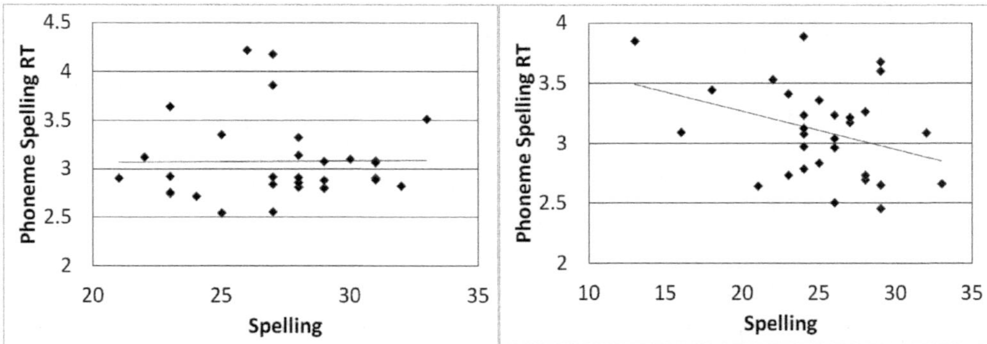

Figure 4. Correlation between phoneme spelling RT and spelling ability among nonphonological spellers, $r(29) = .009$, $p = .960$ (left), compared with correlation between phoneme spelling RT and spelling ability among phonological spellers, $r(28) = -.353$, $p = .056$ two-tailed and .028 one-tailed (right).

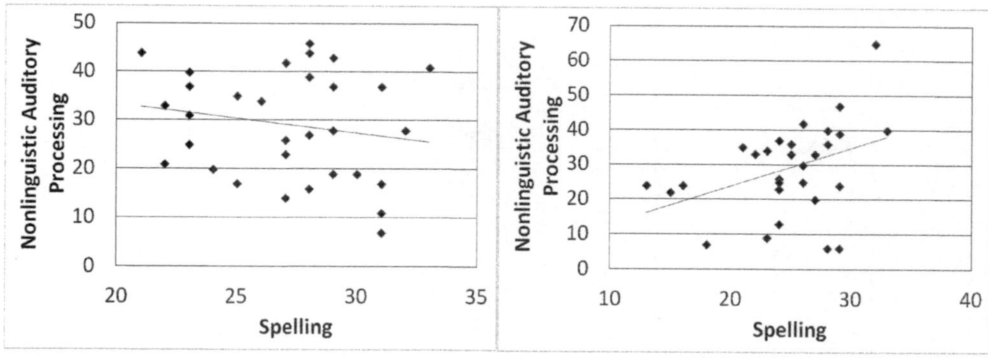

Figure 5. Correlation between nonlinguistic auditory processing accuracy and spelling ability among nonphonological spellers, $r(29) = -.179$, $p = .335$ (left), compared with correlation between nonlinguistic auditory processing accuracy and spelling ability among phonological spellers, $r(29) = .385$, $p = .032$ (right).

finding suggests that some of the conflicts in pre-existing literature may have their roots in different strategy choices among participants. Some researchers, e.g., [36] have reported auditory processing deficits in only sub-groups of individuals with literacy impairments; this research may reflect sub-groups in terms of strategy choice.

Use of Phonology

The significant negative correlation between use of phonology and spelling ability was not surprising. Heavy reliance on phonological strategies into adulthood has been associated with poor spelling and poor reading, e.g., [4], [13–14], [18]. Ideally, spelling ability would be controlled for between groups of phonological and nonphonological spellers; however, among adults, phonological spellers are usually less-accurate spellers. Note that this is not a result we would necessarily expect to replicate among younger spellers.

Conclusions

The main finding of this study is that there appears to be a link between both linguistic and nonlinguistic auditory processing and spelling ability. This link is not as strong as has been reported by researchers who have compared people with disabilities to those whose reading and spelling is typically developing, but it is nevertheless significant in nondisabled spellers. The correlation between auditory processing and spelling ability existed only in the phonological spelling group. Thus, strategy choice appears to be a significant mediating variable, worthy of further investigation. Related to this is the implication that a spelling strategy that is adaptive for one person may not be adaptive for another. Phonological strategies are clearly less adaptive here for individuals with less accurate auditory processing than for those with more accurate auditory processing.

Future Directions

Research to date has focused on improving reading and/or spelling in individuals who are experiencing difficulty. It may be possible, however, to identify individuals before they begin to experience problems. For this reason, replication of this study with children is currently underway. A study is also currently being devised with the intention of following children longitudinally in order to assess spelling achievement in children who have been screened using these auditory processing tasks. The goal would be to determine the usefulness of these auditory processing tasks as screening tools as well as to identify meaningful cutoffs for assessment.

Remediation is another avenue for consideration. If auditory processing is related to spelling for phonological spellers only, it is possible that changing strategies would be useful for people experiencing difficulty with auditory processing. Should individuals who have difficulties with auditory processing be provided with remedial phonics instruction, as they often are? Or should these same individuals receive instruction in alternate spelling strategies? Would individuals benefit from both types of instruction? An in-depth longitudinal study comparing methods of remediation is needed to address and improve methods for helping individuals who are experiencing difficulties with spelling.

Supporting Information

Appendix S1 Tone pairs used in nonlinguistic auditory processing task.

Appendix S2 Phoneme pairs used in phoneme matching task.

Appendix S3 Phonemes and spelling choices used in phoneme spelling task.

Acknowledgments

The authors wish to thank Connie Varnhagen for her assistance with the design of this research, Jason Daniels and Nathan Johnson for their technical support, Megan Duffy for her assistance in collecting data, and Nancy Ogden for her assistance in editing this paper.

Author Contributions

Conceived and designed the experiments: TEK. Performed the experiments: TEK. Analyzed the data: TEK KJB. Contributed reagents/materials/analysis tools: TEK KJB. Contributed to the writing of the manuscript: TEK KJB.

References

1. Amitay S, Ahissar M, Nelken I (2002) Auditory processing deficits in reading disabled adults. Journal of the Association for Research in Otolaryngology 3: 302–320. doi: 10.1007/s101620010093.
2. Amitay S, Ben-Yehudah G, Banai K, Ahissar M (2002) Disabled readers suffer from visual and auditory impairments but not from a specific magnocellular deficit. Brain 125: 2272–2285.
3. Au A, Lovegrove B (2008) The reading ability of good and poor temporal processors among a group of college students. Perception and Psychophysics 70(4): 697–706. doi: 10.3758/PP.70.4.697.
4. Barron RW (1980) Visual and phonological strategies in reading and spelling. In: Frith U, editor. Cognitive processes in spelling. London: Academic Press. pp.195–214
5. Bishop DVM, Bishop SJ, Bright P, James C, Delaney T, et al. (1999) Different origin of auditory and phonological processing problems in children with language impairment: Evidence from a twin study. Journal of Speech, Language & Hearing Research 42: 155–168.
6. Boets B, Ghesquière P, van Wieringen A, Wouters J (2007) Speech perception in preschoolers at family risk for dyslexia: Relations with low-level auditory processing and phonological ability. Brain and Language 101: 19–30. doi: 10.1016/j.bandl.2006.06.009.
7. Boets B, Vandermosten M, Poelmans H, Luts H, Wouters J, et al. (2011) Preschool impairments in auditory processing and speech perception uniquely predict future reading problems. Research in Developmental Disabilities 32: 560–570. doi: 10.1016/j.ridd.2010.12.020.
8. Boets B, Wouters J, van Wieringen A, De Smedt B, Ghesquière P (2008) Modelling relations between sensory processing, speech perception, orthographic and phonological ability, and literacy achievement. Brain and Language 106: 29–40. doi: 10.1016/j.bandl.2007.12.004.
9. Booth JR, Perfetti CA, MacWhinney B, Hunt SB (2000) The association of rapid temporal perception with orthographic and phonological processing in children and adults with reading impairment. Scientific Studies of Reading 4: 101–132.
10. Breier JI, Gray LC, Fletcher JM, Foorman B, Klaas P (2002) Perception of speech and non-speech stimuli by children with and without reading disability and attention deficit hyperactivity disorder. Journal of Experimental Child Psychology 82: 226–250.
11. Bretherton L, Holmes VM (2003) The relationship between auditory temporal processing, phonemic awareness, and reading disability. Journal of Experimental Child Psychology 84: 218–243.
12. Breznitz Z (1997) Enhancing the reading of dyslexic children by reading acceleration and auditory masking. Journal of Educational Psychology 89: 103–113.
13. Bruck M, Waters G (1988) An analysis of the spelling errors of children who differ in their reading and spelling skills. Applied Psycholinguistics 9: 77–92.
14. Bruck M, Waters G (1990) Effects of reading skill on component spelling skills. Applied Psycholinguistics 11: 425–437.
15. Chiappe P, Chiappe DL, Siegel LS (2001) Speech perception, lexicality, and reading skill. (2001). Journal of Experimental Child Psychology 80: 58–74. doi: 10.1006/jecp.2000.2624.
16. Foorman BR, Liberman D (1989) Visual and phonological processing of words: A comparison of good and poor readers. Journal of Learning Disabilities 22(6): 349–355.
17. France SJ, Rosner BS, Hansen PS, Calvin C, Talcott JB, et al. (2002) Auditory frequency discrimination in adult developmental dyslexics. Perception and Psychophysics 64: 169–179.
18. Frith U (1980) Unexpected spelling problems. In: Frith U, editor. Cognitive processes in spelling. London: Academic Press. pp.495–515.
19. Furnes B, Samuelsson S (2009) Preschool cognitive and language skills predicting Kindergarten and Grade 1 reading and spelling: A cross-linguistic comparison. Journal of Research in Reading 32(3): 275–292. doi: 10.1111/j.1467-9817.2009.01393.x.
20. Gilbertson M, Bramlett RK (1998) Phonological awareness screening to identify at-risk readers: Implications for practitioners. Language, Speech, and Hearing Services in Schools 29: 109–116.
21. Guttorm TK, Leppänen PHT, Richardson U, Lyytinen H (2001) Event-related potentials and consonant differentiation in newborns with familial risk for dyslexia. Journal of Learning Disabilities 34(6): 534–544.
22. Guttorm TK, Leppänen PHT Tolvanen AM, Lyytinen H (2003) Event-related potentials in newborns with and without familial risk for dyslexia: Principal component analysis reveals differences between groups. Journal of Neural Transmission 110: 1059–1074. doi: 10.1007/s00702-003-0014-x.
23. Habib M, Rey V, Daffaure V, Camps R, Espesser R, et al. (2002) Phonological training in children with dyslexia using temporally modified speech: A three-step pilot investigation. International Journal of Language and Communication Disorders 37: 289–308.
24. Halliday LF, Bishop DVM (2006) Auditory frequency discrimination in children with dyslexia. Journal of Research in Reading 29(2): 213–228. doi: 10.1111/j.1467-9817.2006.00286.x.
25. Hämäläinen JA, Fosker T, Szücs D, Goswami U (2011) N1, P2, and T-complex of the auditory brain-event related potentials to tones with varying rise times in adults with and without dyslexia. International Journal of Psychophysiology 81: 51–59. doi: 10.1016/j.ijpsyco.2011.04.005.
26. Hammil DD, Larsen SC (2009) Test of Written Language (4th Edition). Austin, Texas: Pro-Ed.
27. Heath SM, Bishop DVM, Hogben JH, Roach NW (2006) Psychophysical indices of perceptual functioning in dyslexia: A psychometric analysis. Cognitive Neuropsychology 23(6): 905–929. doi: 10.1080/02643290500538398.
28. Hill NI, Bailey PJ, Griffiths YM, Snowling MJ (1999) Frequency acuity and binaural masking release in dyslexic listeners. Journal of the Acoustical Society of America 106: 153–158.
29. Kwong TE, Varnhagen CK (2005) Strategy development and learning to spell new words: Generalization of a process. Developmental Psychology 41: 148–159.
30. Leppänen PHT, Hämäläinen JA, Salminen HK, Eklund KM, Guttorm TK, et al. (2010) Newborn brain event-related potentials revealing atypical processing of sound frequency and the subsequent association with later literacy skills in children with familial dyslexia. Cortex 46: 1362–1376. doi: 10.1016/j.cortex.2010.06.003.
31. Leppänen PHT, Pihko E, Eklund KM, Lyytinen H (1999) Cortical responses of infants with and without a genetic risk for dyslexia: II. Group effects. NeuroReport 10(5): 969–973.
32. Leppänen PHT, Richardson U, Pihko E, Eklund KM, Guttorm TK, et al. (2002) Brain responses to changes in speech sound durations differ between infants with and without familial risk for dyslexia. Developmental Neuropsychology 22(1): 407–422.
33. Lewis BA, Freebairn LA, Taylor HG (2002) Correlates of spelling abilities in children with early speech sound disorders. Reading and Writing: An Interdisciplinary Journal 15: 389–407.
34. McAnally KI, Stein JF (1996) Auditory temporal coding in dyslexia. Proceedings of the Royal Society of London, Series B Biological Sciences 263: 961–965.
35. McAnally KI, Stein JF (1997) Scalp potentials evoked by amplitude-modulated tones in dyslexia. Journal of Speech, Language, and Hearing Research 40: 939–945.
36. McArthur GM, Ellis D, Atkinson CM, Coltheart M (2008) Auditory processing deficits in children with reading and language impairments: Can they (and should they) be treated? Cognition 107: 946–977. doi: 10.1016/j.cognition.2007.12.005.
37. Mody M, Studdert-Kennedy M, Brady S (1997) Speech perception deficits in poor readers: Auditory processing or phonological coding? Journal of Experimental Child Psychology 64: 199–231.
38. Morais J, Cluytens M, Algria J (1984) Segmentation abilities of dyslexics and normal readers. Perceptual and Motor Skills 58: 221–222.
39. Pihko E, Leppänen PHT, Eklund KM, Cheour M, Guttorm TK, et al. (1999) Cortical responses of infants with and without a genetic risk for dyslexia: I. Age effects. NeuroReport 10(5): 901–905.
40. Reece C, Treiman R (2001) Children's spelling of syllabic/r/and letter-name vowels: Broadening the study of spelling development. Applied Psycholinguistics 22: 139–165.
41. Richardson U, Thomson JM, Scott SK, Goswami U (2004) Auditory processing skills and phonological representation in dyslexic children. Dyslexia 10: 215–233. doi: 10.1002/dys.276.
42. Rittle-Johnson BR, Siegler RS (1999) Learning to spell: Variability, choice, and change in children's strategy use. Child development 70: 332–348.
43. Robinson KM (2001) The validity of verbal reports in children's subtraction. Journal of Educational Psychology 93: 211–222.
44. Schulte-Körne G, Deimel W, Bartling J, Remschmidt H (1998) Role of auditory temporal processing for reading and spelling disability. Perceptual and Motor Skills 86: 1043–1047.
45. Shrager J, Siegler RS (1998) SCADS: A model of children's strategy choices and strategy discoveries. Psychology Science 9(5): 405–410.
46. Stein JF, McAnally K (1995) Auditory temporal processing in developmental dyslexics. The Irish Journal of Psychology 16: 220–228.
47. Talcott JB, Witton C, Hebb GS, Stoodley CJ, Westwood EA, et al. (2002) On the relationship between dynamic visual and auditory processing and literacy skills; Results from a large primary-school study. Dyslexia 8: 204–225. doi: 10.1002/dys.224
48. Tallal P (1980) Auditory temporal perception, phonics, and reading disabilities in children. Brain and Language 9: 182–198.
49. Tallal P, Miller SL, Bedi G, Byma G, Wang X, et al. (1996) Language comprehension in language-learning impaired children improved with acoustically modified speech. Science 271: 81–84.
50. Tallal P, Stark RE, Mellits ED (1985) Identification of language-impaired children on the basis of rapid perception and production skills. Brain and Language 25: 314–322.
51. Treiman R (2004) Spelling and dialect: Comparisons between speakers of African American vernacular English and White speakers. Psychonomic Bulletin & Review 11: 338–342.
52. Treiman R, Berch D, Tincoff R, Weatherston S (1993) Phonology and spelling: The case of syllabic consonants. Journal of Experimental Child Psychology 56: 267–290.
53. Treiman R, Broderick V, Tincoff R, Rodriguez K (1998) Children's phonological awareness: Confusions between phonemes that differ only in voicing. Journal of Experimental Child Psychology 68: 3–21.

54. Treiman R, Goswami U, Tincoff R, Leevers H (1997) Effects of dialect on American and British children's spelling. Child Development 68: 229–245.
55. Varnhagen CK, Daniels J, Rabiau M, Gillingham TE, Steffler DJ (2000 July) Phoneme perception and children's spelling. Paper presented at the meeting of the Society for Scientific Study of Reading, Stockholm, Sweden.
56. Watson BU (1992) Auditory temporal acuity in normally achieving and learning-disabled college students. Journal of Speech and Hearing Research 35(1): 148–156.
57. Watson BU, Miller TK (1993) Auditory perception, phonological processing, and reading ability/disability. Journal of Speech and Hearing Research 36(4): 850–863.
58. Wilkinson GS (1993) WRAT3: Wide Range Achievement Test administration manual. Wilmington, Delaware: Wide Range, Inc.

18

Episodic Future Thinking in Semantic Dementia: A Cognitive and fMRI Study

Armelle Viard[1,2,3,4]*, Pascale Piolino[5,6], Serge Belliard[1,2,3,4,7], Vincent de La Sayette[1,2,3,4], Béatrice Desgranges[1,2,3,4], Francis Eustache[1,2,3,4]

1 Inserm, U1077, Caen, France, **2** Université de Caen Basse-Normandie, UMR-S1077, Caen, France, **3** Ecole Pratique des Hautes Etudes, UMR-S1077, Caen, France, **4** Centre Hospitalier Universitaire, U1077, Caen, France, **5** Université Paris Descartes, Institut de Psychologie, Memory and Cognition Lab, Paris, France, **6** Inserm UMR S894, Centre de Psychiatrie et Neurosciences, Paris, France, **7** CHU Pontchaillou, Rennes, France

Abstract

Semantic dementia (SD) is characterized by gradual loss of semantic memory. While episodic autobiographical memory seems relatively preserved, behavioral studies suggest that episodic future thinking is impaired. We used fMRI to measure brain activity in four SD patients (JPL, EP, LL, EG) while they envisioned future events and remembered personal past events. Twelve healthy elders served as controls. Episodic quality, emotion, mental imagery and level of consciousness (via remember/know judgements) were checked at debriefing. We analyzed the future compared to the past for each patient. All patients presented lateral temporal atrophy, but varied in terms of frontal and anterior hippocampal atrophy. Patient JPL presented atrophy in bilateral superior medial frontal gyri and left anterior hippocampus and was unable to engage in episodic future thinking, despite hyperactivations in frontal and occipital regions. Patient EP presented no atrophy in the anterior hippocampus, but atrophy in bilateral superior medial frontal gyrus and had difficulties to engage in episodic future thinking. Patient LL presented atrophy in left anterior hippocampus, but hyperactivated its right counterpart for future compared to past thinking, permitting her to project efficiently in the future in an episodic way. Patient EG presented no atrophy in the superior medial frontal gyri or anterior hippocampi and was able to engage in episodic future thinking. Altogether, patients' future projections differed depending on the severity and localization of their atrophy. The functional integrity of bilateral superior medial frontal gyri and anterior hippocampus appear crucial for episodic future thinking: atrophy of both structures strongly impairs future projection, while integrity of these structures or hyperactivation of residual tissue normalizes episodic future projection.

Editor: Jean-Claude Baron, INSERM U894, Centre de Psychiatrie et Neurosciences, Hopital Sainte-Anne and Université Paris 5, France

Funding: This work was supported by the University Hospital Center of Caen, Ecole Pratique de Hautes Etudes (EPHE), Fondation pour la Recherche sur le Cerveau (FRC), Inserm, UCBN (research unit U1077). The funders had no role in study design, data collection and analysis, decision to publish, or preparation of the manuscript.

Competing Interests: The authors have declared that no competing interests exist.

* Email: viard@cyceron.fr

Introduction

Semantic dementia (SD) is a variant of fronto-temporal dementia characterized by a gradual loss of semantic memory [1], with progressive anomia and deterioration of vocabulary [2]). An asymmetrical atrophy of the lateral temporal lobe is generally observed [3] with an antero-posterior gradient, the highest changes located in its anterior portion [4]. A relative preservation of episodic memory is observed [5,6], with intact recent and day-to-day memory. Episodic memory is characterized by a particular self-reflective mental state, termed autonoetic consciousness, which implies that a person recollects his/her personal events with a sense of re-experiencing, by mentally "travelling in time" in the past [7,8]. Converging lines of evidence from different fields of research indicate that remembering the past or envisioning the future share common cognitive [9,10,11] and neural underpinnings [12,13,14,15]. Indeed, past and future thinking build on similar information stored in episodic memory and rely on similar cognitive processes (i.e., self-referential processing, imagery and flexible recombination of stored details). Yet, in semantic dementia, behavioral studies have consistently shown that future thinking is impaired [16,17,18].

Duval et al. [18] examined self-representations and states of consciousness (measured via remember/know judgements) in SD patients for past, present and future periods. The future period elicited poorer performances than the past and present periods in terms of episodic self-representations and autonoetic consciousness. SD patients had difficulties in projecting themselves into the future and had an impaired level of consciousness associated to the future. These findings suggest that personal semantic memory is necessary to imagine one's future self, as confirmed by Irish et al. [16]. Indeed, Irish et al. [16] also indicated that SD patients had difficulties in episodic future simulation, despite a relative preservation of past episodic retrieval. They showed that SD patients' future thinking deficit was driven by their difficulty in providing episodic (specific) details, contrasting with elevated semantic (factual) details. SD patients' phenomenological past experiencing however (measured by subjective ratings of vividness, valence, emotional intensity, personal significance) did not differ from controls. This reveals a disconnect between objective task performances and subjective phenomenological pre-experiencing when generating future events in this population. Irish et al. [17] showed relatively intact episodic retrieval but significant impairments for episodic future thinking in their group of SD patients. Atrophy in areas of the lateral temporal cortex (left inferior temporal gyrus and bilateral temporal pole) was found to correlate with deficits in episodic future thinking. This region is known for its role in semantic processing and thus confirms previous findings that semantic knowledge is critical for the construction of novel future events [19].

Atrophy in the lateral temporal cortex is characteristic of semantic dementia and as indicated above may play a role in SD's episodic future thinking deficit, although other regions are also important (e.g., hippocampus, medial prefrontal cortex). Evidence of hippocampal atrophy is now well documented in SD, even in the early stages of the disease [20,21,22,23,24,25,26,4,27,28,29,6], although some patients were reported to have no hippocampal atrophy [30,6]. The hippocampus supports relational processing [31,32,33], including flexible recombination of details for past and future event construction [34]. Addis and Schacter [35] showed that future-associated activity in the anterior hippocampus was associated with higher demands on recombination of details. Hence, atrophy in this region may strongly affect episodic future thinking. In joint collaboration with the hippocampus, the medial prefrontal cortex is also critical in episodic future thinking. Its anterior part seems more involved in information integration and self-referential thinking, while its dorsal part has a role in generative construction [36].

Studies on future thinking in SD are scarce and no fMRI study is yet available. Neuroimaging studies on future thinking in healthy adults have shown a neural network which has striking similarities with the one recruited during episodic past remembering, including prefrontal and medial temporal cortices, medial parietal (posterior cingulate and retrosplenial cortices), posterior parietal (precuneus and temporo-parietal junction), occipital regions and the cerebellum [12,13,14,15,37,38]. We previously showed that a common network of brain regions was activated for past and future thinking in healthy older adults, reflecting the use of similar cognitive processes [19]. Our results also showed that the episodic nature of future events depended on the inferior frontal and lateral temporal gyri, involved in semantic memory retrieval.

Here, we examined episodic future thinking in four SD patients using fMRI and compared it to past remembering. A group of 12 healthy elders served as a comparison group. In the scanner, upon presentation of a cue-phrase prompting a specific past or future event (obtained by questioning a close family member), patients were asked to mentally recall specific events from the past 12 months and specific plans they intended to pursue in the next 12 months. We also collected several behavioral data to assess the degree of phenomenological (re/pre)experiencing, through ratings of episodic quality, emotional intensity, valence, mental visual imagery, level of consciousness and repetition. Beyond lateral temporal atrophy which was present in all patients and may impact episodic future thinking, each had atrophy in different regions of the episodic future thinking network. We predicted that anterior hippocampal and/or medial prefrontal atrophy would strongly impair episodic future thinking given the crucial role these regions play. We expected that, in the presence of atrophied regions within this network, different processes might arise: either activation in residual tissue, up-regulation of areas within the network or recruitment of additional brain areas.

Materials and Methods

Participants

Patient details. We studied four patients suffering from SD selected according to a codified procedure in French qualified centres by senior neurologists (VDLS & SB) whose major activity is dedicated to the diagnosis and follow-up of patients suffering from neurodegenerative disorders including semantic dementia, in addition to a neuropsychologist and a speech therapist. The four patients all presented the two core features of SD (i.e., impaired picture naming and single-word comprehension) and the three following additional criteria, as specified by Gorno-Tempini et al. [39]: impaired object knowledge, spared repetition, spared speech production (i.e., fluent) and/or surface dyslexia and severe anterior temporal atrophy (see VBM analyses). The clinical and neuropsychological follow-up of our patients, who have been re-examined between 5 to 8 years after their first consultation, has confirmed the initial diagnosis (i.e., predominant semantic memory deficits, and preserved spatial orientation and autonomy). Table 1 summarizes patients' main neuropsychological scores and z-scores. Of note, all participants were scanned within the same week as neuropsychological testing.

JPL, a 62-year-old right-handed male retired cutter with 10 years of formal education, was seen at the University Hospital Center of Caen in November 2006. JPL reported progressive memory loss, particularly involving remembering peoples' names or familiar places, difficulty in word-finding and impaired object knowledge (e.g., he would eat an orange without pealing it). His wife reported a tendency to irritability, lack of initiative and poor conversational interactions, but his day-to-day memory and spatial orientation were preserved. As a leisure activity, he played sudoku. On formal neuropsychological testing, JPL showed relatively well preserved episodic memory (good free recall, but impaired immediate recall) as measured by a procedure derived from the Grober and Buschke test [40] (see Table S9 in File S1 for brief explanation of this test and what it measures). Visuospatial abilities were good as measured by copying and delayed recall of the Rey complex figure [41]. He scored poorly on semantic memory tests, as measured by category (names of animals) and letter (words beginning by letter p) fluency tasks [42] (see Table S9 in File S1 for brief explanation of this test and what it measures). On the Semantic Knowledge Task [43] (see Table S9 in File S1 for brief explanation of this test and what it measures), he was impaired for picture naming and object knowledge, as shown by his difficulty in providing specific attributes of words. He was impaired at recognizing famous faces on the French Celebrities Questionnaire [44] (see Table S9 in File S1 for brief explanation of this test and what it measures). He performed poorly on the Mill Hill test [45], a multiple-choice synonym vocabulary questionnaire which assesses verbal knowledge. His language abilities were tested with the LEXIS battery [46] (see Table S9 in File S1 for brief explanation of this test and what it measures). He produced semantic paraphasias and presented difficulties in picture naming, word-finding, word definitions (e.g., watermelon, deer, hammock, city hall…) and single-word comprehension (e.g., when asked "what is the capital of France?", he would answer: "what does capital mean?" or when asked "in which country is Venice?", he would answer, "what is Venice?"). His speech production was fluent. Repetition, reading of a text and its restitution were spared. He presented no deficit on the Trail Making Test [47].

EP, a 77-year-old right-handed female retired general practitioner with 20 years of formal education, was seen at the University Hospital Center of Caen in April 2008. EP reported difficulties in word-finding and word comprehension, especially

Table 1. Scores on neuropsychological tests for patients JPL, EP, LL, and EG.

Neuropsychological tests	**HE (mean ± s.d.)**	**JPL**	**z-score**	**EP**	**z-score**	**LL**	**z-score**	**EG**	**z-score**
Episodic memory									
Grober and Buschke									
Immediate recall (/16)	15.42±0.99	**12**	**−3.455**	16	0.586	16	0.586	16	0.586
Free recall (/48)	31.75±5.36	24	−1.446	31	−0.140	29	−0.513	30	−0.326
Total recall (/48)	46.67±1.92	**38**	**−4.516**	47	0.172	48	0.693	47	0.172
Delayed recall (/16)	11±2.22	9	−0.901	14	1.351	**6**	**−2.252**	8	−1.351
Rey complex figure									
Copy (sec)	33.90±2.44	36	0.875	36	0.875	36	0.875	33	−0.375
Recall (sec)	16.93±7.33	25	1.101	18	0.146	10.5	−0.877	20	0.419
Semantic memory									
Fluency tasks									
Category fluency (/2 min)	32.64+/−7.9	**17**	**−1.980**	**9**	**−2.992**	**16**	**−2.106**	**9**	**−2.992**
Letter fluency (/2 min)	23.78+/−8.35	**7**	**−2.010**	26	0.266	**8**	**−1.890**	**5**	**−2.249**
Semantic Knowledge Task									
Picture naming (/36)	36+/−0.0	**30**	**pathological**	**32**	**pathological**	**35**	**pathological**	NA	-
Superordinate category (/54)	54+/−0.0	54	OK	54	OK	54	OK	NA	-
Specific attributes (/54)	54+/−0.0	**49**	**pathological**	**50**	**pathological**	**50**	**pathological**	NA	-
BECS-GRECO Semantic Battery									
Words/40)	39.4+/−0.9	NA	-	NA	-	NA	-	**22**	**−19.33**
Pictures (/40)	39.2+/−0.9	NA	-	NA	-	NA	-	**37**	**−2.44**
French celebrities questionnaire (%)	100+/−3.0	**39.1**	**−19.96**		NA	**34.8**	**−21.4**	**2.5**	**−31.17**
Mill Hill (/33)	25.64±5.84	**16**	**−1.651**	29	OK	20	OK	29	OK
Language									
Speech production	NA	Fluent		Fluent		Fluent		Fluent	
Repetition	NA	OK		OK		OK		OK	
Reading	NA	OK		OK		OK		OK	
LEXIS battery									
Picture naming (/80)	72.8±3.28	**55**	**−5.427**	**60**	**−3.902**	NA	-	**47**	**−7.866**
Picture naming (/64)	58.5±3.21	NA	-	NA	-	**47**	**−3.583**	NA	-
Executive functions									
TMT B-A (sec)	76±64	30	−0.719	35	−0.641	63	−0.203	66	−0.156
Other									
MMSE (/30)	28.42±1.38	27	−1.029	29	0.420	**25**	**−2.478**	28	−0.304

Table 1. Cont.

Neuropsychological tests	HE (mean ± s.d.)	JPL	z-score	EP	z-score	LL	z-score	EG	z-score
GDS (/30)	4.83±3.04	7	0.714	5	0.056	9	1.372	7	0.714
Mattis (/144)	142.17±1.34	**132**	**−7.590**	144	1.366	141	−0.873	**120**	**−16.545**

Tests: BECS GRECO Semantic Battery: Merck et al. (2011); French celebrities questionnaire: Belliard et al. (2001); GDS: Yesavage et al. (1983); Grober and Buschke (1987); Mill Hill test: Deltour (1993); Mattis: dementia rating scale (Mattis, 1976); MMSE: Mini-Mental Status Exam (Folstein et al., 1975); Rey complex figure: Rey (1970); Semantic Knowledge Task: Desgranges et al. (1996); Picture naming: LEXIS (de Partz, 2001); TMT: Trail Making Test (Reitan, 1958).
Note: The Semantic Knowledge Task was proposed to patients from Caen (JPL, EP, LL); the BECS GRECO Semantic Battery was proposed to the patient from Rennes (EG). On the Semantic Knowledge Task, performances had to be maximum to be considered unimpaired (i.e., standard deviation in control group equals zero). Hence, if patients did not obtain the maximum score, their performance was impaired (noted "pathological" in the Table). The French celebrities questionnaire was not proposed to EP at the time she participated in this fMRI study.
Results were considered as significant when $z > \pm 1.96$, $p < 0.05$. Pathological scores appear in bold and when no standard deviation was available, pathological performances were noted "pathological" in bold. HE = healthy elders; OK = performance not significantly different from healthy elders; NA = not available.

animal names and geographic locations which she once knew well. She had impaired object knowledge (e.g., for EP, zebras live in French prairies; salads and carrots grow in forests). She continued to have stimulating intellectual activities by reading and attending university senior courses, although she complained not being able to learn efficiently. She was autonomous in daily life and her day-to-day memory was preserved. On formal neuropsychological testing, EP showed relatively well preserved episodic memory on the Grober and Buschke test. Visuospatial abilities were good as measured by copying and delayed recall of the Rey complex figure. Given her high level of education, she scored poorly on semantic memory, as measured by category fluency tasks (names of animals). She produced errors on picture naming and on object knowledge, as shown by her difficulty in providing specific attributes of words on the Semantic Knowledge Task. She performed well on the Mill Hill vocabulary test. Her language abilities, tested with the LEXIS battery, confirmed her difficulties in picture naming. She produced paraphasias (semantic, visual, visuo-semantic), had difficulties on single-word comprehension and in providing word definitions (zebra, hippopotamus, elephant, kiwi…), with many specific attributes being lost. Her speech production was fluent. Repetition and reading were spared. She presented no deficit on the TMT.

LL, a 73-year-old right-handed female retired secretary with 9 years of formal education, was seen at the University Hospital Center of Caen in September 2007. LL reported difficulties in word-finding, object knowledge (e.g., she will cook cucumber and radish; she will put sugar on avocados) and recognizing people. She was fond of logical games (e.g., sudoku). She was autonomous in daily life and her day-to-day memory was preserved. On formal neuropsychological testing, LL had preserved episodic memory (on immediate and free recalls) on the Grober and Buschke test. Visuospatial abilities were good as measured by copying and delayed recall of the Rey complex figure. She scored poorly on semantic memory tests, both on category (names of animals) and letter (words beginning by letter p) fluency tasks. She produced errors on picture naming and on object knowledge (difficulty in providing specific attributes of words) on the Semantic Knowledge Task. She was impaired at recognizing famous faces on the French Celebrities Questionnaire. She performed well on the Mill Hill vocabulary test. Her language abilities, tested with the LEXIS battery confirmed her difficulties in picture naming. She also showed difficulties on single-word comprehension and made errors on word definitions (e.g., bull, kangourou, harp, volcano…). Her speech production was fluent. Repetition, reading of a text and its restitution were spared. She presented no deficit on the TMT.

EG, a 62-year-old right-handed female retired secretary with 9 years of formal education, was seen at the University Hospital Center of Rennes in October 2008. EG reported difficulties in word-finding, names of places and recognizing people. She also showed oral and written comprehension difficulties. Her spatial orientation was good and she mentioned that she frequently consulted atlases to resituate her trip itineraries. She was autonomous in daily life and her day-to-day memory was preserved. Her leisure activities consisted in playing with logical games (e.g., sudoku, video games). On formal neuropsychological testing, EG showed preserved episodic memory (on immediate, free and delayed recalls) on the Grober and Buschke test. Visuospatial abilities were good as measured by copying and delayed recall of the Rey complex figure. She scored poorly on semantic memory tests, both on category (names of animals) and letter (words beginning by letter p) fluency tasks. Being a patient from Rennes (not Caen, like the three other patients), clinicians there proposed the BECS GRECO Semantic Battery [48] to EG, instead of the Semantic Knowledge Task. On the BECS GRECO Semantic Battery, she was impaired on single-word comprehension (difficulty on semantic matching of words) and on object knowledge (difficulty on semantic matching of pictures). She was extremely impaired at recognizing famous faces on the French Celebrities Questionnaire. She presented surface dyslexia (e.g., baptism; note that in French, the [p] is not pronounced). She performed well on the Mill Hill vocabulary test. Her language abilities, tested with the LEXIS battery), confirmed her difficulties in picture naming. Her speech production was fluent. Repetition and reading were spared. She presented no deficit on the TMT.

For all patients, an indicator of disease severity was obtained with the Mini-Mental Status Exam [49] (MMSE; total score/30) which assesses both comprehension and expression abilities through eight different questions. The MMSE has already been used as an indicator of disease severity. Matuszewski et al. [50] subdivided their two groups of SD patients into a mild group (mean score on the MMSE of 26±1.91) and a moderate group (mean score of 21.29±1.07). Based on the MMSE (see Table 1), the four patients (JPL = 27; EP = 29; LL = 25; EG = 28) show high scores, indicative of an early stage of dementia (i.e., mild stage). Note that all patients were autonomous in daily life. Global cognitive functioning was assessed via the Mattis dementia rating scale [51] (total score/144; see Table S9 in File S1 for brief explanation of this test and what it measures). Signs of depression were estimated with the Geriatric Depression Scale [52] (GDS; total score/30). Table 1 summarizes patients' neuropsychological scores and z-scores according to normative data provided for each test.

Healthy elders. Twelve right-handed healthy elders (females, mean age ± s.d. = 67.2±5.2 years; ranging from 60 to 75 years old), mean years of education (11.42±2.81), with no history of psychiatric or neurological disorder were recruited through a senior university, a retirement association or a newspaper advertisement. Participants had no abnormality on their T_1-weighted high-resolution magnetic resonance imaging (MRI). They underwent a battery of neuropsychological tests to assess their cognitive abilities and all performed in the normal range (see Viard et al. [53] for a full description). Each participant resided at home and all were active in cultural pursuits, continuing education or with responsibilities in diverse associations.

The study was approved by the Regional Ethics Committee of Lower Normandy and written informed consent was obtained from all participants prior to their participation in the study. Patients understood the experiment and had full capacity to consent (i.e., no surrogate consent procedure was needed). Data on healthy elders were obtained as part of a broader experiment exploring five past periods previously published [53,54] and a future period [19]. These healthy subjects were scanned with the intention to be compared with the patients. Results of two SD patients (JPL and EP) on a task exploring episodic autobiographical memory retrieval over five past periods have been published previously [6]. Here, we present new results concerning four SD patients on the episodic future thinking task and compare them to the group of healthy elders. Of note, given the rarity of patients with semantic dementia, we were not able to perfectly match each patient to the control group. This group of healthy elders can nonetheless serve as a comparison group to our patients, given that disparities have been controlled for by adding covariates (age and years of education) in statistical analyses (see below).

Task and experimental design

Autobiographical memories from the last 12 months and future plans scheduled in the next 12 months were obtained through an interview with a close family member a week before the scanning session. The family member, in most cases the spouse, was close enough to provide specific personal past memories of the participant and actual future plans that the participant intended to pursue (i.e., events were not made up by family members, but corresponded to actual past or future events in the participant's life). Among events provided by the family member, only those which corresponded to specific (i.e., episodic) events, unique in time and space, were selected. Before scanning, participants were familiarized with the task in a training phase outside of the scanner, using different events than in the experimental task. Special care was taken to explain to the patients the tasks they had to perform. The instructions given to participants for the past period were as follows: "You will see on the screen short sentences which refer to specific past events which happened to you in the last 12 months, followed by a black screen. Press on the button as soon as you can access a specific personal past event, which lasted less than 24 hours, related to the cue and think about all the details that come to mind, until the cross appears. Try to remember the event as if you were reliving it." The instructions given to participants for the future period were as follows: "You will see on the screen short sentences which refer to future plans which you intend to pursue in the next 12 months, followed by a black screen. Press on the button as soon as you can access a specific personal future event, which will last less than 24 hours, related to the cue and think about all the details that come to mind, until the cross appears. Try to envision the event as if you were living it in advance." In the scanner, personal sentence-cues were presented visually in white on a black background, using Superlab software (3.0 version, Cedrus). During the whole experiment, participants were asked to keep their eyes open to be able to read the sentence cues. Upon presentation of the visual cue, participants were instructed to recall or envision a specific detailed event, unique in time and space, that had either occurred in the past 12 months (past period) or was scheduled in the next 12 months (future period). For both past and future events, they were asked to experience the event with as much details as possible. Past and future events were sufficiently different to refrain participants from simply recalling a similar past event when instructed to envision a future event. Two functional runs, one per period, each lasting 5 minutes, were composed of 5 experimental (i.e., 5 events) and 5 control blocks, randomly intermixed across subjects. In the experimental condition, one block consisted of a sentence-cue (5 s) followed by a blank screen (19 s) during which participants had to mentally experience the corresponding specific personal event (e.g., past: "my grandson's last birthday party"; future: "my fifty-third wedding anniversary"). In total, they had to recall five episodic past events and envision five episodic future events. They were asked to press on a button as soon as they gained access to the prompted event. In the control condition, participants were asked to detect the presence of two consecutive letters ("mb") in pseudo-words of six letters (for example, "speugr" or "mbieha") and were instructed to press on a button when "mb" was present in the pseudo-word. Five pseudowords were presented in each control block, each lasting 24 seconds (1 second for cue presentation, followed by 3.8 seconds for the response). All participants were scanned on the same scanner (1.5 tesla) at the University Hospital Center of Caen.

Following the scanning session, the debriefing took place (mean duration = 2,5 hours) in order to verify participants' engagement in the tasks and to identify the nature of the evocations experienced during scanning. Participants were asked to retrieve the five past and five future events again, using the same sentence-cues as in the scanner, but this time aloud in order to check that the events corresponded to the expected cued events and to assess their episodic nature (i.e., specificity and detail). Their episodic nature (or "episodicity") was estimated 1) with "objective" measures, using a 5-point scale (generating overall autobiographical and strictly episodic scores; see below) and 2) with "subjective" measures, by collecting participants' ratings on several behavioral scales (evaluating emotion, mental imagery, level of consciousness and effect of repetition; see below).

First, the specificity of each evocation was measured by the investigators (objective measurement of episodicity) using a fine-grained 5-point scale (0-1-2-3-4) similar to previous episodic scales used with healthy subjects and patients with cerebral diseases [55,56,57,58,59,50,53,19,6]. This scale takes into account the specificity of the content (single or repeated event), the spatiotemporal situation and the presence of details (perceptions, thoughts, feelings). A specific event, situated in time and space, with sensory details is given a score of 4. A specific event with few details, but situated in time and space, scores 3. A generic event (repeated or prolonged over time, situated in time and space) scores 2. A vague event (repeated or prolonged over time, not situated in time and space) scores 1. Absence of memory, or general information about a theme, scores 0 (see Table S10 in File S1). Two different total scores are obtained per period. First, the overall autobiographical score (AS: maximum score per period $4 \times 5 = 20$) includes all the events (specific and generic) and corresponds to the classic episodic memory score used in the well-known Autobiographical Memory Interview [56] (AMI). The AS score is expressed in terms of ratio (i.e., scores obtained for each of the five events per period were summed and divided by the maximum score per period which is 20). Second, the strictly episodic score (ES: maximum score per period $4 \times 5 = 20$) includes only the number of specific and detailed events scoring 4, using a more stringent criterion. ES is expressed in terms of ratio of strictly episodic events per period (i.e., number of strictly episodic events divided by the number of retrieved events). Two independent experts rated each event recalled at debriefing and any difference of opinion between them was discussed until a consensus was reached. A final score was calculated based on the number of episodic (past or future) events experienced by participants in the scanner (e.g., since EP experienced one episodic future event, her score was of one for the future; see Table 2).

Second, subjective measures of episodicity were used to specify the different aspects of the recollective experience. Participants rated their own evocations on several behavioral scales (10-cm lines; self-ratings) known to be crucial to control the degree of episodic (re/pre)experiencing. Emotion is an important phenomenological characteristic of vivid and persistent personal events [60]. Thus, participants were asked to rate their evocations on scales measuring emotional intensity (0 = no emotion to 10 = very strong emotion) and valence (0 = very negative to 10 = very positive). Visual mental imagery is known to increase the recall of specific details [61,62,63]. Several scales were used to measure mental visual imagery: mental strategy used (0 = verbal to 10 = visual), number of images (0 = no images to 10 = over 10 images), image quality (0 = very blurry to 10 = very clear) and perspective of mental images [64] ("field" or "observer" perspectives). Regarding perspective, three choices were proposed: observer (0), field and observer (1) or field (2). The autonoetic and noetic levels of consciousness, which characterize episodic and semantic memory respectively, can be distinguished by the remember or know (R/K) paradigm. Participants were asked to rate their evocations on a scale measuring the level of consciousness between the autonoetic and noetic states (scale range from 0 = knowing to 10 = remembering). Unlike the "knowing" state, the "remembering" state is characterized by phenomenal elements associated with (re/pre)experiencing of specific events (visual images, sensations, feelings). For the future, a "Remember" response indicates that the participant was able to pre-experience future events in advance. Recent reactivation (i.e., was an event evoked recently or not) was evaluated using two scales: (1) the frequency of rehearsal scale (0 = never to 10 = very frequent), to determine how frequently an event was rehearsed, prior to scanning and (2) the last recall scale (0 = today to 10 = over 10 years ago), to determine when each event was last recalled. Unfortunately, for JPL, subjective rating scales for the future are not available due to lost material. However, the subjective rating scales for the past and objective measures for both periods are available.

MRI data acquisition

A blocked functional MRI design was used. Lying in the scanner, participants viewed the display via a mirror to an active matrix video projector. Stimulus onset was synchronized with the acquisition of the first slice. Anatomical and functional MRIs were acquired on a General Electrics Signa 1.5 tesla MRI scanner (GE, BUC, France). First, a high-resolution T1-weighted MRI scan (T1-MRI) was acquired with a three-dimensional inversion recovery spoiled gradient echo sequence (matrix size = $256 \times 256 \times 128$; slice thickness = 1.5 mm). Second, a proton density/T2-weighted MRI scan (PD-MRI, T2-MRI) was acquired with 32 axial slices covering the entire brain and the superior part of the cerebellum (slice thickness = 3.8 mm). Finally, functional images were acquired with echo planar imaging blood oxygen level dependent (BOLD) sequence (repetition time = 6 s, echo time = 60 ms, flip angle = 90°, matrix size = $64 \times 64 \times 32$, 50 volumes, 3.8-mm-thick slices) covering the same field of view as the T2-MRI acquisition.

Construction of an old-adult template

Using voxel-based morphometry [65] (VBM5), each individual T1-MRIs of healthy elders were segmented according to the unified segmentation procedure [66] with spatial normalization included. Mean templates were calculated based on the individual segmented and normalized T1-MRIs, creating three separate old-adult templates according to tissue type (e.g. grey and white matters, cerebro-spinal fluid) which were then spatially smoothed using an 8-mm^3 full width at half maximum (FWHM) Gaussian kernel.

Functional image pre-processing

Functional images were processed and analyzed using the Statistical Parametric Mapping software (SPM5; Wellcome Trust Centre for Neuroimaging, London, United Kingdom; http://www.fil.ion.ucl.ac.uk/spml). The first six volumes of the functional acquisition were discarded, allowing for signal stabilization, and differences in slice acquisition timing were corrected. Images were realigned to correct for interscan movement with the creation of resliced mean functional volumes (mean-fMRI). For inter-modalities registration, rigid registration matrices (mean-fMRI onto T2-MRI, PD-MRI onto T1-MRI, T1-MRI onto the old-adult template) were computed, combined and then applied to fMRI volumes. Individual T1-MRIs were then segmented using the old-adult templates as priors (obtained previously, one for each tissue type; see above) and normalized. In order to set the fMRI volumes into our old-adult space, functional MRI images were resampled using the normalization parameters obtained in the segmentation step. Finally, data were spatially smoothed with an 8-mm^3 FWHM Gaussian kernel.

Table 2. Behavioral ratings for patients JPL, EP, LL, EG and healthy elders (HE) and t values comparing each patient to the control group for each period.

	HE		JPL		EP		LL		EG	
	Past	**Future**	**Past**	**Future**	**Past**	**Future**	**Past**	**Future**	**Past**	**Future**
Episodic scores										
AS score										
Mean ± sd	3.73 (±0.41)	3.17 (±0.57)	3.00	1.20	3.60	2.40	3.80	3.60	3.40	2.60
T			−1.71	**−3.32**	−0.31	−1.29	0.16	0.73	−0.77	−0.96
ES score										
Mean ± sd	3.20 (±1.08)	1.73 (±1.31)	0.80	0.00	2.40	0.80	3.20	2.40	2.40	0.00
T			−2.14	−1.27	−0.71	−0.68	0.00	0.49	−0.71	−1.27
Nb episodic events										
Mean ± sd	4.75 (±0.45)	4.00 (±1.16)	4.00	1.00	5.00	1.00	5.00	4.00	4.00	3.00
t			−1.59	−2.48	0.53	−2.48	0.53	0.00	−1.59	−0.83
Emotion										
Intensity										
Mean ± sd	5.10 (±1.59)	4.80 (±1.72)	8.73	NA	9.50	9.50	2.72	2.66	5.65	2.15
T			2.20	-	**2.66**	**2.63**	−1.44	−1.20	0.33	−1.48
Valence										
Mean ± sd	6.57 (±1.26)	6.75 (±1.05)	8.88	NA	7.80	9.00	6.32	5.70	7.90	4.20
t			1.76	-	0.94	2.06	−0.19	−0.96	1.02	−2.34
Imagery										
Mental strategy										
Mean ± sd	8.65 (±1.83)	8.86 (±1.69)	8.14	NA	10.00	10.00	9.26	5.54	9.30	6.93
t			−0.27	-	0.71	0.65	0.32	−1.89	0.34	−1.10
Image number										
Mean ± sd	5.06 (±2.12)	3.72 (±1.49)	0.80	NA	10.00	10.00	4.40	2.40	1.75	1.50
T			−1.93	-	2.24	**4.06**	−0.30	−0.85	−1.50	−1.43
Image quality										
Mean ± sd	9.13 (±1.25)	8.57 (±1.69)	9.10	NA	9.50	5.00	9.28	6.14	8.25	6.95
T			−0.02	-	0.28	−2.03	0.12	−1.38	−0.68	−0.92
Perspective										
Mean ± sd	1.40 (±0.59)	1.22 (±0.74)	0.42	NA	1.00	1.00	1.00	1.20	2.00	0.00
t			−1.60	-	−0.65	−0.29	−0.65	−0.03	0.98	−1.59
Consciousness										
R/K										
Mean ± sd	9.38 (±0.61)	6.28 (±3.47)	9.56	NA	9.90	5.00	9.24	3.22	9.23	4.15
t			0.28	-	0.82	−0.35	−0.22	−0.85	−0.24	−0.59

Table 2. Cont.

	HE		JPL		EP		LL		EG	
	Past	Future	Past	Future	Past	Future	Past	Future	Past	Future
Repetition										
Rehearsal frequency										
Mean ± sd	5.51 (±1.99)	4.39 (±2.02)	5.82	NA	0.00	9.50	6.32	4.38	3.10	3.90
t			0.15	-	**−2.66**	2.43	0.39	0.00	−1.17	−0.23
Last recall										
Mean ± sd	1.61 (±0.89)	1.46 (±1.49)	0.48	NA	0.50	1.00	2.82	1.82	3.93	4.18
t			−1.22	-	−1.20	−0.30	1.31	0.23	2.50	1.75

Note: Behavioral scales range from 0 to 10 for emotional intensity (0 = no emotion to 10 = very strong emotion), emotional valence (0 = very negative to 10 = very positive), mental strategy used (0 = verbal to 10 = visual), number of mental visual images (0 = no images to 10 = over 10 images), mental visual image quality (0 = very blurry to 10 = very clear), state of consciousness (0 = knowing to 10 = remembering), rehearsal frequency (0 = never to 10 = very frequent), last recall (0 = today to 10 = over 10 years ago). For the perspective, the maximum score is 2 (0 = observer; 1 = field and observer; 2 = field).
Results were considered as significant (in bold) when $t > \pm 2.576$, $p < 0.01$. AS = autobiographical score; ES = strictly episodic autobiographical score; NA = not available; Nb = number; sd = standard deviation; t = t statistic.

Data analyses

Behavioral data analysis. An adjusted t-test intended for single case analyses [67] was used for comparisons between each patient and healthy elders (for autobiographical scores and behavioral scales). Within-subject differences across past and future conditions were conducted using the modified t test [68] which assesses whether the difference between past and future periods in each patient differs significantly from the control group pattern. Results were considered significant at a conservative threshold of $t > \pm 2.576$, $p < 0.01$ to guard against Type 1 errors for multiple comparisons.

VBM analyses. In order to formally assess the extent of atrophy in each SD patient across the whole brain, we compared their structural MRI scans with those of the group of 12 healthy elders using voxel-based morphometry [66] (VBM5). Structural MRI images were analyzed using the optimised VBM procedure implemented in SPM5. Briefly, this involves a number of fully automated preprocessing steps including extraction of brain, spatial normalization into stereotactic (MNI) space, segmentation into grey and white matters and CSF compartments, correction for volume changes induced by spatial normalization (modulation), and smoothing with a 8-mm^3 FWHM isotropic Gaussian kernel. The preprocessing procedures used in SPM5 have been shown to produce good results when matching brains with lesions to standardised templates [69]. We used the optional "modulation of non-linear effects only" which takes into account intracranial volume, hence controlling for differences in brain sizes. Analyses focussed on grey matter. Each patient's structural scan was compared to healthy elders' scans using a two sample t-test to investigate differences in grey matter volume. The significance level was set at $p < 0.05$ FWE corrected for multiple comparisons, $k > 50$ voxels (see Tables S2 to S5 in File S1).

fMRI data analyses. fMRI time series were modelled by a general linear model (GLM) including separate regressors for each of the experimental (past and future periods) and control conditions using SPM5. All regressors were convolved with the canonical hemodynamic response function (HRF). Data were high-pass filtered (cut-off period = 96 s). Coefficients for each regressor were estimated for each participant using maximum likelihood estimates to account for serial correlations in the data. At the first level, linear contrasts of the parameter estimates for each experimental regressor of interest were calculated for each participant, subtracting the corresponding control regressor (resulting in "period minus control task" contrasts). To examine the future thinking network in each patient at the individual level, t-statistic maps were generated for the following contrasts of interest: future minus control task and future minus past period (subtracting for each period the corresponding control regressor) for each participant. The second level random effects analysis was conducted over contrast images obtained at the first level. Each patient was compared to the group of healthy elders (i.e., patients were not grouped together) using the two sample t-test model of SPM5, as recommended by Henson's guidelines (2006; http://www.mrc-cbu.cam.ac.uk//personal/rik.henson/personal/Henson_Singlecase_06.pdf) and previously used to report single case fMRI data, notably in semantic dementia [70,6]. Inter-group subtraction analyses were computed to determine which regions were differentially activated by each patient and healthy elders when comparing past and future periods. The significance level was set at $p < 0.05$ FWE corrected for multiple comparisons, $k > 10$ voxels. Coordinates of brain regions are reported in the MNI space. To control for the age difference between patients and healthy elders, age was included as covariate. EP's duration of education was higher compared to healthy elders. Since education and general intelligence are generally closely inter-related [71], variations due to differences in general intelligence between EP and healthy elders were controlled for by adding years of education as covariate for analyses comparing EP to healthy elders. Finally, to reveal pathophysiological properties of the future thinking brain network in each patient using a different method, plots of activation magnitude were obtained for each patient and average of healthy elders in several regions of interest (ROIs) of the conventional future thinking network (medial frontal gyrus, hippocampus, precuneus). For each participant, mean activation values corresponding to the difference in BOLD activation between the experimental (future period) and control tasks (for Figure S1: control task; for Figure S2: past period; see File S1), were extracted within each ROI using the "anatomical VOI analysis" of the fMRIroi SPM toolbox [54].

Results

Behavioral results

All patients were able to perform the tasks, both recalling past memories and envisioning future events, differences lay in the episodic nature of the events experienced. On the objective measures of episodicity, JPL and EP were able to pre-experience only one episodic future event (rated 3 or 4 on the episodic scale) and four semantic future events (rated 1 or 2). On the contrary, LL was able to pre-experience four episodic future events and one semantic future event. EG was able to pre-experience three episodic future events and two semantic future events. Of note, despite using verbal cues, all patients were all able to read and understand the cues.

Comparisons between each patient and healthy elders showed, on the objective measures of episodicity, significantly lower overall autobiographical score (AS) for the future and a trend for the strictly episodic score (ES) for the past for JPL (see Table 2). Based on the number of episodic events experienced, a trend showed that JPL and EP produced less episodic future events compared to healthy elders. On the subjective rating scales, main results indicated that emotional intensity was greater for the past and the future for EP compared to healthy elders. Concerning mental imagery, EP evoked a greater number of mental images for the future compared to healthy elders, although a trend showed that image quality of future mental images was less clear for EP compared to healthy elders. Within-subject comparisons, using the modified t test procedure [68], did not reveal statistical differences between past and future conditions for each patient (data not shown). Note that adding education as covariate in behavioral analyses for EP, following Crawford et al.'s [72] guidelines, did not change results (see Table S1 in File S1).

VBM results

Results depicted on Figure 1 and Tables S2 to S5 in File S1 reveal areas of grey matter volume loss in JPL, EP, LL and EG compared to healthy elders. All patients present lateral temporal atrophy, predominantly in its anterior portion (see Tables S2 to S5 in File S1). Of the four patients, three have predominant left-lateralized temporal atrophy (JPL, LL, EG) and EP has predominant right-lateralized temporal atrophy. JPL also presented atrophy in the left anterior hippocampus, left amygdala and frontal regions, in particular bilateral superior medial gyri.

Apart from predominantly right-lateralized temporal atrophy, EP also presented atrophy in frontal, in particular bilateral superior medial gyri and parietal regions (bilateral supramarginal, left inferior gyri) (see Table S3). EP showed preservation of anterior hippocampi.

Apart from predominantly left-lateralized temporal atrophy, LL also presented atrophy in left anterior hippocampus, left amygdala and bilateral inferior frontal gyri (see Table S4).

Apart from predominantly left-lateralized temporal atrophy, EG also presented atrophy in frontal regions (bilateral superior, left medial, bilateral inferior gyri) (see Table S5).

Strikingly, VBM analyses reveal that the two patients (JPL and EP) who have difficulties in envisioning the future in an episodic way present atrophy in bilateral superior medial frontal gyri which appears preserved in patients (LL and EG) who can project in the future in an episodic manner. Furthermore, the (left) anterior hippocampus, which is atrophied in JPL (and LL) may additionally explain his difficulties in episodic future projection (LL appears to compensate for this atrophy by hyperactivating the right anterior hippocampus, see below).

fMRI results

Patient JPL. At the individual level, results for the contrast future minus control task for JPL showed an essentially left-lateralized network of regions comprising the left (inferior, middle, superior) frontal gyri, middle temporal gyrus, precuneus, occipital areas and cerebellum (see Table S6). Results for the contrast future minus past period for JPL did not reveal any activation at the given threshold (see Table S7).

At the group level, the past period showed greater activations for JPL than healthy elders mainly in the left middle and inferior frontal gyri, bilateral cuneus and left insula compared to the control task (see Table 3). The future period showed greater activations for JPL than healthy elders mainly in the left calcarine sulcus, inferior and medial frontal gyri compared to the control task (see Table 4, Figure 2). Plots of activation magnitude confirm this medial frontal hyperactivation in JPL compared to healthy elders (see Figure S1). The past period showed greater activations for JPL, compared to healthy elders, in the right middle temporal gyrus compared to the future period (see Table 5). The future period showed no significant activations compared to the past period. No regions were less active in JPL compared to healthy elders.

Patient EP. At the individual level, results for the contrast future minus control task for EP showed activation in the right precuneus (see Table S6). No activation was detected for the contrast future minus past period (see Table S7).

At the group level, the past period showed greater activations for EP than healthy elders in the left middle occipital and precental gyri compared to the control task (see Table 3). No regions were less active in EP compared to healthy elders for this contrast.

The future period showed greater activations for EP than healthy elders in the right middle temporal gyrus compared to the control task (see Table 4, Figure 2). EP showed less activation than healthy elders in the left superior occipital gyrus and right insula for the future period compared to the control task (see Table 4, Figure 2).

The past period revealed greater activations for EP than healthy elders in left middle frontal gyrus compared to the future period (see Table 5). No regions were less active in EP compared to healthy elders for this contrast.

Conversely, the future period showed greater activations in EP than healthy elders in the left parietal gyrus compared to the past period (see Table 6, Figure 3). No regions were less active in EP compared to healthy elders for this contrast.

Patient LL. At the individual level, results for the contrast future minus control task for LL showed activation in the left supplementary motor area (see Table S6). Compared to the past

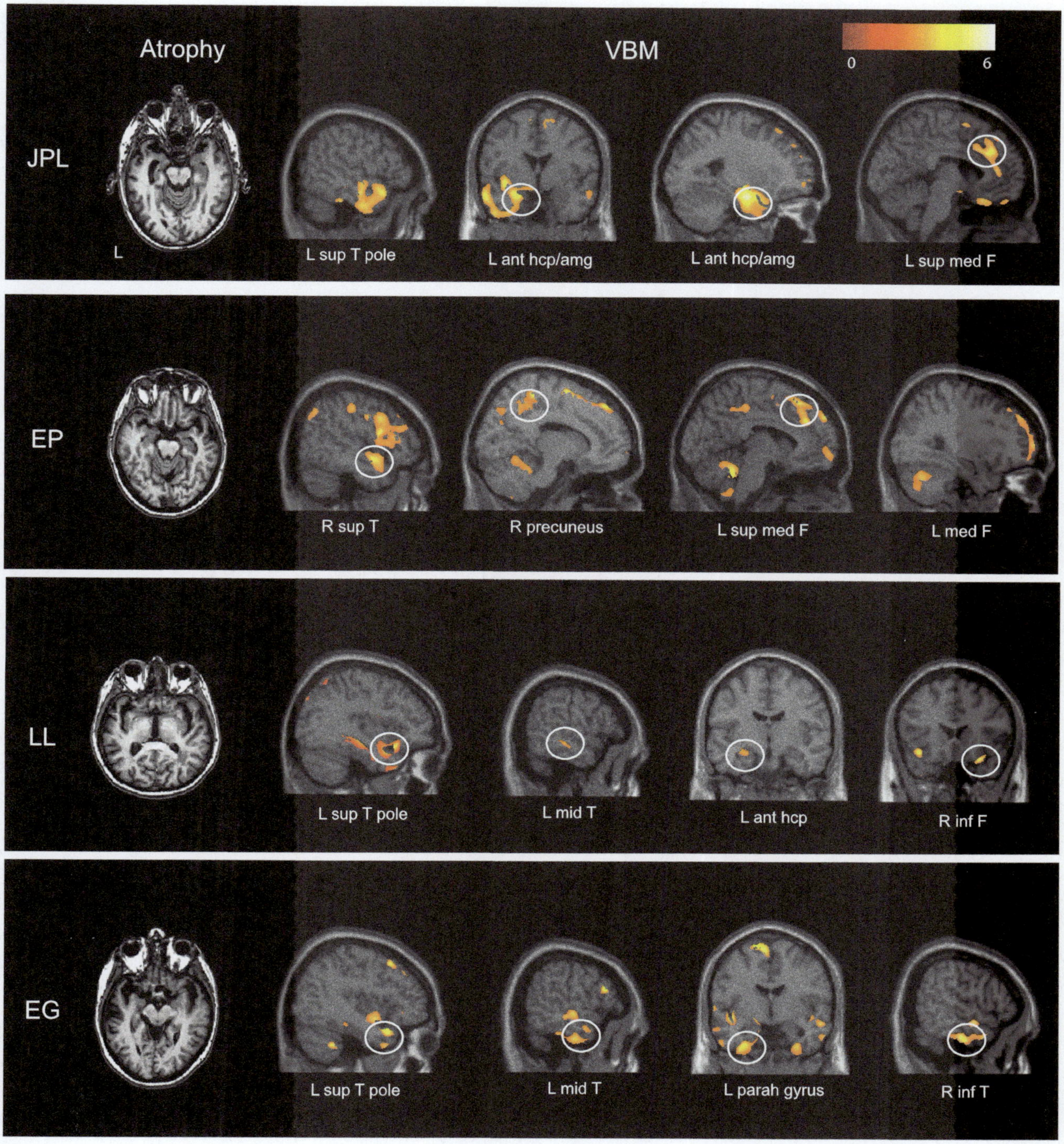

Figure 1. Structural brain scans of the four SD patients. Left panels show coronal sections through the brains of JPL, EP, LL and EG. Right panels show results of the VBM analysis superimposed on MRI scans for each patient at a corrected FWE threshold of $p<0.05$. The pronounced atrophy in superior medial frontal regions is apparent for JPL and EP and atrophy in left anterior hippocampus apparent for JPL and LL. Color scale shows voxel z-scores. See Tables S2 to S5 in File S1 for detailed VBM results. Abbreviations: amg = amygdala; ant = anterior; F = frontal; hcp = hippocampus; inf = inferior; L = left; med = medial; mid = middle; parah = parahippocampal; R = right; sup = superior; T = temporal.

period, the future period showed hyperactivation in the right middle occipital and supramarginal gyri (see Table S7).

At the group level, the past period showed greater activations for LL than healthy elders mainly in the bilateral middle temporal gyri, left middle and inferior frontal gyri, right cuneus and left caudate compared to the control task (see Table 3). LL showed less activation than healthy elders in essentially the right anterior hippocampus, left parahippocampal gyrus, lateral temporal and occipital gyri for the past period compared to the control task (see Table 3).

The future period revealed greater activations for LL than healthy elders mainly in the right supramarginal and left superior

Table 3. Results for the comparisons past>control task for JPL, EP, LL, EG compared to healthy elders (HE) with age and years of education (for EP) as covariates at a corrected FWE statistical threshold of $p<0.05$, $k>10$.

Regions	z-score	k	x	y	z
JPL>HE					
L inferior frontal gyrus	5.83	17	−34	16	28
L middle frontal gyrus	5.48	15	−44	16	40
R cuneus	5.78	21	14	−76	18
L cuneus	5.71	42	−10	−84	12
	5.40	16	−10	−72	22
L insula	5.66	24	−42	−4	−2
HE>JPL					
-	-	-	-	-	-
EP>HE					
L middle occipital gyrus	6.19	32	−46	−80	8
L precentral gyrus	5.59	47	−36	−14	46
HE>EP					
-	-	-	-	-	-
LL>HE					
R middle temporal gyrus	5.94	186	44	−58	8
L middle temporal gyrus	5.42	102	−40	−54	14
	5.13	102	−52	−58	18
L inferior frontal gyrus	5.86	67	−36	14	20
L middle frontal gyrus	5.40	67	−30	16	34
R cuneus	5.46	27	10	−86	28
L caudate	5.90	74	−16	26	2
HE>LL					
R anterior hippocampus	6.87	142	32	−4	−20
L parahippocampal gyrus	5.64	73	−30	−10	−24
R middle temporal gyrus	5.51	142	46	4	−20
R superior temporal pole	5.28	142	38	8	−28
L superior occipital gyrus	6.44	170	−20	−84	36
R superior occipital gyrus	5.66	20	26	−82	26
L middle occipital gyrus	5.37	170	−28	−76	28
	5.09	61	−24	−90	14
	5.41	19	−14	−88	−6
L cuneus	5.29	61	−10	−84	12
R inferior frontal gyrus	5.98	27	26	22	−18
R superior parietal gyrus	5.48	24	48	−38	58
R supramarginal gyrus	5.43	23	50	−34	38
	5.25	11	58	−36	30
R thalamus	5.98	81	16	−14	−2
L thalamus	5.19	64	−12	−14	−2
EG>HE					
L inferior frontal gyrus	6.66	52	−38	8	20
R middle cingulate gyrus	6.26	42	18	8	34
	5.76	29	16	−12	42
L anterior hippocampus	5.35	34	−30	−10	−22
R superior temporal pole	5.44	19	44	8	−22
HE>EG					
-	-	-	-	-	-

L: left, R: right.

Table 4. Results for the comparisons future>control task for JPL, EP, LL, EG compared to healthy elders (HE) with age and years of education (for EP) as covariates at a corrected FWE statistical threshold of p<0.05, k>10.

Regions	z-score	k	x	y	z
JPL>HE					
L calcarine sulcus	5.56	51	−10	−80	10
L inferior frontal gyrus	5.50	53	−48	20	8
L medial frontal gyrus	5.35	28	−4	10	62
HE>JPL					
-	-	-	-	-	-
EP>HE					
R middle temporal gyrus	5.35	10	52	−70	16
HE>EP					
L superior occipital gyrus	5.82	34	−20	−80	28
	5.39	34	−16	−76	36
R insula	5.36	29	36	−4	4
LL>HE					
R supramarginal gyrus	6.57	126	52	−36	38
	5.84	126	60	−36	28
	5.73	18	54	−24	32
L superior parietal gyrus	5.59	19	−26	−54	62
R medial frontal gyrus	5.66	15	10	4	56
	5.66	29	6	−14	66
	5.55	29	12	−10	70
L middle frontal gyrus	5.45	20	−34	6	54
R thalamus	5.78	13	8	−8	−8
HE>LL					
R superior frontal gyrus	5.81	233	26	4	60
L superior frontal gyrus	5.35	19	−20	4	62
	5.11	10	−16	10	58
R middle frontal gyrus	6.40	115	34	40	18
	5.64	115	26	42	22
	5.60	37	32	30	40
L middle frontal gyrus	5.77	25	−32	44	12
	5.41	54	−24	14	42
	5.33	54	−34	18	34
	5.15	54	−36	10	34
R inferior frontal gyrus	5.21	29	34	18	32
R supplementary motor area	5.31	50	8	−22	56
	5.71	31	4	−10	60
	5.28	16	14	18	58
L inferior parietal gyrus	5.79	55	−50	−24	38
R superior parietal gyrus	5.30	16	30	−66	50
L middle cingulate gyrus	5.77	50	0	−30	50
R fusiform gyrus	5.66	18	36	−42	−24
R inferior temporal gyrus	5.65	12	62	−40	−12
R superior temporal gyrus	5.55	22	56	−36	10
L posterior hippocampus	5.49	23	−30	−44	0
L posterior hippocampus	5.20	10	−24	−36	4
R precuneus	5.34	14	12	−54	66
L cuneus	5.82	36	−8	−76	18
R lingual gyrus	5.76	93	30	−48	−6
L middle occipital gyrus	5.15	10	−30	−72	20

Table 4. Cont.

Regions	z-score	k	x	y	z
R middle occipital gyrus	5.11	10	34	−76	26
R insula	5.97	54	34	−18	18
L caudate	6.04	102	−10	12	−8
	5.73	102	−4	6	−8
R caudate	5.17	102	8	10	−10
	5.91	58	14	22	10
R thalamus	5.55	19	2	−14	4
	5.45	27	12	−34	4
R vermis	5.64	36	6	−58	−16
EG>HE					
L superior temporal gyrus	5.64	45	−58	−10	0
	5.60	45	−56	−18	0
L superior parietal gyrus	5.48	16	−30	−66	52
HE>EG					
L superior occipital gyrus	6.96	118	−18	−82	54

L: left, R: right.

parietal gyri, right medial and left middle frontal gyri and right thalamus compared to the control task (see Table 4, Figure 2). LL showed less activation than healthy elders in essentially the left posterior hippocampus, frontal (bilateral superior, middle and right inferior) gyri, right precuneus, lateral parietal gyrus, right lateral temporal and occipital regions for the future period compared to the control task (see Table 4, Figure 2). Plots of activation magnitude confirm the significant lower activation in the left posterior hippocampus and right precuneus in LL compared to healthy elders (see Figure S1).

The past period showed greater activations for LL than healthy elders in the left posterior hippocampus, frontal (bilateral superior medial, middle, left superior and inferior frontal gyri), temporal (right middle, superior and left inferior temporal gyri), occipital (bilateral cuneus, middle and inferior occipital gyri) and parietal regions (angular, inferior parietal and supramarginal gyri, bilateral precuneus) compared to the future period (see Table 5). No regions were less active in LL compared to healthy elders for this contrast.

Conversely, the future period showed greater activations for LL than healthy elders in right anterior hippocampus, bilateral middle occipital gyri, right middle temporal pole and parietal regions (supramarginal and superior parietal gyri) compared to the past period (see Table 6, Figure 3). Plots of activation magnitude confirm this right anterior hippocampal hyperactivation in LL compared to healthy elders (see Figure S2). No regions were less active in LL compared to healthy elders for this contrast.

Patient EG. At the individual level, results for the contrast future minus control task for EG showed an essentially left-lateralized network of regions comprising the left middle frontal and temporal gyri (see Table S6). No activation was detected for the contrast future minus past period (see Table S7).

At the group level, the past period showed greater activations for EG than healthy elders in the left anterior hippocampus, left inferior frontal gyrus, right middle cingulate cortex and superior temporal pole compared to the control task (see Table 3). No regions were less active in EG compared to healthy elders for this contrast.

The future period showed greater activations for EG than healthy elders in the left superior temporal and superior parietal gyri compared to the control task (see Table 4, Figure 2). EG showed less activation than healthy elders in the left superior occipital gyrus for the future period compared to the control task (see Table 4, Figure 2).

The past period showed greater activations for EG than healthy elders in the left superior occipital gyrus compared to the future period (see Table 5). No regions were less active in EG compared to healthy elders for this contrast.

Conversely, the future period showed greater activations for EG than healthy elders in the right middle temporal gyrus and left calcarine sulcus compared to the past period (see Table 6, Figure 3). No regions were less active in EG compared to healthy elders for this contrast.

For sake of clarity, we also added results of the contrast future minus control task in healthy elders (see Table S8 in File S1). Results for the contrast future minus past period in healthy elders have been published previously [19].

Discussion

This work is, to our knowledge, the first fMRI study examining future projection in semantic dementia. While the sparse behavioral studies found that future projection was consistently impaired in SD [18,16,17], here we show that the capability of patients to project into their future largely depends on the structural integrity of certain brain regions, in particular the superior medial frontal cortex and anterior hippocampus. JPL presented atrophy in bilateral superior medial frontal gyri and left anterior hippocampus and had difficulties in experiencing episodic future events and to a certain extent past episodic events. Hyperactivations of neocortical (frontal and occipital) regions appeared inefficient in compensating for his deficit. EP presented atrophy in bilateral superior medial frontal gyri and, like JPL, could pre-experience only one episodic future event, but past episodic remembering was spared. However, behavioral ratings for the future were higher than those of healthy elders (in terms of

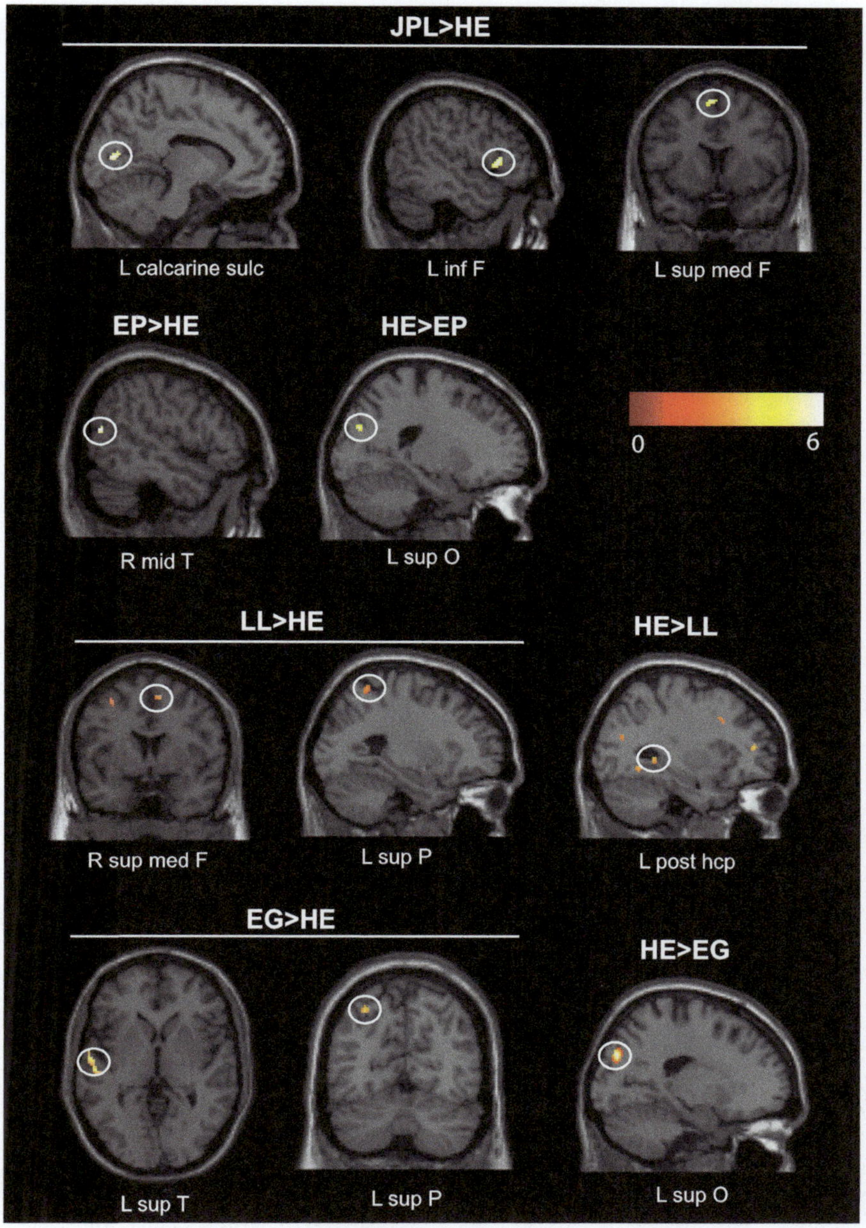

Figure 2. Results of the comparisons between the future period and the control task for EP, LL and EG depicting hyperactivations (Patient>HE) and lower activations (HE>Patient) compared to healthy elders (HE) at a corrected FWE threshold of p<0.05, k>10 voxels. Color scale shows voxel z-scores. See Table 4 for full details. Abbreviations: F = frontal; hcp = hippocampus; sup = superior; inf = inferior; L = left; med = medial; mid = middle; O = occipital; P = parietal; post = posterior; R = right; sulc = sulcus; T = temporal.

emotion and mental imagery), suggesting that EP may have overestimated her capacities to project into the future. On the contrary, LL was able to pre-experience episodic future events. Although she had left anterior hippocampal atrophy, hyperactivation of its right counterpart during future compared to past thinking compensated efficiently for this atrophy. Finally, EG who presented integrity of superior medial frontal gyri and anterior hippocampi was also able to pre-experience episodic future events. Figure 4 depicts summary representations of patients' ability to engage in episodic future thinking (disturbed or spared) depicting sites of atrophy with associated hypothesized function and brain activations for each patient compared to healthy elders. Overall, VBM analyses showed that patients who had difficulties in envisioning the future in an episodic way (JPL and EP) presented specific atrophy in superior medial prefrontal cortex, while this region was relatively preserved in LL and EG who could engage in episodic future projection. Furthermore, JPL and LL presented atrophy in (left) anterior hippocampus, a region known to be crucial for episodic past and future thinking, but LL was able to compensate efficiently by hyperactivation of its right counterpart, while JPL could not. We will mainly focus on these two key regions in the following discussion, distinguishing patients who cannot (JPL and EP) or can (LL and EG) engage in episodic future thinking.

Patients impaired in episodic future projection

JPL presented atrophy mainly in left anterior hippocampus, lateral (middle and inferior) temporal and frontal cortices, including in the bilateral superior medial frontal gyri. Behavioral ratings showed that he was impaired at episodic future projection

Table 5. Results for contrast past>future for JPL, EP, LL, EG compared to healthy elders (HE) with age and years of education (for EP) as covariates at a corrected FWE statistical threshold of p<0.05, k>10.

Regions	z-score	k	x	y	z
JPL>HE					
R middle temporal gyrus	5.62	14	44	−70	14
EP>HE					
L middle frontal gyrus	5.83	52	−34	−6	44
LL>HE					
R superior medial frontal gyrus	6.30	65	10	62	26
	5.46	83	4	66	4
L superior medial frontal gyrus	5.53	142	−4	64	28
	5.15	142	−6	62	20
	5.43	83	−8	62	0
L superior frontal gyrus	5.73	151	−16	58	16
	5.27	151	−20	60	24
	5.48	12	−18	36	52
	5.04	39	−20	48	16
L medial frontal gyrus	5.16	33	−12	50	−6
R medial frontal gyrus	5.41	12	2	−20	56
L middle frontal gyrus	6.19	161	−30	16	36
	6.11	151	−36	58	14
	6.08	52	−30	44	10
	5.45	29	−46	30	30
	5.40	39	−20	48	26
R middle frontal gyrus	6.00	34	32	16	54
	5.99	162	42	14	42
	5.69	34	32	10	48
L inferior frontal gyrus	5.15	17	−56	18	30
	5.26	12	−46	28	16
L posterior hippocampus	6.07	108	−26	−40	−2
	5.83	108	−24	−38	6
R parahippocampal gyrus	5.82	308	36	−38	−12
R middle temporal gyrus	5.66	51	54	−54	8
	5.23	51	44	−56	10
	5.39	42	18	−74	58
R superior temporal gyrus	5.56	40	58	−34	10
L inferior temporal gyrus	5.35	21	46	−68	8
	5.29	12	−46	−60	−12
R fusiform gyrus	5.34	35	26	−78	−6
R cuneus	6.08	59	12	−88	30
L cuneus	5.72	21	−10	−78	20
L middle occipital gyrus	5.98	48	−36	−74	24
	5.35	55	−24	−58	32
	5.14	80	−38	−78	36
R inferior occipital gyrus	5.43	35	34	−86	−4
	5.15	12	38	−76	−4
R angular gyrus	6.55	180	40	−62	40
	6.01	180	46	−72	36
L angular gyrus	5.57	55	−34	−54	36
L inferior parietal gyrus	5.67	60	−52	−24	38
	5.51	80	−32	−78	42
R inferior parietal gyrus	5.39	39	56	−52	46

Table 5. Cont.

Regions	z-score	k	x	y	z
	5.19	39	56	−44	44
R supramarginal gyrus	5.55	19	52	−22	22
R precuneus	5.74	35	12	−50	44
	5.48	13	8	−56	56
L precuneus	5.62	66	−12	−56	40
L anterior cingulate gyrus	5.43	20	−6	44	6
L middle cingulate gyrus	5.76	58	−4	−42	46
R thalamus	5.64	29	12	−32	4
	5.44	20	18	−20	14
R cerebellum	6.44	205	12	−62	−16
	5.75	205	18	−64	−22
	5.53	13	34	−42	−26
EG>HE					
L superior occipital gyrus	6.29	28	−16	−84	34

No regions were less active by patients compared to healthy elders for this contrast. L: left, R: right.

and past remembering. The overall autobiographical score (AS) for the future and a trend for the strictly episodic autobiographical score (ES) for the past were significantly lower compared to healthy elders, indicating that JPL had difficulties in providing episodic details for future and past periods. A trend also showed that he produced less episodic future events compared to healthy elders. Irish et al. [16] showed that the future thinking deficit in SD was driven by a difficulty to provide "internal" details (i.e., episodic details, central to the event), while "external" details (i.e., semantic facts) were more numerous. With JPL, we confirm behavioral studies showing that SD patients are impaired at projecting into the future in an episodic way [18,16,17] and provide the neural correlates of these cognitive findings. JPL presented atrophy in bilateral superior medial frontal gyri (approximately corresponding to Brodmann areas 8 and 9). This area has been previously reported in episodic prospection studies [73,74,75,36] and has a role in processing coherent contexts [36] (BA9), manipulating processes in working memory [76] (BA8),

Table 6. Results for contrast future>past for JPL, EP, LL, EG compared to healthy elders (HE) with age and years of education (for EP) as covariates at a corrected FWE statistical threshold of $p<0.05$, $k>10$.

Regions	z-score	k	x	y	z
JPL>HE					
-	-	-	-	-	-
EP>HE					
L inferior parietal cortex	6.90	91	−52	−34	46
	6.54	91	−44	−42	52
LL>HE					
L middle occipital gyrus	6.77	130	−22	−82	36
R middle occipital gyrus	5.72	12	26	−92	6
R supramarginal gyrus	6.68	262	52	−36	38
	6.28	262	60	−36	30
	6.11	262	54	−22	32
L superior parietal gyrus	5.44	15	−24	−54	60
R posterior hippocampus	5.80	23	24	−44	4
R anterior hippocampus	5.42	21	30	−4	−20
R middle temporal pole	5.28	15	46	4	−18
EG>HE					
R middle temporal gyrus	5.52	21	60	−52	8
L calcarine sulcus	5.35	14	−6	−90	−6

No regions were less active by patients compared to healthy elders for this contrast. L: left, R: right.

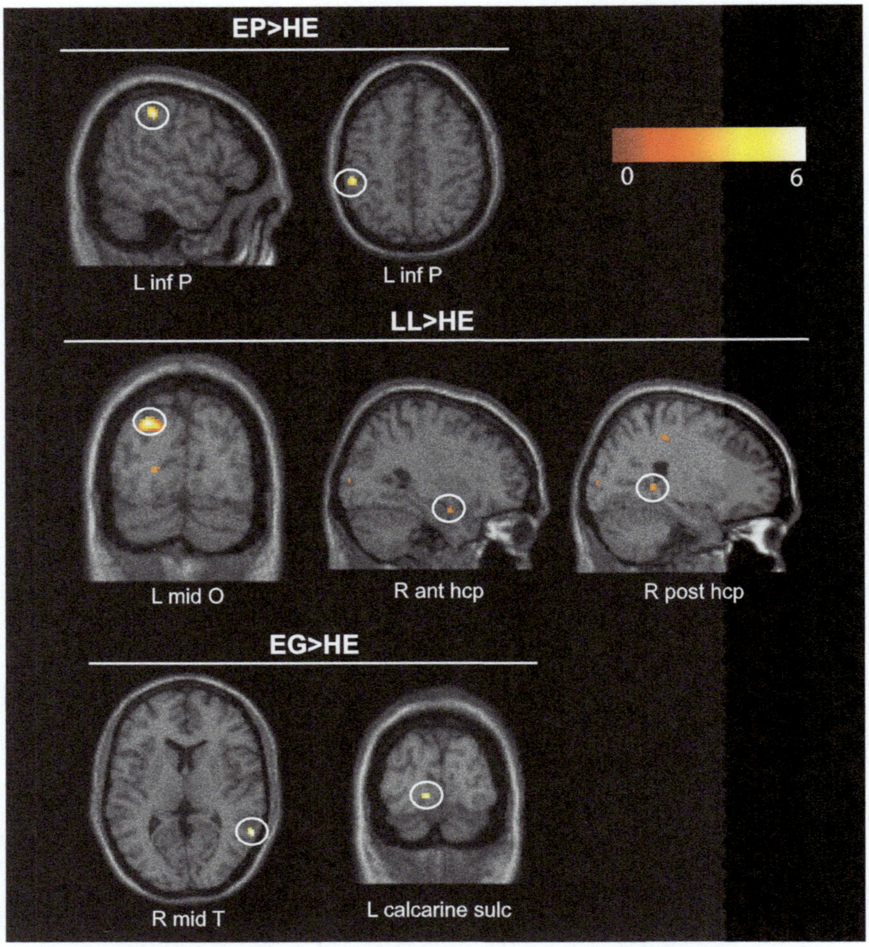

Figure 3. Results of the comparisons between the future and past periods for JPL, EP, LL and EG compared to healthy elders (HE) at a corrected FWE threshold of $p<0.05$, $k>10$ voxels. See Table 6 for full details. Abbreviations: ant = anterior; hcp = hippocampus; inf = inferior; L = left; mid = middle; O = occipital; P = parietal; post = posterior; R = right; sulc = sulcus; T = temporal.

creative story generation [77] (BA8) and autonoetic consciousness [8,37], essential to pre-experience episodic future events. Bilateral atrophy in this region may also have been responsible for JPL's inability to project into the future. JPL also presents atrophy in the left anterior hippocampus. We previously showed that anterior hippocampal integrity in SD is crucial for episodic past remembering [6,70]. Here, we expand these findings to episodic future thinking which also requires anterior hippocampal integrity. The anterior hippocampus supports relational processing [31,32,33], including flexible recombination of details for past and future event construction [34]. Addis and Schacter [35] showed that future-associated activity in the anterior hippocampus was associated with higher demands on recombination of details. Left atrophy in this region may be in part responsible for JPL's inability to project into the future in an episodic way. Thus, we confirm that atrophy in crucial regions of the future thinking network (e.g., superior medial frontal gyrus and anterior hippocampus), overlapping with the autobiographical memory network, impairs episodic future projection. Examination of activation patterns at the individual level indicated that JPL failed to activate the core episodic future thinking network observed in healthy elders (reported in Table S8 and Viard et al. [19]), although several regions may show similar activation patterns across patient and healthy elders (e.g., precuneus, middle cingulate gyrus). Compared to healthy elders, JPL hyperactivated left (medial and inferior) frontal and occipital regions during future thinking compared to the control task. Plots of activation magnitude confirmed hyperactivation in the medial frontal gyrus in JPL compared to healthy elders. Yet, these hyperactivations did not efficiently compensate for atrophied regions, since he was unable to pre-experience episodic future events, as shown by behavioral results.

EP also presented atrophy in frontal cortices, including bilateral superior medial frontal gyri, and lateral (middle and superior) temporal cortices, but sparing of anterior hippocampi. EP was able to pre-experience only one episodic future event, most being semantic. Indeed, like JPL, a trend showed that EP produced less episodic future events compared to healthy elders. She was however not impaired at episodic past remembering. It appears that integrity of anterior hippocampi may have permitted EP to remember episodic past memories, but atrophy of bilateral superior medial frontal gyri may have been in part responsible for EP's deficit in episodic future thinking. Examination of activation patterns at the individual level indicated that, except for the right precuneus, EP failed to activate the core future thinking network observed in healthy elders (Table S8; [19]). Direct comparisons with healthy elders showed that EP hyperactived the inferior parietal and middle temporal cortices for the

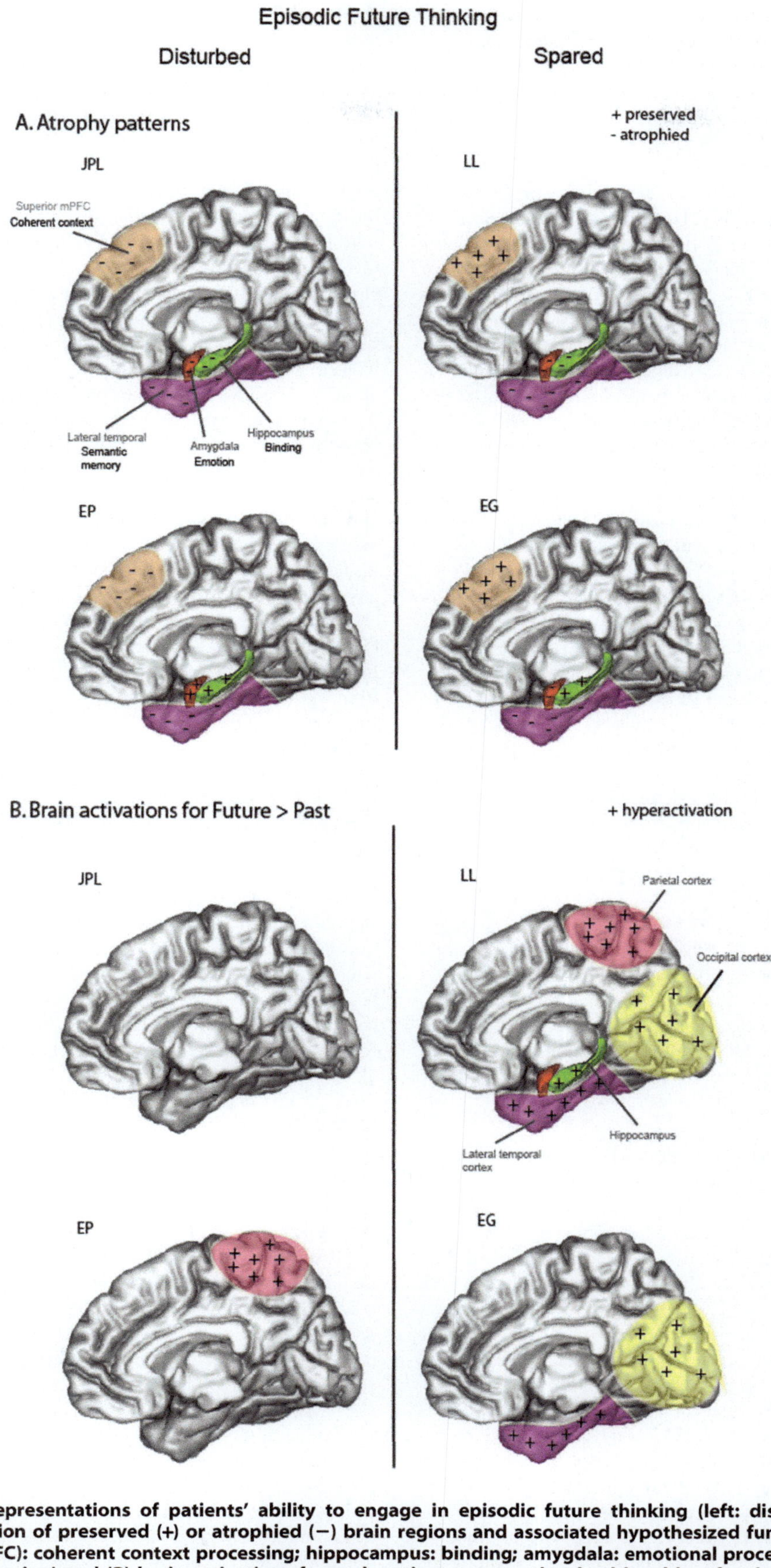

Figure 4. Summary representations of patients' ability to engage in episodic future thinking (left: disturbed; right: spared) depicting (A) localization of preserved (+) or atrophied (−) brain regions and associated hypothesized function (superior medial prefrontal cortex (mPFC): coherent context processing; hippocampus: binding; amygdala: emotional processing; lateral temporal cortex: semantic processing) and (B) brain activations for each patient compared to healthy elders for the contrast Future>Past thinking (see results on Table 6).

future compared to the past period, or to the control task, which appeared inefficient in compensating for her deficit, since she could pre-experience only one episodic future event.

EP had higher ratings on the scale of emotional intensity compared to healthy elders for the past and the future. Conversely, Irish et al. [78] found impaired emotion processing in a group of SD patients during past remembering and suspected that atrophy in the amygdala, generally reported in such patients, might explain their emotional processing deficit. Here, EP's bilateral amygdala were not atrophied compared to healthy elders, but she showed less activation than healthy elders in the right insula for the future compared to the control task, a region known to be implicated in emotional processing [79,80,81]. Hence, EP seems to evaluate the phenomenological nature of her mental evocations inadequately and may tend to exaggerate or overestimate her emotions on behavioral self-ratings. This may be paralleled with Irish et al.'s [16] findings of a disconnect between "objective" task performances (as shown here by scores on the episodic scale) and "subjective" phenomenological pre-experiencing (as shown here by self-ratings) when generating future events in SD. An early report by Snowden et al. [82] had already indicated that SD patients showed "exaggerated reactions to sensory stimuli" which fits with the present results.

Decreased activity in the occipital cortex for the future period compared to the control task was observed for EP compared to healthy elders. This decreased activity in a visuospatial area for the future contradicts EP's behavioral self-ratings on visual imagery which indicate a greater number of mental images for the future for EP compared to healthy elders. Yet, a trend showed that EP's image quality of future events was less clear compared to healthy elders. Overall, as for ratings of emotional intensity, EP may have overestimated the number of images she visualized.

Overall, JPL and EP both presented atrophy in bilateral superior medial prefrontal cortices, in addition to their lateral temporal atrophy, and were impaired at projecting into the future in an episodic way. JPL, unlike EP, was also impaired at remembering the past and presented atrophy in left anterior hippocampus. Thus, joint atrophy in bilateral superior medial prefrontal cortices and anterior hippocampi may have prevented episodic thinking in the past and the future (as observed in JPL). Atrophy in bilateral superior medial prefrontal cortices, but preservation of anterior hippocampal structures, appear to preserve past episodic recollection, at least to a certain extent, but impairs episodic future thinking (as observed in EP).

Patients capable to engage in episodic future thinking

LL presented atrophy mainly in left anterior hippocampus, frontal (superior, inferior) and lateral (middle and superior) temporal cortices. LL was able to pre-experience episodic future events. Examination of activation patterns at the individual level showed that LL failed to activate the core future thinking network observed in healthy elders (Table S8; [19]), although several regions (e.g., occipital and parietal cortices) showed similar activation patterns across her and healthy elders. Nevertheless, she was able to engage in episodic future thinking and pre-experience future plans. Thus, at the neural level, she was able to develop different strategies from those of healthy elders which proved successful at the behavioral level since she was able to perform the future thinking task by envisionning several episodic future events. Indeed, hyperactivation in the right anterior hippocampus was detected for future compared to past thinking, confirmed by plots of activation magnitude. This right anterior hippocampal activation probably compensated for atrophy in its left counterpart. Addis et al. [74] showed that future event construction uniquely engaged the right hippocampus, possibly as a response to the novelty of these events. Beyond its role in relational processing in memory [83], this structure also has the capacity to bind disparate event details for novel future scenarios. Of note, out of the four patients, LL was the one who showed the most reductions in the pattern of neural activity compared to healthy adults, essentially in occipital regions for the past and occipital and frontal regions for the future. These reductions, however, appeared to be sufficiently compensated by hyperactivations in LL (in occipital cortex for the past and frontal cortex for the future) compared to healthy adults, since she was able to efficiently engage in episodic past and future thinking.

EG was able to engage in episodic past and future thinking in spite of atrophy in lateral temporal areas (superior, middle, inferior) gyri and poles and frontal (superior, middle) regions. Irish et al. [17] showed that atrophy in lateral temporal (inferior temporal cortex and temporal pole) correlated with deficits in episodic future thinking in their group of SD patients. Here, although correlations were not possible since we report single cases, we show that EG and LL, who were both able to engage in episodic future thinking, hyperactivated remnant tissue in lateral temporal lobes for the future compared to the past. Hence, our results corroborate Irish et al.'s [17] findings which suggest that lateral temporal cortex, strongly implicated in semantic memory, is critical for the construction of novel future events. Altogether, we extend Irish et al.'s [17] findings by showing that lateral temporal hyperactivation in addition to the integrity of superior medial frontal cortex and anterior hippocampus promote episodic future thinking in SD patients.

Overall, two patients out of four (LL and EG) were able to engage in episodic future thinking, unlike what has been reported in the behavioral literature [16,17,18]. Methodological differences may explain these discrepancies. Here, we used highly personalized cues derived from an interview with the spouse. These personally-relevant stimuli directly point to a specific event. Previous studies, instead, used single words which the patient should use to imagine a plausible future event. These stimuli may not immediately direct to a unique personally-relevant event which has already been planned by the participant. Hence, constructing personally-relevant sentences may be more helpful to trigger episodic future thinking in patients with semantic dementia who present integrity of superior medial prefrontal cortices and anterior hippocampus. Moreover, the group analysis approach used in previous studies may have obscured preservation of function that might have been evident in some (but not all) patients, which we highlighted here by using a case study approach.

Limits

Albeit the clinical and theoretical relevance of the present findings, some potential limits should be mentioned. Given the rarity of patients with semantic dementia, we were not able to perfectly match each patient to the control group. Thus, results may have been influenced by differences in age and years of education (only EP) between each patient and the group of healthy elders. Yet, these variables were added as covariates in the analyses to attenuate any confound between patients and healthy elders. Adding a second covariate to control for differences in education between EP and healthy elders may have underestimated brain activations in EP. Yet, even with a higher education level compared to healthy elders, EP had difficulties in episodic future thinking. Hence, brain activations which may have been underestimated in the analyses (due to the addition of covariates) could not have been sufficient anyway to compensate for EP's deficit in episodic future thinking, since she was able to pre-experience only one episodic future event.

Another potential bias is that a male (JPL) was compared to a group of healthy females. Semantic dementia affects similarly males and females [84,85] and no studies have shown a gender effect in this pathology. However, some studies have observed gender differences favouring women on episodic-memory tasks requiring verbal processing, but favouring men when requiring visuospatial processing [86,87,88]. Yet, the gender difference between JPL and the group of healthy elders may have played only a marginal role in the present results as mental retrieval of past memories and future projection involve both verbal and visuo-spatial processing.

Finally, unlike some studies in the future thinking field that use the cue-word technique with generic stimuli [16,17,74], the task used here was not to simulate or imagine a plausible fictitious future event, but to pre-experience an actual future event that was really supposed to happen in the next twelve months, prompted from a personally-relevant cue. In other words, future events had not happened yet, but were going to happen. Hence, since future events were actual projects that participants really intended to pursue in the future, these were planned in the past. Of note, in everyday life, this kind of future thinking is very frequent, probably the most frequent concerning the recent future. Thus, retrieval processes may have happened in the future thinking condition. Results from behavioral scales evaluating recent reactivation can indicate if each event was evoked recently or not. On the frequency of rehearsal scale, LL and EG obtained scores below 4.5 indicating that they did not frequently rehearse their future plans in the past. EP obtained a score of 9.5, suggesting that she frequently rehearsed her future plans. Yet, EP envisioned only one episodic future event (the four other events being semantic). Thus, she was probably able to envision this unique future plan in an episodic way because she had frequently rehearsed it. On the last recall scale, EP, LL and EG obtained scores indicating that, on average, they last recalled their future plans a sufficiently long time ago, minimizing a possible retrieval effect. It is nevertheless possible that by presenting cues referring to actual future plans, a retrospective thinking effect may have happened. However, unlike some future thinking studies in which participants are asked to imagine plausible future events (which are not necessarily going to happen) using generic cues, here we chose to study the self-projecting aspect of future thinking in which future actions are planned beforehand [12]. It would be interesting to study the purely imaginative aspect, as some studies have already explored [89].

Conclusion

Altogether, this study aimed at examining the neural correlates of future projection in SD compared to past remembering. Main results indicated that episodic future projection in patients with lateral temporal atrophy largely depends on the integrity of superior medial prefrontal cortices and anterior hippocampi. With atrophy in the bilateral superior medial frontal gyri and left anterior hippocampus, JPL was unable to engage into past or future episodic thinking, in spite of neocortical hyperactivity which appeared inefficient in compensating for atrophy within these key regions. EP presented atrophy in bilateral superior medial frontal gyri and was, like JPL, able to pre-experience only one episodic future event, but past remembering appeared relatively preserved. On the contrary, LL despite atrophy in the left anterior hippocampus, was able to efficiently compensate for the deficit by hyperactivating its right counterpart during episodic future thinking. EG, who did not show atrophy in the superior medial frontal gyrus nor anterior hippocampus, was able to envision episodic future events. Altogether, these findings suggest that patients' ability to envision the future in an episodic way largely depends on the severity and localization of their atrophy, in addition to their lateral temporal atrophy. Our results indicate that the integrity of the superior medial frontal gyri and anterior hippocampi, in addition to the use of personally-relevant cues, are essential to trigger episodic future thinking.

Supporting Information

File S1 Contains the following files: **Table S1**: Behavioral ratings comparing EP and healthy elders (HE) for past and future periods with years of education added as covariate. Significant results appear in bold ($p<0.05$). AS = autobiographical score; ES = strictly episodic autobiographical score; Nb = number; p = probability; sd = standard deviation. **Table S2**: Areas of grey matter volume loss in JPL vs. 12 healthy elders at a corrected FWE statistical threshold of $p<0.05$. L: left, R: right. **Table S3**: Areas of grey matter volume loss in EP vs. 12 healthy control participants at a corrected FWE statistical threshold of $p<0.05$. L: left, R: right. **Table S4**: Areas of grey matter volume loss in LL vs. 12 healthy elders at a corrected FWE statistical threshold of $p<0.05$. L: left, R: right. **Table S5**: Areas of grey matter volume loss in EG vs. 12 healthy control participants at a corrected FWE statistical threshold of $p<0.05$. L: left, R: right. **Table S6**: Results for the contrast future>control task for JPL, EP, LL and EG at a corrected FWE statistical threshold of $p<0.05$, $k>10$. **Table S7**: Results for the contrast future>past period for JPL, EP, LL and EG at a corrected FWE statistical threshold of $p<0.05$, $k>10$. L: left, R: right. **Table S8**: Results for the contrast future>control task for healthy elders at a corrected FWE statistical threshold of $p<0.05$, $k>10$. L: left, R: right. SMA = supplemental motor area. **Figure S1**: plots of activation magnitude for each patient (JPL, EP, LL and EG) and average of healthy elders (Ctl) in the bilateral medial frontal gyri, hippocampi and precuneus for the contrast future>control task. **Table S9**: Brief explanation of the neuropsychological tests used to test participants and what they measure. **Table S10**: Specificity scoring chart of past and future episodic tasks, performed at debriefing.

Acknowledgments

Thanks to Brigitte Landeau, Karine Lebreton, Vanessa Matuszewski, Alice Pélerin and Alan Young for their help in this study.

Author Contributions

Conceived and designed the experiments: AV PP BD FE. Performed the experiments: AV PP VdLS. Analyzed the data: AV. Contributed reagents/materials/analysis tools: AV. Wrote the paper: AV. Patient recruitment: VdLS SB.

References

1. Snowden JS, Goulding PJ, Neary D (1989) Semantic dementia: A form of circumscribed cerebral atrophy. Behav Neurol 2: 167–182.
2. Neary D, Snowden JS, Gustafson L, Passant U, Stuss D, et al. (1998) Frontotemporal lobar degeneration: a consensus on clinical diagnostic criteria. Neurology 51: 1546–1554.

3. Hodges JR, Patterson K (2007) Semantic dementia: a unique clinicopathological syndrome. Lancet Neurol 6: 1004–1014.
4. Desgranges B, Matuszewski V, Piolino P, Chételat G, Mézenge F, et al. (2007) Anatomical and functional alterations in semantic dementia: a voxel-based MRI and PET study. Neurobiol of Aging 28: 1904–1913.
5. Hodges JR, Graham KS (2001) Episodic memory: insights from semantic dementia. Philos Trans R Soc Lond B Biol Sci 356: 1423–1434.
6. Viard A, Desgranges B, Matuszewski V, Lebreton K, Belliard S, et al. (2013) Autobiographical memory in semantic dementia: New insights from two patients using fMRI. Neuropsychologia 51: 2620–2632.
7. Tulving E (2001) Episodic memory and common sense: how far apart? Philos Trans R Soc Lond B Biol Sci 356: 1505–1515.
8. Wheeler MA, Stuss DT, Tulving E (1997) Toward a theory of episodic memory: the frontal lobes and autonoetic consciousness. Psychol Bull 121: 331–354.
9. D'Argembeau A, Van der Linden M (2004) Phenomenal characteristics associated with projecting oneself back into the past and forward into the future: influence of valence and temporal distance. Conscious Cogn 13: 844–858.
10. D'Argembeau A, Van der Linden M (2006) Individual differences in the phenomenology of mental time travel: The effect of vivid visual imagery and emotion regulation strategies. Conscious Cogn 15: 342–350.
11. Gamboz N, Brandimonte MA, De Vito S (2010) The role of past in the simulation of autobiographical future episodes. Exp Psychol 57: 419–428.
12. Buckner RL, Carroll DC (2007) Self-projection and the brain. Trends Cogn Sci 11: 49–57.
13. Hassabis D, Maguire EA (2007) Deconstructing episodic memory with construction. Trends Cogn Sci 11: 299–306.
14. Hassabis D, Maguire EA (2009) The construction system of the brain. Philos Trans R Soc Lond B Biol Sci 364: 1263–1271.
15. Schacter DL, Addis DR (2007) The cognitive neuroscience of constructive memory: remembering the past and imagining the future. Philos Trans R Soc Lond B Biol Sci 362: 773–786.
16. Irish M, Addis DR, Hodges JR, Piguet O (2012a) Exploring the content and quality of episodic future simulations in semantic dementia. Neuropsychologia 50: 3488
17. Irish M, Addis DR, Hodges JR, Piguet O (2012b) Considering the role of semantic memory in episodic future thinking: evidence from semantic dementia. Brain 135: 2178
18. Duval C, Desgranges B, de La Sayette V, Belliard S, Eustache F, et al. (2012) What happens to personal identity when semantic knowledge degrades? A study of the self and autobiographical memory in semantic dementia. Neuropsychologia 50: 254–265.
19. Viard A, Chételat G, Lebreton K, Desgranges B, Landeau B, et al. (2011) Mental time travel into the past and the future in healthy aged adults: an fMRI study. Brain Cogn 75: 1–9.
20. Chan D, Fox NC, Scahill RI, Crum WR, Whitwell JL, et al. (2001) Patterns of temporal lobe atrophy in semantic dementia and Alzheimer's disease. Ann Neurol 49: 433–442.
21. Good CD, Scahill RI, Fox NC, Ashburner J, Friston KJ, et al. (2002) Automatic differentiation of anatomical patterns in the human brain: validation with studies of degenerative dementias. NeuroImage 17: 29–46.
22. Rosen HJ, Gorno-Tempini ML, Goldman WP, Perry RJ, Schuff N, et al. (2002) Patterns of brain atrophy in frontotemporal dementia and semantic dementia. Neurology 58: 198–208.
23. Boxer AL, Rankin KP, Miller BL, Schuff N, Weiner M, et al. (2003) Cinguloparietal atrophy distinguishes Alzheimer disease from semantic dementia. Arch Neurol 60: 949–956.
24. Davies RR, Graham KS, Xuereb JH, Williams GB, Hodges JR (2004) The human perirhinal cortex and semantic memory. Eur J Neurosci 20: 2441–2446.
25. van de Pol LA, Hensel A, van der Flier WM, Visser PJ, Pijnenburg YA, et al. (2006) Hippocampal atrophy on MRI in frontotemporal lobar degeneration and Alzheimer's disease. J Neurol Neurosurg Psychiatry 77: 439–442.
26. Nestor PJ, Fryer TD, Hodges JR (2006) Declarative memory impairments in Alzheimer's disease and semantic dementia. NeuroImage 30: 1010–1020.
27. Lehmann M, Douiri A, Kim LG, Modat M, Chan D, et al. (2010) Atrophy patterns in Alzheimer's disease and semantic dementia: a comparison of FreeSurfer and manual volumetric measurements. NeuroImage 49: 2264–2274.
28. Acosta-Cabronero J, Patterson K, Fryer TD, Hodges JR, Pengas G, et al. (2011). Atrophy, hypometabolism and white matter abnormalities in semantic dementia tell a coherent story. Brain 134: 2025–2035.
29. La Joie R, Perrotin A, de La Sayette V, Egret S, Doeuvre L, et al. (2013) Hippocampal subfield volumetry in mild cognitive impairment, Alzheimer's disease and semantic dementia. NeuroImage Clin 3:155–162.
30. Mummery CJ, Patterson K, Price CJ, Ashburner J, Frackowiak RS, et al. (2000) A voxel-based morphometry study of semantic dementia: relationship between temporal lobe atrophy and semantic memory. Ann Neurol 47: 36–45.
31. Chua EF, Schacter DL, Rand-Giovannetti E, Sperling RA (2007) Evidence for a specific role of the anterior hippocampal region in successful associative encoding. Hippocampus 17: 1071–1080.
32. Davachi L, Mitchell JP, Wagner AD (2003) Multiple routes to memory: distinct medial temporal lobe processes build item and source memories. Proc Natl Acad Sci U S A 100: 2157–2162.
33. Jackson O 3rd, Schacter DL (2004) Encoding activity in anterior medial temporal lobe supports subsequent associative recognition. NeuroImage 21: 456–462.
34. Preston AR, Shrager Y, Dudukovic NM, Gabrieli JD (2004) Hippocampal contribution to the novel use of relational information in declarative memory. Hippocampus 14: 148–152.
35. Addis DR, Schacter DL (2008) Constructive episodic simulation: temporal distance and detail of past and future events modulate hippocampal engagement. Hippocampus 18: 227–237.
36. Abraham A, Schubotz RI, von Cramon DY (2008) Thinking about the future versus the past in personal and non-personal contexts. Brain Res 1233: 106–119.
37. Nyberg L, Kim AS, Habib R, Levine B, Tulving E (2010) Consciousness of subjective time in the brain. Proc Natl Acad Sci U S A 107: 22356–22359.
38. Viard A, Desgranges B, Eustache F, Piolino P (2012) Factors affecting medial temporal lobe engagement for past and future episodic events: an ALE meta-analysis of neuroimaging studies. Brain Cogn 80: 111–125.
39. Gorno-Tempini ML, Hillis AE, Weintraub S, Kertesz A, Mendez M, et al. (2011) Classification of primary progressive aphasia and its variants. Neurology 76:1006–1014.
40. Grober E, Buschke H (1987) Genuine memory deficits in dementia. Dev Neuropsychol 3: 13–36.
41. Rey A (1970) Test de mémorisation d'une série de 15 mots. In: Rey A, editor. L'examen clinique en psychologie. Paris: PUF.
42. Cardebat D, Doyon B, Puel M, Goulet P, Joanette Y (1990) [Formal and semantic lexical evocation in normal subjects. Performance and dynamics of production as a function of sex, age and educational level]. Acta Neurol Belg 90: 207–217.
43. Desgranges B, Eustache F, Rioux P, de La Sayette V, Lechevalier B (1996) Memory disorders in Alzheimer's disease and the organization of human memory. Cortex 32: 387–412.
44. Belliard S, Perron M, Rouyer F, Golfier V, Sartori E, et al. (2001) [Présentation d'une batterie franç aise de personnes célèbres. Résultats auprès de patients atteints de démence sémantique]. Revue Neurologique 157:10–14.
45. Deltour JJ (1993) Echelle de vocabulaire de Mill Hill de JC Raven. Adaptation française et normes européennes du Mill Hill et du Standard Progressive Matrices de Raven. Braine-le-Chateau: Editions l'application des techniques modernes.
46. de Partz MP, Bilocq V, De Wilde V, Seron X, Pillon A (2001) LEXIS: Tests pour l'évaluation des troubles lexicaux chez la personne aphasique. Marseille: Solal.
47. Reitan R (1958) Validity of the Trail Making Test as an indicator of organic brain damage. Percept Mot Skills 8: 271–276.
48. Merck C, Charnallet A, Auriacombe A, Belliard S, Hahn-Barma V, et al. (2011) The GRECO neuropsychological semantic battery (BECS GRECO): Validation and normative data. Rev Neuropsychol 3: 235–255.
49. Folstein MF, Folstein SE, McHugh PR (1975) Mini -mental state. A practical method for grading the cognitive state of patients for the clinician. J Psychiatr Res 12: 189–198.
50. Matuszewski V, Piolino P, Belliard S, de la Sayette V, Laisney M, et al. (2009) Patterns of autobiographical memory impairment according to disease severity in semantic dementia. Cortex 45: 456–472.
51. Mattis S (1976) Mental status examination for organic mental symptoms in elderly patients. In: Bellak L, Karatsu TB, editors. Geriatric psychiatry: a handbook for psychiatrists and primary care physicians. New York: Grune et Stratton. pp. 77–121.
52. Yesavage JA, Brink TL, Rose TL, Lum O, Huang V, et al. (1983) Development and validation of a geriatric depression screening scale: a preliminary report. J Psychiatr Res 17: 37–49.
53. Viard A, Piolino P, Desgranges B, Chételat G, Lebreton K, et al. (2007) Hippocampal activation for autobiographical memories over the entire lifetime in healthy aged subjects: An fMRI study. Cereb Cortex 17: 2453–2467.
54. Viard A, Lebreton K, Chételat G, Desgranges B, Landeau B, et al. (2010) Patterns of hippocampal-neocortical interactions in the retrieval of episodic autobiographical memories across the entire life-span of aged adults. Hippocampus 20: 153–165.
55. Graham KS, Hodges JR (1997) Differentiating the roles of the hippocampal complex and the neocortex in long-term memory storage: evidence from the study of semantic dementia and Alzheimer's disease. Neuropsychology 11: 77–89.
56. Kopelman MD, Wilson BA, Baddeley AD (1989) The autobiographical memory interview: a new assessment of autobiographical and personal semantic memory in amnesic patients. J Clin Exp Neuropsychol 11:724–744.
57. Piolino P, Desgranges B, Belliard S, Matuszewski V, Lalevée C, et al. (2003a) Autobiographical memory and autonoetic consciousness: triple dissociation in neurodegenerative diseases. Brain 126: 2203–2219.
58. Piolino P, Belliard S, Desgranges B, Perron M, Eustache F (2003b) Autobiographical memory and autonoetic consciousness in a case of semantic dementia. Cogn Neuropsychol 20: 619–639.
59. Piolino P, Giffard-Quillon G, Desgranges B, Chételat G, Baron JC, et al. (2004) Re-experiencing old memories via hippocampus: a PET study of autobiographical memory. NeuroImage 22: 1371–1383.
60. Brewer W (1988) Memory for randomly sampled autobiographical events. In: Neisser U, Winograd E, editors. Remembering reconsidered: ecological and

traditional approaches to the study of memory. Cambridge: Cambridge University Press. pp. 21–90.
61. Dewhurst SA, Conway MA (1994) Pictures, images, and recollective experience. J Exp Psychol Learn Mem Cogn 20: 1088–1098.
62. Brewer W (1996) What is recollective memory? In: Rubin DC, editor. Remembering our past: studies in autobiographical memory. Cambridge: Cambridge University Press. pp. 19–66.
63. Rubin DC, Schrauf RW, Greenberg DL (2003) Belief and recollection of autobiographical memories. Mem Cognit 31: 887–901.
64. Nigro G, Neisser U (1983) Point of view in personal memories. Cogn Psychol 15: 467–482.
65. Good CD, Johnsrude IS, Ashburner J, Henson RN, Friston KJ, et al. (2001) A voxel-based morphometric study of ageing in 465 normal adult human brains. NeuroImage 14: 21–36.
66. Ashburner J, Friston KJ (2005) Unified segmentation. NeuroImage 26: 839–851.
67. Crawford JR, Garthwaite PH, Azzalini A, Howell DC, Laws KR (2006) Testing for a deficit in single-case studies: effects of departures from normality. Neuropsychologia 44: 666–677.
68. Crawford JR, Garthwaite PH (2002) Investigation of the single case in neuropsychology: confidence limits on the abnormality of test scores and test score differences. Neuropsychologia 40:1196–1208.
69. Crinion J, Ashburner J, Leff A, Brett M, Price C, et al. (2007) Spatial normalization of lesioned brains: performance evaluation and impact on fMRI analyses. Neuroimage 37:866–875.
70. Maguire EA, Kumaran D, Hassabis D, Kopelman MD (2010) Autobiographical memory in semantic dementia: a longitudinal fMRI study. Neuropsychologia 48: 123–136.
71. Deary IJ, Johnson W (2010) Intelligence and education: causal perceptions drive analytic processes and therefore conclusions. The International Journal of Epidemiology 39:1362–9.
72. Crawford JR, Garthwaite PH, Ryan K (2011) Comparing a single case to a control sample: testing for neuropsychological deficits and dissociations in the presence of covariates. Cortex 47: 1166–1178.
73. Okuda J, Fujii T, Ohtake H, Tsukiura T, Tanji K, et al. (2003) Thinking of the future and past: the roles of the frontal pole and the medial temporal lobes. NeuroImage 19: 1369–1380.
74. Addis DR, Wong AT, Schacter DL (2007) Remembering the past and imagining the future: common and distinct neural substrates during event construction and elaboration. Neuropsychologia 45: 1363–1377.
75. Szpunar KK, Watson JM, McDermott KB (2007) Neural substrates of envisioning the future. Proc Natl Acad Sci U S A 104: 642–647.
76. Cabeza R, St Jacques P (2007) Functional neuroimaging of autobiographical memory. Trends Cogn Sci 11: 219–227.
77. Howard-Jones PA, Blakemore SJ, Samuel EA, Summers IR, Claxton G (2005) Semantic divergence and creative story generation: an fMRI investigation. Brain Res Cogn Brain Res 25: 240–250.
78. Irish M, Hornberger M, Lah S, Miller L, Pengas G, et al. (2001) Profiles of recent autobiographical memory retrieval in semantic dementia, behavioural-variant frontotemporal dementia, and Alzheimer's disease. Neuropsychologia 49: 2694–26702.
79. Ochsner KN, Gross JJ (2005) The cognitive control of emotion. Trends Cogn Sci 9: 242–249.
80. Holland AC, Kensinger EA (2010) Emotion and autobiographical memory. Phys Life Rev 7: 88–131.
81. Craig AD (2009) How do you feel now? The anterior insula and human awareness. Nat Rev Neurosci 10: 59–70.
82. Snowden JS, Bathgate D, Varma A, Blackshaw A, Gibbons ZC, et al. (2001) Distinct behavioural profiles in fronto temporal dementia and semantic dementia. J Neurol Neurosurg Psychiatry 70:323–332.
83. Eichenbaum H (2001) The hippocampus and declarative memory: cognitive mechanisms and neural codes. Behav Brain Res 127:199–207.
84. Belliard S, Bon L, LeMoal S, Jonin PY, Vercelletto M, et al. (2007) [Démence sémantique]. Psychol Neuropsychiatr Vieil 5:127–138.
85. Thompson SA, Patterson K, Hodges JR (2003) Left/right asymmetry of atrophy in semantic dementia: behavioral-cognitive implications. Neurology 61: 1196–1203.
86. Herlitz A, Nilsson LG, Bäckman L (1997) Gender differences in episodic memory. Mem Cognit 25: 801–811.
87. St Jacques PL, Conway MA, Cabeza R (2011) Gender differences in autobiographical memory for everyday events: retrieval elicited by SenseCam images versus verbal cues. Memory 19: 723–732.
88. Andreano JM, Cahill L (2009) Sex influences on the neurobiology of learning and memory. Learn Mem 16: 248–266.
89. Summerfield JJ, Hassabis D, Maguire EA (2009) Cortical midline involvement in autobiographical memory. Neuroimage 44:1188–1200.

The Effect and Mechanism of Growth Hormone Replacement on Cognitive Function in Rats with Traumatic Brain Injury

Hao Zhang[1], Mengqi Han[2], Xiaonian Zhang[1], Xinting Sun[1], Feng Ling[3]*

1 China Rehabilitation Research Center, Capital Medical University, Beijing, China, **2** Beijing Jishuitan Hospital, Beijing, China, **3** Beijing Xuanwu Hospital, Capital Medical University, Beijing, China

Abstract

Objective: The effects of growth hormone on cognitive dysfunction were observed in a controlled cortical impact (CCI) rat model and the underlying mechanism was explored.

Method: Three-month-old male SD rats were randomly divided into sham (n = 10), control (n = 10), and CCI groups (n = 40) The parameters were set as follows: striking speed, 3.5 m/s; impact depth, 1.5 mm; and dwell time, 400 msec. Eight and ten weeks post-injury, the GH levels were measured the water maze test and novel object recognition test were performed. CCI rats were divided into normal and decreased GH groups, and further randomly divided into two sub-groups (rhGH treatment and saline vehicle groups). All rats were tested for SYN, BDNF, and TrkB mRNA in the prefrontal cortex and hippocampus by RT-PCR.

Results: CCI rats 8 weeks post-injury had cognitive dysfunction regardless of the GH level ($P<0.05$). rhGH treatment improved cognitive function in CCI rats. There was a positive correlation between the expression of prefrontal BDNF and SYN mRNA in CCI rats after rhGH therapy and the water maze test score ($r = 0.773$ and 0.534, respectively; $P<0.05$). Furthermore, the expression of BDNF, TrkB, and SYN mRNA in the hippocampus was negatively correlated with the water maze test score ($r = 0.602$, 0.773, 0.672, and 0.783, respectively; $P<0.05$). There was a difference in the expression of hippocampal and prefrontal BDNF, TrkB, and SYN mRNA ($P<0.05$)

Conclusion: rhGH treatment had a positive effect on cognitive function, which was more evident in GH-deficient rats. The increased expression of hippocampal and prefrontal BDNF and TrkB mRNA is implicated in rhGH therapy to improve cognitive function. Changes in the expression of hippocampal SYN mRNA following rhGH therapy may also play a role in improving cognitive function.

Editor: Sergio T. Ferreira, Federal University of Rio de Janeiro, Brazil

Funding: The special basic research fund for Chinese central public research institutes (2011CZ-6,2012CZ-5) http://www.most.gov.cn/ztzl/gjzctx/ptzckjtr/200802/t20080222_59209.htm. The funders had no role in study design, data collection and analysis, decision to publish, or preparation of the manuscript.

Competing Interests: The authors have declared that no competing interests exist.

* Email: crrck3@sina.com

Introduction

Traumatic brain injury (TBI) is a medical condition with high morbidity worldwide, and leading mortality and disability rates [1]. Cognitive impairment is one of the most common symptoms in patients with moderate-to-severe TBI. Patients with varying degrees of TBI may develop cognitive impairment, causing a significant impact on daily life, which impedes a patient returning to society. Endocrine dysfunction after a TBI may be due to primary or secondary lesions in the hypothalamus and pituitary. Any degree of TBI can cause varying changes in pituitary hormone levels [2], the most prominent of which is growth hormone (GH) deficiency. GH is important to the development of the central nervous system, especially in promoting the maturation of the brain, myelin formation, glial cell differentiation, and cognitive function. The relationship between the GH level and cognitive function has been studied in Alzheimer's disease (AD) [3–5] and patients with growth hormone deficiency (GHD) [6,7]. The relationship among TBI, GH, and recombinant human growth hormone (rhGH) therapy has been the focus of clinical epidemiologic studies [8]; however, there are few experimental studies and the underlying mechanism is unclear.

In 1986 the genetic synthesis of rhGH, which is identical to the natural structure and function of human GH, was reported for the treatment of GHD [9]. There are also some reports of TBI patients with GH deficiency who had neurologic improvement and quality of life after being treated with rhGH [10–12]. The lesion sites in TBI primarily involve the frontal and temporal lobes, basal ganglia, and hippocampus, all of which can cause cognitive disorders. Among the cranial structures affected by a TBI, the hippocampus is the most common site for lesions.

A controlled cortical impact (CCI) is considered to be an accurate TBI model, which can control the cerebral hemodynamic parameters, including striking speed, dwell time, impact depth, and site. Therefore, the CCI model can replicate different degrees of brain damage with greater reproducibility and less affected by individual differences [13,14]. Rats have low price, abundant source and pure strains than other animals, model making procedure is simple, the survival rate is high; and rats have the similar cerebral vascular anatomy and physiology to humans, so easy to study anatomy; and social ethics are more likely to be accepted than other large mammals, so choose SD rats to make the TBI model. The mechanism implicated in long-term GH deficiency caused by CCI is ill-defined, and cannot explain the neuroprotective effects in TBI settings. Currently, the neuroendocrine changes associated with cognitive impairment in patients with TBI have become a research hotspot.

Brain-derived neurotrophic factor (BDNF) is a class of secreted proteins that affect nervous system plasticity and is closely associated with synaptic activity. The synaptic function of all neurotrophins is adjusted by Trk receptors via binding. BDNF does not only maintain neuronal survival, but also has an extremely important impact on synaptic development [15]. At present, controversy exists regarding the effect of BDNF and TrkB on hippocampal neurons and cognitive function after TBI. Miladi et al. [16] reported that cognitive impairment in rats addicted to morphine is likely to be mediated through the TrkB molecular pathway. Synaptophysin (SYN) is the phosphorylated protein connected with the synaptic vesicle, which is the specific protein on the synaptic vesicle membrane involved in synaptic vesicle import, transit, and neurotransmitter release [17]. Teny et al. [18] reported that the immunoreactivity of SYN is related to the degree of cognitive impairment in patients with AD, and furthermore, hippocampal synaptophysin immunohistochemical staining was significantly reduced in aged rats with memory impairment compared to those with normal memory.

There are few studies that have investigated the effect of rhGH treatment following TBI. Because of limitations in clinical research, our project was focused on the relationship between decreased GH following TBI and cognitive dysfunction. In addition, we investigated the relationships after rhGH treatment from the genetic level to determine the underlying mechanism for the clinical use of rhGH.

Subjects and Methods

1.1 Subjects and groups

All procedures were performed in accordance with the Chinese Capital Medical University Animal Welfare guidelines and approved by the Institutional Animal Care and Use Committee of the Chinese Capital Medical University. Sixty 3-month-old healthy, clean, male SD rats, weighing 275±25 g (purchased from the PLA Academy of the Military Medical Experimental Animal Center), were used in this study. We performed the animal experiments in strict compliance with medical laboratory animal management implementation rules and other relevant laws and regulations. The rearing conditions were as follows: temperature, 21±1°C; light/dark cycle, 12 h/12 h; and illumination time, 0700–1900. Sufficient water and food were given daily before and after surgery; the rats fasted for 8 hours pre-operatively. The rodents were randomly divided into three groups, as follows: normal control group (n = 10); sham group (n = 10); and CCI group (n = 40). Based on the GH level 8 weeks post-surgery, the rats in the CCI group were further divided into two subgroups (CCI-N and CCI-D groups). Each rats was pierced in ear to number, experiments were proceed by number order.

1.2 Brain injury model

All of the following animal experiments were carried out in the course of SPF animals laboratory. We used the eCCI-6.3 device (New York University) as previously described [19]. Rats were administered 10% chloral hydrate (0.3 ml/100 g ip), (Chloral hydrate is relatively safe, easy to control dose and no respiratory damage.) then underwent a bilateral frontal craniotomy, and the lesion site was set 3 mm anterior and lateral to the bregma. The diameter of the bone window was ≥5 mm. A CCI impactor was used to cause the cortical injury, and the parameters were set as followed: striking speed, 3.5 m/s; blow depth, 1.5 mm; and dwell time, 400 msec [20]. The whole procedure lasts 15 to 20 min, maintain body temperature all the time, after the surgery, rats were placed on a warm blanket in an hour and then returned to their own cages. The normal control group received no intervention, and the sham group underwent craniotomies without a striking blow [21].

1.3 Determination of growth hormone

Tail blood was collected before the CCI, 8 weeks after the CCI, and 10 weeks (rhGH replacement therapy for 2 weeks) after CCI. The volume of blood was 1.5–2.0 ml, and after centrifugation, the upper serum fraction was tested by radioimmunoassay (provided by the Di Ann Medical Testing Center) for GH. The unit of GH was ng/ml.

1.4 Administration of recombinant human growth hormone

The rhGH was provided by Changchun Kinsey Pharmaceutical Company [Changchun, China]. The dose was 30 IU/ml. The administration of rhGH was via subcutaneous cervical injection at a dose of 200 μg/kg [22]. The same dose of saline was given to the control group. These injections were administered once a day at 8:00 am [23] for 2 consecutive weeks.

1.5 Water maze test

All rats were tested in a water maze at baseline. At 8 and 10 weeks (rhGH replacement therapy for 2 weeks) post-injury, the water maze test was performed (MWM model XR-XM101, Shanghai Xinruan Technology Co., Ltd., Shanghai, China). The water temperature was controlled at 28±1°C, and melanin was added to the water to visualize the underwater platform clearly and reduce the impact on the positioning of underwater structures [23]. For the navigation test, the platform was located in one quadrant and 2 cm below the water surface. The rat was put in the maze facing the maze wall. If the rat could not find the hidden platform within 60 seconds, the rat was guided to the platform by the experimenter, where the rat remained for 10 seconds. During 3 consecutive days, rats were trained 4 times a day in the platform, and the interval of time between the two training session was 15–20 minutes. The latency time was recorded [24]. For the space exploration experiment, followed the navigation test, the rat would be put into the opposite quadrant, and the percentage of total time spent in the original quadrant within 60 seconds was recorded.

1.6 Novel object recognition test

Baseline of novel object recognition of all rats were measured one day before the CCI test. Object recognition experiments were repeated in rats at the end of 8 and 10 weeks after CCI (i.e. 2 weeks after rhGH replacement therapy) respectively. The rats were first exposed to the empty arena (60*60*45 cm, made of black PVC, XR-XX117, Shanghai Xinruan Technology Co., Ltd., Shanghai, China) for 5 min (day 0) under bright light, to minimize stress related to a novel environment. After the first hour, the rats were allowed to interact with two identical objects for 5 min. The rats were then re-introduced into the arena for 3 min after the second hour, with one familiar and one novel object this time. The position of the objects remained the same in the arena to remove any spatial memory component from the task. The animals were filmed with a camera (Shanghai Xinruan Technology Co., Ltd., Shanghai, China) and the interaction time(nose at 2 cm or less in the object's direction)with the novel and familiar objects, and distance traveled(cm) were analyzed with the TopScan2.0 tracking software(Shanghai Xinruan Technology Co., Ltd., Shanghai, China). The above experiments were also recorded by cameras. The time rats explore the old object (object A) and the new one (object B) were recorded by Stopwatch Software (TimeLeft3) respectively, and the discrimination index (DI) were calculated. The formula for is $DI = (N-F)/(N+F) \times 100\%$. N referes to the time the rats used to explore the new objects. F refers the time the rats to explore the old objects.

1.7 Detection of BDNF, TrkB, and SYN mRNA levels by real-time PCR

After the behavioral test, each rat was sacrificed and the brain was removed. The brain tissue was placed on ice; the hippocampus and prefrontal brain tissue were isolated and frozen in liquid nitrogen. The total RNA was extracted for RT- PCR analysis. GADPH was used as the internal reference, and the gene sequence is shown in Table 1. Primers were synthesized by Beijing Reagan Biotechnology Co., Ltd. (Beijing, China). The TL988 PCR instrument detection system [INESA Instrument, Shanghai, China] was used for quantitative RT-PCR analysis, and 5′ -3′ exonuclease activity was amplified by Taq polymerase. The PCR conditions were as follows: 95°C for 2 min; 94°C for 30 s, 54°C fir 30 s, and 72°C for 30 s; and the fluorescence value was read at 72°C. Altogether, there were 45 cycles. The $2^{-\Delta\Delta ct}$ value method was used to calculate the relative ratio of the Ct value with the TL988 PCR instrument software acquisition (PCR software analysis system).

1.8 Statistical analysis

Data were analyzed using SPSS 16.0 software. Ordinal data are expressed as the absolute value and percentage, and measurable data are presented as the mean ± standard deviation ($\bar{x} \pm s$). GH values were compared with paired t-tests. The data from the MWM were analyzed by repeated-measures ANOVA, and space exploration data from the same time point were compared among groups using one-way ANOVA, with *post hoc* LSD for the comparison between groups. The latency period was translated into scores for each group (highest = 60 points and lowest = 1 point) corresponding to the time spent. Then, the result was averaged for 3 days, as a result of cognitive function [25]. The data from the novel object recognition test were analyzed by ANOVA test and group comparisons were analyzed by the LSD *post hoc* test. The data from CCI-N and CCI-D were analyzed by paired T-test. Correlations were determined for BDNF, Trk, and SYN mRNA in different parts of the brain and cognitive function test scores the by rank-sum test. When the difference was statistically significant, the LSD test was used. A $P<0.05$ was considered statistically significant.

Results

2.1 GH levels at different time points

Fig. 1 shows that the GH level changed 8 weeks post-CCI and the effect of rhGH treatment(including 5 death and 19 GH level reduced, the death reason maybe flatulence and malnutrition). There was no significant difference in the GH level between 8 and 10 weeks post-injury ($P>0.05$). Whether or not the GH level was decreased, rhGH treatment increased the GH level in CCI rats ($P<0.01$).

2.2 Result of the water maze test

Fig. 2(a) and 2(b) show that, at 8 weeks post-injury, there was a significant difference among the four groups ($P<0.05$); after 2 weeks of treatment, there was also a significant difference among the four groups ($P<0.05$). The latency after rhGH treatment was less than before treatment.

2.3 Results of spatial memory in the water maze test

Shown in Fig. 3, at 8 weeks post-CCI, the time spent in the targeted quadrant was significantly different among the 4 groups ($P = 0.001$). After 2 weeks of treatment with rhGH, there was no significant difference between the CCI-D and CCI-N groups ($p = 0.100$). As shown in the bar graph, regardless of the level of GH reduction, the time spent in the targeted quadrant increased after rhGH treatment.

2.4 The results of novel object recognition test

Shown in Table 2 and Fig. 4(a)(b), total exploration time in CCI-D group (rhGH treatment for 2 weeks) can be seen significant difference statistically compared with control rats. But there is no statistical significance about total exploration time in CCI-N group (rhGH treatment for two weeks) compared with control. Before and after the rhGH treatment for CCI-D and CCI-N group, the significant differences about discrimination index were not be seen.

Table 1. Real-time PCR Primer Sequence.

Gene size (bp)		Primer
BDNF	Upstream: 5′- ctgcgcccatgaaagaag- 3′ Downstream: 5′- attcctccagcagaaaga -3′	291
TrkB	Upstream: 5′- acggagtaccacggctg-3′ Downstream: 5′-gcaatcaccaccacggca-3′	299
SYN	Upstream: 5′- ctgcgcccatgaaagaag- 3′ Downstream: 5′- attcctccagcagaaaga -3′	188
GAPDH	Upstream: 5′- gctggcattgctctcaatg - 3′ Downstream: 5′- cctctcttgctctcag -3′	163

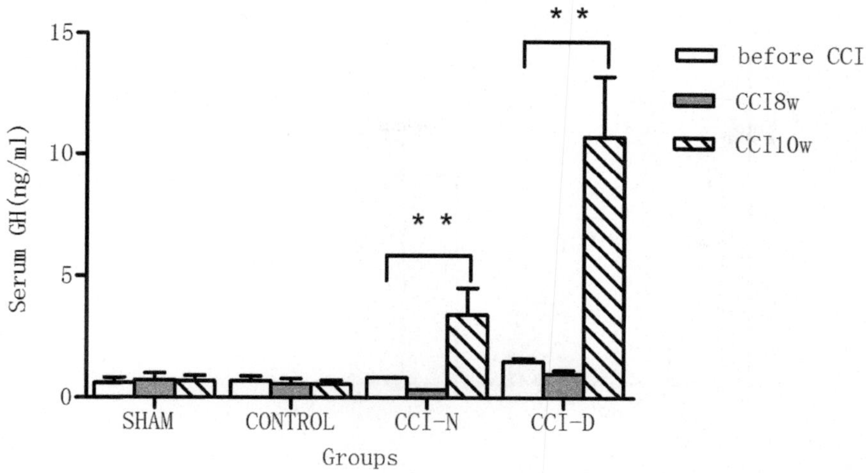

Figure 1. GH levels at different time points. Note: ** indicated as p<0.01 between different time points.

2.5 The correlation between transmitter mRNA expression at different sites with results of water maze testing (shown in Table 3 and 4)

2.6 Effect of rhGH treatment on gene expression at different sites

Shown in Fig. 5(a)–(c), the results of real-time PCR demonstrated that there were significant differences in the expression of hippocampal and prefrontal Trk, BDNF, and SYN mRNA between the groups (P<0.05). Furthermore, the expression of hippocampal and prefrontal TrkB mRNA was also different between the CCI-N and CCI-D groups (p = 0.004 and 0.005, respectively). The expression of hippocampal BDNF and SYN mRNA was also significantly different between the CCI-N and CCI-D groups (p<0.05).

Discussion

3.1 Effect of long-term GH level on cognitive function following TBI in rats

According to the clinical imaging data, approximately 30% of patients with TBIs develop morphologic changes in the pituitary in the acute stage [26]. Any degree of TBI can cause varying changes in pituitary hormone levels, and 3 months after the TBI, the most common is a GH deficiency [27]. A study has shown that the GH level is lower in TBI rats 8 weeks post-injury [28]. In the current study, we increased the subject sample and set the control group, and further confirmed the fact that the GH level decreased 8 weeks post-TBI, with an incidence rate of 54.28%.

In recent years, a number of clinical studies have shown that secondary hypopituitarism occurs in patients with moderate-to-severe TBIs, and the reduced GH level is associated with cognitive impairment in these patients [2,29–31]. From Figure2(a), our results showed that the control and sham groups 8 weeks after the incubation period demonstrated a decreased latency time, indicating a good spatial learning ability in rats. After 8 weeks, whether or not the GH level was decreased, the latency time in the water maze test was significantly reduced in all rats. The latency time in the CCI-D group was significantly longer than the control and sham groups, indicating that reduced GH following TBI affected the spatial learning ability in TBI rats. Similarly, the CCI-D group had the shortest time in the space exploration experiment, with a significant difference between the different groups, indicating that a reduced GH level following TBI would also affect spatial memory in TBI rats. In GH-deficiency and AD models, a reduced GH level could extend the latency time in the water maze test with impaired cognitive function [6,32]. Leon et al. [10] studied 11 cases with reduced GH levels after TBIs and showed decreased attention, executive function, memory, and mood disorders compared with TBI patients with normal GH levels. Our study was consistent with previous clinical findings

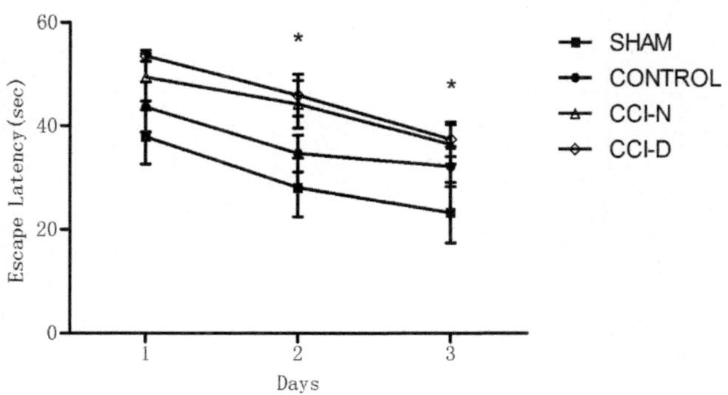

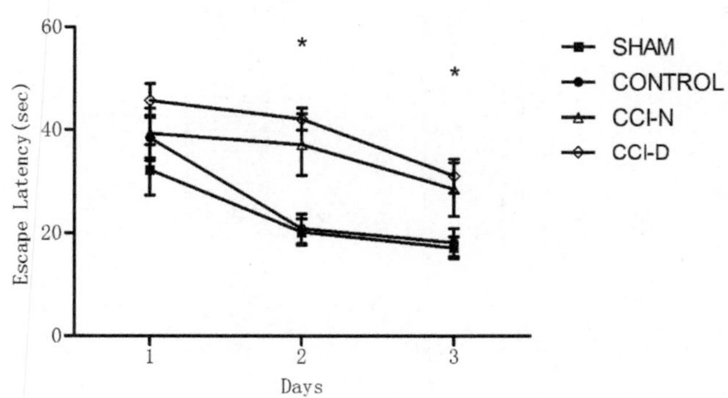

Figure 2. The changes of latency time. (a). 8 weeks after CCI (left). (b). 2 weeks after rhGH treatment (right). Note: *difference of P<0.05 between the four groups at the same time point.

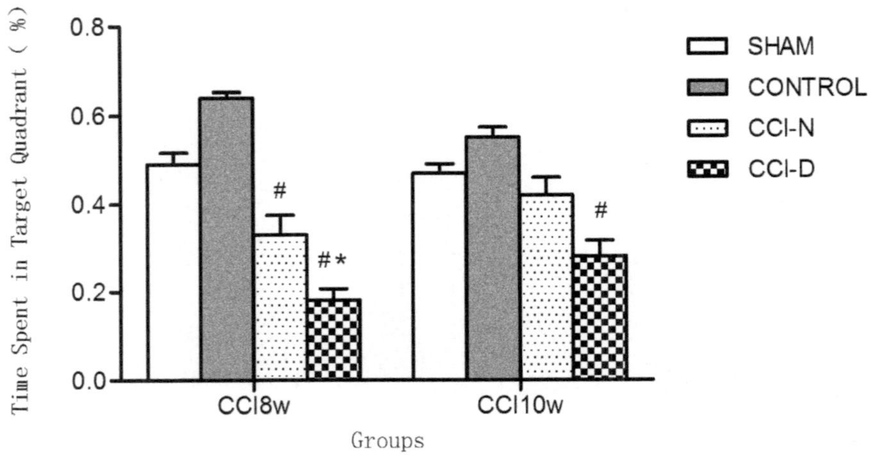

Figure 3. Time spent in the targeted quadrant after 2 weeks of rhGH treatment. Note: * P<0.05 compared to the sham group; # P<0.05 compared to the control group.

showing that the GH level declined in the chronic stage of TBIs and patients with more severe cognitive dysfunction had lower GH levels [33].

3.2 Long-term rhGH treatment on cognitive function following TBI

In 1985, scientists in the United States synthesized rhGH, which is identical to the natural structure and function of human GH. Recent studies have shown that rhGH has some neuroprotective and angiogenic effects, thus improving cognitive function in a variety of diseases. Clinical studies have shown that patients with GH deficiency treated with subcutaneous physiologic requirement of GH can increase the GH concentrations in cerebrospinal fluid, and further improve their attention and memory. Whether or not adults or children are GH-deficient, rhGH therapy can improve cognitive function [34–37]. In animal experiments, it has been confirmed that both GH and GHRH can promote long-term memory in young rats, and prolong the reaction time in young and aged rats during fear subside experiments [36].

Shown in Figure 2(b), in contrast, the latency time in the two groups decreased after 10 weeks of feeding, and there was still a shorter latency time in the CCI-D group compared to the CCI-N group. After rhGH treatment, the latency time was shortened compared to that at 8 weeks and the time spent in the CCI-D group was longer than the CCI-N group. This indicated the positive effect of rhGH treatment on spatial learning function, which clearly occurred in the CCI-D group. As shown in Figure 3, whether or not the GH level is reduced, rhGH treatment increased the time spent in the targeted quadrant. This finding also indicated that rhGH therapy improved spatial memory in rats. In clinical studies it has been suggested that rhGH treatment for >1 year improves patient memory, attention, executive function, abstract thinking, and quality of life [8,11,38,39]; however, these clinical studies were limited due to the small sample size and large variability between individuals, and because of the ethical limitations and clinical research. Thus, rhGH treatment is not an option for patients with normal GH levels and there are few studies regarding this clinical situation experimentally. In the current study, the effect of rhGH treatment on cognitive function not limited to TBI rats with reduced GH levels is reported for the first time.

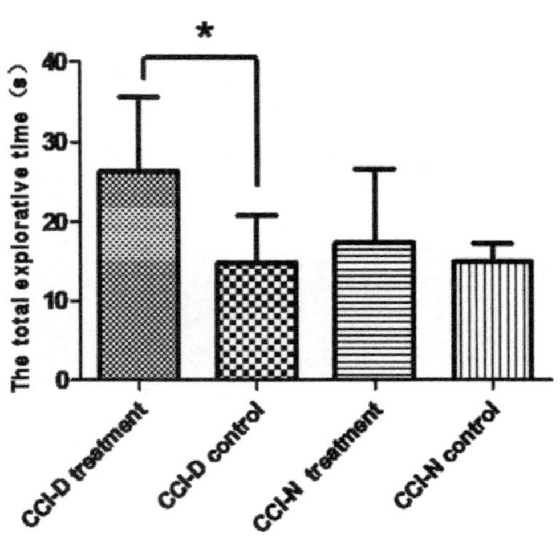

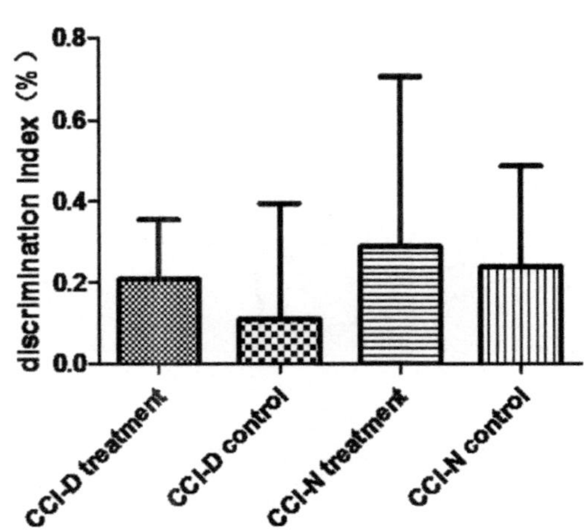

Figure 4. The total exploration time and discrimination index after rhGH treatment. (a) total exploration time (left). (b). discrimination index (right). Note: * P<0.05 between the two groups.

Table 2. The results of novel object recognition test before rhGH treatment.

Group	Number of rats	Total exploration time (s)	DI (%)
Control	10	34.83±8.77	20.23±7.87
Sham-operated	10	30.42±3.93	15.52±3.78
CCI-N	20	**16.71±4.15***	18.86±3.96
CCI-D	20	**17.08±3.13***	17.71±5.41

*P<0.05 compared to control group.

3.3 Possible mechanisms underlying the effect of GH treatment on cognitive function

It has been shown that several brain structures are related to cognitive function, such as the hippocampus, striatum, basal forebrain, and neocortical structures. It has also been reported that the hippocampus, thalamus, putamen, and choroid plexus are associated with the expression of GH [40]. In addition, lesions in the hippocampus and prefrontal lobes exhibit cognitive deficits, and parietal damage does not cause aa deficit [41]. Therefore, we selected the hippocampus and prefrontal cortex for analysis in our study. Currently, the mechanism underlying the effect of GH treatment on cognitive function remains unclear. Some studies have shown that the mechanism underlying the effect of GH treatment on cognitive function is associated with a neuroprotective effect, inhibition of the inflammatory response [42], and promotion of angiogenesis [43] or promotion of cell growth via IGF-1 [44] and relevant neuroprotection [45].

3.4 Effect of GH on TrkB and BDNF

BDNF was extracted and purified from swine brain as decribed by Barde et al. in 1982 [15]. BDNF was shown to have a molecular weight of 13 ku, and an isoelectric point of 9.99. BDNF is mainly synthesized in the brain, and has a wide distribution in the central nervous system, especially in the cortex and hippocampus. Recent animal and clinical studies have shown that BDNF treatment after TBI has a neuroprotective effect [46]. The roles of BDNF include neutralizing high concentrations of amino acid which lead to neurotoxicity [47], down-regulation of the NMDA receptor, and inducing the expression of calcium-binding proteins to stabilize the intracellular Ca^{2+} concentration, thus reducing the generation of free radicals [48], inhibition of apoptosis [49], and reducing hypoxic-ischemic brain damage and promoting regeneration of damaged neurons. BDNF is a cerebral protection factor that contributes to the repair of brain damage and has a protective effect on neurons. BDNF can combine with the TrkB receptor to initiate autophosphorylation and activate other signaling pathways, and thus facilitates the synthesis and release of neurotransmitters involved in learning and memory, thereby playing a role in promoting learning and memory. Shown in Table 2、3 and Figure4(b), our study showed that hippocampal and prefrontal TrkB mRNA levels were significantly different before and after rhGH therapy, with an increasing trend after rhGH treatment. In addition, the hippocampal TrkB mRNA level was negatively correlated with the water maze test score, suggesting that rhGH treatment can increase the expression of TrkB mRNA in rat brain after TBI and shortens the time spent for spatial exploration during the water maze test. Other experiments have confirmed that BDNF mRNA is correlated with cognitive function, thus the change in the gene alone has some significance. In adult TBI rats, decreased BDNF mRNA expression was correlated with the decline in cognitive function [50]. From Figure 1 and Figure 5(a), our study showed that regardless of decreased or normal GH, rhGH treatment following TBI could increase the serum GH level. Combined with genetic testing, it has been shown that exogenous rhGH replacement can also increase the expression of brain BDNF mRNA, secretion of GH, and ultimately affect the expression of BDNF and TrkB related to cognitive function in brain areas and improve cognitive function [46]. Shown in Figure 5(a) and 5(b), in our study, we also found there was a significant difference in the hippocampal mRNA levels of BDNF and TrkB between the CCI-N and CCI-D group. In the prefrontal area, only the TrkB mRNA level was significantly different between the two groups, suggesting that rhGH treatment has a more obvious effect on the regulation of neurotransmitters in the hippocampus. We observed a long-term change post-injury; although rhGH replacement therapy

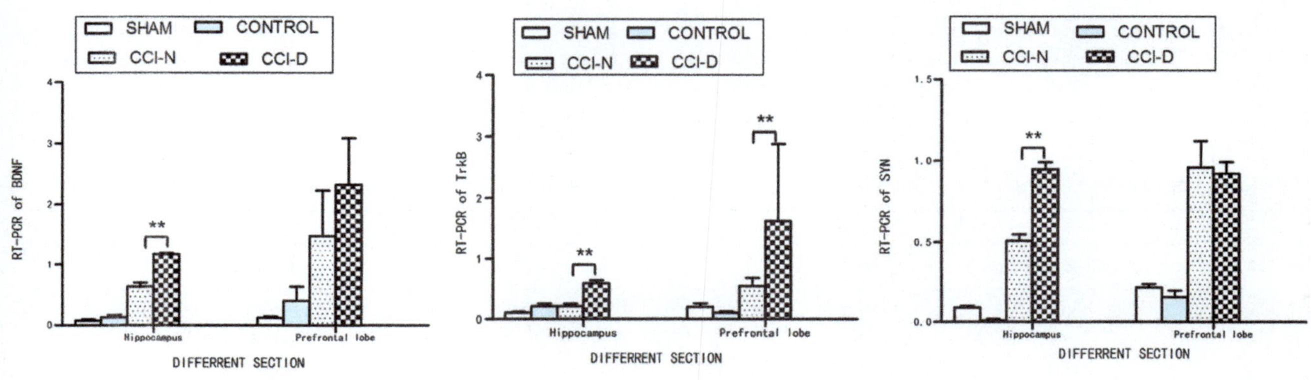

Figure 5. The effect on mRNA levels after rhGH treatment. (a). BDNF mRNA levels (left). (b). TrkB mRNA levels (middle). (c). SYN mRNA levels (right). Note: ** indicated as P<0.05 between the two groups.

Table 3. Correlation between prefrontal transmitter mRNA expression and water maze testing.

mRNA	Pearson coefficient	P value
BDNF	−0.458	**0.001**
TrkB	−0.974	0.224
SYN	−0.101	**0.010**

The linear correlational study showed that after rhGH treatment, the expression of prefrontal BDNF and SYN mRNA in CCI rats was significantly correlated with the results of water maze testing ($r=0.77$ and 0.534, respectively; $P<0.05$), while the expression of prefrontal TrkB mRNA was not significantly associated with the results of water maze testing ($r=0.270$; $P>0.05$).

improved cognitive function, it lasted for only 2 weeks, which was too short for regulation of BDNF changes requiring TrkB, and also because there was a large number of inflammatory cytokines released in the prefrontal cortex, which had an effect on the expression of TrkB with a corresponding effect on BDNF expression.

The mechanism by which GH regulates BDNF to improve cognitive function may be via the basal forebrain cholinergic system to release acetylchloine (Ach) through positive feedback, affecting synaptic plasticity, adjusting learning and memory, and increasing Ach activity through enhanced phosphorylation of the NMDA receptor, regulating hippocampal synaptic transmission, and inducing long-term potentiation(LTP), thereby enhancing learning and memory.

3.5 The role of GH on SYN

SYN is a calcium-binding glycoprotein widely present in the presynaptic vesicle membrane, synthesized in the neuron cell body, and transmitted to the axon terminals. SYN is specifically located in the presynaptic axon terminals to the membrane vesicles and closely related to synaptic structure and function. The phosphorylation of SYN has a significant role in the neurotransmitter releasing process, which consists of a fast and efficient regulation system for neurotransmitter release. In recent years, studies have shown that synaptic change in morphology and function is one of the most important pathologic causes in learning and memory dysfunction. SYN, as a calcium-binding glycoprotein, is widely present in the membrane of presynaptic vesicles, and is closely related to synaptic structure and function. SYN modulates the release of neurotransmitters through phosphorylation and dephosphorylation, and gets involved in the import, transport, recycling, and synaptogenesis of synaptic vesicles, which plays a role in synaptic plasticity. Therefore, SYN is one of the important molecules in learning and memory processes. SYN has been the focus in a large number of studies; SYN is also involved in the release of Ca^{2+}-dependent neurotransmitters, such as Ach and glutamate, and the circulation of synaptic vesicles and synaptic remodeling. SYN also affects the stability and mobility of synaptic vesicle through its redox state [51,52]. Therefore, the amount of SYN protein may reflect the level of synaptic function, the transmission of synaptic information, and neurotransmitter release.

Brain synaptic plasticity undergoes major changes following TBI, and the synaptic reorganization plays an important role in the recovery of anatomy, physiology, and function. Shojo et al. [53] used a fluid percussion injury animal model of TBI to study the change in cortical SYN 2–30 days post-injury for mild, moderate, and severe brain injury. Shojo et al. [53]reported, with an increase in impact time and degree, cortical SYN increased, but the total SYN did not significantly change within the brain, and the increase in SYN at the lesion site was thought to be due to the inhibition of synaptic vesicles and the dysfunction of the synapse and transduction. Pyramidal neurons and synapses in hippocampal CA1 are thought to be the structural basis of learning and memory. Overseas studies have shown that the expression of SYN is increased in the model of learning and memory and the LTP phenomenon occurs in the hippocampus, which results in a 6-fold increase in SYN expression, while the expression of SYN is decreased in rats with cognitive dysfunction [54], indicating that the amount of SYN expression was positively correlated with learning and memory. We achieved the same results in our study. Previous studies have also shown that synaptic dysfunction and failure occur in the early stage of AD, and the decline in the synapse is the best pathologic basis to explain cognitive dysfunction, and SYN can regulate synaptic function [55]. Therefore, we suggest that the mechanism underlying improved cognitive function following rhGH treatment to be via SYN, which increases synaptic function and has a role in synaptic transmission and the release of the synaptic vesicle. In addition, GH can increase the release of excitoxic glutamate through SYN, maintain the LTP, improve message transmission, processing, and storage, and ultimately improve learning and memory.

Eastwood et al. [56] reported that in the dentate and parahippocampal gyri of the human brain, SYN is positively correlated with SYN mRNA, indicating that the expression of SYN is regulated by the encoded gene. Shown in Table 3,4 and

Table 4. Correlation between the expression of hippocampal transmitter mRNA with results of water maze testing.

mRNA	Pearson coefficient	P value
BDNF	−0.458	**0.001**
TrkB	−0.066	**0.008**
SYN	−0.370	**0.001**

The linear correlational study showed that after rhGH treatment, the expression of hippocampal BDNF, TrkB, and SYN mRNA in CCI rats was significantly correlated with the results of water maze testing ($r=0.773$, 0.672 and 0.783, respectively; $P<0.05$).

Fig.5(c), our study showed that treatment with rhGH can significantly increase the SYN mRNA levels in the hippocampus and prefrontal area, and SYN mRNA is negatively correlated with water maze test scores, suggesting that rhGH treatment can increase SYN mRNA expression, which is associated with a shortened water maze navigation time. Therefore, we speculated that the improved cognitive function may be caused by up-regulating SYN mRNA. Shown in Figure 5(c), in the current study we also found a significant difference in the SYN mRNA in the hippocampus between the CCI-N and CCI-D groups. This indicated that whether or not GH is reduced, rhGH therapy can improve SYN mRNA expression. In combination with cognitive function test results, this illustrated that rhGH therapy improves cognitive function in TBI rats through up-regulation of the expression of hippocampal SYN mRNA.

Conclusion

Our study confirmed that GH deficiency damages spatial learning and spatial exploration abilities in TBI rats. Whether or not GH is reduced, rhGH treatment has a positive effect on cognitive function. The increased expression of BDNF and TrkB mRNA in the hippocampus and prefrontal region might be the basis for improved memory function following rhGH therapy. Changes in hippocampal SYN mRNA following rhGH therapy may also play a role in improving memory function. The experiment did not carry out the dynamic observation of GH level at different time poin, so the GH curve is still not clear, larger sample size and dynamic observation of GH level is needed; Because rhGH administration and dosage may have an impact on cognitive function, so the next experiment should thoroughly investigate the cognitive impairment in rats after TBI and the role of rhGH administration and dosage. In order to provide a theoretical basis for the clinical application of rhGH, and one day rhGH replacement therapy will be used in clinical and help more patients.

Author Contributions

Conceived and designed the experiments: HZ FL. Performed the experiments: HZ MH. Analyzed the data: HZ XZ FL. Contributed reagents/materials/analysis tools: MH XS. Wrote the paper: HZ MH FL.

References

1. Bruns JJ, Hauser WA (2003) The epidemiology of traumatic brain injury: a review. Epilepsia USA 44 Suppl 10: 2–10.
2. Urban RJ (2006) Hypopituitarism after acute brain injury. Growth Horm Igf Res SCO 16: S25–S29.
3. Kinney BA, Coschigano KT, Kopchick JJ, Steger RW, Bartke A (2001) Evidence that age-induced decline in memory retention is delayed in growth hormone resistant GH-R-KO (Laron) mice. Physiol Behav USA 72: 653–660.
4. Wass JA, Reddy R (2010) Growth hormone and memory. J Endocrinol ENG 207: 125–126.
5. Thornton PL, IngramRL, Sonntag WE (2000) Chronic D-Ala2.-growth hormone-releasing hormone administration attenuates age-related deficits in spatial memory. J Gerontol A Biol Sci Med Sci USA 55: B106–B112.
6. Nieuwpoort IC, Drent ML (2008) Cognition in the adult with childhood-onset GH deficiency. Eur J Endocrinol ENG 159: S53–S57.
7. Morselli LL, Bogazzi F, Cecconi E, Genovesi M, Martino E, et al. (2008) Hypopituitarism (GHD) and neurodegenerative diseases. J Endocrinol Invest ITA 31: 39–43.
8. Bhagia V, Gilkison C, Fitts RH, Zgaljardic DJ, High WJ, et al. (2010) Effect of recombinant growth hormone replacement in a growth hormone deficient subject recovering from mild traumatic brain injury: A case report. Brain Inj ENG 24: 560–567.
9. Zhou JP (2007) The influence of GnRH analogues on the expression of oxytocin in hypothalamus-pituitary-gonad axis and effect of learning and memory. CHN: Northwest A&F University 2007.
10. Leon-Carrion J, Leal-Cerro A, Cabezas FM, Atutxa AM, Gomez SG, et al. (2007) Cognitive deterioration due to GH deficiency in patients with traumatic brain injury: a preliminary report. Brain Inj ENG 21: 871–875.
11. Moreau OK, Cortet-Rudelli C, Yollin E, Merlen E, Daveluy W, et al. (2013) Growth hormone replacement therapy in patients with traumatic brain injury. J Neurotrauma USA 30: 998–1006.
12. Beca SG, High WJ, Masel BE, Mossberg KA, Urban RJ (2012) What are critical outcome measures for patients receiving pituitary replacement following brain injury? Pituitary USA 15: 10–19.
13. Ommaya AK (1995) Head injury mechanisms and the concept of preventive management: a review and critical synthesis. J Neurotrauma USA 12: 527–546.
14. Lippert-Gruner M, Maegele M, Pokorny J, Angelov DN, Svestkova O, et al. (2007) Early rehabilitation model shows positive effects on neural degeneration and recovery from neuromotor deficits following traumatic brain injury. Physiol Res CZE 56: 359–368.
15. Tong L, Prieto GA, Kramar EA, Smith ED, Cribbs DH, et al. (2012) Brain-derived neurotrophic factor-dependent synaptic plasticity is suppressed by interleukin-1beta via p38 mitogen-activated protein kinase. J Neurosci USA 32: 17714–17724.
16. Miladi-Gorji H, Rashidy-Pour A, Fathollahi Y, Akhavan MM, Semnanian S, et al. (2011) Voluntary exercise ameliorates cognitive deficits in morphine dependent rats: the role of hippocampal brain-derived neurotrophic factor. Neurobiol Learn Mem USA 96: 479–491.
17. Hao LY, HaoXQ, Li SH, Li XH (2010) Prenatal exposure to lipopolysaccharide results in cognitive deficits in age-increasing offspring rats. Neuroscience ENG 166: 763–770.
18. VanGuilder HD, Farley JA, Yan H, Kirk CA, Mitschelen M, et al. (2011) Hippocampal dysregulation of synaptic plasticity-associated proteins with age-related cognitive decline. Neurobiol Dis USA 43: 201–212.
19. Dixon CE, Clifton GL, Lighthall JW, Yaghmai AA, Hayes RL (1991) A controlled cortical impact model of traumatic brain injury in the rat. J Neurosci Methods NED 39: 253–262.
20. Guseva MV, Hopkins DM, Scheff SW, Pauly JR (2008) Dietary choline supplementation improves behavioral, histological, and neurochemical outcomes in a rat model of traumatic brain injury. J Neurotrauma USA 25: 975–983.
21. Cole JT, Yarnell A, Kean WS, Gold E, Lewis B, et al. (2011) Craniotomy: true sham for traumatic brain injury, or a sham of a sham? J Neurotrauma USA 28: 359–369.
22. Kwak MJ, Park HJ, Nam MH, Kwon OS, Park SY, et al. (2009) Comparative study of the effects of different growth hormone doses on growth and spatial performance of hypophysectomized rats. J Korean Med Sci KOR 24: 729–736.
23. Morris GM (2008) Morris water maze. Scholarpedia USA 3: 6315.
24. D'Hooge R, Deyn PP (2001) Applications of the Morris water maze in the study of learning and memory. Brain Res Brain Res Rev NED 36: 60–90.
25. Griesbach GS, Sutton RL, Hovda DA, Ying Z, Gomez-Pinilla F (2009) Controlled contusion injury alters molecular systems associated with cognitive performance. J Neurosci Res USA 87: 795–805.
26. Maiya B, Newcombe V, Nortje J, Bradley P, Bernard F, et al. (2008) Magnetic resonance imaging changes in the pituitary gland following acute traumatic brain injury. Intensive Care Med USA 34: 468–475.
27. Ommaya AK (1995) Head injury mechanisms and the concept of preventive management: a review and critical synthesis. J Neurotrauma USA 12: 527–546.
28. Kasturi BS, Stein DG (2009) Traumatic brain injury causes long-term reduction in serum growth hormone and persistent astrocytosis in the cortico-hypothalamo-pituitary axis of adult male rats. J Neurotrauma USA 26: 1315–1324.
29. Kelly DF, McArthur DL, Levin H, Swimmer S, JR Dusick, et al. (2006) Neurobehavioral and quality of life changes associated with growth hormone insufficiency after complicated mild, moderate, or severe traumatic brain injury. J Neurotrauma USA 23: 928–942.
30. Quik EH, Valk GD, Drent ML, StalpersLJ, Kenemans JL, et al. (2012) Reduced growth hormone secretion after cranial irradiation contributes to neurocognitive dysfunction. Growth Horm Igf Res SCO 22: 42–47.
31. Popovic V(2005) GH deficiency as the most common pituitary defect after TBI: clinical implications. Pituitary USA 8: 239–243.
32. Doulah AH, Rohani AH, Khaksari HM, Motamedi F, Farbood Y, et al. (2009) The effect of peripheral administration of growth hormone on AD-like cognitive deficiency in NBM-lesioned rats. Neurosci Lett IRL 466: 47–51.
33. Falleti MG, Maruff P, Burman P, Harris A (2006) The effects of growth hormone (GH) deficiency and GH replacement on cognitive performance in adults: a meta-analysis of the current literature. Psychoneuroendocrino ENG 31: 681–691.
34. Oertel H, Schneider HJ, Stalla GK, Holsboer F, Zihl J (2004) The effect of growth hormone substitution on cognitive performance in adult patients with hypopituitarism. Psychoneuroendocrino ENG 29: 839–850.
35. Deijen JB, Boer H, Veen EA (1998) Cognitive changes during growth hormone replacement in adult men. Psychoneuroendocrino ENG 23: 45–55.
36. Pathipati P, Surus A, Williams CE, Scheepens A (2009) Delayed and chronic treatment with growth hormone after endothelin-induced stroke in the adult rat. Behav Brain Res NED 204: 93–101.
37. Creyghton WM, Dam PS, Koppeschaar HP (2004) The role of the somatotropic system in cognition and other cerebral functions. Semin Vasc Med USA 4: 167–172.

38. Maric NP, Doknic M, Pavlovic D, Pekic S, Stojanovic M, et al. (2010) Psychiatric and neuropsychological changes in growth hormone-deficient patients after traumatic brain injury in response to growth hormone therapy. J Endocrino Invest ITA 33: 770–775.
39. High WJ, Briones-Galang M, Clark JA, Gilkison C, Mossberg KA, et al. (2010) Effect of growth hormone replacement therapy on cognition after traumatic brain injury. J Neurotrauma USA 27: 1565–1575.
40. Lai Z, Roos P, Zhai O, Olsson Y, Fholenhag K, et al. (1993) Age-related reduction of human growth hormone-binding sites in the human brain. Brain Res NED 621: 260–266.
41. Granon S, Poucet B (1995) Medial prefrontal lesions in the rat and spatial navigation: evidence for impaired planning. Behav Neurosci USA 109: 474–484.
42. Dou Y, Zhang Q, Zhang X, Dong JY, Tang JJ, et al. (2009) Effect of different immunomodulation on inflammatory response in burn rats with sepsis. Zhonghua Shao Shang Za Zhi CHN 25: 275–280.
43. Ying XG, Wu BC, Zhang YM, Shao JH (2004) Recombinant human growth hormone on acute effects of coronary collateral circulation in rats with myocardial infarction. J Clin Cardiovascu Dis CHN 10: 613–615.
44. Christophidis LJ, Gorba T, Gustavsson M, Williams CE, Werther GA, et al. (2009) Growth hormone receptor immunoreactivity is increased in the subventricular zone of juvenile rat brain after focal ischemia: a potential role for growth hormone in injury-induced neurogenesis. Growth Horm Igf Res SCO 19: 497–506.
45. Isgaard J, Aberg D, Nilsson M (2007) Protective and regenerative effects of the GH/IGF-I axis on the brain. Minerva Endocrinol ITA 32: 103–113.
46. Kuribara M, Hess MW, Cazorla M, Roubos EW, Scheenen WJ, et al. (2011) Brain-derived neurotrophic factor stimulates growth of pituitary melanotrope cells in an autocrine way. Gen Comp Endocrinol USA 170: 156–161.
47. Rocha M, Martins RA, Linden R (1999) Activation of NMDA receptors protects against glutamate neurotoxicity in the retina: evidence for the involvement of neurotrophins. Brain Res NED 827: 79–92.
48. Brandoli C, Sanna A, Bernardi MA, Follesa P, Brooker G, et al. (1998) Brain-derived neurotrophic factor and basic fibroblast growth factor downregulate NMDA receptor function in cerebellar granule cells. J Neurosci USA 18: 7953–7961.
49. Leeds P, Leng Y, Chalecka-Franaszek E, Chuang DM (2005) Neurotrophins protect against cytosine arabinoside-induced apoptosis of immature rat cerebellar neurons. Neurochem Int ENG 46: 61–72.
50. Schober ME, Block B, Requena DF, Hale MA, Lane RH (2012) Developmental traumatic brain injury decreased brain derived neurotrophic factor expression late after injury. Metab Brain Dis USA 27: 167–173.
51. Tarsa L, Goda Y (2002) Synaptophysin regulates activity-dependent synapse formation in cultured hippocampal neurons. Proc Natl Acad Sci USA 99: 1012–1016.
52. Crispino M, Stone DJ, Wei M, Anderson CP, Tocco G, et al. (1999) Variations of synaptotagmin I, synaptotagmin IV, and synaptophysin mRNA levels in rat hippocampus during the estrous cycle. Exp Neurol USA 159: 574–583.
53. Shojo H, Kibayashi K (2006) Changes in localization of synaptophysin following fluid percussion injury in the rat brain. Brain Res NED 1078: 198–211.
54. Ferrer I (1999) Neurons and their dendrites in frontotemporal dementia. Dement Geriatr Cogn Disord SUI 10 Suppl 1: 55–60.
55. Hao LY, Hao XQ, Li SH, Li XH (2010) Prenatal exposure to lipopolysaccharide results in cognitive deficits in age-increasing offspring rats. Neuroscience ENG 166: 763–770.
56. Eastwood SL, Cairns NJ, Harrison PJ (2000) Synaptophysin gene expression in schizophrenia. Investigation of synaptic pathology in the cerebral cortex. Br J Psychiatry ENG 176: 236–242.

Permissions

All chapters in this book were first published in PLOS ONE, by The Public Library of Science; hereby published with permission under the Creative Commons Attribution License or equivalent. Every chapter published in this book has been scrutinized by our experts. Their significance has been extensively debated. The topics covered herein carry significant findings which will fuel the growth of the discipline. They may even be implemented as practical applications or may be referred to as a beginning point for another development.

The contributors of this book come from diverse backgrounds, making this book a truly international effort. This book will bring forth new frontiers with its revolutionizing research information and detailed analysis of the nascent developments around the world.

We would like to thank all the contributing authors for lending their expertise to make the book truly unique. They have played a crucial role in the development of this book. Without their invaluable contributions this book wouldn't have been possible. They have made vital efforts to compile up to date information on the varied aspects of this subject to make this book a valuable addition to the collection of many professionals and students.

This book was conceptualized with the vision of imparting up-to-date information and advanced data in this field. To ensure the same, a matchless editorial board was set up. Every individual on the board went through rigorous rounds of assessment to prove their worth. After which they invested a large part of their time researching and compiling the most relevant data for our readers.

The editorial board has been involved in producing this book since its inception. They have spent rigorous hours researching and exploring the diverse topics which have resulted in the successful publishing of this book. They have passed on their knowledge of decades through this book. To expedite this challenging task, the publisher supported the team at every step. A small team of assistant editors was also appointed to further simplify the editing procedure and attain best results for the readers.

Apart from the editorial board, the designing team has also invested a significant amount of their time in understanding the subject and creating the most relevant covers. They scrutinized every image to scout for the most suitable representation of the subject and create an appropriate cover for the book.

The publishing team has been an ardent support to the editorial, designing and production team. Their endless efforts to recruit the best for this project, has resulted in the accomplishment of this book. They are a veteran in the field of academics and their pool of knowledge is as vast as their experience in printing. Their expertise and guidance has proved useful at every step. Their uncompromising quality standards have made this book an exceptional effort. Their encouragement from time to time has been an inspiration for everyone.

The publisher and the editorial board hope that this book will prove to be a valuable piece of knowledge for researchers, students, practitioners and scholars across the globe.

List of Contributors

Håvard Loras
Sør-Trøndelag University College, Trondheim, Norway

Hermundur Sigmundsson
Sør-Trøndelag University College, Trondheim, Norway
Norwegian University of Science and Technology, Trondheim, Norway

Ann-Katrin Stensdotter
Norwegian University of Science and Technology, Trondheim, Norway

Joel B. Talcott
Aston Brain Centre, School of Life and Health Sciences, Aston University, Birmingham, United Kingdom

Zhao Sun, Shanshan Shao and Ranran Song
Department of Maternal and Child Health, School of Public Health, Tongji Medical College, Huazhong University of Science and Technology, Wuhan, China

Li Zou
Department of Maternal and Child Health, School of Public Health, Tongji Medical College, Huazhong University of Science and Technology, Wuhan, China
Department of Epidemiology and Biostatistics and MOE Key Lab of Environment and Health, School of Public Health, Tongji Medical College, Huazhong University of Science and Technology, Wuhan, China

Rong Zhong, Juntao Ke, Xuzai Lu and Xiaoping Miao
Department of Epidemiology and Biostatistics and MOE Key Lab of Environment and Health, School of Public Health, Tongji Medical College, Huazhong University of Science and Technology, Wuhan, China

Jiajia Zhang
Department of Epidemiology and Biostatistics, Arnold School of Public Health, University of South Carolina, Columbia, South Carolina, United States of America

Shengnan Mo
Office of Administration, Renmin Hospital of Wuhan University, Wuhan, China

Maaike Callens, Wim Tops and Marc Brysbaert
Department of Experimental Psychology, University of Ghent, Ghent, Belgium

Janosch Linkersdörfer and Sven Lindberg
Center for Individual Development and Adaptive Education of Children at Risk, Frankfurt, Germany
German Institute for International Educational Research, Frankfurt, Germany

Marcus Hasselhorn
Center for Individual Development and Adaptive Education of Children at Risk, Frankfurt, Germany
German Institute for International Educational Research, Frankfurt, Germany
Institute for Psychology, Goethe-University Frankfurt, Germany

Christian J. Fiebach
Center for Individual Development and Adaptive Education of Children at Risk, Frankfurt, Germany
Institute for Psychology, Goethe-University Frankfurt, Germany
Donders Institute for Brain, Cognition and Behaviour, Radboud University Nijmegen, The Netherlands

Jan Lonnemann
German Institute for International Educational Research, Frankfurt, Germany
Institute for Psychology, Goethe-University Frankfurt, Germany

Manuel Perea
ERI-Lectura and Departament de Metodologia, Universitat de Valéncia, Valencia, Spain

Pablo Gomez
Psychology Department, DePaul University, Chicago, Illinois, United States of America

Frédérique Bielle
Centre Référent de Diagnostic des Troubles du Langage et des Apprentissages, Pôle Couple-Enfant, Centre Hospitalier Universitaire, Grenoble, France

Rachel Zoubrinetzky and Sylviane Valdois
Centre Référent de Diagnostic des Troubles du Langage et des Apprentissages, Pôle Couple-Enfant, Centre Hospitalier Universitaire, Grenoble, France
Laboratoire de Psychologie et NeuroCognition, CNRS, UMR 5105, Université Grenoble Alpes, Grenoble, France

Gayathri Chandrasekar, Liselotte Vesterlund and Isabel Tapia-Páez
Center for Biosciences, Department of Biosciences and Nutrition, Karolinska Institutet, Huddinge, Sweden

Kjell Hultenby
Clinical Research Center, Department of Laboratory Medicine, Karolinska Institutet, Stockholm, Sweden

Juha Kere
Center for Biosciences, Department of Biosciences and Nutrition, Karolinska Institutet, Huddinge, Sweden
Folkhälsan Institute of Genetics, Helsinki and Molecular Neurology Program, Research Programs Unit, University of Helsinki, Helsinki, Finland
Science for Life Laboratory, Karolinska Institutet, Stockholm, Sweden

Iris Berent
Department of Psychology, Northeastern University, Boston, Massachusetts, United States of America

Vered Vaknin-Nusbaum
Western Galilee College, Akko & Univeristy of Haifa, Haifa, Israel

Evan Balaban
Department of Psychology, McGill University, Montreal, Canada

Albert M. Galaburda
Department of Neurology, Division of Cognitive Neurology, Harvard Medical School, Beth Israel Deaconess Medical Center, Boston, Massachusetts, United States of America

William T. Adler, Maryann P. Platt, Alison J. Mehlhorn, Joshua L. Haight, Timothy A. Currier, Mikel A. Etchegaray, Albert M. Galaburda and Glenn D. Rosen
Department of Neurology, Beth Israel Deaconess Medical Center, Boston, Massachusetts, United States of America

Franz Fazekas
Department of Neurology, Medical University of Graz, Graz, Austria

Daniela Gebauer
Department of Neurology, Medical University of Graz, Graz, Austria
Department of Psychology, Karl-Franzens-University Graz, Graz, Austria

Christian Enzinger
Department of Neurology, Medical University of Graz, Graz, Austria
Department of Radiology, Medical University of Graz, Graz, Austria

Andreas Fink and Karl Koschutnig
Department of Psychology, Karl-Franzens-University Graz, Graz, Austria

Reinhard Kargl and Christian Purgstaller
Institute for Reading and Spelling, Graz, Austria

Gernot Reishofer
Department of Radiology, Medical University of Graz, Graz, Austria

Tracy M. Centanni, Crystal T. Engineer, Andrew M. Sloan, Robert L. Rennaker and Michael P. Kilgard
School of Behavioral and Brain Sciences, University of Texas at Dallas, Richardson, Texas, United States of America

Fuyi Chen, Anne M. Booker and Joseph J. LoTurco
Physiology and Neurobiology, University of Connecticut, Storrs, Connecticut, United States of America

Troy A. W. Visser
School of Psychology, University of Western Australia, Perth, Western Australia, Australia

Yuping Zhang, Jun Li, Bingjie Shi and Hua Shu
State Key Laboratory of Cognitive Neuroscience and Learning, Beijing Normal University, Beijing, China

Twila Tardif
Department of Psychology, University of Michigan, Ann Arbor, Michigan, United States of America

Sandra M. Villafuerte
Molecular and Behavioral Neuroscience Institute, University of Michigan, Ann Arbor, Michigan, United States of America,
Department of Psychiatry, University of Michigan, Ann Arbor, Michigan, United States of America

Margit Burmeister
Molecular and Behavioral Neuroscience Institute, University of Michigan, Ann Arbor, Michigan, United States of America,
Department of Psychiatry, University of Michigan, Ann Arbor, Michigan, United States of America
Department of Human Genetics, University of Michigan, Ann Arbor, Michigan, United States of America

Catherine McBride-Chang
Department of Psychology, The Chinese University of Hong Kong, Hong Kong, China

Hong Li
Department of Psychology, Beijing Normal University, Beijing, China

Weilan Liang and Zhixiang Zhang
Peking University First Hospital, Beijing, China

Dror Kraus
Department of Pediatric Neurology, Cincinnati Children's Hospital Medical Center, Cincinnati, Ohio, United States of America

Tzipi Horowitz-Kraus
Pediatric Neuroimaging Research Consortium, Cincinnati Children's Hospital Medical Center, Cincinnati, Ohio, United States of America
Edmond J. Safra Brain Research Center for the Study of Learning Disabilities, Faculty of Education, University of Haifa, Haifa, Israel

Emilie Réhault
UMR Unité 825, Faculté Paul Sabatier, IFR 96, Toulouse, France

Franck-Emmanuel Roux and Jean-François Démonet
UMR Unité 825, Faculté Paul Sabatier, IFR 96, Toulouse, France
Pole Neurosciences, Centres Hospitalo-Universitaires, Toulouse, France

Marion Reddy
Pole Neurosciences, Centres Hospitalo-Universitaires, Toulouse, France

Jean-Baptiste Durand
Centre de Recherche Cerveauet Cognition, Toulouse, France

Mélanie Jucla
UMR Unité 825, Faculté Paul Sabatier, IFR 96, Toulouse, France
U.R.I. Octogone-Lordat 4156, Université de Toulouse II, Toulouse, France

Maria Pia Bucci and Naziha Nassibi
Laboratoire de Psychologie et Neuropsychologie Cognitives, FRE 3292 CNRS - Université Paris Descartes, Boulogne Billancourt Cedex, France

Christophe-Loic Gerard
Service de Psychopathologie de l'enfant et de l'adolescent, Hôpital Robert Debré, Paris, France

Emmanuel Bui-Quoc
Service d'Ophtalmologie, Hôpital Robert Debré, Paris, France

Magali Seassau
e(ye)BRAI, Ivry-sur-Seine, France

Tru E. Kwong and Kyle J. Brachman
Department of Psychology, Mount Royal University, Calgary, Alberta, Canada
Armelle Viard, Vincent de La Sayette, Béatrice Desgranges and Francis Eustache
Inserm, U1077, Caen, France
Université de Caen Basse-Normandie, UMR-S1077, Caen, France
Ecole Pratique des Hautes Etudes, UMR-S1077, Caen, France
Centre Hospitalier Universitaire, U1077, Caen, France

Serge Belliard
Inserm, U1077, Caen, France
Université de Caen Basse-Normandie, UMR-S1077, Caen, France
Ecole Pratique des Hautes Etudes, UMR-S1077, Caen, France
Centre Hospitalier Universitaire, U1077, Caen, France
CHU Pontchaillou, Rennes, France

Pascale Piolino
Université Paris Descartes, Institut de Psychologie, Memory and Cognition Lab, Paris, France
Inserm UMR S894, Centre de Psychiatrie et Neurosciences, Paris, France

Hao Zhang, Xiaonian Zhang and XintING Sun
China Rehabilitation Research Center, Capital Medical University, Beijing, China

Mengqi Han
Beijing Jishuitan Hospital, Beijing, China

Feng Ling
Beijing Xuanwu Hospital, Capital Medical University, Beijing, China

Index

A
Adolescent, 23, 32, 35, 129, 157, 163
Allophonic, 88
Ameliorated, 85, 90, 108, 121
Angiogenic, 202
Anomalies, 41, 74, 99, 121, 163
Apoptosis, 69, 203, 206
Arabinoside, 206
Articulatory, 34, 40, 89-90
Atrophied, 177, 184, 192-194
Autonoetic, 176, 181, 192, 196

B
Bilingual, 64, 135, 155
Binocular, 48, 157-159, 162-164
Biological, 16, 18, 36, 41, 65, 67, 77, 88-89, 100, 116, 122, 135, 146, 174
Bravaccio, 74, 136
Brysbaert, 19, 21, 31-32, 164

C
Calcarine, 184, 187-188, 191
Carbonnel, 63-64, 129
Catherine, 130, 155
Centrosome, 73, 75
Cerebrospinal, 72, 202
Chlamydomonas, 73, 75
Chromosome, 17, 67, 74, 91, 98, 122, 130
Ciliogenesis, 66, 69, 72-73, 75
Clinicopathological, 155, 196
Comorbidity, 6-8, 17, 19, 31, 52, 111
Cytoarchitectonic, 41, 99, 154, 156
Cytoskeletal, 73, 75, 99

D
Degeneration, 195-196, 205
Dendritic, 65, 99, 121
Dephosphorylation, 204
Depression, 128, 180, 196
Diagnosis, 6-7, 19, 21, 23, 29, 32, 40, 85, 121, 128, 146, 166, 177
Diaminobenzidine, 92
Disturdyslexia, 155
Donnadieu, 63, 129
Doublecortin, 97, 99, 121-122
Dysfunction, 1, 33-34, 36-37, 39, 41, 57, 64, 72, 75, 108, 121, 138, 157, 164, 198-199, 202, 204-205
Dyslexics, 7, 16, 21, 27-28, 31-39, 41, 43, 49-50, 53, 56-58, 60, 76-85, 89, 98, 108-109, 114, 116, 122, 129, 146, 157-159, 161, 174

E
Electrode, 118, 140-141, 143-144, 146-149
Electroporation, 91-93, 95, 98, 110
Embryonic, 65, 67-68, 74, 91, 93-95, 97-98, 121-122
Epidemiology, 9, 197, 205
Episodicity, 181, 184
Etchegaray, 91, 98, 122
Excitability, 118, 122, 155
Exogenous, 1, 129, 203
Extracurricular, 10, 12

G
Glutamate, 204, 206
Glycoprotein, 204

H
Haplotype, 74, 98, 122, 130, 132, 136
Hemodynamic, 183, 198
Heritability, 89, 116, 130
Heterogeneity, 34, 42, 50, 52, 59, 61-62, 64
Hydrocephalus, 65, 67, 69, 71-73, 75
Hypopituitarism, 201, 205

I
Illumination, 158, 164, 199
Immunoreactivity, 199, 206
Instrucphonological, 173
Integration, 36, 41, 89, 105, 177
Intellectual, 31, 76, 90, 131, 179
Intracellular, 75, 97, 203
Isotropic, 103, 183

K
Kiaauditory, 115, 118

L
Lexicosemantic, 147, 155
Lipopolysaccharide, 205

Logographeme, 135

M
Malformations, 37, 65, 74, 92, 99, 148, 155
Maturation, 6, 37, 61, 146, 198
Mechanism, 16, 75, 98, 110, 112, 118, 137-138, 146, 148, 158, 163, 198-199, 203-204
Microelectrode, 120
Microscopy, 67, 72, 74, 94-95
Microtubule, 65, 72-73, 97
Montgomery, 98, 121-122, 136
Morphology, 1, 8, 23, 25-26, 28, 42, 89, 99, 108, 121, 204
Multivariate, 9, 11-12, 16, 125
Myllyluoma, 74, 98, 136

N
Neocortex, 65, 73-75, 91-98, 110, 121, 196
Nephronophthisis, 72, 75
Neurolinguistics, 8, 108, 156
Neurology, 10, 41, 65, 76, 91, 99-100, 108, 137, 146, 155, 195-197
Neuropsychol, 63-64, 89, 108, 129, 164, 196
Neurotoxicity, 203, 206

O
Olfactory, 65-68, 70-73
Orthographic, 8, 18, 21, 24, 32-33, 36, 38, 41, 49-51, 57-60, 62-64, 85, 89, 108, 122, 130-136, 146-148, 155, 169, 174
Orthoptic, 158, 162-163
Oscillations, 122

P
Pathology, 92, 195, 206
Perisylvian, 34, 37, 42, 147-148, 150, 154
Photomicrograph, 94-95
Pituitary, 198, 201, 205-206
Polycystic, 72, 75, 97
Polymorphisms, 98, 121-122
Precuneus, 34, 103-104, 106-108, 177, 184, 187-188, 191-192, 195
Psychopathologie, 157, 163

R
Rehabilitation, 198, 205

S
Sensorimotor, 33, 39, 77, 90, 121

T
Tetratricopeptide, 65, 74, 98
Therapeutic, 52, 109, 116

V
Vernacular, 165, 174
Visuospatial, 20, 129, 177, 179, 194-195
Volumetric, 34, 41, 196